Mind, State and Society

Mind, State and Society

Social History of Psychiatry and Mental Health in Britain 1960–2010

Edited by

George Ikkos
Royal National Orthopaedic Hospital

Nick Bouras
King's College London

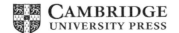

CAMBRIDGE
UNIVERSITY PRESS

University Printing House, Cambridge CB2 8BS, United Kingdom

One Liberty Plaza, 20th Floor, New York, NY 10006, USA

477 Williamstown Road, Port Melbourne, VIC 3207, Australia

314–321, 3rd Floor, Plot 3, Splendor Forum, Jasola District Centre,
New Delhi – 110025, India

79 Anson Road, #06–04/06, Singapore 079906

Cambridge University Press is part of the University of Cambridge.

It furthers the University's mission by disseminating knowledge in the pursuit of
education, learning, and research at the highest international levels of excellence.

www.cambridge.org
Information on this title: www.cambridge.org/9781911623717
DOI: 10.1017/9781911623793

First published 2021

Printed in the United Kingdom by TJ Books Limited, Padstow Cornwall

A catalogue record for this publication is available from the British Library.

Library of Congress Cataloging-in-Publication Data
Names: Ikkos, George, editor. | Bouras, Nick, editor.
Title: Mind, state and society : social history of psychiatry and mental health in Britain 1960–2010 / edited by George Ikkos,
Nick Bouras.
Description: Cambridge ; New York, NY : Cambridge University Press, 2021. | Includes bibliographical references and
index.
Identifiers: LCCN 2020055195 (print) | LCCN 2020055196 (ebook) | ISBN 9781911623717 (hardback) | ISBN
9781911623793 (ebook)
Subjects: LCSH: Mental health services – Great Britain – History – 20th century. | Mental health services – Great Britain –
History – 21st century. | Psychiatry – Great Britain – History – 20th century. | Psychiatry – Great Britain – History – 21st
century.
Classification: LCC RA790.7.G7 M55 2021 (print) | LCC RA790.7.G7 (ebook) | DDC 362.20941–dc23
LC record available at https://lccn.loc.gov/2020055195
LC ebook record available at https://lccn.loc.gov/2020055196

ISBN 978-1-911-62371-7 Hardback

....

Contents

Foreword

Since the 1930s, the adjective 'social' has become a popular qualifier of historical writings. Familiarity has banalized the adjective and a title like a 'Social History of X' draws little attention. What once was an interesting and controversial term[1] seems now to have lost its qualifying force and become a mere rhetorical adjunct. During the last few decades, the social sciences have undergone a 'cultural turn',[2] and this has threatened to engulf social history into the new 'cultural history'.[3] Therefore, it is important to rescue the adjective 'social' by reaffirming what it adds (or should add) to a historical writing.[4]

The Social

Since the seventeenth century, the meaning of 'social' has mirrored successive definitions of 'society'.[5] More interestingly, it has also broadened its remit: in addition to naming an abstract property (sociality), it has for some time also named a noun (the social).[6] This multivocality caused confusion when, during the first half of the twentieth century, 'social' started to be used to qualify a new type of historical writing ('social history').[7] The resulting ambiguity remains unresolved.

Social History

According to country and political tradition, this historiographical approach has been interpreted differently. A well-known definition states that it is a 'Historical writing that concentrates on the study of social groups, their interrelationships, and their roles in economic and cultural structures and processes; often characterized by the use of social science theory and quantitative methods.'[8] That is, it is less interested in traditional state and political history and does not organise itself around the contributions of 'great men'.

Since the 1920s, social history in Great Britain has been seen as resulting from an abiding interest in the contribution to history of the 'common people' as expressed in the work of historians such as R. H. Tawney and E. P. Thompson, who, for a time, worked outside the university system. 'However, more important than its physical location was social history's intellectual and methodological *raison d'être*. Although obviously shaped by time, institutions, and national intellectual traditions, the professional practice of social history has been dominated by two historical sociologists, Karl Marx and Max Weber.'[9] The Marxist influence became clear later in the writings on social history of the British historian Eric Hobsbawm.[10]

P. N. Stearns, an American social historian and founder of the *Journal of Social History*, wrote:

> one of the central and enduring impulses of the new social history involves the insistence on the active agency for the groups under examination; the past is no longer a pattern of leadership (benign or exploitative) shaping a passive population mass. On virtually any topic, from formal politics to the working of insane asylums or slave plantations, interaction becomes the key, as the presumably powerless play a definite historical role.[11]

The French view is closely associated with the *Annales* School, by common agreement considered as the main intellectual source of social history. In 1929, in Strasbourg, Lucien Febvre and Marc Bloch started a Journal entitled *Annales d'histoire économique et sociale* which was 'founded on a sharing of problems and a borrowing of concepts, methods, and data' where 'more often than not history found itself in the position of having to ask the social sciences for what it wanted. At bottom the idea was that a common fund of ideas and techniques existed among the social disciplines, from which each one was free to help itself.'[12]

These multinational definitions carry disparate ideologies, aims and methodologies. Can commonalities be found so that the style of 'social history' that has inspired the name of this book can be identified? The obstacle is to be found in the instability of the subaltern definitions, on how the 'social', 'economic', 'quantitative', 'qualitative' and so on are conceived of and, most importantly, how they are applied to the objects of psychiatry (hospitals, institutions, professional associations, parliamentary acts, diseases, biological treatments, political trends, patient groups, etc.).

Not only are subaltern concepts defined differently, but they are also prioritised and knitted differently into the warp and weft of history. For example, although the *Annales* School emphasises the economic structures, in the end most variables are included in their analysis, thereby giving rise to a form of 'total history'.[13] As mentioned, in Great Britain, Hobsbawm and followers offered a Marxist interpretation of the relationship between economic and cultural structures. In the United States, Stearns favoured a quantitative approach to manage the relationship between economic and social measurement and insisted on a 'bottom-up' approach.[14] In Germany, Jürgen Kocka[15] claims that, in contrast to traditional history, 'social history stressed the importance of social and economic factors, while simultaneously striving to connect the social, political, and cultural spheres. In contrast to traditional history, social history also emphasised the importance of collective factors in history and downplayed the role of the individual.'[16]

This Book

How should these professional perspectives bear upon a book of 'social history' intent on exploring the last fifty years of psychiatry? Ideally, they should provide a methodology and compass by means of which the reader can evaluate the historiographical intentions of both editors and contributors. The first two part titles ('Social and Institutional Contexts' and 'The Cogwheels of Change') suggest that the guiding idea has been one of contextualised 'social causation', that is, making use of a new way of explicating the changes (Part III: 'Implications in Practice') putatively undergone by British psychiatry.

Social Causality

'Causality' in the social sciences and in social history is a field where angels fear to tread.[17] In earlier years, it was assumed that the causality models used in mechanics and the natural sciences (considered then as a sign of mature scientificity) should also be used in the social sciences and in social history. In the period between the two world wars, and in both the natural and social sciences, these hopes were abandoned and replaced by a form of probabilistic causation.[18] Since then, philosophers of history have worried as to whether even probabilistic causality itself may be too strong a mechanism to aspire to in social history.[19] The debate continues.[20]

A Prequel

The historiographical approach that has inspired this book differs from the one that guided *150 Years of British Psychiatry: 1841–1991* (fifty-seven chapters in two volumes), a book published in 1991 by the Royal College of Psychiatrists to celebrate an institutional anniversary of British psychiatry.[21] At the time, there had been no comprehensive historical study of biographies, clinical themes, biological treatments, institutions and so on, relating to British psychiatry since it had been institutionalised during the nineteenth century.[22]

The driving force behind the production of those two volumes was the original incarnation of the Royal College of Psychiatrists (RCPsych) Interest Group for the History of Psychiatry, and the intellectual stimulus came from the late Hugh Freeman (then also editor of the *British Journal of Psychiatry*), Thomas Bewley and Henry Rollin, whose knowledge of things past acted as the bridge between the College and the Medico-Psychological Association.

Different times require different books. Interestingly, although thirty years apart, these works have both relied upon the help of professional historians and clinicians with historical interest. Equally interesting (and worth of celebration) is the fact that the names of some of the contributors to the 1991 volumes also appear in this present book. All national psychiatries require periodic auditing and recording and the book in hand should well satisfy this need during the early twenty-first century.

A Sequel?

'British psychiatry', since its construction during the nineteenth century, has been rather different from the psychiatry developed in other European countries (Germany, France, Italy, Spain, etc.). Its main originality and contribution are to be found in the institutional and legislative fields rather than in nosology or psychopathology.[23] Likewise, and perhaps due to its *sui generis* organisation, British psychiatry was less affected (as was Germany psychiatry)[24] by rivalries between academic and institutional factions. Yet another difference can be found in its susceptibility to abstract ideas: for example, it was far less permeable to the influence of Jacksonian ideas,[25] which were important to French psychiatry and psychology, and to psychoanalysis.[26]

Although no longer extant, these international differences still need historical explanation. It would be too easy to accept the ongoing globalisation of psychiatry (including the gradual convergence of the ICD and DSM listings)[27] as the only cause for the disappearance of international differences. In the same way, globalisation itself should not simply be seen as the result of the triumph of value-neutral neuroscience. This is a good bone for social history to get its teeth into.

Because not enough is yet known about what makes people mad, the absolute predominance of one point of view is not epistemologically healthy; indeed, psychiatric creativity can be negatively affected by effectively curtailing other explanatory options. Once again, it is a job of the social history of psychiatry to examine the mechanisms and pressures underlying these decisions.

The size of the field in which psychiatry claims expertise has expanded dramatically since the nineteenth century when alienists only dealt with madness (renamed psychosis after the 1860s), epilepsy and some organic disorders.[28] As is well known, it was other medical specialists that looked after anxieties, panics, hypochondriasis, obsessions, compulsions, hysteria, secondary depressions and so on (sufferings that, after the 1890s, were grouped under the new 'neuroses').[29]

From the early twentieth century on, alienists started claiming exclusive expertise in the management of these new 'neuroses' and also of a variety of new behavioural deviancies (soon called 'personality disorders').[30] Enlightened alienists soon perceived that the language of description and brain-related explanations used for madness did not work well for these new 'clinical' additions.[31] Many remained reluctant to use psychological explanations;[32] others, particularly those with large private practices, searched around for alternative narratives and happened upon psychoanalysis.[33] This knowledge gap encouraged Henry Maudsley to bequeath £30,000 to the London County Council to help with the treatment of 'acute' mental disorders and 'neurosis'.[34]

The list of mental disorders is still growing. The official position is that these additions are 'evidence-based'. However, there has been little research into the decision (particularly covert) mechanisms involved. The claim that the human brain is the same the world over, and hence the results of neuroscientific research must be valid in all possible worlds, has had various consequences. A negative one has been that countries bereft of economic wherewithal have become passive recipients of the nosological views and expensive treatments developed in leading countries. In a world fully governed by scientific and ethical integrity, this disparity may be acceptable. However, in the complex realities of today, client countries cannot be blamed for worrying about their subaltern status.

This is another field where social history can contribute, particularly because, since the time of the *Annales* School, one of its strengths has been the serious analysis of economic variables. Social history possesses methodologies apt for the exploration both of the world of concepts and values and of the dark forest of economic interests. It would be of great help to psychiatry to know how these factors affect neuroscientific research.

This book may be pointing to another useful way of doing history of psychiatry. Its findings should add to the periodic documentation required by British psychiatry. I am grateful to the editors for giving me the opportunity to make these points.

G. E. Berrios
Emeritus Professor of the Epistemology of Psychiatry
Robinson College
University of Cambridge

Notes

1. G. Himmelfarb, 'The writing of social history: Recent studies of 19th century England', *Journal of British Studies* (1971), 11: 148–70.

2. K. Nash, 'The cultural turn in social theory', *Sociology* (2001), 35: 77–92; D. Chaney, *The Cultural Turn*. London: Routledge, 1994; V. Depkat, 'The "cultural turn" in German and American historiography', *American Studies* (2009), 54: 425–50.

3. P. Burke, *What Is Cultural History* (2nd ed.). Cambridge: Polity Press, 2008; L. Hunt, ed., *The New Cultural History*. Berkeley: University of California Press, 1989; M. Bentley, 'The arrival of cultural history', in M. Bentley, ed., *Companion to Historiography*. London: Routledge, 2006, pp. 312–22.

4. P. N. Stearns, 'Social history present and future', *Journal of Social History* (2003), 37: 9–19; M. M. Smith, 'Making sense of social history', *Journal of Social History* (2003), 37: 165–86.

5. On the changing meaning of the concept of society: R. Williams, *Key Words: A Vocabulary of Culture and Society*. Oxford: Oxford University Press, 1983, pp. 291–5; M. Dean, 'Society', in T. Bennett, L. Grossberg and M. Morris, eds, *New Key Words: A Revised Vocabulary of Culture and Society*. Oxford: Blackwell, 2005, pp. 326–9.

6. On the history of 'the social': P. Joyce, 'What is the social in social history?', *Past and Present* (2010), 206: 213–48; J. Terrier, *Visions of the Social*. Leiden: Brill, 2011; J. Terrier, 'Social: The history of the concept', in J. D. Wright, ed., *International Encyclopedia of the Social and Behavioral Sciences*, Vol. 22 (2nd ed.), New York: Elsevier, 2015, pp. 827–32; W. Sewell, *Logics of History*. Chicago: University of Chicago Press, 2005, chapter 10; B. Latour, *Reassembling the Social*. Oxford: Oxford University Press, 2005.

7. P. N. Stearns, *Encyclopedia of Social History*. New York: Garland, 2006; P. N. Stearns, *Encyclopedia of European Social History*, 2 vols. Detroit: Charles Scribner's Sons, 2001.

8. H. Ritter, *Dictionary of Concepts in History*. New York: Greenwood, 1986, p. 408.

9. G. Lewis, 'Social history', in K. Boyd, *Encyclopedia of Historians and History Writing*, 2 vols. London: Fitzroy Dearborn Publishers, 1999, p. 1110.

10. E. Hobsbawm, 'From social history to the history of society', *Daedalus* (1971), 100: 20–45; G. Elliott, *Hobsbawm: History and Politics*. London: Pluto Press, 2010; J. E. Cronin, 'Memoir, social history and commitment: Eric Hobsbawm's "interesting times"', *Journal of Social History* (2003), 37: 219–31.

11. P. N. Stearns, *Encyclopedia of Social History*. New York: Garland, 2006, p. 893.

12. J. Revel, 'The *Annales* School', in L. D. Kritzman, *The Columbia History of Twentieth-Century French Thought*. New York: Columbia University Press, 2006, p. 12.

13. S. Clark, ed., *The Annales School, Vol. 1: History and Overviews*. London: Routledge, 1999; P. Burke, *The French Historical Revolution: The Annales School*. Cambridge: Polity Press, 1990; J. Tendler, *Opponents of the Annales School*. London: Palgrave, 2013.

14. P. N. Stearns, 'Towards a wider vision: Trends in social history', in M. Kammen, ed., *The Past Before Us*. Ithaca, NY: Cornell University Press, 1980, pp. 205–30.

15. J. Kocka, *Sozialgeschichte. Begriff, Entwicklung, Probleme* (2nd ed.). Göttingen: Vandenhoeck & Ruprecht, 1986; J. Kocka, 'Losses, gains and opportunities: Social history today', *Journal of Social History* (2003), 37: 21–8.

16. C. Lorenz, 'Jürgen Kocka', in K. Boyd, *Encyclopedia of Historians and History Writing*. London: Fitzroy Dearborn Publishers, 1999, p. 650.

17. J. Woodward, *Making Things Happen: A Theory of Causal Explanation*. Oxford: Oxford University Press, 2003; H. Beebee, C. Hitchcock, P. Menzies et al., eds, *The Oxford Handbook of Causation*. Oxford: Oxford University Press, 2009.

18. G. Gigerenzer, Z. Swijtink, T. Porter et al., *The Empire of Chance*. Cambridge: Cambridge University Press, 1989.

19. H. Kincaid, 'Causation in the social sciences', in Beebee et al. *The Oxford Handbook of Causation*; A. Reutlinger, *A Theory of Causation in the Social and Biological Sciences*. London: Palgrave, 2013.

20. C. C. Ragin, *The Comparative Method: Moving Beyond Qualitative and Quantitative Strategies* (2nd ed.). Oakland: University of California Press, 2014.

21. G. E. Berrios and H. Freeman, eds, *150 Years of British Psychiatry 1841–1991*. London: Gaskell, 1991, pp. 79–88; H. Freeman and G. E. Berrios, eds, *150 Years of British Psychiatry, Vol. 2: The Aftermath*. London: Athlone Press, 1996.

22. Before 1991, there had, of course, been many studies of private madhouses, eighteenth-century psychiatry, specific institutions, diseases, hospitals and so on, but no comprehensive approach to a historical object called 'British Psychiatry' had been attempted.

23. An illustration of international differences can be found in the many entries of D. H. Tuke, *A Dictionary of Psychological Medicine*, 2 vols. London: J and A Churchill, 1892; W. F. Bynum, 'Tuke's dictionary and

psychiatry at the turn of the century', in G. E. Berrios and E. Freeman, eds, *150 Years of British Psychiatry 1841–1991*. London: Gaskell, 1991, pp. 163–79.

24. This issue is well explored in K. Jaspers, *General Psychopathology*, trans J. Hoenig and M. W. Hamilton. Manchester: Manchester University Press, 1963; see also E. Engstrom, *Clinical Psychiatry in Imperial Germany: A History of Psychiatric Practice*. Ithaca, NY: Cornell University Press, 2003.

25. G. E. Berrios, 'The factors of insanities', *History of Psychiatry* (2001), 12: 353–73; G. E. Berrios, 'Henri Ey, Jakcosn et les idées obsédantes', *L'Evolution Psychiatrique* (1977), 52: 685–99.

26. Works on the reception of psychoanalysis in specific countries abound, e.g. F. Allodi, 'History of psycho-analysis in Spain', *Acta Española de Psiquiatría* (2012), 40: 1–9; N. G. Hale, *The Rise and Crisis of Psychoanalysis in the United States: Freud and the Americans, 1917–1985*. Oxford: Oxford University Press, 1995; D. Rapp, 'The reception of Freud by the British press: General interest and literary magazines, 1920–1925', *Journal of the History of the Behavioral Sciences* (1988), 24: 191–205; S. Alexander, 'Psychoanalysis in Britain in the early twentieth century', *History Workshop Journal* (1998), 45: 135–43; M. Pines, 'The development of the Psychodynamic Movement', in G. E. Berrios and H. Freeman, eds, *150 Years of British Psychiatry 1841–1991*. London: Gaskell, 1991, pp. 206–31; H. Decker, *Freud in Germany: Revolution and Reaction in Science, 1893–1907*. New York: International Universities Press, 1977; A. De Mijolla, *La France et Freud*. Paris: Presses Universitaires de France, 2012. However, fewer works comparing the relevant countries seem to have been published.

27. P. Tyrer, 'A comparison of DSM and ICD classifications of mental disorder', *Advances in Psychiatric Treatment* (2014), 20: 280–5; D. Stein, C. Lund, R. M. Nesse et al., 'Classification systems in psychiatry: Diagnosis and global mental health in the era of DSM-5 and ICD-11', *Current Opinion in Psychiatry* (2013), 26: 493–7.

28. There are many published nineteenth-century clinical tabulations and classifications. See some references in G. E. Berrios, 'Baillarger and His Essay on a classification of different genera of insanity', *History of Psychiatry* (2008), 19: 358–73. For access to British archival material, see the National Archives online guide on how to look for records of 'Asylums, psychiatric hospitals and mental health': www.nationalarchives.gov.uk/help-with-your-research/research-guides/mental-health.

29. J. M. López Piñero, *Historical Origins of the Concept of Neurosis*, trans. D. Berrios. Cambridge: Cambridge University Press, 1983; J. M. López Piñero and J. M. Morales Meseguer, *Neurosis y psicoterapia: Un estudio histórico*. Madrid: Espasa-Calpe, 1970.

30. G. E. Berrios, 'European views on personality disorders: A conceptual history', *Comprehensive Psychiatry* (1993), 34: 14–30.

31. G. E. Berrios, 'British psychopathology since the early 20th century' in G. E. Berrios and H. Freeman, eds, *150 Years of British Psychiatry 1841–1991*. London: Gaskell, 1991, pp. 232–44.

32. M. J. Clark, 'A rejection of psychological approaches to mental disorder in late nineteenth century British psychiatry', in A. Scull (ed.), *Madhouses, Mad-doctors and Madmen* (Philadelphia: University of Pennsylvania Press, 1981), pp. 271–312.

33. R. D. Hinshelwood, 'Psychodynamic psychiatry before World War I', in Berrios and Freeman, *150 years of British Psychiatry*, pp. 197–205.

34. P. Allderidge, 'The foundation of the Maudsley Hospital', in Berrios and Freeman, *150 years of British Psychiatry*, pp. 79–88; E. Jones et al., 'The Maudsley Hospital: Design and strategic direction, 1923–1939', *Medical History* (2007), 51: 357–78.

Acknowledgements

The present work emerged from more than a decade of conversations, co-organising events and co-authoring articles. Much of this has taken place through the Royal Society of Medicine (RSM) Psychiatry Section activities, especially at its programme on Psychiatry in Dialogue with Neuroscience Medicine and Society. The Section has been fortunate to enjoy the support of the Lambert Endowment Fund, which has enabled the invitation of distinguished overseas speakers to its events, and now has funded fully the open electronic access to this publication. We are grateful to Mr Simon Lambert FRCS for his generosity and support.

The Royal College of Psychiatrists (RCPsych) has also played a crucial part and not only through its decisive impact on our professional formation. In recent years, we have continued our collaboration through the History of Psychiatry Special Interest Group (HoPSIG). RCPsych is investing increasingly in the history of psychiatry and we are grateful to Dr Adrian James, formerly Registrar and now President, Professor Peter Tyrer, former Editor-in-Chief, and Dr Claire Hilton, co-founding Chair of HoPSIG and now Historian in Residence at RCPsych for their initiatives and support.

Advice from our psychiatrist colleagues Baroness Elaine Murphy, Professor George Szmukler and Dr Nori Graham has served to improve both the formulation and the execution of our project, as similarly have reviews of our original proposal by the RCPsych Publications Committee referees. The chapter authors have been a pleasure to collaborate with. Professors Tom Burns, Allen Frances and Behrooz Morvaridi, Dr Paul St John Smith and Mr David Gilbert have helped with our editing. At Cambridge University Press, we have enjoyed ready availability and support. To all we extend our thanks. The result is our responsibility.

Contributors

Esther Ansah-Asamoah completed an MSc Natural Sciences degree at Lancaster University, with a focus in Psychology, Chemistry, Microbiology and Biomedicine. Esther is particularly interested in mental health care within the black, Asian and minority ethnic (BAME) community and hopes to be able to work in the mental health sector in the future.

Annie Bartlett is Professor of Offender Healthcare at St George's Hospital Medical School, University of London. She worked clinically as a forensic psychiatrist in secure hospital and other settings, most recently in HMP/YOI Holloway prior to its closure. Her research background is in social anthropology; her doctoral thesis was published as a monograph on the lives of staff and patients in high secure hospital care. She was Clinical Director of Central and North West London NHS Trust's Offender Care services in London and the South East until 2016. Her research career has been varied and has included investigation into the relationship between the LGBT community and psychiatry.

Arnon Bentovim is a child and adolescent psychiatrist. He trained at the Maudsley Hospital and as a psychoanalyst and family therapist. He was a consultant at the Great Ormond Street Children's Hospital and the Tavistock Clinic, an honorary senior lecturer at the Institute of Child Health University of London and is a visiting professor at the Royal Holloway University of London. At Great Ormond Street, he shared responsibility for child protection,

initiated the first sexual abuse assessment and treatment service and was a member of the group who developed family therapy in the UK. He established the Child and Family Practice and the Child and Family Training organisation.

Peter Beresford OBE is Professor of Citizen Participation at the University of Essex, Co-Chair of Shaping Our Lives, the national disabled people's and service users' organisation and network, and Emeritus Professor of Social Policy at Brunel University London. He is a long-term user of mental health services and has a long-standing background of involvement in issues of participation as a writer, researcher, activist and teacher. He is a co-editor of *Madness, Violence and Power: A Critical Collection* (2019) and *The Routledge Handbook of Service User Involvement in Human Services Research and Education* (2020).

G. E. Berrios is Emeritus Professor of Psychiatry at Cambridge University where he occupied the first chair of the Epistemology of Psychiatry. He read Philosophy, Psychology and Physiology at Corpus Christi College, Oxford University and trained in Neurology and Psychiatry at the then Oxford United Hospitals. He is Fellow and Honorary Fellow of the Royal College of Psychiatrists. In 1989, with Roy Porter, he founded the international journal *History of Psychiatry*, of which he remains the editor. His research has centred on the psychiatric complications of neurological disease and the history, structure and epistemological power of descriptive psychopathology. In 2020, ex-students and other members of the Cambridge Epistemology Group published a Festschrift in his honour.

Allan Beveridge is History and Humanities Editor of the *Journal of the Royal College of Physicians of Edinburgh*, Editor of *Psychiatry in Pictures* and joint Book Review Editor of the *British Journal of Psychiatry*. He is an honorary fellow at the Department of the History of Medicine, Edinburgh University. He has written extensively on the history of psychiatry and on the medical humanities. Until his retirement, he was a consultant psychiatrist at the Queen Margaret Hospital, Dunfermline.

Kamaldeep Bhui is Professor of Psychiatry at the Department of Psychiatry University of Oxford, Honorary Consultant Psychiatrist at East London NHS Foundation Trust, and Editor-in-Chief of the *British Journal of Psychiatry*. He studied Pharmacology (BSc) at University College London (UCL) and Medicine (MBBS) at United Medical and Dental Schools of Guys and St Thomas' (now King's College), qualifying in 1988. He holds postgraduate qualifications in psychiatry, mental health studies, epidemiology and psychotherapy. His first consultant appointment was in 1999, followed in 2000 and 2003 by consultant/ senior lecturer and consultant/professorial posts in East London Foundation Trust and Queen Mary University of London.

Emily Blackshaw is employed at Mind as CEO Office and Business Development Team Assistant. She has been undertaking a PhD at the University of Roehampton since 2016, carrying out a psychometric evaluation of the Young Person's Clinical Outcomes in Routine Evaluation (YP-CORE). She studied Psychology at the University of Warwick, before working for

three years at the Institute of Psychology, Psychiatry and Neuroscience at King's College London. Most of her prior research experience involves quantitative research designs with a focus on community-based projects and adolescent mental health. Her research publications include contributions to child and adolescent mental health and health services and delivery research.

Jed Boardman is Senior Lecturer in Social Psychiatry at the Institute of Psychiatry and Senior Policy Adviser at the Centre for Mental Health. Throughout his career, he has worked mainly in social and community psychiatry and was Consultant Psychiatrist at South London and Maudsley Trust until 2016. He is now the lead for Social Inclusion at the Royal College of Psychiatrists, where he advises on employment, poverty, welfare reform, personalisation and recovery.

Nick Bouras is Emeritus Professor of Psychiatry at King's College London, Institute of Psychiatry, Psychology and Neuroscience. He worked as consultant psychiatrist for thirty years initially at Guy's hospital and then at the South London and the Maudsley NHS Foundation Trust where he also became clinical director. His research has centred on the psychiatric ward environments, community psychiatry and the mental health of people with intellectual disabilities. He led the research programme in one of the first community mental health centres in the UK and played an important role in the development of the first community-based mental health service in the UK for people with intellectual disabilities. He systematically studied the re-provision of services, following the closure of institutions. He initiated and developed the Estia Centre, an innovative concept combining clinical services, training and research. He has published extensively in community psychiatry and mental health aspects of people with intellectual disabilities including the textbook *Psychiatric and Behavioral Disorders in Intellectual and Developmental Disabilities* (2016) and an autobiographical account: *Reflections on the Challenges of Psychiatry in the UK and Beyond* (2017). Several of his publications have been translated into different languages.

Joanna Bourke is Professor of History at Birkbeck, University of London, and Fellow of the British Academy. She is the Principal Investigator on an interdisciplinary Wellcome Trust–funded project entitled SHaME or Sexual Harms and Medical Encounters (shame.bbk.ac.uk). She is the prize-winning author of fourteen books, including histories on modern warfare, military medicine, psychology and psychiatry, the emotions, what it means to be human, and rape, as well as more than 100 articles in academic journals. Her most recent book is *The Story of Pain: From Prayer to Painkillers* (2014). Her books have been translated into Chinese, Russian, Spanish, Catalan, Italian, Portuguese, Czech, Turkish and Greek.

Liz Brosnan has been a user/survivor activist and researcher for more than twenty years. In 2013, she completed a PhD in medical sociology examining the dynamics surrounding user involvement/ engagement. Her research interests also include psychosocial disability rights and the UNCRPD, survivor epistemology and, latterly, change methodologies in mental health services. After ten years in academia as a survivor researcher, she has returned to practise in Irish services to enhance the inclusion of the voices of lived experience in service planning design and evaluation.

Tom Burns is Professor Emeritus of Social Psychiatry at the University of Oxford. His research was predominantly health services research in community psychiatry, particularly complex interventions. He has published 6 books and more than 300 papers, including randomised controlled trials (RCTs) of case management, vocational rehabilitation and Community Treatment Orders (CTOs). These CTOs appear to be utterly ineffectual but are currently being introduced worldwide. His book *Our Necessary Shadow: The Nature and Meaning of Psychiatry* (2014) is on psychiatry for the general reader. He was awarded the CBE in 2006 for services to mental health care.

Peter Byrne is a consultant liaison psychiatrist at the Royal London Hospital in east London. He graduated with a master's degree in film studies from University College Dublin in 1994 and taught film studies there for eight years. He has written many articles on the representation of people with mental health problems in film and programmed the UK's first mental health film festival in January 2002 at Riverside Studios, London. He also helped to programme films for the *Reel Madness* Film Festival (London, 2004) and for the Scottish Mental Health Arts Festival (www.mhfestival.org) beginning in 2007. His principal research interest is the stigma of mental health problems and the effects of prejudice and discrimination. He was appointed Director of Public Education for the Royal College of Psychiatrists for five years from 2007; in 2013, he became RCPsych Associate Registrar for public mental health.

Peter Carpenter is Honorary Consultant Psychiatrist at Avon and Wiltshire Mental Health Partnership NHS Trust. He was a consultant psychiatrist in Learning Disabilities for Hanham Hall Hospital for ten years before it became the last large hospital to close in the Bristol area. He has had a lifelong interest in history, saving the records of the psychiatric hospitals of Leicester before collecting the surviving records for intellectual disability in Avon. He was a long-term trustee of Glenside Hospital Museum and has written extensively on various aspects of the history of psychiatry and intellectual disability. His current interests are the private madhouses of Avon and the work of the Burdens.

Peter Carter OBE is an independent health care consultant and visiting professor at Anglia Ruskin, Canterbury Christchurch, Chester and King's College universities. He is a registered nurse and has a PhD and MBA from the University of Birmingham. He is a fellow of the Royal College of Nursing (RCN) and an honorary fellow of the Royal College of General Practitioners as well as an ad eundem of the Royal College of Surgeons in Ireland. He was awarded the inaugural medal of the President of the Royal College of Psychiatrists in 2011. He is the former CEO of the Central and North West London NHS Trust and the RCN.

Hedy Cleaver is Professor Emeritus at Royal Holloway College, University of London. Her experience as a social worker and child psychologist informs her research on vulnerable children and their families and the impact of professional interventions. The guiding principle underpinning her work is a desire to improve the quality of life for children living in circumstances that place them at risk of abuse and neglect. Recent research focuses on perinatal death and the support available for grieving parents. Findings from her research have impacted UK policy, in respect to children and families, for more than thirty years.

Christopher C. H. Cook is Professor of Spirituality, Theology and Health and

Director of the Centre for Spirituality, Theology and Health at Durham University. He is a fellow of the Royal College of Psychiatrists, with research doctorates in medicine and theology. Ordained as a priest in 2001, he is an honorary chaplain for Tees, Esk and Wear Valleys NHS Foundation Trust. His books include *Spirituality, Theology and Mental Health* (2013), *Spirituality and Narrative in Psychiatric Practice: Stories of Mind and Soul* (edited with Andrew Powell and Andrew Sims, 2016), *Hearing Voices, Demonic and Divine* (2018) and *Christians Hearing Voices* (2020).

Tom K. J. Craig is Emeritus Professor of Social Psychiatry at the Institute of Psychiatry, Psychology and Neuroscience, King's College, London, and past president of the World Association of Social Psychiatry. He qualified in medicine at the University of the West Indies and trained in psychiatry in Nottingham, UK. He was appointed as Professor of Community Psychiatry in 1990, based in the South London and Maudsley NHS Trust and was the psychiatric lead for the closure of Tooting Bec Hospital. His research includes services for first episode psychosis and current studies of the AVATAR therapy for auditory hallucinations.

Ilana Crome is Emerita Professor of Addiction Psychiatry at Keele University, Honorary Consultant Psychiatrist at Midlands Partnership Foundation Trust and Visiting Professor at St George's University of London. Ilana has experience in providing comprehensive addiction services for all substances across the life cycle and played an active role in the addiction field in service development, research, training and policy. She has published extensively and had many national and international leadership roles, including Chair of Trustees of Drug

Science. Her ongoing research interests in addiction include mental and physical comorbidity, decision-making, suicide and training for health professionals.

Paul Farmer has been Chief Executive of Mind, the leading mental health charity working in England and Wales since May 2006. He is Chair of the NHS England Independent Oversight and Advisory Group, which brings together health and care leaders and experts to oversee the current mental health long-term plan for the NHS in England. He co-authored *Thriving at Work* (2017) for the government, setting out how to transform mental health in workplaces. Paul is a commissioner at Historic England. He has an honorary Doctor of Science from the University of East London, is an honorary fellow of St Peter's College, Oxford, and the Royal College of Psychiatrists and was awarded a CBE in the New Year's Honours 2016.

Sarah-Jane Fenton is a lecturer in mental health policy in the Institute for Mental Health (IMH) at the University of Birmingham. Sarah-Jane completed her doctoral research in 2016, graduating with a dual award degree from the University of Birmingham (2016) and the University of Melbourne (2017). The PhD used a comparative study design to explore mental health policy and service delivery for adolescents and young people aged sixteen to twenty-five years of age in the UK and Australia. Sarah-Jane has particular expertise in youth, adolescence, mental health, health policy, realist and qualitative research.

Jon Glasby is Professor of Health and Social Care in the Department of Social Work and Social Care at the University of Birmingham. A qualified social worker by background, Jon specialises in research,

teaching, consultancy and policy advice around joint working between health and social care, personalisation and community care services. He has previously served as the editor-in-chief of the *Journal of Integrated Care* and is currently a non-executive director of University Hospitals Birmingham NHS Foundation Trust and of the Birmingham Children's Trust. Jon is the author of numerous health and social care textbooks, including *Mental Health: Policy and Practice* (2015).

Lawrence O. Gostin is University Professor, Georgetown University's highest academic rank, and Founding O'Neill Chair in Global Health Law. He directs the World Health Organization (WHO) Center on National and Global Health Law. He is Professor of Medicine at Georgetown University and Professor of Public Health at Johns Hopkins University. Before leaving for Harvard, he was Legal Director of Mind, where he worked on mental health law reform and advocacy for the rights of persons with mental disabilities.

Kevin Gournay is Emeritus Professor at the Institute of Psychiatry, Psychology and Neuroscience, King's College London. He is a registered nurse, registered psychologist and chartered scientist with wide-ranging clinical, research and training experience. He is an honorary professor at the Matilda Centre, University of Sydney, where he continues to pursue his interest in comorbidity. He was appointed CBE in the New Year's Honours 1999. He is a fellow of the Academy of Medical Sciences, a fellow of the Royal College of Nursing and an honorary fellow of the Royal College of Psychiatrists. He was USA Psychiatric Nurse of the year in 2004.

John Gunn is Emeritus Professor of Forensic Psychiatry, King's College

London, Maudsley Hospital graduate and foundation member, one-time Chairman of the Faculty of Forensic Psychiatry, Honorary Fellow 2010 and currently elected trustee of the Royal College of Psychiatrists. As consultant forensic psychiatrist at the Maudsley, 1972–2002, he developed a large postgraduate teaching scheme for forensic psychiatry. His research has included epidemiological studies of prisoners, the workings of Grendon Prison and violence studies. He is Founder of the Effra Trust for ex-prisoner patients and Co-founder of the Ghent Group for European Psychiatrists. He was also a member of the Parole Board from 2006 to 2015, the co-editor of the textbook *Forensic Psychiatry: Clinical, Legal and Ethical Issues* (2014) and Founder of Crime in Mind, a research charity.

Jamie Hacker Hughes is a clinical psychologist and neuropsychologist. After a commission in the Army and five years in sales and marketing, Jamie studied at University College London (UCL), Cambridge and Surrey universities. After five years in the NHS, he returned to the Ministry of Defence (MoD), becoming a defence consultant advisor and head of clinical psychology before establishing the Veterans and Families Institute at Anglia Ruskin University. Jamie has been both British Psychological Society (BPS) President and Minister Provincial for Europe of the Third Order Franciscans. He is a committed campaigner against mental health stigma and is very open about his own twenty-year experience of bipolar disorder.

John Hall is Visiting Professor of Mental Health and Senior Research Associate at the Centre for Medical Humanities, Oxford Brookes University. He was formerly Head of NHS Clinical Psychology Services for Oxfordshire and Senior Clinical Lecturer in Clinical Psychology at Oxford University. He was Consultant Adviser in Clinical Psychology to the Department of Health for six years and received a Lifetime Achievement Award from the British Psychological Society (BPS) Professional Practice Board in 2011. He was the lead editor for *Clinical Psychology in Britain: Historical Perspectives*, published by the BPS in 2015, and is currently writing on the histories of the mental health professions.

Ahmed Hankir is Academic Clinical Fellow in General Adult Psychiatry at King's College London and Senior Research Fellow at the Centre for Mental Health Research in association with Cambridge University. His research interests include global and Muslim mental health and pioneering and evaluating innovative programmes that challenge mental health–related stigma. He is passionate about public engagement and education and empowering and dignifying people with lived/living experience of mental health difficulties. He is the recipient of the Royal College of Psychiatrists Foundation Doctor and Core Psychiatric Trainee of the Year awards.

David Healy is a professor in the Department of Family Medicine, McMaster University, Canada, having previously been a professor of Psychiatry at Cardiff and Bangor universities. His historical work has centred on the discovery of physical treatments in mental health, the problems these treatments can cause and methods to evaluate treatments, leading to publications such as *The Antidepressant Era* (1999) and *The Creation of Psychopharmacology* (2004).

Louise Hide is a social historian of psychiatry and its institutions. She is a Wellcome Trust Fellow in Medical Humanities (Grant Reference: 205417/Z/

16/Z) and based in the Department of History, Classics and Archaeology at Birkbeck, University of London. Her research project is titled 'Cultures of Harm in Residential Institutions for Long-term Adult Care, Britain 1945–1980s'. She co-edited a special issue of the *Social History of Medicine* (2018) and has published on the histories of pain, delusions and institutional cultures. Her first monograph, *Gender and Class in English Asylums, 1890–1914*, was published in 2014.

Claire Hilton trained in psychiatry in Manchester and was a consultant old age psychiatrist in North West London from 1998 to 2017. Her MD was on psychiatric complications of sickle cell disease, with the data collected in Jamaica. Her PhD was on the history of old age psychiatry in England, *c.*1940–89. Her published work includes three history monographs as well as academic papers on history, policy, old age psychiatry and transcultural psychiatry. She is currently Historian in Residence at the Royal College of Psychiatrists.

Peter Hughes is an NHS consultant psychiatrist at Springfield University Hospital, London. He is Chair of the London Division of the Royal College of Psychiatrists. He founded the Volunteering and International Psychiatry Special Interest Group of the Royal College of Psychiatrists. He has worked as a mental health specialist for the past fifteen years globally, including in humanitarian emergencies and refugee settings. He has worked with the World Health Organization (WHO), other UN organisations and non-governmental organisations (NGOs).

George Ikkos is Honorary Fellow and Chair of the History of Psychiatry Special Interest Group (HoPSIG) of the Royal College of Psychiatrists. He was the first

president of the Pain Medicine Section at the Royal Society of Medicine (RSM) and President of the Psychiatry Section as well as Honorary Visiting Research Professor at London South Bank University. Working with Barnet Voice for Mental Health from 1999 to 2006, he pioneered consistent co-production of interview and communication skills in UK postgraduate psychiatric training through a weekly seminar and clinical simulation workshop. This also had a profound impact on his own practice. The year 2021 marks forty years of work for the NHS, where he continues to practise as a consultant liaison psychiatrist at the Royal National Orthopaedic Hospital. He has been the clinical lead in the development of the Stanmore Nursing Assessment of Psychological Status (SNAPS); medical advisor to the Scotsman Fringe First award-winning play *The Shape of the Pain*, which was directed by an expert by experience; and delivered invited plenary lectures at meetings of the British Pain Society and the International Association for the Study of Pain. A qualified group analytic psychotherapist, he has published on psychosomatic, psychodynamic, interpersonal and social aspects of psychiatry.

Edgar Jones is Professor of the History of Medicine and Psychiatry at the Institute of Psychiatry, Psychology and Neuroscience, King's College London. He originally studied history, completing a doctorate at Nuffield College, Oxford, but subsequently trained in clinical psychopathology at Guy's Hospital and as a psychodynamic psychotherapist. He has written on shell shock, somatic symptoms associated with post-traumatic stress disorder (PTSD), the cultural representation of psychiatric casualties and moral injury experienced by veterans. He is the course director of King's MSc in War and Psychiatry.

Doreen Jones is a BAME survivor. She has been a campaigner, advocate, trainer, lecturer and writer on race, mental health and faith. She worked for Rethink, Mental Health Foundation, Mind, Sainsbury's Centre for Mental Health, Mellow Campaign and Social Action for Health. She co-founded and ran her own advocacy service (charity) Black & Ethnic Minorities Advocacy & Counselling Service. She was a BAME representative on London Clinical Network for Mental Health and a member of NHS England Black Voices Network. She was a Race Equality Cultural Competence trainer in East London. She has published widely and is passionate about improving mental experiences for BAME people.

Cornelius Katona is Medical Director of the Helen Bamber Foundation – a human rights charity that works with asylum seekers and refugees – and is Honorary Professor in the Division of Psychiatry at University College London (UCL). He is the Royal College of Psychiatrists' lead on Refugee and Asylum Mental Health. He was a member of the committee that recently updated NICE guidelines on post-traumatic stress disorder (PTSD). He has published more than 250 peer-reviewed papers and written or edited sixteen books. In 2019, he was awarded the Royal College of Psychiatrists' Honorary Fellowship, the College's highest honour, for his 'outstanding service to psychiatry'.

Stephen Lawrie hails from St Andrews, studied medicine in Aberdeen and, after a sojourn in Glasgow, has worked in Edinburgh for more than thirty years. He completed basic psychiatry training at the Royal Edinburgh Hospital. Following six months as a Wellcome Research Fellow, he was Lecturer and then Senior Clinical Research Fellow/Reader in the Department of Psychiatry in Edinburgh. As an honorary consultant psychiatrist with NHS Lothian,

he works as a general adult psychiatrist in south-west Edinburgh. As an academic, his research is primarily focused on understanding and treating schizophrenia. Stephen is also enthusiastic about public engagement, training, clinical and evidence-based psychiatry.

Paul McCrone is a health economist at the University of Greenwich. He was previously at the Institute of Psychiatry, Psychology and Neuroscience at King's College London), where he worked for twenty-seven years after having previously worked at the University of Kent. He has worked on many economic studies in health and social care. He also teaches health economics to Master's-level students, supervises PhD students and has published widely in peer-reviewed journals. He is involved in policy discussions around health funding and is part of the Mental Health Policy Research Unit funded by the National Institute for Health Research (NIHR).

Elaine, Baroness Murphy has been a crossbench life peer since May 2004, taking an interest in mental health and social care legislation in the House of Lords. From 1983 to 1997, she was Foundation Professor of Psychiatry of Old Age at Guy's (now part of King's College London). She was also, for a time, a district general manager in the London NHS and later chaired NHS trusts and health authorities in London. She was Vice Chairman of the Mental Health Act Commission from 1987 to 1994, Chief Medical Officer's personal advisor in her field and a UK advisor to the World Health Organization (WHO). In retirement, she researches local history in East Anglia.

David Nutt is a psychiatrist and the Edmond J. Safra Professor of Neuropsychopharmacology in the Division of Brain Science, Imperial College London. He was previously President of the European Brain Council, British Association of Psychopharmacology, British Neuroscience Association and European College of Neuropsychopharmacology. He is currently Founding Chair of DrugScience. org.uk and holds visiting professorships at the Open University and the University of Maastricht. In 2013, he won the John Maddox Prize from Nature/Sense about Science for standing up for science and, in 2017, a Doctor of Laws honoris causa from the University of Bath.

David Pilgrim is Honorary Professor of Health and Social Policy at the University of Liverpool and Visiting Professor of Clinical Psychology at the University of Southampton. His recent publications include *Understanding Mental Health: A Critical Realist Exploration* (2015); *Key Concepts in Mental Health* (5th ed., 2019); *Child Sexual Abuse: Moral Panic or State of Denial?* (2018); and *Critical Realism for Psychologists* (2020).

Rob Poole is Professor of Social Psychiatry at Bangor University, where he co-directs the Centre for Mental Health and Society. He trained at St George's Hospital, London, and in Oxford before working as an NHS community psychiatrist in Liverpool and in North Wales for twenty-one years. His clinical and research interests centre on the social determinants of mental health. He has written extensively, including scientific papers, book chapters and several books. In 2009, the Critical Psychiatry blog described him as 'an old-fashioned radical'. He received the Royal College of Psychiatrists' Lifetime Achievement Award in 2017.

Gianetta Rands achieved six A levels and a degree in Experimental Psychology at Oxford University before embarking on medical training at the Royal Free Hospital Medical School. She trained as a general practitioner and as a psychiatrist. She worked in the NHS for thirty-four years and held many roles as consultant psychiatrist, tutor and training programme director and actively contributed to Royal College of Psychiatrists committees. She now has an independent practice specialising in complex assessments of dementias, brain injuries and mental capacity judgements. She is concerned about the effects on the brain of current in-flight cabin environments and the persistence of so many inequalities affecting women's lives.

Miles Rinaldi is Head of Strategic Development at South West London and St George's Mental Health NHS Trust. He pioneered the implementation of the Individual Placement and Support approach in the UK within community mental health services, first episode psychosis teams and primary care mental health services. He implemented a recovery-focused approach across his organisation, including establishing the first Recovery College in the UK. He also developed mental health policy at the Office of the Deputy Prime Minister, Department of Health, Cabinet Office and Department for Work and Pensions. He is the author of more than thirty peer-reviewed publications.

Catherine Robinson is Professor of Social Care Research. She is Co-director of the Institute for Health Policy and Organisation and leads the Social Care and Society research group at the University of Manchester. Catherine is also an associate director of the National Institute for Health Research (NIHR) School for Social Care Research. Her research interests include global mental health, adult social care and the prevention of suicide and self-harm.

Anne Rogers is Professor of Medical Sociology and Health Systems Implementation at the University of Southampton. Her current interests include research and knowledge translation in the sociological aspects of mental health and illness, users' experiences of health care, health need and demand for care and how patients adapt to and incorporate new technologies into their everyday lives. Currently she is focused on addressing how personal and social networks and relationships in domestic and community settings act as a conduit for accessing resources and support for managing health and illness.

Wendy Rose OBE has a background in social work practice and social services management and was a senior civil servant in England advising on children's policy. As a senior research fellow at the Open University and later an honorary research fellow at Cardiff University, she was an advisor to the Scottish Government on developing its children's policy and subsequently to the Welsh Government on safeguarding reforms. She has worked extensively on national and international projects. Major themes of her work are improving child and family well-being, developing and implementing change and evaluating outcomes for children.

Graham Scambler is Emeritus Professor of Sociology at University College London (UCL) and Visiting Professor of Sociology at Surrey University. He has written extensively on social theory, health, health inequality and stigma. His latest books are *Sociology, Health and the Fractured Society: A Critical Realist Account* (2018); *A Sociology of Shame and Blame: Insiders Versus Outsiders* (2020); and, with Aksel Tjora, *Communal Forms: A Sociological Exploration of the Concept of Community* (2020). He was a founding editor of the international journal *Social Theory and* *Health* and is a fellow of the Academy of Social Sciences, UK.

Andrew Scull is Distinguished Research Professor at the University of California, San Diego. He was educated at Balliol College, Oxford University, and Princeton University and completed a postdoctoral fellowship in the history of medicine at University College London (UCL). He is past president of the Society for the Social History of Medicine and the author of more than a dozen books on this history of psychiatry, including *Decarceration* (1977, 1984); *Museums of Madness* (1979); *Social Order/Mental Disorder* (1989); *The Most Solitary of Afflictions* (1993); *Madhouse* (2005); *Hysteria* (2010); *Madness in Civilization* (2015); and *Psychiatry and Its Discontents* (2019).

Edward Shorter is a Harvard-trained social historian who has held the Hannah Professorship in the History of Medicine at the University of Toronto since 1991. In 1996, he was cross-appointed as Professor of Psychiatry in recognition of his contributions to the history of the discipline. He is the author of numerous books on aspects of psychiatric history, including *A History of Psychiatry* (1997); *Before Prozac* (2009); and *What Psychiatry Left Out of the DSM-5* (2015). His latest book is *The Madness of Fear: A History of Catatonia* (2018), co-written with Dr Max Fink, Professor Emeritus of Psychiatry and Neurology at SUNY-Stony Brook.

Thomas Stephenson is a trainee psychiatrist working in South London and Maudsley NHS Trust with a clinical and research interest in mental health among people in prison. Thomas is an active member of the Royal College of Psychiatrists' History of Psychiatry Special Interest Group (HoPSIG) executive committee.

George Szmukler is Emeritus Professor of Psychiatry and Society at the Institute of

Psychiatry, Psychology and Neuroscience. King's College London. He was previously Consultant Psychiatrist at the South London and Maudsley NHS Foundation Trust; Medical Director of the Bethlem and Maudsley NHS Trust; Dean of the Institute of Psychiatry, King's College London; Visiting Professor at the Department of Sociology, London School of Economics; and Associate Director of the National Institute for Health Research (NIHR) – Mental Health Research Network. He is currently Chair of the Special Committee on Human Rights of the Royal College of Psychiatrists.

Pamela Taylor was trained in general adult and forensic psychiatry in the UK and United States. Roles include the Special Hospitals' Service Authority's Head of Medical Services (1990–5); Inner London Probation Service Executive Board member (1992–2002); special hospital personality disorder unit lead (1995–2004); Chair RCPsych Forensic Psychiatry Faculty (2017–20); editor-in-chief of *Criminal Behaviour and Mental Health*; and trustee of the *Howard League for Penal Reform, Crime in Mind*. Taylor's publications include more than 200 peer-reviewed papers and edited books: *Forensic Psychiatry: Clinical, Legal and Ethical Issues* (1993, 2014); *Violence in Society* (1993); *Couples in Care and Custody* (1999); and *Personality Disorder and Serious Offending: Hospital Treatment Models* (2006).

Jerry Tew is Professor of Mental Health and Social Work School of Social Policy at the University of Birmingham. Following his graduation from Cambridge University, Jerry worked as a specialist mental health social worker before moving into an academic role where he has written and researched on social approaches in mental health, mental health policy, recovery and 'whole family' approaches. He is currently a co-investigator in an NIHR-funded trial of

the Open Dialogue approach and is a senior fellow of the NIHR School for Social Care Research, for whom he is currently leading a research project on the implementation of asset-based and capacity-building approaches in social care and mental health.

Philip Timms trained in medicine and, subsequently, in psychiatry at Guy's Hospital, London. In the late 1980s, he helped to set up and run the Psychiatric Team for Single Homeless People, the first mental health outreach team for homeless people in the UK. He subsequently led the START team for homeless people, which engaged patients on the streets and across other homeless milieu. He edited the RCPsych brochures for the public for twenty years. He is currently a consultant psychiatrist at the National Psychosis Unit. He has published on homelessness, information for patients and the use of jargon in mental health.

Trevor Turner attained his MBBS in 1976 at Barts Hospital in London, trained in psychiatry at the Maudsley Hospital and obtained his MRCPsych in 1981 and his MD at London University in 1990. He was a general adult consultant based at Barts, Hackney and then Homerton Hospital between 1987 and 2013, working as a medical director and a clinical director. He chaired the North Thames and then one of the London Divisions of the Royal College of Psychiatrists and was Vice-President in 2004–6. He has written more than ninety papers and five books, including *Community Mental Health Care: A Practical Guide to Outdoor Psychiatry*. He remains an honorary consultant at the East London Foundation Trust.

Peter Tyrer is Emeritus Professor of Community Psychiatry in the Division of Psychiatry in Imperial College, having previously been a head of department and a professor at Imperial College since 1991. He received the Lifetime Achievement Award of the Royal College of Psychiatrists in 2015; has chaired NICE guideline groups for borderline personality disorder (2009), substance misuse and psychosis (2012) and management of imminent aggression (2015); and has written 41 books and more than 650 original articles. He was the editor of the *British Journal of Psychiatry* between 2003 and 2013, and between 2001 and 2006 headed a research group to evaluate components of the DSPD programme.

Introduction: Mind State and History in Britain 1960–2010

George Ikkos and Nick Bouras

'The need to lend a voice to suffering is a condition of all truth.'

T. W. Adorno[1]

At the end of the Second World War in 1945, Britain emerged victorious, with the largest industrial base in Europe and its empire intact; but it was also in debt to the United States, which led to continuing food rationing and a decade of austerity. Nevertheless, by the end of the 1950s the economy had recovered, setting in motion a doubling of gross domestic product (GDP) between 1950 and 1975, a feat not matched between 1975 and 2000. This despite, or perhaps because, the fact that the empire began to recede from the late 1940s. By the mid-1960s, it had been lost for good.

The period 1960–2010 coincides with major changes in UK politics, the economy, society and health care. Legislation such as the Abortion and Sexual Relations Acts in 1967, the Race Relations Act 1968 and the Equal Pay Act 1970 illustrates the direction of reform. Since 1979, the successive electoral triumphs of Margaret Thatcher (and the acceptance by New Labour of the general thrust of her policies – particularly in health care) fundamentally changed the nation's orientation but did not reverse the liberalising trends. For example, with respect to diversity, positive change has advanced regardless, even if it is still short of natural justice.

It was also a period of major transformation in the international operating environment. Events such as the Oil Crisis of 1973, the collapse of the Soviet Union in 1989 and the 'War on Terror' since 1991 have weighed heavily on internal matters. For example, while the communist Soviet Union had continued to give the impression of a living European ideological alternative to Western liberal democracies, dominant centre-right and centre-left UK politicians had been reluctant to allow inequality and social exclusion to flourish. Later market-oriented libertarians have had no such qualms. Even a senior New Labour figure achieved notoriety by proclaiming himself as 'intensely relaxed about people getting filthy rich', adding 'as long as they pay their taxes'.

During this period, the UK has moved from a narrow post-war social conservativism, through liberalism and social welfare, towards libertarianism, free market fundamentalism and trade globalisation. However, at a time of significant growth in inflation-adjusted GDP, these changes, though questioning of the role of the state, did not prevent the proportion of GDP expenditure on health rising from 3.1 per cent in 1960 to 7.5 per cent in 2010 (see also Chapter 11). Yet, by contemporary European standards, it should have been more.

Among the biggest transformations have been those of deinstitutionalisation and community care in psychiatry and mental health. Challenged by the marketisation of the National Health Service (NHS), the early community care reformers might hardly recognise

1

the current landscape. Evolving technology has also had an enormous impact, though less so in psychopharmacology than had been hoped. Since 1990, the explosion in big data and new social media has brought us to a radically different phase, perhaps a fourth industrial revolution dominated by artificial intelligence. In Greek, 'meta' means 'after' and we have argued that we have now entered a new era of 'meta-community' psychiatry and mental health care.[2] This, coupled with the shock of the financial crisis of 2008, makes it timely to look back to the half-century 1960–2010 and reflect on changes during those decades.

The motivating questions behind this volume are, what have citizens' attitudes towards mental ill health been? How have those with mental ill health and their families or other informal and formal carers fared? And what has changed for mental health professionals? In exploring these questions, we have tried to avoid the pitfall of restricting ourselves to themes of deinstitutionalisation and community care and to shine the light more broadly.[3] Our intentions have been to bear witness, inform and stimulate curiosity and research but not be exhaustive in detail.

As editors, we have been determined to steer a course between self-sufficiency in each chapter and the structural integrity of the whole volume. Many of the contributors have been protagonists of psychiatry and mental health care, some experts by experience. Their chapters will reflect these experiences and personal opinions. We believe these add depth. However, as well as addressing a range of more narrowly defined facets of psychiatry and mental health services, the volume is also enriched by historical, sociological and political contributions. As ideological considerations have had and are likely to continue to have influence, complementary or discordant perspectives should help refine debate and advance policy and practice.[4] Though each chapter may be read on its own, we believe that those who read the volume as a whole will benefit most. We have thought carefully about whether the title of the book should refer to British or UK history. There are a handful of references to Northern Ireland but not to clinical services. Therefore, we decided to refer only to Britain in the title.

Readers will find that some ideas, events, institutions, policies and so on recur through different chapters. This is because of the cardinal position of certain constellations during this period which merit repeated illumination. As Walter Benjamin observed:

> One only knows a spot once one has experienced it in as many dimensions as possible. You must have approached a place from all four cardinal points if you want to take it in, and what's more, you also have to have left it from all these points. Otherwise it will quite unexpectedly cross your path three or four times before you are prepared to discover it.[5]

Notes

1. T. W. Adorno, *Negative Dialectics*, trans E. B. Ashton. London: Routledge, 1973, p. 17.

2. N. Bouras, G. Ikkos and T. Craig, From community to meta-community mental health care. *International Journal of Environmental Research and Public Health* (2018) 15: 806, https://doi.org/10.3390/ijerph15040806

3. J. Turner, R. Hayward, K. Angel et al., The history of mental health services in modern England: Practitioner memories and the direction of future research. *Medical History* (2015) 59: 599–624, 600.

4. N. Bouras and G. Ikkos, Ideology, psychiatric practice and professionalism. *Psychiatriki* (2013) 24(1): 17–27.

5. W. Benjamin, *Moscow Diary*, trans R. Sieburth. Cambridge, MA: Harvard University Press, 1986, p. 25.

Chapter

Historical Perspectives on Mental Health and Psychiatry

Joanna Bourke

Introduction

Robairt Clough was a long-term patient at Holywell Psychiatric Hospital in Antrim (Northern Ireland). In the Christmas 1972 edition of the patients' magazine, he wrote the following verses:

> Little drops of medicine,
> Little coloured pills,
> Cure us of all ailments,
> Cure us of all ills.
>
> Doctors with a stethoscope,
> Doctors with a bag,
> Make us fit and healthy,
> Cheer us when we flag.
>
> Pretty little nurses
> Nurses bold and strong,
> Nurses with a banjo,
> Nurses sing a song.
>
> Wardsmaids with the dinner,
> Wardsmaids with the tea,
> Keep our tummies happy,
> Until the day we're free.[1]

This little ditty from 1972 draws attention to some of the dominant themes in the social history of mental health and psychiatry in Britain from the 1960s to the 2010s. These include the championing of psychopharmacology (those 'little coloured pills'), symbolic representations of psychiatric authority (stethoscope and medicine bag), the emotional management of patients ('pretty little nurses' with their songs), cultures of conviviality (keeping tummies happy) and, of course, the ominous mood instilled by disciplinary practices and environments (they wait 'Until the day we're free'). The ditty acknowledges the *social* meanings generated when psychiatric patients and health professionals meet. Each participant brings to the encounter a multitude of identities based on gender, class, ethnicity, sexuality, generation, age, religion and ideological dogmas as well as memories of past encounters, sensual perceptions and embodied knowledges. As a result, any overview of the history of British psychiatry needs to grapple with the tension between temporally fluid *societal* contexts and the sensual intimacy of very *personal* human

3

encounters (i.e. seeing the Other, touching, stories only partly heard, bodily smells, the metallic taste of pills).

The historiographical literature on mental health and psychiatry from the 1960s to the end of the first decade of the twenty-first century is exceptionally detailed in terms of policy and politics. Scholars have drawn on Foucault's 'great confinement' (particularly his book *Madness and Civilization*), Roy Porter's patients' perspectives, material culture and the powerful themes of discipline, power and social construction.[2] In contrast to these grand political and theoretical themes, this chapter seeks to explore some of the most significant changes in the lived experiences of mental health and psychiatry. It pays attention to social encounters between medical professionals and patients.

It is important to acknowledge, however, that the medical professionals discussed in this chapter are not the main caregivers. People identified as having 'mental health issues' engage in their own practices of self-care. They often have strong familial networks (especially those sustained by mothers, grandmothers, daughters and sisters). They routinely seek advice from health-oriented journalists, radio and television programmers, teachers, police, pharmacists and doctors' receptionists, not to mention herbalists, tarot card readers, astrologers, psychics and faith healers. Since the 1960s, Britain has undoubtedly become more secular, but distressed people continue to seek the laying on of hands. As I argue in my book *The Story of Pain: From Prayer to Painkillers*, secularisation is honoured more in rhetoric than reality.[3] The same people who attend consultations with cognitive behavioural therapy (CBT) therapists eventually return home where they call out to their gods for relief of mental suffering.

Psychiatric professionals, however, claim to provide a *superior* tier of help to people who identify themselves, or are identified by others, as experiencing mental health problems. In the period from the 1960s to 2010, there are six major shifts in encounters between these professionals and their patients: deinstitutionalisation, changes in diagnostic nomenclature, anti-psychiatry, patients' movements, evidence-based medicine and the privileging of psychopharmacology, neurochemistry and neurobiology. These themes overlap to varying degrees.

Deinstitutionalisation

The first theme is deinstitutionalisation (see also Chapter 31). The closure of the Victorian public asylum system and its replacement with community-based psychiatric services is the greatest social shift for patients and professionals since the 1960s. Although the movement had a long history and was by no means confined to Britain, a decisive moment for British practices occurred in 1961 when Enoch Powell, the minister of health, gave a speech at the annual conference of the National Association for Mental Health (now called Mind). In it, Powell predicted that, within fifteen years, 'there may well be needed not more than half as many places in hospitals for mental illness as there are today'. He described the Victorian asylums as standing 'isolated, majestic, imperious, brooded over by the gigantic water-tower and chimney combined, rising unmistakable and daunting out of the countryside'. These asylums 'which our forefathers built with such immense solidity to express the notions of their day' were now outdated. He maintained that it was necessary for 'the medical profession *outside* the hospital service . . . to accept responsibility for more and more of that care of patients which today is given *inside* the hospitals'. They had to be 'supported in their task' by local authorities.[4] In the years that followed Powell's speech, mentally ill people moved repeatedly between hospitals, care centres, other local facilities and family homes, as well as within a growing sector of 'for-profit' care. The belief that welfare dependency was obsolete and morally corrupting grew; the mentally ill were not only encouraged but *required* to become independent and autonomous.

Deinstitutionalisation had major societal effects. Attacks on the welfare state by the governments of Margaret Thatcher and John Major contributed to the stigmatisation of the poor and mentally ill. Asylums were emptied and converted into luxury homes, parks and other public centres. In the 1950s, there were 150,000 psychiatric beds in England; by 2006, this had fallen to 34,000.[5] The underfunding of mental health services, especially when compared to physical health facilities, plagues the entire field.[6]

The emergence of therapeutic communities in the 1950s led by Maxwell Jones encouraged other psychiatrists such as John Wing, director of the Medical Research Council's Social Psychiatry Research Unit between 1965 and 1989, to propagate the concept of 'rehabilitation'. Prior to this period, 'rehabilitation' had primarily referred to assistance to people who were *physically* injured, especially ex-servicemen, but it was reworked as a way of providing mentally unwell patients with the skills necessary for independent living.[7] Prescriptions for drugs skyrocketed. Prisons, too, had to deal with soaring numbers of inmates diagnosed with mental illnesses, although it is unclear if this was due to the 'psychiatrisation' of criminality or a greater recognition of mental illness more generally.[8]

There is no consensus about whether deinstitutionalisation has been a good or bad thing. Was it an enlightened move, facilitated by the introduction of more effective drugs and seeking to give greater autonomy to the mentally ill? Or was it a component of right-wing policies determined to slash public spending, irrespective of the effects on vulnerable members of society?

Few commentators, though, dispute the fact that deinstitutionalisation did create many new problems. A lot of people who needed support lost contact with mental health services altogether.[9] There was often inadequate or non-existent community provision in the first place. After all, in 1959, there were only twenty-four full-time psychiatric social workers employed by local authorities throughout England. This problem was exacerbated by the balance-of-payment crisis and inflation in the 1970s, which left local authorities struggling to cope.[10] Even Frank Dobson, secretary of state for health between 1997 and 1999, admitted that 'care in the community has failed'. He observed that

> people who are mentally ill, their carers and the professional staff responsible for their welfare have suffered from ineffective practices, an outdated legal framework and lack of resources ... Discharging people from institutions has brought benefits to some. But it has left many vulnerable patients to try to cope on their own ... Too many confused and sick people have been left wandering the streets and sleeping rough.[11]

Deinstitutionalisation was a particular problem for the most severely and chronically ill who required long-term care. One group that was most ruthlessly affected was older people. They often suffer from complex, overlapping psychiatric conditions, including disorders such as depression, chronic degenerative brain disorders and lifestyle crises resulting from isolation and bereavement.[12] Despite this, mentally ill older people were relegated to a lowly position within the hierarchy of psychiatry patients. As late as the 1940s, there were *no* specialist services in England for people with senile dementia.[13] The first international conference on the subject only took place in London in 1965.[14] Even at the end of the 1970s, only half of health service districts provided specialist services for older people with mental health issues.[15] Older men and women were increasingly and disproportionately represented in psychiatric institutions. For example, in the early 1970s, around 9 per cent of the population of England and Wales were over sixty-five years of age, but they occupied 47 per cent of the psychiatric beds.[16] In the words of the psychiatrist W. Alwyn Lishman, who worked in the late 1950s,

> Every large mental hospital has a secret large ward tucked away – perhaps three or four . . . which were not much visited because they were full of old demented people. Because there was no interest in them, it fell to the most junior doctor to go there once a week to see if any one needed to have their chest listened to. The most neglected parts of any mental hospital were the old age wards.[17]

Deinstitutionalisation and 'community care' made these older patients' situation even worse (see also Chapter 22). Families struggled to cope. Despite the obvious dependence of older people on the state, little investment was forthcoming. Ageism and prejudiced beliefs that nothing could be done to improve their well-being hampered positive responses. In 1973, J. A. Whitehead, consultant psychiatrist at Bevendean Hospital in Brighton, bluntly declared that psychiatric services were 'loath to deal with [older] patients'. He added that, when this neglect was 'coupled with society's fear of mental illness and the ambivalent attitudes to older people in general, the mentally ill old person is in a dismal position'.[18]

Anti-psychiatry

If the first theme is deinstitutionalisation, with its negative effects on the most vulnerable members of society, including older people, the second is anti-psychiatry (see also Chapter 20). Although the German physician Bernhard Beyer first used the term 'anti-psychiatry' in 1912, David Graham Cooper (a South African psychiatrist who trained and worked in London) popularised it in his book *Psychiatry and Anti-Psychiatry* (1967). In it, Cooper accused psychiatry of being 'in danger of committing a well-intentioned act of betrayal of those members of society who have been ejected into the psychiatric situation as patients'.[19] The movement was led by global figures such as Michel Foucault, Erving Goffman, Ken Kesey and Thomas Szasz and, in Britain, by R. D. Laing, Cooper and, from 1966, the Institute of Phenomenological Studies.[20] These anti-psychiatrists were embedded in wider countercultural movements. They maintained political links with global liberationist movements and were attracted by existential psychiatry and phenomenology.

They were a diverse group but all rejected the 'whiggish' approach to psychiatry – that is, the 'rise and rise' of psychiatric knowledge and power. Instead, they developed damning critiques of the profession, arguing that it was damaging people's lives. As Laing explained in *The Voice of Experience* (1982), asylums were total institutions, like concentration camps. When patients enter psychiatric care, he contended, they 'are mentally dismembered. Raw data go into the machine, as once raw human meat into the mouth of Moloch' (i.e. the Canaanite god associated with child sacrifice).[21]

For anti-psychiatrists, *society* not biology was the cause of mental distress. Laing's highly influential work on schizophrenia strengthened their belief that even major disturbances could be understood as intelligible responses to environments and relationships. Both Laing and Cooper were also highly critical of the bourgeois family, warning that it fostered psychic abuse. For many anti-psychiatrists, mental illness did not even exist. As the scholar Michael

Staub explains in *Madness Is Civilization* (2018), anti-psychiatrists believed that only 'good fortune and chance' stood between insanity and mental health.[22]

Anti-psychiatrists insisted that mental health could be better achieved by the establishment of therapeutic communities (such as Cooper's Shenley Hospital for young schizophrenics between 1962 and 1967) that were anti-hierarchical, people-led, positive and open to the worlds of psychotics. Laing even argued that severe psychotic illnesses could be healing, enabling a person to travel into a mystical world and return with greater insight. He established the Kingsley Hall therapeutic community for people with psychotic afflictions in 1965, eradicating hierarchies between patients and doctors.[23]

The long term assessment of anti-psychiatry is divided. The movement drew attention to abuses of power and the need to give people control over their own lives. Yet, as the historian Andrew Scull concluded, it also encouraged two views. The first was the 'romantic notion' that madness was nothing more than a 'social construction, a consequence of arbitrary labeling'. The second was that 'existing mental hospitals were so awful that *any* alternative must somehow represent an improvement. Sadly, "it just ain't so".'[24]

However, anti-psychiatry gained support from a wide range of people who were becoming critical of what was increasingly seen as the abuse of power by psychiatrists. Lobotomy, insulin coma therapy, drug-induced convulsions and electroconvulsive therapy (ECT) treatments were dubbed instruments of oppression, designed not to heal but to coerce people into behaving in particular ways. The treatment of homosexuals was exposed as particularly repellent. Not only were homosexuals given religious counselling and psychoanalysis in an attempt to 'cure' them of their sexual orientation but they were also prescribed oestrogen treatments to reduce libido,[25] and between the early 1960s and the early 1970s, they were subjected to behavioural aversion therapy with electric shocks. Many were given apomorphine (which causes severe nausea and vomiting) as an aversive stimulus (see also Chapter 34).[26]

Revelations of psychiatric abuses swung support behind anti-psychiatrists. Particularly important were Barbara Robb's *Sans Everything: A Case to Answer* (1967); a 1968 *World in Action* documentary; reports that ECT was being given without anaesthetic or muscle relaxant at Broadmoor Hospital; and exposés of abuses at Ely (1969), Farleigh (1971), Whittingham (1972), Napsbury (1973), South Ockendon (1974) and Normansfield (1978) hospitals. One of the consequences of the earlier scandals was the setting up of the Health Service Commissioner (Ombudsman) in 1972. Dr Louise Hide discusses these scandals in Chapter 7 in this volume.

Patients' Movements

Scandals, coupled with rising numbers of *voluntary* patients (who had been admitted to mental hospitals from 1930), resulted in the third major shift in the social history of mental health and psychiatry in Britain after the 1960s. This was the rise of parents' and then patients' movements (see also Chapters 13 and 14).

There was a range of reasons for the frustration felt by people being treated for psychiatric ailments but the dominant one was linked to debates about informed consent. The 1959 Mental Health Act had not even *mentioned* consent to treatment. By the early 1970s, the Medical Defence Union endorsed the need for consent but there was a lack of clarity about *how* medical professionals were expected to ensure that their patients understood the nature, purpose and risks of treatments.[27]

By the 1983 Mental Health Act (England and Wales), however, consent was a prominent feature. Part of the credit for this change goes to the rise and growing influence of mental health charities and activist groups, including the National Association for Mental Health (now Mind). When it was established in 1946, Mind brought together professionals, relatives and volunteers to lobby for the improved care of children and adults with psychiatric problems. There was also an abundance of other user-movements, including the Mental Patients' Union, the Community Organisation for Psychiatric Emergencies, Protection for the Rights of Mental Patients in Treatment, Campaign Against Psychiatric Oppression, Survivors Speak Out and the United Kingdom Advocacy Network. Other groups, styling themselves (initially) as charities included the National Autistic Society, which sought to draw the public's attention to the specific needs of autistic children, while also castigating the medical establishment for stigmatising them. From only a dozen such organisations in the 1980s, there were more than 500 by 2005, partly due to the establishment of the NHS and the Community Care Act of 1990.[28] By banding together, the families of people designated 'mentally ill' could share information, provide encouragement and lobby for improved facilities.[29] In 1970, a major battle was won when the government passed the Education (Handicapped Children) Act, which gave all children with disabilities the right to education.

From the 1970s, activists began drawing on the language of *human rights* to make their case. In contrast to *parents'* movements, which tended to lobby for more and better biomedical research into the causes and cures of mental illness, an abundance of *patient-led* organisations sprang up. These groups repudiated the paternalism inherent in charity status, together with the implication that they needed to be 'cured'. As patients, they insisted that *they* were the ones with the authority to adjudicate on the meaning of their situation and the appropriate responses (which may or may not include treatment). They emphasised health rather than illness.[30] These patients' movements sought to draw attention to the positive aspects of being 'different'; they insisted on the complexity of their lives; and they reminded people of the contributions they made to society.[31]

Patients' movements were encouraged by the rise of the Internet, which enabled people with mental health problems to communicate with each other much more easily. Mental health blogging greatly facilitated the development of therapeutic communities outside institutional ones. Unfortunately, the positive aspects of these forms of communications have also been exploited by unscrupulous commercial companies, quacks and advertisers.

In more recent decades, the 'rights' discourse has been supplanted by one emphasising individual 'choice'. As the historian Alex Mold boldly states, patients 'have been made into consumers', in which the main language is choice and autonomy.[32] The Labour government from 1997 to 2010 transformed the NHS into a 'market', which unfortunately has exacerbated inequalities based on race, region, class, gender and age (see also Chapters 3, 10 and 11). Mold concludes that 'It is difficult to see how patient-consumers can overcome completely the power imbalance with health professionals' and 'the tension between individual demands and collective needs also persists'.[33]

Diagnostic Nomenclature

The fourth shift involves the fabrication as well as demolition of diagnostic categories. These processes provide important insights into how knowledge is created, spread, consolidated and shrunk (see also Chapter 17).

There have always been dramatic shifts in medical nomenclature, the most written about one being the rise of hysteria as a diagnostic category in the Victorian period and then its falling from grace in the twentieth century, as documented by Mark Micale.[34] In the period from the 1960s to the 2010, the most notable change has been the 1973 removal of homosexuality from the category of a mental illness (although transsexuality has been introduced as an item of interest to psychiatrists).

Another new diagnostic category that has been introduced is attention deficit hyperactivity disorder. It has proved controversial, however, on the grounds that it pathologises children and leads to over-medicalisation. These critiques were linked to wider debates about the 'medicalisation' of everyday problems. Social anxiety disorder, for example, has been said to be an example of medicalising shyness, giving rise to the 'therapeutic state' that psychologises every aspect of people's lives and is inherently pathologising. There has also been the growth of transcultural psychiatry, recognising that diagnostic categories, symptoms and measuring instruments might not be valid for the twenty-two different ethnic groups with populations of more than 100,000 living in the UK (see also Chapters 35 and 36).[35]

Evidence-Based Medicine

The fifth shift is more administrative but had a major impact on patients and mental health professionals. This is the revolution in evidence-based medicine, with the standardisation of evaluation methods, as well as the formalisation of quality assurance, efficiency metrics, interdisciplinary teams and randomised controlled trials (see also Chapter 17).[36] In the 1960s, drug trials had simply meant clinical observations. As one psychiatrist involved in early trials of drugs for schizophrenia recalled,

> There was no blinding and no randomization. Informed consent was unnecessary. There were no institutional review boards. Initially, there were no rating scales, and results were reported in a narrative fashion.[37]

This all was swept away. As Ann Donald in an article in *Culture, Medicine, and Psychiatry* argues, one result was the introduction of 'algorithms of care' or 'Wal-Marting'. Instead of individualised, personalised treatments, physicians turn to population-based databases. This 'epistemological change results in the development of a clinical knowledge patterned along algorithmic pathways', Donald explains, 'rather than subjective understanding. An increased and more rapidly rationalization of psychiatry is the result.'[38]

Psychopharmacology, Neurochemistry and Neurobiology

The final shift is one that has affected each of the five themes discussed in this chapter. Since 1900, psychiatric thought has been divided between what have (in very broad strokes) been called biomedical versus psychosocial models (see also Chapters 4 and 17). Is psychiatric ill health primarily physiological or psychosocial? Of course, in reality, nearly everyone (except some anti-psychiatrists) agree that the answer is 'a bit of both'; the dispute is over the *balance* of impacts. From the 1960s, however, the neurochemical and neurobiological origins of mental illness were privileged over the psychodynamic and sociological. New pharmaceutical products such as anti-anxiety and anti-depressant compounds have also revolutionised treatments. With 'big pharma' has come the increased role of mental health insurance industries. Crucial to this shift was the synthetisation of chlorpromazine (Largactil) in 1952, the 'new wonder drug for psychotic illness'.[39] As G. Tourney observed in 1968,

> We are in the great age of psychopharmacology, in which industry has great stakes … The physician has become increasingly dependent on brochures from drug companies rather than formal scientific reports.[40]

Freudian therapies, in particular, were stripped from medical training as well as practice. In the words of one commentator, the last half of the twentieth century saw the 'disappearance of the couch'; the Freudian fifty minutes of therapeutic time has been cut to only fifteen minutes of CBT.[41]

Psychopharmacology has been boosted by a massive investment of capital in neurology, other brain sciences and chemistry. The prominent neuropsychiatrist Henry A. Nasrallah argues that the 'future of psychiatry is bright, even scintillating'. He maintains that 'psychiatric practice will be transformed into a clinical neuroscience that will heal the mind by replacing the brain'. In particular, he mentions new technologies, including 'cranial electrical stimulation (CES), deep brain stimulation (DBS), epidural cortical stimulation (ECS), focused ultrasound (FUS), low-field magnetic stimulation (LFMS), magnetic seizure therapy (MST), near infrared light therapy (NIR), and transcranial direct current stimulation (TDCS)'.[42] What this will mean for patients is still unknown.

Conclusion

This chapter began with the patient Robairt Clough's ditty, published in the 1972 Christmas edition of the patients' magazine of Holywell Psychiatric Hospital in Antrim:

> Little drops of medicine,
> Little coloured pills,
> Cure us of all ailments,
> Cure us of all ills.

A year after Robairt Clough wrote these words, the Christmas edition of the magazine was to be the last edition. In-patient numbers at the Holywell Psychiatric Hospital were in decline. Faculties were 'generally cramped', occupational therapy was 'substandard' and the entire health service was being restructured.[43] With deinstitutionalisation, 'communities of suffering' moved elsewhere; diagnostic categories expanded dramatically with the growth of the therapeutic state; anti-psychiatry morphed into patient activism; and those 'little coloured pills' continued to be popped into the open mouths of patients like Robairt Clough who waited for 'the day we're free'.

Summary Key Points

- This chapter draws attention to social encounters between medical professionals and patients.
- Deinstitutionalisation, changes in diagnostic nomenclature, anti-psychiatry, patients' movements, evidence-based medicine and advances of psychopharmacology, neurochemistry and neurobiology are among the main encounters between professionals and patients from the 1960s to the 2010s.

- Discipline, power and social construction have been prominent in the policy and politics of psychiatry.
- Deinstitutionalisation is perhaps the most important social experiment of the last century.
- The mental health needs of older people, homosexuality and consent are among the major themes underlined during the fifty years under consideration.

Notes

1. R. Clough, Holywell Rhymes. *Speedwell* (1972) 22: 29.

2. V. Hess and B. Majerus, Writing the history of psychiatry in the 20th century. *History of Psychiatry* (2011) 22: 139–45, 140; R. Porter, *Patients and Practitioners: Lay Perceptions of Medicine in Pre-Industrial Society.* Cambridge: Cambridge University Press, 1985.

3. J. Bourke, *The Story of Pain: From Prayer to Painkillers.* Oxford: Oxford University Press, 2016.

4. J. E. Powell, 'Enoch Powell's Water Tower Speech 1961', www.studymore.org.uk/xpowell.htm.

5. B. Cooper, British psychiatry and its discontents. *Journal of the Royal Society of Medicine* (2010) 103: 397–402, 394.

6. J. Turner, R. Hayward, K. Angel et al., The history of mental health services in modern England: Practitioner memories and the direction of future research. *Medical History* (2015) 59: 599–624, 604.

7. V. Long, Heading up a blind alley? Scottish psychiatric hospitals in the era of deinstitutionalization. *History of Psychiatry* (2017) 28: 115–28, 117.

8. D. Double, The limits of psychiatry. *The British Medical Journal* (April 2002) 324: 900–4, 901.

9. I. Shaw, A short history of mental health. In I. Shaw, H. Middleton and J. Cohen, eds, *Understanding Treatment without Consent: An Analysis of the Work of the Mental Health Act Commission*, 3–12. Aldershot: Ashgate, 2007, p. 8.

10. R. Porter, Two cheers for psychiatry!: The social history of mental disorder in twentieth century Britain. In H. Freeman and G. E. Berrios, eds, *150 Years of British Psychiatry: Volume 2: The Aftermath*, 383–406. London, Athlone Press, 1996.

11. BBC, Dobson outlines mental health plans, *BBC News*, 29 July 1998, http://news.bbc.co.uk/1/hi/health/141 651.stm.

12. C. Hilton, Psychiatrists, mental health provision, and 'senile dementia' in England, 1940s–1979. *History of Psychiatry* (2015) 26: 182–99, 182.

13. Ibid., 185.

14. *Psychiatric Disorders in the Aged: Report of the Symposium Held by the World Psychiatric Association at the Royal College of Physicians, London, September 28th–30th, 1965*, Manchester: Geigy, 1965.

15. Hilton, Psychiatrists, mental health provision, and 'senile dementia' in England, 185.

16. Ibid., 190.

17. Ibid., 183. See also The Oral History of Geriatrics as a Medical Specialty Collection, Oral History Collections, British Library, BL C512/39/01.

18. J. A. Whitehead, *Psychiatric Disorders in Old Age: A Handbook for the Clinical Team.* Aylesbury: Harvey Miller and Medcalf, 1974, p. 5.

19. D. G. Cooper, *Psychiatry and Anti-Psychiatry.* London: Tavistock Publications, 1967, p. x.

20. O. Wall, *The British Anti-Psychiatrists: From Institutional Psychiatry to the Counter-Culture, 1960–1971.* London: Routledge, 2018.

21. R. D. Laing, *The Voice of Experience: Experience, Science and Psychiatry*. London: Allen Lang, 1982.

22. M. E. Staub, *Madness Is Civilization: When the Diagnosis Was Social, 1948–1980*. Chicago: University of Chicago Press, 2011.

23. M. Barnes and J. Berke, *Mary Barnes: Two Accounts of a Journey Through Madness*. Harmondsworth: Penguin Books, 1973.

24. A. Scull, Mental patients and the community: A critical note. *International Journal of Law and Psychiatry* (1986) 9: 383–92.

25. G. Smith, A. Bartlett and M. King, Treatments of homosexuality since the 1950s – an oral history: The experience of patients. *The British Medical Journal* (February 2004) 328: 427–29, 428.

26. Ibid.

27. Medical Defence Union, *Consent to Treatment*. London: Medical Defence Union, 1971.

28. P. Campbell, From little acorns: The mental health service user movement. In A. Bell and P. Lindley, eds, *Beyond the Water Towers: The Unfinished Revolution in Mental Health*, 73–82. London: Sainsbury Centre for Mental Health, 2005.

29. M. Waltz, *Autism: A Social and Medical History*. Basingstoke: Palgrave Macmillan, 2013.

30. N. Crossley, Transforming the mental health field: The early history of the National Association for Mental Health. *Sociology of Health and Illness* (1998) 20: 458–88.

31. Waltz, *Autism*.

32. A. Mold, *Making the Patient-Consumer: Patient Organisations and Health Consumerism in Britain*. Manchester: Manchester University Press, 2015.

33. Ibid., p. 204.

34. M. S. Micale, On the 'disappearance' of hysteria: A study in the clinical deconstruction of a diagnosis. *ISIS* (1993) 84: 496–526.

35. British Medical Journal, The search for a psychiatric Esperanto. *British Medical Journal* (1976) 2: 600–1.

36. G. Eghigian, Deinstitutionalizing the history of contemporary psychiatry. *History of Psychiatry* (2011) 22: 201–14.

37. M. V. Seeman, Forty-five years of schizophrenia: Personal reflections. *History of Psychiatry* (2006) 17: 363–73.

38. A. Donald, The Wal-Marting of American psychiatry: An ethnography of psychiatric practice in the late-twentieth century. *Culture, Medicine, and Psychiatry* (December 2001) 25: 467–72.

39. P. Fennell, *Treatment without Consent: Law, Psychiatry, and the Treatment of Mentally Disordered People Since 1845*. London: Routledge, 1996, p. 156.

40. Quoted in ibid., p. 158.

41. M. S. Micale, The ten most important changes in psychiatry since World War II. *History of Psychiatry* (2014): 25: 485–91; D. Healy, *The Creation of Psychopharmacology*. Cambridge, MA: Harvard University Press, 2002.

42. H. A. Nasrallah, Transformative advances unfolding in psychiatry. *Current Psychiatry* (2019) 18: 10–12.

43. P. Prior and G. McClelland, Through the lens of the hospital magazine: Downshire and Holywell psychiatric hospitals in the 1960s and 1970s. *History of Psychiatry* (2013) 24: 399–414.

Chapter 2

The International Context

Edward Shorter

Introduction

There is a distinctive British tradition of psychiatry that goes back to the earliest days embodied in such institutions as the York Retreat. What is the definition of 'insanity'?, asked James Sims in 1799. It is, he said, 'the thinking, and therefore speaking and acting differently from the bulk of mankind, where that difference does not arise from superior knowledge, ignorance, or prejudice'.[1] It is a definition that has never been surpassed.

The late 1950s and early 1960s were a period of dynamic change in British psychiatry. The Mental Health Act in 1959 saw a vast expansion of outpatient care and made it possible for clinicians to admit patients without the intervention of the magistrate. Eliot Slater, editor-in-chief of the *British Journal of Psychiatry* and head psychiatrist at the National Hospital at Queen Square London, said in 1963, 'Rehabilitation and new treatments are already reducing the bed numbers throughout the country, allowing many of the old "asylums" built in the last century to close within the next 10 to 15 years.'[2]

Michael Shepherd stated in 1965, 'The term "social psychiatry" has come to designate a distinctly British contribution, much as "psychodynamic psychiatry" has characterized American thinking.' Shepherd flagged such British innovations as the 'open-door' system, the 'therapeutic community' and the emphasis on rehabilitation.[3]

Seen in international perspective, British psychiatry is best set against the American. This is the fundamental difference between American and British psychiatry: American psychiatry is for those who can afford it unless they receive forensic referrals. Maxwell Jones, instrumental in creating the 'therapeutic community', commented in 1963 after a guest stay at a mental hospital in Oregon, 'About 50 million people in the United States have no health insurance whatever, mostly because they cannot afford it.'[4] In Britain, psychiatry, of course, is funded by the state.

Equally crucial in the United States has been the evolution of psychopharmacology. In pharmacotherapeutics, the palette went from a supply of genuinely effective agents around 1960 to a limited handful of drugs around 2010 that are now either of disputed efficacy, such as the selective serotonin reuptake inhibitors (SSRIs) 'antidepressants', or toxic when used inappropriately or in children and the elderly, such as the so-called atypical antipsychotics (or second-generation antipsychotics (SGAs)). In diagnosis, US psychiatry went from an eclectic group of indications that had accumulated over the years to the 'consensus-based' system of the *Diagnostic and Statistical Manual of Mental Disorders* (DSM). The result in the United States was that the psychiatry of 2010 was scientifically in a much more parlous state than in 1960.

Travellers between the UK and the United States

In the mid-1970s, the American psychiatrist Jay Amsterdam, later head of the depression unit at the University of Pennsylvania, spent a year training at the Maudsley Hospital in London. He said, 'Back then, my Maudsley teachers called their diagnostic process a "phenomenological" approach, and rarely seemed to have difficulty distinguishing folks with true, melancholic, biological, cognitive, physical depression from other types of depression. In London, it all seemed so obvious and "Schneiderian" to me, it just seemed like the correct way to diagnose physical from mental disorders.' What a shock when he re-entered the world of psychoanalysis in the United States. 'It seemed so, well, undisciplined to me, compared to my days at the Maudsley!'[5]

Yet the traffic went both ways. In 1955–6, Michael Shepherd, a senior psychiatrist at the Maudsley Hospital, spent a year travelling across the United States. He was overcome by the differences from British psychiatry. The American world lived and breathed psychoanalysis. 'In the U.S.A. a remarkable attempt has been made in many centres to inject the whole system, python-like, into the body of academic opinion.' By contrast, 'In Great Britain psychoanalysis has been in contact with, rather than part of, academic psychiatry; its concepts have been transmitted through a semi-permeable membrane of critical examination and testing, and the rate of absorption has been slow.'[6] This was a gracious way of putting the substantial rejection of psychoanalysis on the part of British psychiatry. Medical historian Roy Porter concluded, 'The British medical community as a whole long remained extremely guarded towards psychoanalysis.'[7]

David Goldberg contrasted in 1980 typical hospital visits to a psychiatrist in Britain and the United States. In the latter, 'He will wait for his interview in a comfortably furnished waiting area usually complete with armchairs, fitted carpets, and luxurious potted plants. He will be interviewed by an unhurried psychiatrist who will be sitting in an office which looks as little like a hospital clinic as he can make it.' Eighty-six per cent of such patients will receive psychotherapy, drugs are prescribed in only 25 per cent. In Britain, by contrast, the patient will be interviewed in an office 'which looks most decidedly like a hospital clinic. He is relatively more likely to be physically examined and then to have blood tests and X-rays.' About 70 per cent of British psychiatry patients will receive drugs.[8]

In retrospect, it is hard for British clinicians to imagine the hold which psychoanalysis once exercised on US psychiatry. The psychoanalyst, or 'my shrink', became the standard go-to figure for any mental issue. The parents of Jason, age eight, feared that he might be gay and took him to the 'psychoanalyst', where he remained in treatment for his purported homosexuality for four years.[9] These were all private practitioners.

Shepherd noted with wonder the large amounts of funding available to psychiatric research in the United States. Yet the National Institute of Mental Health (NIMH) had barely opened its doors, and shortly enormous amounts of money would start sloshing across academic psychiatry in the United States. British psychiatrists comforted themselves with their beggar's pittance. Aubrey Lewis said, 'To buy a little piece of apparatus costing £5 was a matter which one had to discuss at length and go to the highest authority in order to get approval.'[10]

Finally, Shepherd found curious the American fixation upon 'mental health', which seemed more a hygienic than a medical concept. The British, at that point, felt more comfortable with the notion of mental pathology than mental health, and even though

Aubrey Lewis preached the ethics and sociology of social and community psychiatry, in Britain the study of psychopathology had a high priority.[11]

Jumping ahead fifty years, in understanding 'the British mental health services at the beginning of the twenty-first century', certain perspectives have been lacking: 'The scope and rapidity of change has left many developments in social policy, legislation, medico-legal practice, service design, service delivery and clinical practice without systematic historical analysis.'[12] In studying the history of psychiatry in Britain from 1960 to 2010, a most interesting question is, to what extent did the British escape the American disaster?

Diagnosis

At the beginning of the period, there were striking international differences in diagnosis. As Swiss psychiatrist Henri Ellenberger noted in 1955,

> The English call almost any kind of emotional trouble 'neurosis'. The French apply the diagnosis of feeble-mindedness very liberally; in Switzerland we demand much more serious proof before using it ... Child schizophrenia is a rare diagnosis in Europe, but a rather frequent one in America; Americans diagnose schizophrenia in almost all those cases of children whom we would call 'pseudo-debiles'.[13]

Yet as early as the 1960s, psychiatry in Britain was alive with innovative thinking about diagnosis. There were a number of systems in play, and in 1959 émigré psychiatrist Erwin Stengel in Sheffield classified them.[14] It was a *mise au point* of the richness of the international offering. Michael Shepherd led efforts to foster an 'experimental approach to psychiatric diagnosis'. The Ministry of Health published in 1968 a 'glossary of mental disorders' that presented in concrete terms the nosology of the eighth edition of the *International Classification of Diseases* by the World Health Organization (WHO) (which made it apparent how inadequate the diagnoses of DSM-II were).[15]

This innovation came to an end with the American Psychiatric Association's publication of the third edition in 1980 of the DSM, which erected gigantic monolithic diagnoses such as 'major depression' and, in later editions, 'bipolar disorder', while retaining the hoary age-old 'schizophrenia'. The Americans soon came to dominate the world diagnostic scene with DSM-III. This represented an extraordinary demonstration of the prescriptive power of American psychiatry: that a consensus-based (not a science-based) nosology such as DSM could have triumphed over all these other systems.

There has always been an academic tradition in England of distrust of abstract diagnostic concepts, such as manic depression, in favour of the clinically concrete. This would be in contrast to the Americans' initial fixation on psychoanalysis, which they then re-exported back to Europe. Following the psychoanalysis vogue came the wholesale US plunge into psychopharmacology. The British were resistant to both these trends. In 1964, E. Beresford Davies, in Cambridge, urged colleagues to switch out disease thinking in favour of just noting symptoms and their response.[16]

Cautiousness in the face of novelty can spill over into a stubborn resistance to innovation. Catatonia, for example, has for decades ceased to be considered a subtype of schizophrenia;[17] but not in the Maudsley Prescribing Guidelines, the 2016 issue of which continues to include catatonia in the chapter on schizophrenia. Melancholia, a diagnosis that goes back to the ancients and has experienced a recent revival, is not even mentioned in the index.[18]

Other distinctively British approaches have also battled to preserve themselves. One was, in contrast to the DSM tendency to treat the clinical picture as the diagnosis, a British reluctance to leap directly from current presentation to diagnostic determination. As Felix Brown, a child psychiatrist in London, pointed out in 1965, 'I have seen many patients who have given an early history of neurosis and they have appeared twenty years later with a really severe depression.' Syndromes, he said, were valuable: 'But I do not believe that they necessarily represent disease entities, especially as the syndromes vary at different times in the lives of the patients.'[19]

Epidemiology

Lest it be thought that Great Britain was limping along behind some mighty US power-house, there were areas where the US NIMH squandered hundreds of millions of dollars, such as the very modestly helpful at best trials of SSRI 'antidepressants' in the Sequenced Treatment Alternatives to Relieve Depression (STAR*D) study. In contrast, at the same time, on much smaller amounts of funding, British investigators made significant progress in areas that mattered in patient care, such as the amount of psychiatric morbidity in general practice. In 1970, David Goldberg and Barry Blackwell assessed with the General Health Questionnaire some 553 consecutive attenders in a general practitioner's surgery. They found that 20 per cent of these patients had previously undiagnosed psychiatric morbidity. This study became an international epidemiological landmark.[20]

Goldberg was among Britain's leading psychiatric epidemiologists; but here, there was a deep bench. Myrna Weisman, a social worker turned leading US psychiatric epidemiologist, commented from her ringside seat, 'The UK led in psychiatric epidemiology. In America we didn't think you could make diagnoses in the community ... The leaders in the field were all English. There was John Wing, who developed the Present State Examination, Norman Kreitman and Michael Shepherd. These were giants in the field.'[21]

Therapeutics

At a certain point, the therapeutics baton is passed from the UK and France to the United States. In the 1960s and 1970s, the Americans were still enmeshed in psychoanalysis and the English had more or less free run internationally. Malcolm Lader, a psychopharmacologist at the Institute of Psychiatry said, 'The United States was not interested in drugs. I was lucky, we had almost a 30-year clear run in the 1960s and 1970s when the Americans were not doing much psychopharmacology. It was only then that they finally gave up their flirtation with psychoanalysis and moved into psychopharmacology, and of course with their resources they've swamped the subject.'[22]

There is one other area of psychopharmacology where there seem to be, alas, few international differences and that is the influence of the pharmaceutical industry over education and practice in psychiatry (see also Chapter 17). One would not be far afield in speaking of the 'invasion' of psychiatry by Pharma, given the companies' influence over Continuing Medical Education and over 'satellite' sessions at academic meetings. Joanna Moncrieff deplored industry's influence on both sides of the Atlantic, on the grounds that it led to over-biologizing psychiatric theory and over-prescribing psychotropic drugs. Moncrieff concluded, not unjustly, that 'Psychiatric practice is now firmly centred around drug treatment, and millions of other people, who have no contact with a psychiatrist, are receiving psychotropic drugs in general practice.'[23]

Yet in terms of the classes of psychotropic medications prescribed, there are international differences, and there have been major changes over the fifty-year period. The conservatism of British clinicians with regard to new diagnoses extended towards new medications. In contrast to Germany, where prescriptions of new drugs in 1990 amounted to 29 per cent of total prescriptions, it was in the UK about 5 per cent (down from 10 per cent in 1975).[24] (Yet English clinicians were not actually shy about prescribing psychotropic medication; as one observer noted, 'In 1971, in order to make patients feel happy, keep calm, sleep or slim, about 3,000,000,000 tablets or capsules of psychotropic drugs were prescribed by general practitioners in England and Wales.')[25]

In the central nervous system (CNS) area, there was once quite a bit of divergence between the UK and the United States. In the years 1970–88, only 39.4 per cent of drugs were introduced in both countries, one of the lowest overlap figures for any therapeutic class.[26] Later, this divergence narrowed as the pharmaceutical industry became more international.

Successive Mental Health Acts of 1983 and 2007 in England largely addressed psychiatry's custodial and coercive functions and will not be considered here, except that the 2007 Act stipulated that electroconvulsive therapy (ECT) must not be administered to patients who had the capacity to refuse to consent to it, unless it is required as an emergency. This continued the stigmatisation of convulsive therapy that has governed British psychiatry over the years: when you must *not* use it. In contrast, in the United States, ECT legislation, if any, is decreed at the state level, and here the tendency has been towards a growing acceptance of ECT as the most powerful treatment that psychiatry has on offer. A NICE Guidance in 2003 begrudgingly consented that ECT might be useful in certain circumstances (after 'all other alternatives had been exhausted'), but its use must not be increased above current levels (imposing a ceiling on it, in other words). Of maintenance ECT there was to be no question.[27] (An update in 2009 moderated only slightly this forbidding approach.) These recommendations contravened international trends in this area.[28]

Research

Before the Second World War, with the exception of the psychiatry unit at the National Hospital in Queen Square and perhaps the Maudsley, there was virtually no psychiatric research in England. Even at the Maudsley, Aubrey Lewis, who declared a pronounced interest in social rehabilitation, kept aloof from drug research. The phrase 'Maudsley psychiatry' meant social psychiatry, epidemiology and statistical methods.[29] It did not refer to a special approach to clinical care or pharmacotherapeutics.[30]

The first real step forward in psychiatric research originated after Eliot Slater's arrival in 1931 at Queen Square. There he was soon joined by several eminent émigré German psychiatrists of international reputations. Otherwise there was silence on the British psychiatric research. (However fabulous Aubrey Lewis might have been as a teacher at the Maudsley, he was not a researcher, and his famous paper on the unitary nature of depression got the story exactly wrong.)[31]

The basic medical sciences were, however, another story, and the history of British psychopharmacology must be seen in the context of a long history of interest in neurophysiology at Oxford and Cambridge. The work of Charles Sherrington, Richard Adrian and Henry Dale attracted worldwide attention. Derek Richter discovered monoamine oxidase at Cambridge, and John Gaddum at Edinburgh thought that serotonin might play a role in mood regulation.[32]

The big British leaps in this area were achieved at Oxford and Cambridge but also at the established 'red-brick' universities in Birmingham, Manchester and Liverpool as well as at London. In 1954, Charmian Elkes and Joel Elkes in Birmingham at the Department of Experimental Psychiatry – the world's earliest dedicated laboratory for research in psychopharmacology – reported the first randomly controlled trial for chlorpromazine.[33] In 1970, Hannah Steinberg became Professor of Psychopharmacology at University College London, the first woman in the world to occupy such a chair. She pioneered research on the effect of drug combinations on the second-messenger system in the brain.[34] The work of Malcolm Lader at the Institute of Psychiatry, Martin Roth at Newcastle upon Tyne and Eugene Paykel as Professor of Psychiatry at Cambridge, helped lay the foundations of clinical psychopharmacology. The efforts of Alec Coppen, Max Hamilton and others led to the foundation of the British Association for Psychopharmacology in 1974.

In sum, British contributions to drug discovery and development in CNS were immense. As a joint government–industry task force reported in 2001, 'Companies based here maintain a significant presence in all the major markets in the world and the UK has consistently "punched well above its weight" since the 1940s ... In terms of overall competitiveness, the UK is second only to the US and well ahead of its main European competitors.'[35]

Deinstitutionalisation and Community Care

Among the most dramatic international differences is that, in Britain, services were transferred from the asylum to local hospitals and, in the United States, from the asylum to the prison system (see also Chapters 1, 23, 30).

In Britain, the locus of care was shifting from the old mental hospital 'bins' to general hospitals. This process began before the Second World War as the Maudsley set up clinics in three big London hospitals.[36] It continued with the District General Hospitals created by Enoch Powell's 'Hospital Plan' in 1962. No longer mere waystations before the transfer to the asylum, the general hospital departments provided comprehensive care. An early innovator here in the 1960s was the Queen's Park Hospital in Blackburn a borough in Lancashire. Its 100 beds were divided into three sections: emergency, ambulatory-chronic and acute. The acute section was divided between male and female. All sections were 'open' and the hospital provided lunch for the emergency and ambulant-chronic patients. Maurice Silverman, the consultant psychiatrist, noted with some pride in 1961, 'This has been largely due to the pioneering work of the Regional Hospital Board in forging ahead with comprehensive psychiatric units in general hospital centres throughout the region.'[37] In contrast to Britain, in the United States 'The overall proportion of the population with mental disorders in correctional facilities and hospitals together is about the same as 50 years ago. Then, however, 75% of that population were in mental hospitals and 25% incarcerated; now, it is 5% in mental hospitals and 95% incarcerated'.[38]

The Psychiatrist of the Past versus the Psychiatrist of the Future

It is training that stamps the clinician's whole mindset, and here the change in training objectives has been dramatic and resulting UK/US differences wide.

A UK survey in the mid-1960s established the teachers' principal learning objectives for their students: 'scientific attitude regarding behavior', 'factual knowledge about psychiatric illnesses' and 'treatment skills'. For example, within the category of scientific study of behaviour, the lecturers were asked to rank various attainments. 'Students must be taught psychopharmacology and neurophysiology as an essential part of their psychiatric training' was number one; systematic history-taking and 'methodical examination of the mental state' was number two; and learning the 'importance of diagnosis and systematic classification for effective practice of psychological medicine' was number three.[39]

Now, no training programme would ever ignore any of these objectives, but we see how the goals sought for trainees have changed today. In 2008, one observer at the Institute of Psychiatry listed the attributes of the future psychiatrist.[40] It was a list that would have made Aubrey Lewis, the earlier professor and himself an advocate of community care, blink:

'Working in partnership' – this was long thought to have been self-understood.

'Respecting diversity' – diversity was a newcomer to the list.

'Challenging inequality' – this gave psychiatry a decided political spin.

'Providing patient-centred care' – Aubrey Lewis, rightly or wrongly, believed that he and his colleagues at the Maudsley offered such care, in that competent treatment in the community was inevitably 'patient-centred'; yet it was the physician's intuitive sense of ethics, values and professional responsibility that decided what was patient-centred, not a climate of opinion that demanded it.

On the other side of the coin, we have surveys of the reasons students *don't* chose psychiatry. One survey of the literature concluded, 'The major factors that appeared to dissuade medical students/trainees from pursuing psychiatry as a career included: an apparent lack of scientific basis of psychiatry and work not being clinical enough, perception that psychiatry is more concerned about social issues.'[41] In Aubrey Lewis's generation there were complaints that psychiatry was *too medical*, with its insistence on seeing illness as brain disease (treatable with electroshock, phenothiazines and tricyclic antidepressants); in the current generation, there are complaints that psychiatry is *not medical enough*, with views of the field as an extended arm of social work.

In the 1960s, the term 'diversity' was as yet on no one's lips, but concern was already stirring about the low number of women in psychiatric training. One tabulation showed the percentage of female trainees as low as zero in the Welsh National School of Medicine, 0.3 per cent in St Thomas's Hospital and 0.4 at Leeds. (The maximum was 2 per cent at Bristol.)[42]

The putative deterioration in NHS services and decline in psychiatric care became a major theme. Brian Cooper wrote in 2010, 'British psychiatry, it appears, flourished as long as the NHS remained secure and in good hands, but then, despite ongoing scientific progress, it has gone into decline since the national service infrastructure began to disintegrate under sustained political pressures.'[43]

Interestingly, US training has developed in a quite different direction. Rather than emphasising a progressive agenda, as in Britain, the accent in the United States has been on 'professionalism', not necessarily as a humanitarian objective but as a defensive posture. Several observers at Emory University wrote in 2009, 'Most medical educators would agree that learning how to deliver care in a professional manner is as necessary as learning the core scientific data'. Here, the themes of diversity, equality and partnership are completely absent, although, if queried, the authors might have agreed to the importance of these as well. What was really on their minds, however, was that 'Patient complaints, malpractice lawsuits, and media stories that depict the inequity and high costs in the U.S. health care system' are the real agenda.[44]

Conclusion

Roy Porter noted that, 'Deep irony attends the development of psychiatry within twenti-eth-century British society. The public became more receptive towards the fields of psychiatry and psychology.' The asylum was dismantled; new modes of care more congenial to 'service-users' were conceived. 'Yet the longer-term consequence', continued Porter, 'has not been growing acclaim, but a resurgence of suspicion.'[45] The challenge of the future will be demonstrating that psychiatry really is capable of making a difference in people's lives.

Key Summary Points

- British psychiatry is almost entirely publicly funded; in the United States, a tradition of well-remunerated private practice has prevailed.
- Despite similar therapeutics and nosology, psychiatry in Britain and the United States has developed in strikingly different ways.
- Psychoanalysis once dominated US psychiatry; in a big swing of the pendulum, it has been almost entirely replaced by psychopharmacology.
- In Britain, the research tradition in the past was weak; in the United States, it has been fuelled by large amounts of government funding. A British hesitancy about embracing large abstract theories has no US counterpart.
- In terms of training, a progressive agenda has been emphasised in Britain, more defensive postures in the United States.

Notes

1. J. Sims, Pathological remarks upon various kinds of alienation of mind. *Memoirs of the Medical Society of London* (1799) 5: 372–406, 374.

2. E. Slater, British psychiatry. *American Behavioral Scientist* (May 1963): 43.

3. M. Shepherd, Psychiatric education in the United States and United Kingdom: Similarities and contrasts. In M. Shepherd, ed., *The Psychosocial Matrix of Psychiatry*, 217–7. London: Tavistock Publications, 1983, p. 224. This essay was initially published in *Comprehensive Psychiatry* in 1965.

4. M. Jones, Some common trends in British and American mental hospital psychiatry. *Lancet* (1963) 1: 433–4.

5. Jay Amsterdam, personal communication to Edward Shorter, 17 December 2016. Kurt Schneider described 'First Rank Symptoms of Schizophrenia' which he considered diagnostic.

6. M. Shepherd, An English view of American psychiatry. *American Journal of Psychiatry* (1957) 114: 417–20.

7. R. Porter, Two cheers for psychiatry!: The social history of mental disorder in twentieth century Britain. In H. Freeman and G. E. Berrios, eds, *150 Years of British Psychiatry, Volume 2: The Aftermath*, 383–406. London: Athlone Press, 1996, p. 389.

8. D. Goldberg and P. Huxley, *Mental Illness in the Community: The Pathway to Psychiatric Care*. London: Tavistock Publications, 1980, 120–1.

9. T. Bergling, *Sissyphobia: Gay Men and Effeminate Behavior*. New York, Harrington Press, 2001, p. 41.

10. Psychiatric Bulletin, Interview with Sir Aubrey Lewis by Professor Michael Shepherd. *Psychiatric Bulletin* (1966) 17: 738–44, 745.

11. Shepherd, An English view of American psychiatry.

12. J. Turner, R. Hayward, K. Angel et al., The history of mental health services in modern England: Practitioner memories and the direction of future research. *Medical History* (2015) 59: 599–624, 600.

13. H Ellenberger, A comparison of European and American psychiatry. *Bulletin of the Menninger Clinic* (1955) 19: 43–52, 48.

14. E. Stengel, Classification of mental disorders. *WHO Bulletin* (1959) 21: 601–883.

15. See J. R. M. Copeland, Classification and the British Glossary of Mental Disorders: Some experience of its use. *British Journal of Psychiatry* (1971) **119**: 413–18.

16. See the discussion with E. Beresford Davies in J. Marks and C. M. B. Pare, eds, *The Scientific Basis of Drug Therapy in Psychiatry: A Symposium at St. Bartholomew's Hospital in London, 7th and 8th September, 1964.* Oxford: Pergamon, 1965, p. 182.

17. E. Shorter and M. Fink, *The Madness of Fear: A History of Catatonia*, Oxford: Oxford University Press, 2018.

18. D. Taylor, C. Paton and S. Kapur, *The Maudsley Prescribing Guidelines in Psychiatry*, 12th ed. Chichester: Wiley, 2016, pp. 105–9.

19. See the discussion with F. Brown in F. A. Jenner, ed., *Proceedings of the Leeds Symposium on Behavioural Disorders 25–27 March 1965.* Dagenham: May & Baker, 1965, p. 197.

20. D. P. Goldberg and B. Blackwell, Psychiatric illness in general practice. *British Medical Journal* (1970) 1: 439–43.

21. See the M. Weisman interview in D. Healy, ed., *The Psychopharmacolgists*, Vol. 2. London: Chapman and Hall, 1998, p. 539.

22. See the M. Lader interview in D. Healy, ed., *The Psychopharmacologists*, Vol. 1. London: Chapman and Hall, 1996, p. 467.

23. E. Shorter, *How Everyone Became Depressed*. New York: Oxford University Press, 2013.

24. G. I. Spielmans, Atypical antipsychotics: Overrated and overprescribed. *The Pharmaceutical Journal* (February 2015). www.pharmaceutical-journal.com/news-and-analysis/opinion/comment/atypical-antipsychotics-overrated-and-overprescribed/20067929.article?firstPass=false.

25. UK Patients Denied New Medicines? *Scrip* Aug 7 1992: 2.

26. P. A. Parish, discussion in The medical use of psychotropic drugs: A report of a symposium sponsored by the Department of Health and Social Security and held at University College, Swansea on 1–2 July, 1972. Supplement, *Journal of the Royal College of General Practitioners* (1973) S2: 23: 57.

27. NICE (National Institute for Health and Care Excellence), *Guidance on the Use of Electroconvulsive Therapy*, 26 April 2003. www.nice.org.uk/guidance/ta59/resources/guidance-on-the-use-of-electroconvulsive-therapy-pdf-2294645984197.

28. E. Shorter and D. Healy, *Shock Therapy: A History of Electroconvulsive Treatment in Mental Illness*. New Brunswick: Rutgers University Press, 2007; M. Fink, Challenges to British practice of electroconvulsive therapy. *Journal of ECT* (2006) 22: 30.

29. Psychiatric Bulletin, Interview with Sir Aubrey Lewis by Dr D. L. Davies [1967]. *Psychiatric Bulletin* (1994) 18: 410–17, 414–15.

30. Fink, Challenges to British practice of electroconvulsive therapy, 30.

31. A. J. Lewis, Melancholia: A clinical study of depressive states. *Journal of Mental Science*, (1934) 80: 277–378.

32. See D. Healy, The history of British psychopharmacology. In Freeman and Berrios, *150 Years of British Psychiatry, Volume 2: The Aftermath*, pp. 61–88.

33. Charmian Elkes's trial was first reported by Willi Mayer-Gross in October 1955 at Jean Delay's big conference in Paris on chlorpromazine. He gave her full credit. See W. Mayer-Gross, Intervention. In J. Delay, ed.,

Colloque International sur la Chlorpromazine et les Médicaments Neuroleptiques en Thérapeutique Psychiatrique, Paris, 20, 21, 22 Octobre 1955, 776–8. Paris: Doin, 1956.

34. See E. Shorter, *Historical Dictionary of Psychiatry.* New York: Oxford University Press, 2005, pp. 311–12.

35. *Pharmaceutical Industry Competitiveness Task Force. Final Report March 2001*:19; www.doh.gov.uk/pictf/pictf.pdf

36. Psychiatric Bulletin, Interview with Sir Aubrey Lewis by Michael Shepherd [1966]. *Psychiatric Bulletin* (1993) 17: 738–44, 744.

37. M. Silverman, A comprehensive department of psychological medicine. *British Medical Journal* (1961) 2: 698–701.

38. N. Bark, Prisoner mental health in the US. *International Psychiatry* (2014) 3: 53–5.

39. H. Walton, Aims of teachers of psychiatry in five medical schools. *British Journal of Psychiatry* (1968) 114: 1417–23, 1419.

40. D. Bhugra, Psychiatric training in the UK: The next steps. *World Psychiatry* (2008) 7: 117–18.

41. A. Choudry and S. Farooq, Systematic review into factors associated with the recruitment crisis in psychiatry in the UK: Students', trainees' and consultants' views. *Psychological Bulletin* (2017) 41: 345–52, 350.

42. P. Brook, Where do psychiatrists come from? The influence of United Kingdom medical schools on the choice of psychiatry as a career. *British Journal of Psychology* (1976) 128: 313–17, 315. Statistics for 1961–70.

43. B. Cooper, British psychiatry and its discontents. *Journal of the Royal Society of Medicine* (2010) 103: 397–402, 402.

44. A. C. Schwartz, R. J. Kotwicki and W. M. McDonald, Developing a modern standard to define and assess professionalism in trainees. *Academic Psychiatry* (2009) 33: 442–50.

45. Porter, Two cheers for psychiatry, 403.

Liberty's Command: Liberal Ideology, the Mixed Economy and the British Welfare State

Graham Scambler

Introduction

The immediate period after the Second World War and lasting until the 1960s was an unusual one for capitalism. It was characterised not only by steady economic growth, not to be matched since, but also by a cross-party political consensus on the desirability of a strong safety net in the form of a welfare state. The period has often been termed 'welfare state capitalism' by commentators. It was an era that came to a fairly abrupt end in the mid-1970s. If the oil crisis of that time provided a marker, the election of Margaret Thatcher in 1979 was to usher in a new phase of what we might call 'financial capitalism'. In this chapter, I trace the origins and course of this transition up to and including the global financial crash of 2008–9. It was a transition that was as cultural as it was structural, leading to new and exacerbated forms of individualism and fragmentation as well as material and social inequality. The generalised commitment to the provision of state welfare gave way to a ubiquitous, near-global ideology of neoliberalism.

I start with a necessarily abbreviated consideration of the history of the British welfare state in general and the emergence of the National Health Service (NHS) in particular. The present, we need to remind ourselves, involves both past and future, the former being the present's precursor, the latter its vision of what is to come.

Origins of the Welfare State and NHS

In fact, Britain was slow off the mark with welfare provision. The first direct engagement was via the National Health Insurance Act of 1911. Prompted by concerns about high rates of work absenteeism and lack of fitness for war duty among working men, this Act protected a segment of the male working class from the costs of sickness. It drew contributions from the state, employers and employees, and it entitled beneficiaries to free primary care by an approved panel doctor (a local GP) and to a sum to compensate for loss of earning power due to sickness. Better paid employees, women, children and older people were excluded and had either to choose fee-for-service primary as well as secondary health care or resort to a limited and fragmented system of 'public' (state-funded) or 'voluntary' (charitable) care. The Act covered 27 per cent of the population in 1911, and this had only expanded to 45 per cent by the beginning of the Second World War.

Pressure, most notably from the expanding middle class, grew during the 1920s and 1930s to extend the reach of health care services. An overhaul eventually took place during the Second World War, evolving out of Beveridge's (1942) painstaking blueprint for an all-out assault on the 'five giants' standing in the way of social progress: Want, Disease, Ignorance, Squalor and Idleness. In retrospect, it seems clear that this initiative marked the end of liberal capitalism, the consolidation and expansion of state intervention and the commencement of welfare state capitalism. The Beveridge Report incorporated plans for a National Health Service. The displacement of Churchill's wartime government by Attlee's Labour Party in 1945 not only realised the concept of a welfare state but, following the National Health Service (NHS) Act of 1946 – a skilled piece of midwifery by Health Minister Aneurin Bevan – the birth of the NHS in 1948. The NHS was based on the principles of collectivism, comprehensiveness, universalism and equality (to which should be added professional autonomy). The state was thereafter committed to offer primary and secondary care, free at the point of service for anyone in need. These services were to be funded almost exclusively out of central taxation.

The 1946 Act was a compromise with history and the medical profession. GPs avoided what they saw as salaried control and became independent contractors paid capitation fees based on the number of patients on their books; the prestigious teaching hospitals won a substantial degree of autonomy; and GPs and, more significantly, hospital consultants won the 'right' to continue to treat patients privately. The survival of private practice has been judged important: 'the NHS was weakened by the fact that the nation's most wealthy and private citizens were not compelled to use it themselves and by the diluted commitment of those clinicians who provided treatment to them.'[1]

Evolution of the Welfare State and the NHS to 2010

It is not possible in this short contribution to do justice to the development of the post–Second World War welfare state in Britain, but a brief mention of changes in social security, housing and education is important. The terms 'welfare' and 'social security' are often treated as synonyms, and state interventions in welfare provision in Britain date back to the introduction of the Poor Law (and Work Houses) in 1536. What is known as the 'welfare state', however, has its origins in the Beveridge Report. Beveridge recommended a national, compulsory flat-rate insurance that combined health care, unemployment and retirement benefits. This led to the passing of the National Assistance Act (1948), which saw the formal ending of the Poor Law; the National Insurance Act (1946); and the National Insurance (Industrial Injuries) Act (1946). There have been many changes to this legislative package since, most having the character of piecemeal social engineering, but there has been a growing tendency towards cutting welfare benefits in post-1970s financial capitalism. By 2010, expenditure on state pensions amounted to 45 per cent of the total welfare bill, with housing benefit coming a distant second at 11 per cent. Then came the decade of austerity and much more savage cuts.

As far as housing is concerned, the average home in 1960 cost £2,507, while by 2010 this had risen to £162.085. Incomes failed to keep up with property prices everywhere, although there were strong regional differences. The type of housing also changed dramatically. Between 1945 and 1964, 41 per cent of all properties built were semi-detached, but after 1980 this fell to 15 per cent. The number of bungalows also declined. Detached houses, however, which were 10 per cent of stock built between 1945 and 1964, accounted for 36 per cent of new builds after 1980. The peak year for house building was in 1968. Private renting made a comeback after years of decline, reflecting a growth in buy-to-let investing, while home ownership slipped back from a peak of 70 per cent in 2004 to 68 per cent by 2010. Thatcher's right-to-buy legislation meant that the number of people renting from their local council fell from 33 per cent in 1961 to 14 per cent in 2008.[2]

The Education Act of 1944 introduced a distinction between primary and secondary schooling and was followed by the introduction of the eleven-plus examination that determined the type of secondary education a child received. One in four passed the eleven-plus and attended grammar schools (or more rarely technical grammar schools), while the remainder attended secondary modern schools and were typically destined to end up in manual jobs. The private sector continued, including the major 'public schools', and these institutions still tutor the political and social elite. In 1965, Crosland in Wilson's Labour Cabinet brought in mixed ability or 'comprehensive state education', which expanded to become the national norm. This system remained largely in place until Thatcher's Education Act of 1988, which emphasised 'school choice' and competition between state schools. In the years since, 'successive governments have sought to reintroduce selection or selective processes under different guises'.[3]

The evolution of the NHS is covered more fully in other chapters of this volume, so brevity is in order. A political consensus on the 'character' of the NHS held steady through much of the era of welfare state capitalism. Moreover, its 'tripartite' structure – involving divisions between GP, hospital and local authority services – remained largely intact into the 1960s. By the close of that decade, however, the increasing number of people with long-term and disabling conditions in particular provoked calls for a more integrated as well as a more efficient service. The result in 1974 was a bureaucratic reorganisation of the NHS initiated by Heath's Conservative government.

The recession of the 1970s saw the advent of financialised capitalism and a renewed focus on cost containment in health care. In its first year of stability in spending, 1950/1, the NHS had absorbed 4.1 per cent of gross domestic product (GDP); this percentage fell steadily to 3.5 per cent by the mid-1950s; by the mid-1960s, it had regained and passed the level of 1950/1; and by the mid-1970s, it had risen to 5.7 per cent of GDP (see also Chapter 11). In fact, total public expenditure as a percentage of GDP peaked in 1975, accounting for nearly half. The Wilson and Callaghan Labour administrations from 1974 to 1979 felt compelled to take steps to contain public expenditure, including that on the health service. Faced with the prospect of stagflation, Labour retreated from its traditional, socio-democratic stance, most notably with the beginnings of fiscal tightening announced in Healey's 1975 budget. While the 'centre-left technocratic agenda' was not abandoned, impetus was certainly lost.[4]

When Thatcher was elected in 1979, she brought to office a set of convictions fully in tune with the idea that the welfare state was in crisis. She took advantage of Galbraith's (1992) observation that bureaucracy had long been more conspicuous in public than in private institutions.[5] In 1983, she invited Griffiths (from Sainsbury's supermarket chain) to conduct an enquiry into NHS management structures (see also Chapter 12). The result was the end of consensus management and its replacement by a new hierarchy of managers on fixed-term contracts.

Against a background of a continuing political rhetoric of crises of expenditure and delivery, in 1988 Thatcher announced a comprehensive review of the NHS. A White Paper, *Working for Patients*, followed a year later. The notion of an internal market was the most significant aspect of the NHS and Community Care Act of 1990 that followed. I have argued that 'it sat on a spectrum somewhere between a bureaucratic command and control economy and a private free market'.[6] Key was the separation of 'purchaser' and 'provider' in what was described as 'managed competition' (see also Chapter 9).

It was Thatcher's successor as Conservative leader, John Major, who introduced the Private Finance Initiative (PFI). This paved the way for the private sector to build, and own, hospitals and other health care facilities that they then leased back to the NHS, often at exorbitant rents. This was a convenient arrangement for government since PFI building and refurbishment did not appear on government books: they represented an investment of private not public capital. Nevertheless, by the time of Major's departure from office in 1997, expenditure on the NHS had topped 7 per cent of GDP.

Labour prime ministers Blair and Brown were in office up to the end of the period of special relevance to this volume. Both embraced PFIs, despite warnings that many trusts were destined to fall heavily into debt as a consequence. As Allyson Pollock predicted in 2005,[7] the chickens would one day come home to roost. There was in fact considerable continuity between the Thatcher/Major and Blair/Brown regimes. Blair, too, saw the welfare state as encouraging dependency, adversely affecting self-esteem and undermining ambition and resolve. Labour's 'third way' afforded cover for the sticking with the Thatcher experiment.

In 2000, Blair announced that spending on the NHS would increase by 6.1 per cent annually in real terms over a four-year period. In the same year, 'The NHS Plan' was published. These moves showed a degree of continuity with the Thatcher project rather than a halting of or rowing back from it.

This brief sketch or timeline covers the period of relevance to this discussion, though it will be important to refer to changes to the NHS post-2010 in what follows. It is time now to turn to the nature of the underlying societal shifts that help us to understand and explain these NHS 'reforms' in the half-century from 1960 to 2010.

Parameters of Societal Change

Given the limited space available, it will be expedient here to identify and focus on select themes. The first of these might be termed the 'financialisation of capitalism'. The decade from the mid-1960s to the mid-1970s saw a slow-burning transition from the relatively benign era of post–Second World War welfare state capitalism to a much harsher era of financial capitalism. If it was Thatcher, along with Reagan in the United States, who symbolised and was the principal political champion and beneficiary of this shift, it must be added that in doing so she was surfing much deeper social structures.

It was the American abrogation of Bretton Woods and the rise of the Eurodollar – which freed up money capital from national regulation by central banks – that marked the advent of financial capitalism. The international recession brought banks further and deeper into the global arena. Banks became internationalised and developed closer relations with transnational corporations. References to financialisation grew more common, summing up not only the phenomena of deregulation and internationalisation but also a shift in the distribution of profits from productive to money capital (accompanied by an increase in the external financing of industry). Industrial capital more and more resembled financial capital.

Pivotal for financial capitalism as it developed was a revision of the 'class/command dynamic'.[8] This refers to the relations between what I have termed the 'capital executive', namely that mix of financiers, rentiers and major shareholders and CEOs of largely transnational corporations that comprise today's dominant capitalist class, and the political elite at the apex of the nation state. The key point here is that those who make up the capital executive in Britain are essentially global operators: they have been described as 'nomads' who no longer belong or identify their interests with their nation of origin. They, like their capital, can resituate at a rapid and alarming pace. The American historian David Landes once remarked that 'men (*sic*) of wealth buy men of power'.[9] What the class/command dynamic asserts, in a nutshell, is that they get more for their money during financial capitalism than they did during welfare state capitalism. This can be interpreted as follows: *capital buys power to make policy*. This is a critical insight for anyone wanting to understand and explain the ramping up of the assault on the principles and practices of the welfare state in general, and the NHS in particular, from Thatcher onwards.

A second theme concerns material and social inequality. Health inequalities are not simply a function of the nature of a health care system, important though this is. Rather, they reflect the distribution of material, social and cultural goods or assets in the population served.[10] I have articulated this elsewhere in terms of 'asset flows',[11] arguing that strong flows of biological, psychological, social, cultural, spatial, symbolic and, especially, material asset flows are conducive to good health and longevity, while weak flows are associated with poor health and premature death. Moreover, there tend to be strong and weak 'clusters' of asset flows. Having said this, compensation can occur across asset flows: there is evidence, for example, that a strong flow of social or cultural assets can compensate for a weak flow of material assets.

The transition to financial capitalism, characterised by its newly distinctive class/command dynamic, has witnessed growing levels of material and social inequalities, with elevated rates of health inequalities following closely in their wake. At the time of writing this chapter, this is being reflected in the specific patterning of the Covid-19 pandemic in the UK and elsewhere.[12] It is not coincidental that attempts to 'reform' the NHS post-Thatcher have occurred alongside deepening material, social and health inequalities. The tacit model for these health care reforms, tentative at first but growing in conviction and potency post-2010, is the United States, where commercial interests predominate and yield rich returns. The putative 'Americanisation' of the NHS is very much on the agenda (to reiterate, capital buys power to make policy).

To push this point home, it is necessary for a moment to go beyond the timeline of this chapter. The 2010 General Election resulted in a Cameron–Clegg Conservative-led coalition government. Almost instantly this government reneged on a pre-election promise not to initiate any further top-down reorganisations of the NHS. Health Minister Lansley published a White Paper called *Liberating the NHS* a mere sixty days after the election, having consulted widely with private providers beforehand.[13] This led to the Health and Social Care Act of 2012, a piece of legislation that opened the door for a root-and-branch privatisation of health care in England. There was considerable opposition to the passing of this Act from both inside and outside of the medical profession, but perhaps few realised its likely longer-term ramifications. A decade later this was clearer: what the Act made possible, namely a rapid privatisation of clinical and other services, was underway.[14]

In short, social processes of health care 'reform' that started around the beginning of the period under consideration here, 1960–2010, have gathered pace since and come to regressive fruition. It will be apparent that this statement has application beyond health care. It is pertinent to physical and mental health alike that ideological assaults on the welfare state have been major contributors to growing material and social inequalities. Like those on the NHS itself, these assaults have accelerated post-2010, culminating in years of political austerity and welfare cuts via devices like Universal Credit. In fact, social security payments in 2020 were proportionally the lowest since the formation of the welfare state back in the time of the Attlee government. Formal social care has been decimated. The advent of the

Covid-19 pandemic in 2020 has exposed these properties of what has been called the 'fractured society'.[15]

There emerged cultural shifts alongside structural social change through the years 1960 to 2010. In the arts, humanities and social sciences, these were sometimes characterised as 'postmodern'. One aspect was certainly the foregrounding of individualism, which fed into political and economic ideologies of personal responsibility: remember Thatcher's insistence that 'there is no such thing as society'. Another aspect of the cultural shift has been the 'postmodernisation' or 'relativisation' of culture itself. The French theorist Lyotard put it well when he argued that *grand* narratives had given way to a multitude of *petit* narratives.[16] What he meant was that overarching philosophies or theories of history or progress, or visions or blueprints of the good society, had been seen to fail and consequently been abandoned. Now people had been emancipated: they were free to choose their own identities, projects and futures as discrete individuals. New identity politics had displaced the old politics of distribution associated with welfare statism.

While some commentators and others celebrated this newfound freedom, others labelled it a form of neoconservatism. Habermas, for example, maintained that the announcement of the death of the *grand* narrative was not only philosophically premature but also politically convenient.[17] After all, it followed that no rationally compelling case might now be made for challenging the (conservative) status quo.

The right of the individual to choose – their identities, orientations and practices – has become firmly established in the culture of financial capitalism. It is a major theme running through accounts of 'neoliberal epidemics'.[18] If individuals can be presumed responsible for their behaviour, then they can be held culpable for any medically defined conditions, physical or mental, that can be associated with *lifestyle choices*. If, for example, obesity is causally linked to diabetes and heart disease, and possibly Covid-19, too, then the obese must surely accept some personal responsibility for indulging in 'risk behaviours'. The point here is a political one: it is not that individuals are not responsible for their health but rather that (1) their health and their behaviours are also a function of, often inherited, circumstance and (2) a governmental emphasis on risk behaviours allows for cutbacks in spending and support. Furthermore, given that during the fifty years under consideration here the implicit rationing of health care services has transmuted into explicit rationing, it is only reasonable that 'behavioural conditionality' be factored into decisions about priorities for treatment and care.

This argument has potency beyond health and health care. The political contraction of the welfare state as a whole, together with the spread of 'precarity' in employment via zero-hours contracts and the undermining of work conditions, sick pay and pensions, has been facilitated by a recasting of personal responsibility.[19] Distinguishing between 'stigma', referring to infringements against norms of shame, and 'deviance', denoting infringements against norms of blame, I refer to a *stigma/deviance dynamic* and maintain that 'blame has been heaped upon shame' in the era of neoliberalism. What I mean by this is that citizens are now being held responsible (blamed) for what was previously regarded as non-conformance rather than non-compliance with cultural prescriptions. Thus, people who are disabled are now treated as if this is in some way their fault and similarly with many departures from mental health. If blame can be effectively appended to shame, the thesis suggests, then people are rendered 'abject', permitting governmental sanctions, even punishments, without public protest. The disabled have been among those hit hardest by welfare cuts enabled by the calculated political 'weaponising of stigma'. If these processes have only become tangible post-2010, their DNA establishes their origins in Thatcher's 1980s.

A Welfare and Health Care System Unravelling

The years from 1960 to 2010 reflect major social change. During that period, the exceptionally benign phase of post–Second World War welfare state capitalism came to an end, to be succeeded by a much harsher regime of financial capitalism. While the New Labour years of 1997 to 2010 to some degree saw a stalling of the deindustrialisation, financial deregulation and the programmes of privatisation of the Thatcher/Major years, and a corresponding decrease in the rate of growth of material inequality, this has been no abandonment of neoliberalism.

Financial capitalism has witnessed an accelerating rate of mental as well as physical health problems in line with the fracturing of society. Health inequalities already entrenched by the 1960s have since expanded.[20] This was especially true in the 1980s, when Thatcher's policies of state-enforced neoliberal individualism led to a surge in rates of morbidity and premature mortality among poor segments of the population.

The period 1960–2010 set the scene for what many at the time of writing (2020) see as a severe crisis in welfare and health care. The years of austerity, coupled with a sustained political effort to get citizens to obey the capitalist 'imperative to work' as well as to privatise as wide a range of public sector services as possible, have precipitated an 'Americanisation' of British society. Cultural cover has been provided for these policies by a populist rhetoric of individualism and 'freedom of choice'. Scant regard has been paid to the distinction between 'formal' and 'actual' freedom, in other words between what people are formally free to do (e.g. buy their own house or send their children to fee-paying schools) and what they are actually free to do (i.e. in the absence of the requisite capital and/or a reasonable income).

Conclusion

Starting with a highly abbreviated chronology of the evolution of the welfare state, this chapter has gone on to discuss core structural and cultural mechanisms that have shaped the policy shifts that have occurred, concentrating on the period 1960–2010. The case has been made that policy shifts are often functions of deeper social processes. It is in this context that the class/command and stigma/deviance dynamics have been explored. Discourses, too, typically have ideological components that reflect structural and cultural dynamics. This complicates simple historical chronologies of social institutions like the NHS, as it does debates about improving welfare support and the delivery of good health care. Not infrequently policy-based evidence is substituted for evidence-based policy. Another level of complexity has been added of late, which is largely cultural. This was apparent by 2010 and has been characterised in this chapter as a relativisation of perspectives and modes of thinking. Progeny of this tendency include present analyses of 'post-truth' and 'fake news', linked to but trespassing beyond social media, each rendering rational judgements based on available evidence harder both to make and to evaluate.

Key Summary Points

- The decade from the mid-1960s to the mid-1970s saw a slow-burning transition from the relatively benign era of post–Second World War welfare state capitalism to a much harsher era of financial capitalism. Scant regard has been paid to the distinction between 'formal' and 'actual' freedom.

- The recession of the 1970s saw the advent of financialised capitalism and a renewed focus on cost containment in health care. At the same time, new identity politics had displaced the old politics of distribution associated with the welfare state. The political contraction of the welfare state as a whole, together with the spread of 'precarity' in employment via zero-hours contracts and the undermining of work conditions, sick pay and pensions, has been facilitated by a recasting of personal responsibility.
- Strong flows of biological, psychological, social, cultural, spatial, symbolic and, especially, material asset flows are conducive to good health and longevity, while weak flows are associated with poor health and premature death.
- Ideological assaults on the welfare state have been major contributors to growing material and social inequalities. Financial capitalism has witnessed an accelerating rate of mental as well as physical health problems in line with the fracturing of society.
- The period 1960–2010 set the scene for what many at the time of writing (2020) see as a severe crisis in welfare and health care.

Notes

1. L. Doyal and L. Doyal, The British National Health Service: A tarnished moral vision. *Health Care Analysis* (1999) 7: 263–76.

2. P. Collinson, Fifty years on: House prices outstrip earnings but toilets move inside. *The Guardian*, 20 January 2010.

3. D. Scott, Education, education, education. In D. Scott, ed., *Manifestos, Policies and Practices: An Equalities Agenda*. London: UCL Press, 2019.

4. J. Tomlinson, Economic policy. In A. Crines and K. Hickson, eds, *Harold Wilson: The Unprincipled Prime Minister?* London: Biteback Publishing, 2016.

5. K. Galbraith, *The Culture of Contentment*. London: Sinclair-Stevenson, 1992.

6. G. Scambler, *Sociology, Health and the Fractured Society: A Critical Realist Account*. London: Routledge, 2018.

7. A. Pollock, *The NHS Plc: The Privatisation of Our Health Care*. London: Verso, 2005.

8. Scambler, *Sociology, Health and the Fractured Society*; G. Scambler, *A Sociology of Shame and Blame: Insiders Versus Outsiders*. London: Palgrave Macmillan, 2020.

9. D. Landes, *Wealth and Poverty of Nations*. London: Little, Brown & Co., 1998.

10. M. Marmot, J. Allen, T. Boyce, P. Goldblatt and J. Morrison, *Health Equity in England: The Marmot Review Ten Years On*. London: Institute of Health Equity, 2020.

11. Scambler, *Sociology, Health and the Fractured Society*.

12. M. Marmot, Society and the slow burn of inequality. *The Lancet* (2020) 395: 1413–14.

13. C. Leys and S. Player, *The Plot against the NHS*. London: Merlin Press, 2011.

14. G. Scambler, The Labour Party, health and the National Health Service. In D. Scott, ed., *Manifestos, Policies and Practices: An Equalities Agenda*. London: UCL Press, 2019.

15. G. Scambler, Covid-19 as a 'breaching experiment': Exposing the fractured society. *Health Sociology Review* (2020).

16. J.-J. Lyotard, *The Postmodern Condition*. Manchester: Manchester University Press, 1984.

17. J. Habermas, *The New Conservatism*. Cambridge: Polity Press, 1989.

18. T. Schrecker and C. Bambra, *How Politics Makes Us Sick: Neoliberal Epidemics*. London: Palgrave Macmillan, 2015.

19. G. Scambler, Heaping blame on shame: 'Weaponising stigma' for neoliberal times. *Sociological Review* (2018) 66: 766–82.

20. D. Black, *Inequalities in Health: The Black Report*. London: Penguin Books, 1982; Landes, *Wealth and Poverty of Nations*.

Social Theory, Psychiatry and Mental Health Services

Rob Poole and Catherine Robinson

Introduction

This chapter describes the development of social concepts within psychiatry and mental services between 1960 and 2010 and the impact of the new ideas developed within social sciences at the time. Concepts and movements considered include deinstitutionalisation; therapeutic communities; Community Mental Health Teams (CMHTs); social constructionism; labelling theory; social functionalism; paradigm shift; stigma; the service user movement; and the social determinants of mental health. There was tension between new postmodernist ideas and the positivist-scientific model that underpinned both social psychiatry of the period and confident, and ultimately hubristic, advocacy of the primacy of neuroscience in psychiatry during 'the Decade of the Brain'. Although some new ideas were eventually assimilated by psychiatry, the tension was unresolved in 2010.

Social Thinking in Psychiatry in 1960

In 1960, the social perspective was prominent within British mental health services. A subdiscipline of social psychiatry had been forming for some time and many of its enduring themes were already evident. British psychiatry had needed to change rapidly as a consequence of the social, political and economic impact of the Second World War and its aftermath. Mental hospitals, which previously had been the responsibility of local authorities, were absorbed into the new National Health Service (NHS) in 1948 and deinstitutionalisation commenced almost immediately, alongside changes in organisation, staffing and attitudes to treatment.

During the Second World War, psychological reactions to combat were regarded as a medical problem rather than as a matter of military discipline. A relatively small pool of psychiatrists was called upon to treat large numbers of service personnel suffering from 'battle fatigue' or 'effort syndrome', leading to pragmatic experimentation with group treatments. Necessity proved to be a virtue and new group-based social therapeutic modalities followed. At the Maudsley Hospital, Maxwell Jones developed the idea that the entire experience of living together could be therapeutic and, at Northfield Military Hospital, Tom Main coined the term 'therapeutic community', which became a banner under which many later reforms were made to inpatient care (sometimes less stridently labelled the 'therapeutic milieu').

There was a growing belief that, with support, people with chronic psychosis could have better lives in the community. There was optimism about new biomedical treatments, such as antipsychotic and antidepressant drugs, and electroconvulsive treatment. A degree of therapeutic heroism meant that there were some awful therapeutic mistakes too, such as deep sleep therapy (continuous narcosis) and insulin shock, which, when properly evaluated, were found to be dangerous and ineffective. Nonetheless, at the time there seemed to be a realistic possibility that NHS psychiatrists would soon be able to work from day hospitals (developed by Joshua Bierer at the Marlborough Day Hospital in London) and outpatient clinics, avoiding mental hospital admission altogether.

Social psychiatry was also ascendant in academia under the pervasive influence of Sir Aubrey Lewis at the Maudsley Hospital. Lewis was a social psychiatrist who had undertaken early anthropological research among Aboriginal Australians. He was influenced by Adolf Meyer's work in Baltimore (see also Chapter 2). The Institute of Psychiatry was formed at the Maudsley in 1946 under his leadership and in 1948 he became the first director of the Medical Research Council (MRC) Social Psychiatry Unit there. He retired in 1966, but his influence persisted long after he had gone, as did his brand of social psychiatry.

As the 1960s started, and for many years thereafter, organised British medicine, including social psychiatry, followed a theoretical model that went back to scientific medicine's Enlightenment origins. It was based upon the belief that positivism, reductionism and empiricism were the most powerful and meaningful ways of understanding mental disorders and that science itself was intrinsically subject to continuous progress. Fundamental causes of mental disorders were believed to be biological or psychological but social factors were recognised to influence their expression, course and outcome. Social psychiatry research mainly concerned itself with quantifying the impact of social environment and social interventions on mental illnesses, without challenging the fundamental assumptions of what came to be labelled 'the medical model'. Classic studies of the time (e.g. Wing and Brown's Three Hospitals study)[1] exemplified social psychiatry's research approach; patients' symptoms and their social environment were assessed using operationalised criteria, the beginning of a long tradition of quantification through the use of symptom and social interaction rating scales.

A seminal 1963 study by Goldberg and Morrison addressed the possibility that social adversity might cause psychosis.[2] It appeared to convincingly demonstrate that people with a diagnosis of schizophrenia drifted down the hierarchy of social class after they became ill, while unaffected family members did not. For many years, this 'social drift' was taken to account for known differences in prevalence between prosperous and deprived areas. It was not until the mid-1990s that new research methods started to shift the balance of evidence by showing that a variety of childhood adversities consistently increased the risk of adult psychosis. Psychiatry's resistance to the idea that social adversity might cause mental illness was such that, even in 2010, there was little sign that British psychiatrists were changing their thinking in response to the implications of newer research findings.

The positivist but eclectic scientific stance of mainstream British psychiatry meant that it readily adopted the biopsychosocial model proposed by Engel in the late 1970s and a version of it remained the explicit stance of organised British psychiatry until 2010 and beyond.[3] Although a broad church of scientific and clinical orientations flourished within British psychiatry, psychiatrists remained highly protective of their status as leaders of mental health services and of research. They encouraged growth and development in mental health nursing, social work and clinical psychology, but they were insistent that their own profession was uniquely equipped to be in charge.[4] A reluctance to take on new ideas about relative professional standing eventually weakened psychiatry's position when, from 1979 onwards, neoliberal politicians increasingly forced change upon it.

Pilgrim and Rogers have suggested that, in 1960, psychiatry and sociology were in alliance with each other, using empiricism to understand the impact of social context on mental health.[5] However, everything in social science was about to change. While empirical sociology never disappeared, a rift opened between the disciplines that was only just beginning to close again in 2010.

New Social Theories and the Reaction of British Psychiatry

In Chapter 20, Burns and Hall refer to four books published in 1960/1 (Foucault's *Madness and Civilisation*; Laing's *The Divided Self*; Szasz's *The Myth of Mental Illness* and Goffman's *Asylums*) which were collectively the founding texts of so-called anti-psychiatry (a term rejected by the authors and later contested within social theory as serving to dismiss and marginalise valid critiques of psychiatry). They set out many of the themes that dominated social theory about mental health over the subsequent decades.

The new social theories had diverse origins and many variations developed. Those of the left came to be lumped together under the umbrella of 'postmodernism' (another label that was not wholeheartedly embraced by all of those it was applied to). The key theoretical positions about mental health were social functionalism, social constructionism and social labelling theory. Postmodernism tended to be concerned with the way that power is exercised and with privilege sustained through social and cultural institutions, language and ownership of knowledge. Many ideas were developed within a framework of neo-Marxism (in particular, the work of Gramsci), but psychoanalytic ideas as applied to social interaction were also important. Few post–Second World War social theories ignored psychiatry, because many social scientists came to understand it as a key way in which society managed 'deviance' (in other words, the breaking of social rules).

Erving Goffman stood alone as a critic of mental health services who was well received by a significant proportion of psychiatrists. According to Goffman, mental hospitals were 'total institutions' where every aspect of life, activity and human interaction served to maintain control and subjugation of the patients. Far from being therapeutic, they were intrinsically oppressive and marginalising. This characterisation distressed some psychiatrists, who saw themselves as benign and caring, but an influential minority felt that Goffman had described something that concerned them too and that his ideas were helpful to programmes of deinstitutionalisation that they were leading.

Goffman's next project was on 'the spoiled identity' or stigma. According to social labelling theory, the ways that words that are used by psychiatry and society to describe mental illness, and the people so diagnosed, have a profound impact on both social attitudes to them and their sense of self. New concepts of stigma had an extensive and enduring impact, leading to successive campaigns for the use of less negative forms of language for mental illnesses and the people diagnosed with them (sometimes disparagingly labelled by opponents as 'political correctness'). The importance of stigma, and of reducing it, influenced mainstream psychiatry to the point where, in 1998, the Royal College of Psychiatrists mounted a five-year anti-stigma campaign.

Other new social theories proved more difficult for psychiatry to accept. Postmodernism held that mental illness had no existence independent of psychiatrists. It was seen as a social construct, which had developed to maintain order in the new urbanised society of the Industrial Revolution, justifying the sequestration of disruptive people in mental hospitals. This process was labelled 'the Great Confinement' by Foucault. British psychiatry rejected this as a denial of scientific facts and of human suffering and by 2010 had not reconciled itself to the idea.

The belief that the things that people diagnosed with schizophrenia said were intrinsically bizarre and non-understandable was a key element in Karl Jaspers's phenomenological approach to psychopathology, a cornerstone of British descriptive psychopathology. Laing and others strongly challenged this, insisting that the things people with psychosis said were intelligible if you took the trouble to understand the social and family context they existed within. Jaspers's influence weakened from the 1990s, mainly because of the application of cognitive behavioural ideas to the psychopathology of psychosis. Almost without acknowledgement, some of Laing's early ideas eventually gained acceptance (see also Chapter 20).

According to postmodernism, psychiatric practice, diagnosis and treatment could not be separated from the oppressive values of those who controlled society, especially sexism, racism and homophobia. Activists pointed out that women, people of black and other minority ethnic heritage, and gay people were more likely to receive a psychiatric diagnosis than male, white and heterosexual people. Professional ideologies were seen as intrinsically sexist, racist and homophobic. Diagnoses such as 'hysterical personality disorder' were condemned as sexist caricatures. Aversion therapies to change sexual orientation and the attribution of high rates of psychosis among black people to an intrinsic racial characteristic (rather than to social adversities, such as racism) were seen as value-laden and oppressive. From the mid-1990s, these ideas did begin to exert an influence on the way that psychiatry thought about itself, particularly as some urban CMHTs (see the section 'Developments in Social Thinking In Psychiatry') developed links with the communities they served. There was also increasing evidence from psychiatric research that these critiques were valid.

To the four key books of 1960/1 identified by Burns and Hall (see Chapter 20) can be added Thomas Kuhn's *The Structure of Scientific Revolutions*,[6] which was published in 1962. This highly influential book had nothing specific to say about psychiatry but it had implications for the certainty with which psychiatry defended its positivistic roots. Kuhn's central thesis was that science does not progress smoothly following immutable and irreducible principles. Instead, 'normal science' operates within a constructed meta-model or paradigm. Over time, conflicting evidence accumulates that cannot be reconciled within the paradigm and eventually there is a paradigm shift, whereby all previous assumptions and ways of thinking about scientific problems are revised or dismissed, with the formation of an entirely new paradigm of greater explanatory power. 'Normal science' then proceeds within the new paradigm until it, in turn, is replaced. The implication for psychiatry was that its methods and models of science (and, by extrapolation, the profession's status) were neither timeless nor self-evident. Kuhn lent support to the postmodernist concept that psychiatry found most unpalatable: the suggestion that the objectivity of psychiatric science was illusory and rested upon a medical model that was a poor fit for psychological distress. The medical model could only, it was suggested, reflect psychiatrists' perception of 'truth'. Psychiatrists' understanding of mental disorder had no intrinsic claim to greater legitimacy than their patients' or anybody else's. By 2010, this concept was still fiercely resisted by psychiatry, despite a growing acceptance, at least theoretically, that there was value in social science qualitative research techniques that captured lived experience.

As postmodernism became increasingly influential, the gap between sociology and psychiatry widened. The scope of critiques of the medical model became greater, particularly after the publication of Ivan Illich's *Medical Nemesis: Limits to Medicine* in 1976.[7] The book opened with the statement 'The medical establishment has become a major threat to health' and went on to suggest that this involved three different types of iatrogenesis: clinical, social and cultural. The first referred to direct adverse effects of treatment, the second and third to a wider impact that has the effect of undermining people's ability to manage their own health.

In the later period, social theorists were especially influenced by Foucault. Pierre Bourdieu, widely considered the most influential social theorist of his time, built on Foucault's ideas to develop concepts about social and cultural capital that were relevant to the understanding of mental disorders.[8] Unlike Foucault, Bourdieu regarded empirical evidence as important. Nonetheless, his ideas only influenced a small minority of social psychiatrists. Later still, Nikolas Rose developed Foucault's concept of governmentality to explore the impact of the 'psy disciplines' beyond people diagnosed with mental disorder.[9] He suggested that these disciplines (or industries) had had a profound role in forming general ideas about self, autonomy, control and authority for the entire population. Through the whole of our period of interest, UK psychiatry reacted negatively to postmodern critiques. Eventually, the relationship between sociology and psychiatry was distant, if not actively hostile.

The social theories of the new left challenged all the institutions of liberal democracy, but they were not the only intellectual movements that did so. Szasz, for example, was a rightwing libertarian who objected to the restriction of individual liberty by the state. To Szasz, compulsion had no role in helping people who were emotionally distressed. Indeed, the state itself had no legitimate role. The only legitimate relationship between psychiatrist and patient was an individual commercial transaction, freely entered into by both parties. Similarly, in economics, a challenge to the institutions of liberal democracy was forming on the right from neoliberals influenced by political economists such as Friedrich Hayek and Milton Friedman.[10] In its purest form, neoliberalism came to see post–Second World War social welfare provision as a structural impediment to the workings of a free market which, if unfettered, would resolve social problems through perfectly expressed individual self-interest. These free market libertarian concepts became the economic orthodoxy of the second half of our period. They had a vicarious impact on psychiatry through the progressive marketisation of British health care following the NHS reforms of 1990 (see also Chapter 12).

Developments in Social Thinking in Psychiatry

While there was tacit acceptance of elements of new social theories in the later period, organised psychiatry mostly stood aloof and saw little reason to examine its own legitimacy. Postgraduate curricula and standard textbooks made scant reference to the new social theories. In 1976, a young Irish psychiatrist working at the Maudsley Hospital, Anthony Clare, published a book in defence of psychiatry, *Psychiatry in Dissent*.[11] The book sought to refute anti-psychiatry and the new social theories on empirical grounds. To the profession, the exercise was satisfying and successful, but to psychiatry's critics, Clare missed the point. Having rejected the primacy of positivist science, a defence on that basis could not be convincing to them. On the other hand, academic mental health nursing, which developed rapidly from the mid-1980s onwards, embraced the new theories much more readily. Over time, nurses came to dominate mental health service management. By this route, postmodernist ideas came to have an impact on psychiatry from within services but from outside of the profession.

Despite resistance to postmodernism, from 1960 to 2000 service innovation was led by social psychiatry. From 1962, Maxwell Jones applied therapeutic community principles to the entire mental health service at Dingleton Hospital in Scotland (see also Chapter 2). The result was the earliest version of the CMHTs. Twenty years later, alongside efforts to suppress the use of stigmatising language, specialist services started to emerge for women, for black and other minority ethnic groups and (mainly in response to the HIV epidemic) for gay people. These new services tended to accept that systematic disadvantage and discrimination were relevant to people's mental health and actively acknowledged this. Psychiatrists started to actively engage with these communities and more collaborative approaches developed. As usual, these developments were piecemeal and many services remained unreconstructed. Attitudes among younger psychiatrists changed, but this was probably a consequence of shifts in values among the educated middle class in general.

A major factor that eventually influenced all of the mental health professions was the mental health service user movement (see also Chapter 13). This had roots outside of health services and universities. It developed in the wake of the other liberation movements as part of the radical 'underground' of the 1960s and 1970s. It was a broad movement that varied in its attachment to critiques of, and hostility towards, psychiatry. Despite marked differences, the movement had some generally agreed-upon objectives: that service users should have choices in, and agency over, their treatment; that they should be involved in planning services and in developing research; that mental health assessment should take into account their full circumstances; that talking therapies should be as available as medication; that mental disorder should not be regarded as lifelong; that the aim of treatment should be recovery, defined by the patient; and that services should avoid stigmatising its users. By 2010, few service users felt that these objectives had been achieved, but they were accepted as legitimate and desirable by most mental health service managers and psychiatrists. From the 1990s, psychiatrists were pressed by governmental policies such as the Care Programme Approach and National Service Frameworks to conform to some of the service user movement's demands. In the later period, this led to major changes in the way that psychiatry was practised in the UK. For example, in 2010, many services claimed to follow 'the Recovery Model', albeit amid some controversy over ownership of 'recovery'.

'The Decade of the Brain'

Prompted by industry lobbying in the wake of the huge success of a new antidepressant, Prozac (fluoxetine), US president George H. W. Bush declared the 1990s to be 'the Decade of the Brain'. This had international ramifications and academic social psychiatry went into sharp decline. There was a massive biomedical research and development effort and new medications appeared that were claimed to be more effective, with fewer side effects, than the older ones. Advances in molecular genetics and brain imaging technologies created an expectation that the limitations of psychiatric treatment would be overcome by reference to 'fundamental' brain processes. New diagnostic categories appeared, generating suspicions that new markets were being created. There was less money available for social research in mental health and most of it was directed at trials of complex manualised community interventions such as 'assertive outreach'.

Optimism about biological advances in 'the Decade of the Brain' proved ill-founded. The new drugs proved no more effective and just as problematic as the old ones. Molecular genetics and new imaging techniques generated much new knowledge, but by 2000 there was no sign of any implementable technologies that might revolutionise psychiatric treatment. In fact, psychiatry had unwittingly confirmed some aspects of postmodernist critiques. It stood accused of having a deep and corrupt relationship with the pharmaceutic industry. Although organised psychiatry worked hard from the late 1990s onwards to distance itself from the industry, it was too late to undo the reputational damage. Intense attention to 'fundamental' biological processes had proven as fruitless as postmodernism had predicted.

Postmodernism did influence psychiatry in other parts of the world. For example, in Italy, neo-Marxist and Foucauldian theories underpinned Franco Basaglia's Psichiatria Democratica movement. Basaglia was a professor of psychiatry in Trieste. He was influenced by visiting Dingleton in the 1960s, and in 1978 his movement was successful in getting Law 180/78 enacted throughout Italy, banning mental hospital admissions and introducing a system of community care. The UK saw no corresponding positive response to new social theories until, in 2001, Bracken and Thomas heralded the development of a postmodern psychiatry (which they labelled 'post-psychiatry') with an article in the *British Medical Journal* (*BMJ*).[12] Bracken and Thomas were part of the broader Critical Psychiatry Network, a group of radical psychiatrists. Unlike the medically qualified anti-psychiatrists of the 1960s, they insisted that they remained within the umbrella of the psychiatric mainstream, but the impact of their various conceptual threads varied. Their concerns over the medicalisation of life were widely shared, but post-psychiatry per se enjoyed little general support, possibly because of its use of the dense and unfamiliar language of postmodernism.

Other Social Theory Developments

From 2000, disillusionment with the claims of 'the Decade of the Brain' set in and social psychiatry gradually revived. Interest started to grow in the social determinants of mental health, due to the work of empirical researchers from public health and sociology such as Michael Marmot and Richard Wilkinson and the emerging epidemiological evidence that childhood deprivation related to psychosis more as a causal factor than a confounding factor.[13] These findings implied the possibility of preventing mental ill health through social and public health intervention. Linked to this, there was increasing interest in global mental health, whereby international socio-economic factors were seen to have a disproportionate impact on the mental health of people in low- and middle-income countries, who were the majority of humanity.

A range of other social theories were little noticed by mainstream psychiatry but had some impact on specific therapies. For example, cybernetics and systems theory were applied to systemic family therapy. This was seen to be a powerful technique but attracted little interest beyond child and adolescent psychiatry. New ways of understanding social networks developed but they were rarely adopted in psychiatric research, and similarly concepts concerning social capital had little impact on psychiatry's understanding of inequality.

There are other examples, but the point is clear. Complex ways of understanding inequality and social context were hard to absorb into psychiatry's medical model, despite signs of a renaissance of interest in social factors by 2010. Writing at the end of the period, we pointed out that the biopsychosocial paradigm could not accommodate the contradictions in the evidence about mental health problems and that we appeared to be awaiting a scientific paradigm shift.[14]

Conclusion

While postmodernism and other social theories had a limited direct impact on the way that organised psychiatry understood social context and its own role in society, an indirect impact was felt as the years passed. This was due mainly to external influences such as the service user movement and assertive nurse-led management of mental health services. Later empirically based work had some traction on psychiatry, but at the end of our period, notwithstanding signs of revival, social psychiatry remained significantly less influential than it had been fifty years earlier.

Key Summary Points

- This chapter describes the development of social concepts within psychiatry and mental services between 1960 and 2010. This occurred against the backdrop of the emergence of new social theories concerned with psychiatry, medicine, science and other institutions of liberal democracy from the very beginning of the period.
- Attacks on the legitimacy of psychiatry came from postmodernists on the left and neoliberals on the right and coincided with a distancing between psychiatry and sociology.
- Organised psychiatry reacted defensively to most, but not all, of its critics and had difficulty assimilating even those new social theories that appeared neutral regarding the professional and scientific status of psychiatrists.
- From the 1990s, mental health nursing become dominant in a newly empowered NHS management, and the service user movement was successful in its campaigns to have key demands included in national and local government policy. These external influences forced change upon psychiatry.
- In the last decade of the period, empirical evidence regarding social determinants of mental health, together with the failure of biomedical technology to deliver on promises of better treatments, led to the beginnings of a revival of interest in social factors within academic psychiatry.

Notes

1. J. K. Wing and G. W. Brown, Social treatment of chronic schizophrenia: A comparative survey of three mental hospitals. *Journal of Mental Science* (1961) 107: 847–61.

2. E. M. Goldberg and S. L. Morrison, Schizophrenia and social class. *British Journal of Psychiatry* (1963) 109: 785–802.

3. G. L. Engel, The need for a new medical model: A challenge for biomedicine. *Science* (1977) 196(4286): 129–36.

4. N. Craddock, D. Antebi, M.-J. Attenburrow et al., A wake up call for British psychiatry. *British Journal of Psychiatry* (2008) 193: 6–9.

5. D. Pilgrim and A. Rogers, Social psychiatry and sociology. *Journal of Mental Health* (2005) 14(4): 317–20.

6. T. S. Kuhn, *The Structure of Scientific Revolutions.* Chicago: University of Chicago Press, 1962.

7. I. Illich, *Limits to Medicine: Medical Nemesis: The Expropriation of Health.* London: Maryon Boyars, 1976.

8. P. Bourdieu, The forms of capital. In J. Richardson, ed., *Handbook of Theory and Research for the Sociology of Education*, 241–58. New York: Greenwood, 1986.

9. N. Rose, *Inventing Our Selves: Psychology, Power and Personhood*. Cambridge: Cambridge University Press, 1996.

10. F. A. Hayek, *The Road to Serfdom*. London: George Routledge & Sons, 1944.

11. A. Clare, *Psychiatry in Dissent*. London: Tavistock Publications, 1976.

12. P. Bracken and P. Thomas, Postpsychiatry: A new direction in mental health. *BMJ* (2001) 322: 724–7.

13. M. Marmot and R. Wilkinson, *Social Determinants of Health*. Oxford: Oxford University Press, 1999.

14. R. Poole, R. Higgo and C. Robinson, *Mental Health and Poverty*. Cambridge: Cambridge University Press: 2014.

A Sociological Perspective on Psychiatric Epidemiology in Britain

5

David Pilgrim and Anne Rogers

Introduction

The relationship between psychiatry and sociology has been both 'troubled' and collaborative.[1] Social psychiatry represents a reconciliation between positivist labelling in the profession (diagnoses) and social causations, as an alternative to bio-determinism. Either side of the Second World War, social psychiatry had emerged in the United States, influenced by Adolf Meyer's work, the ecological wing of the Chicago School of sociology and, subsequently, the development of the biopsychosocial model by George Engel.

In Britain, during the twentieth century 'environmentalism' or 'the social' was evident in the treatment of shellshock and in the development of therapeutic communities as well as in the emergence of attachment theory and social epidemiology.[2] The last of these offered us a 'bio-social' model of common mental disorders, deleting the 'psychological' from the biopsychosocial model.[3] Before looking at the ways in which this legacy influenced psychiatric research, we consider the influence of the nearby British sociological work of George Brown and his colleagues.

The Social Origins of Depression

Originally Tirril Harris, George Brown and colleagues aspired to examine the link between social class and depression. The title *The Social Origins of Depression* signalled that intention.[4] However, on grounds of methodological pragmatism it became celebrated mainly as a study of female depression; women were more available to participate and so only they were interviewed. Accordingly, the subtitle of the book became *A Study of Psychiatric Disorder in Women*. Brown and Harris considered that their work demonstrated the exposure of working-class women in 'urban industrialised communities' to depression-inducing stressors, which reflected social inequalities and a 'major social injustice'.

What the study brought to light were the biopsychosocial dimensions expected within the Meyerian legacy, in which the team developed a model of depression that included three groups of aetiological factors. These referred to biographical vulnerability, provoking agents and symptom formation factors. Subsequently, the model was elaborated to include more on childhood adversity and social defeat (negative 'life events') and a breakdown in the interpersonal bonds that sustain a confident sense of self. Brown and colleagues concluded that the probability of depression increases not necessarily with loss or threatened loss per se but with the coexistence of humiliation and entrapment and the meanings that they incur for incipient patients.[5]

The research started an interest in adverse childhood events, which we now know increase the possibility of mental health problems in general and are not diagnosis-specific. Around a third of the women studied by the research team had experienced neglect or physical or sexual abuse during childhood. This subgroup had twice the chances of becoming depressed in one year, compared to those without such adverse antecedents,[6] which also predicted anxiety symptoms. Bifulco and colleagues' work elaborated the original model to mark a convergence with attachment theory,[7] setting the scene for a 'trauma-informed' approach to mental health work.

The Harris, Brown and colleagues research was augmented in Camberwell by psychiatrists, but this focused on the follow-up of discharged hospital patients with a diagnosis of unipolar depression.[8] This time, men were included in the sample but were still in a minority. This team concluded that gender, not class, does predict depression and that life events were important. This project was different from the community surveys of the Harris and Brown group, as its focus was on a particular clinical population and their families, with a view to disaggregating the salience of nature and nurture.

This research group embodied equivocation within British psychiatry about 'the social', as the search for the salient role of biogenetics continued as part of the work. This can be contrasted, for example, with the work of Brown and colleagues or that of Goldberg and Huxley, who were more interested in how social factors, as immediate stressors, may impact on somatic systems.[9] The sampling and theoretical differences in these studies raised questions about the sociological competence on the part of psychiatrists. As will be clear now, their engagement of the 'sociological imagination' was sparse but not always absent.[10] For reasons of space, our summary of the topic is guided by examples given from British contributions to the main international social psychiatric journal, *Social Psychiatry and Social Epidemiology*. This brings us to consider how 'the social' was framed and represented in papers from British psychiatry.

British Articles in *Social Psychiatry and Social Epidemiology*

When we looked at the articles from the UK in the journal *Social Psychiatry and Social Epidemiology* (which began life in 1966 as *Social Psychiatry*), we traced three overlapping framings of 'the social', which for heuristic convenience here we have called 'the micro', 'the meso' and 'the macro'. We provide illustrative examples of this tracing exercise in what follows.

The Micro Version of 'the Social': The Biological Undertow and Clinical Focus

Adelstein and colleagues reported an epidemiological study from Salford, which described the clinical characteristics of newly diagnosed patients.[11] A series of correlates were reported about sex, class, age and marital status. The authors opted to compare 'functional' mental disorders to Huntington's chorea, noting that the 'resemblance is great, and these data therefore provoke serious consideration of the existence of genetic susceptibility to schizophrenia and psychoneurosis, although there are good reasons for seeking multiple causes including social causes'.

Social psychiatric research set in that period remained wedded to the hospital as an institution, reflected in the reliance and focus on the use of *service-based* data (rather than community, nonclinical samples) to map out mental disorders in society. Cooper argued for the 'need to look outside hospital' to primary care.[12] He identified that women were over-represented in the latter but not the former, but no sociological hypothesis was raised about its reason (e.g. about risky male conduct requiring control). The author did note, however, that more research was required on 'the general population'.

Later, this focus on individual characteristics in clinical samples began to define 'the social', as an outcrop of patient pathology or deficit. For example, Platt and colleagues reported on the development of the 'Social Behaviour Assessment Schedule', to measure 'the patient's disturbed behaviour, the patient's social performance, and the adverse effects on the household'.[13] Another example of making 'the social' a *patient* characteristic was the investigation of the problematic conduct of those abusing alcohol in Scotland.[14]

The Meso Level of 'the Social': The Focus on Immediate Relationships

The reporting of social disability as a product of patient pathology continued but overtime was now augmented by an interest in family life. As we noted earlier, one motive for this was to test the nature/nurture question. The role of family life in *relapse* but not causation (eschewing a possible implication of British 'anti-psychiatry') came to the fore in the study of 'expressed emotion'.[15] Speculating more generally about intimacy, Birtchnell and Kennard posed the question, does marital maladjustment lead to mental illness?[16]

The interpersonal field was reflected in the emerging epidemiological picture of the overrepresentation of black and ethnic minority patients (mainly African-Caribbean). Family and cultural features of these groups became a focus of interest, along with a consideration about stressors linked to migration and community; not just clinical samples were investigated.[17]

Up until the mid-1990s the social 'deficits' assumed to be flowing *from* mental illness continued to be of interest,[18] as well as an exploration of the racialised picture of admissions, with a particular interest in why rates of psychosis were higher in second generation Afro-Caribbean people.[19] Also, the biogenetic assumption from the 1960s persevered in studies looking at social factors.[20]

With that continued assumption, premorbid deficits implied an endogenous source for current social disability. An example of the continuing biological undertow was the suggestion that immigrant mental illness might be caused by a virus in their host country. This preference for a putative biological cause is noteworthy given the clear prevalence of both poverty and racism in society.

An alternative exploration of significant others was offered by Morley and colleagues,[21] who suggested that the relatives of patients are wary of services and this shapes admission decisions of African-Caribbean patients. Also, the continuation of the research on how 'high expressed emotion' in the families of psychotic patients contributed to relapse continued; the relapse focus thereby allowed the biogenetic assumption to be retained.[22]

There was a continuing focus on clinical routines. For example, Tunnicliffe and colleagues were interested in tracing how ethnic background predicted compliance levels with depot medication.[23] 'The social' then was a profession-centred resource in the research and not a window into sociological understanding. For example, the depot question could have been discussed in terms of psychiatrists as being agents of social control in open settings, in anticipation of the controversy about Community Treatment Orders (see also Chapter 8).

The discursive picture in this period of social psychiatric research is one in which patient characteristics (i.e. symptoms and deficits, with embedding biogenetic assumptions) and service utilisation processes define what is meant by 'the social'. The latter might be extended to family context, as a source of relapse and possible gene pool of aetiology. The

Camberwell Depression study mentioned in the section 'The Social Origins of Depression' was of this type.

The Macro Level of 'the Social': A Shift Back to Social Causation

The insights of the ecological wing of the Chicago School of sociology were seemingly unrecognised or acknowledged in the abovementioned published research. However, gradually a fuller account of social causation emerged, along with more methodological sophistication and some willingness to explore the sociological imagination. The latter dawning was evident in a paper by Rodgers looking at the social distribution of neurotic symptoms in the population.[24] The role of poverty became evident and the author commented (we assume without irony) that previous studies 'may have underestimated the importance of financial circumstances'. Similarly, Gupta showed significant statistical correlations between mental disorder, occupation and urbanicity.[25] The powerful causal combination of poverty and city living was now being re-vindicated.

Those signs in the 1990s of a recognition of the macro level have been more evident recently. For example, resonating in part with the sociological notion of intersectional disadvantage, the older pattern of racialised admissions was now revisited with the added question of class. Brugha and colleagues found that 'ethnic grouping was strongly associated with: unemployment; lone parent status; lower social class; low perceived social support; poverty (indicated by lack of car ownership) and having a primary social support group of less than three close others'.[26]

By the turn of this century, the taken-for-granted diagnostic categories used by social psychiatrists were subject to critical questioning. The weak construct validity of schizophrenia was conceded and a broader notion of *psychosis* as the medical codification of madness (i.e. socially unintelligible conduct) emerged.[27] This marked a recognition that social constructivist arguments might now be relevant to explore, when and if dubious diagnostic concepts were the dependent variable in epidemiology (i.e. *what* exactly was being studied?). This small shift should not be over-drawn, though; except for querying 'schizophrenia', there was no apparent rush to abandon psychiatric diagnosis in social psychiatric research.

Samele and colleagues found that occupational (but not educational) status predicted psychotic symptoms.[28] In line with these newer macro-focused studies, Mallett and colleagues found that 'unemployment and early separation from both parents distinguish African-Caribbeans diagnosed with schizophrenia from their counterparts of other ethnic groups as well as their normal peers, and imply that more attention needs to be focussed on socio-environmental variables in schizophrenia research'.[29] A similar point was made by Marwaha and Johnson about the role of employment in recovery from psychosis.[30] The focus on black and minority ethnic (BME) patients remained present in the literature but within that there was a return to a focus on the impact of migration,[31] though with a continuing interest in British-born BME groups as well.[32]

By the start of the present century, there had also been a return to community-based rather than clinical sampling. For example, King and colleagues examined psychotic symptoms in the BME general population and concluded that prevalence rates 'were higher in people from ethnic minorities, but were not consistent with the much higher first contact rates for psychotic disorder reported previously, particularly in Black Caribbeans'.[33] This return to the general population rather than clinical samples also applied to depressive and anxiety symptoms, with links being made explicitly to them being inflected by social inequality.[34]

During the first decade of this century there was a continuing service-centred concern but now it was explicitly in relation to the context of deinstitutionalisation, especially when substance misuse amplified the risky conduct of psychotic patients in the community.[35] Other new trends included a small shift to well-being rather than mental disorder,[36] as well as a concern with self-harm and suicide, especially in relation to middle-class groups.[37]

Discussion

We noted that the sociological work of Tirril Harris, George Brown and colleagues was of a different character to that led by psychiatrists, as it was explicitly about social inequality and its implied social injustice (defying the fact-value separation of the positivist tradition). During the 1960s, British social psychiatrists at first tended to discuss 'the social' as an attribute of patients to be measured, taking it for granted that their illness made them socially impaired and that this placed a social burden on others. This gave way to one in which family determinants, especially about relapse or service contact, took on a greater salience. These micro and meso depictions of 'the social' always carried with them the strong presumption of bio-determinism. Eventually, there was a return to a macro-social interest; socio-economic conditions were now causally relevant and community, not clinical, samples regained their importance.

Looking at the literature of the period of interest, apart from this pattern about the framing of 'the social', another observation is the uneven ecology of the research itself. Most of the work is derived from the Institute of Psychiatry in London, augmented by a minority of studies from Scotland and the English provinces. Accordingly, one immediately convenient locality (Camberwell) has been investigated disproportionately. It may well be that Camberwell reflected the UK-wide picture of what was being researched in the past few decades, but we will never know. The dominance of the work in South London may have had the effect of marginalising the impact of attachment theory from the rival Tavistock Clinic, north of the Thames;[38] and within the London-based quantitative research, the relevant correlations were derived from varying sample sizes. For example, the clinical sample in the Camberwell Depression study in the 1980s was of 130 patients, whereas the community sample from King and colleagues in 2005 was of 4,281 face-to-face interviews.

By the turn of this century, British social psychiatric research was still largely medically led, although the faltering integration of health and social care prompted some social worker leadership.[39] We also noted some work on assessment tools that was led occasionally by psychologists (e.g. Slade and Kuipers) or sociologists (e.g. Platt). Epistemologically, medical dominance extended to the ongoing reliance on diagnostic groups as dependent variables. However, we noted a cautious shift, for some, from 'schizophrenia' to 'psychosis'. This ambivalence within social psychiatry about reifying diagnoses is an old trope, traceable to Meyerian psychiatry.

At the start of the chapter, we noted that it had provided the basis for a potential collaboration between the psychiatric profession and sociology. The material covered suggests that the latter has not had a consistent impact on the former, with the sociological imagination being in poor supply at times, though occasionally contributions from sociologists were evident.[40] We mention this separation because sociologists themselves have produced their own research on mental health and illness, which *does* cite the psychiatric (and psychological) literature. We have summarised this intermittently in the past thirty years.

Conclusion

British social psychiatry has tended to start with the anchor point of clinical concerns and diagnoses and their presupposed underlying biological causation. It then moves out tentatively to interpersonal settings and societal stressors. By contrast, sociologists are more likely to start at the other end of the telescope. Their focus is on groups of people in their social context not pathology, which then comes into focus because of sociological reflection more widely. Their alternative agenda inter alia includes medical dominance and the social control role of psychiatry in society, eugenics, political economy, lay views, especially from service users, and metaphysical debates about social causationism and social constructivism. A life-course approach predominates, for example, with considerations about childhood adversity and mental health in old age. These topics, drawing upon wider sociological work, might have helped social psychiatrists to develop their sociological imagination.

No discipline has a monopoly of understanding about this topic and so the interdisciplinary potential of social psychiatry, broadly conceived, remains an opportunity for all. However, for its potential to be realised, interdisciplinarity needs to be fully respected by all. The shortcomings about the sociological imagination, which we drew attention to in this chapter, might have been avoided had this point been recognised in the mid-1960s in British social psychiatry. Psychiatric wariness of sociology was one likely source of this shortcoming, along with the self-referential norm in the medical literature reinforcing a uni-disciplinary silo.

Key Summary Points

- Either side of the Second World War, social psychiatry had emerged in the United States, influenced by Adolf Meyer's work, the ecological wing of the Chicago School of sociology and, subsequently, the development of the biopsychosocial model by George Engel. The sociological imagination in British social psychiatry was sparse but not always absent.
- Most of the work in UK is derived from the Institute of Psychiatry in London, augmented by a minority of studies from Scotland and the English provinces.
- By the turn of the present century, the taken-for-granted diagnostic categories used by social psychiatrists were subject to critical questioning. The weak construct validity of schizophrenia was conceded and a broader notion of *psychosis* as the medical codification of madness (i.e. socially unintelligible conduct) emerged.
- No discipline has a monopoly of understanding about this topic and so the interdisciplinary potential of social psychiatry, broadly conceived, remains an opportunity for all. However, for its potential to be realised, the principle of interdisciplinarity needs to be fully respected by all. British psychiatry has been wary of sociology and has had a tendency, like other medical specialities, to be self-referential in its published outputs, thereby producing a largely uni-disciplinary silo.

Notes

1. D. Pilgrim and A. Rogers, The troubled relationship between psychiatry and sociology. *International Journal of Social Psychiatry* (2005) 51: 228–41.

2. T. Main, The hospital as a therapeutic institution. *Bulletin of the Menninger Clinic* (1946) 10: 64–71; M. Jones, The treatment of personality disorders in a therapeutic community. *Psychiatry* (1957) 20: 211–20; J. Bowlby, *Maternal Care and Mental Health*. Geneva: World Health Organization, 1951; D. Goldberg and P. Huxley, *Common Mental Disorders: A Bio-social Model*. London: Tavistock and Routledge, 1992.

3. G. Engel, The clinical application of the biopsychosocial model. *American Journal of Psychiatry* (1980) 137: 535–44.

4. G. W. Brown and T. O. Harris, *The Social Origins of Depression: A Study of Psychiatric Disorder in Women*. London: Tavistock, 1978.

5. G. W. Brown, T. O. Harris and C. Hepworth, Loss, humiliation and entrapment among women developing depression: A patient and non patient comparison. *Psychological Medicine* (1995) 25: 7–21.

6. A. Bifulco, T. O. Harris and G. W. Brown, Mourning or inadequate care? Reexamining the relationship of maternal loss in childhood with adult depression and anxiety. *Development and Psychopathology* (1992) 4: 119–28.

7. A. Bifulco, P. M. Moran, P. Ball et al., Adult attachment style. I: Its relationship to clinical depression. *Social Psychiatry and Psychiatric Epidemiology* (2002) 37: 50–9.

8. P. Bebbincton, T. Brugha, T. B. McCarthy et al., The Camberwell Collaborative Depression Study – I: Depressed probands: Adversity and the form of depression. *British Journal of Psychiatry* (1988) 152: 754–65; P. McGuffin and P. Bebbington, The Camberwell collaborative depression study – II: Investigation of family members. *British Journal of Psychiatry* (1988): 766–74; P. McGuffin, R. Katz and P. Bebbington, The Camberwell collaborative depression study – III: Depression and adversity in the relatives of depressed probands *British Journal of Psychiatry* (1988) 152: 775–82.

9. Goldberg and Huxley, *Common Mental Disorders*.

10. C. W. Mills, *The Sociological Imagination*. New York: Oxford University Press, 1959.

11. A. M. Adelstein, M. Downham, Z. Stein et al., The epidemiology of mental illness in an English city: Inceptions recognized by Salford psychiatric services. *Social Psychiatry and Psychiatric Epidemiology* (1968) 3: 47–9.

12. B. Cooper, Psychiatric disorder in hospital and general practice. *Social Psychiatry* (1966) 1: 7–10.

13. S. Platt, A. Weyman, S. Hirsch et al., The Social Behaviour Assessment Schedule (SBAS): Rationale, contents, scoring and reliability of a new interview schedule. *Social Psychiatry and Psychiatric Epidemiology* (1980) 15: 43–55.

14. M. A. Plant and F. Pirie, Self-reported alcohol consumption and alcohol-related problems: A study in four Scottish towns. *Social Psychiatry and Psychiatric Epidemiology* (1979) 14: 65–73.

15. L. Kuipers Expressed emotion in 1991. *Social Psychiatry and Psychiatric Epidemiology* (1992) 27: 1–3.

16. J. Birtchnell and J. Kennard, Does marital maladjustment lead to mental illness? *Social Psychiatry and Psychiatric Epidemiology* (1983) 18: 79–88.

17. E. Hurry, P. Sturt, P. Bebbington and C. Tennant, Socio-demographic associations with social disablement in a community sample. *Social Psychiatry and Psychiatric Epidemiology* (1983) 18: 3113–21.

18. T. S. Brugha, J. Wing and J. C. Brewin, The relationship of social network deficits in social functioning in long term psychiatric disorders. *Social Psychiatry and Psychiatric Epidemiology* (1993) 28: 218–24.

19. D. McGovern and R. Cope, First psychiatric admission rates of first and second generation Afro Caribbeans. *Social Psychiatry and Psychiatric Epidemiology* (1987) 22: 139–49; D. McGovern and R. Cope, Second generation Afro-Caribbeans and young whites with a first admission diagnosis of schizophrenia. *Social Psychiatry and Psychiatric Epidemiology* (1991) 26: 95–9.

20. R. Mallett, J. Leff, D. Bhugra et al., Social environment, ethnicity and schizophrenia. *Social Psychiatry and Psychiatric Epidemiology* (2002) 37: 229–335.

21. R. Morley, T. Wykes and B. MacCarthy, Attitudes of relatives of Afro-Caribbean patients: Do they affect admission? *Social Psychiatry and Psychiatric Epidemiology* (1991) 26(1): 87–193.

22. R. G. McCreadie, The Nithsdale schizophrenia surveys. *Social Psychiatry and Psychiatric Epidemiology* (1992) 27: 40–5.

23. S. Tunnicliffe, G. Harrison and P. J. Standen, Factors affecting compliance with depot injection treatment in the community. *Social Psychiatry and Psychiatric Epidemiology* (1992) 27: 230–3.

24. B. Rodgers, Socio-economic status, employment and neurosis. *Social Psychiatry and Psychiatric Epidemiology* (1991) 26: 104–14.

25. S. Gupta, Can environmental factors explain the epidemiology of schizophrenia in immigrant groups? *Social Psychiatry and Psychiatric Epidemiology* (1993) 28: 263–6.

26. T. S. Brugha, R. Jenkins, P. Bebbington et al., Risk factors and the prevalence of neurosis and psychosis in ethnic groups in Great Britain. *Social Psychiatry and Psychiatric Epidemiology* (2004) 39: 939–46.

27. J. Van Os, P. Jones, P. Sham et al., Risk factors for onset and persistence of psychosis. *Social Psychiatry and Psychiatric Epidemiology* (1998) 33: 596–605.

28. C. Samele, J. van Os, K. McKenzie et al., Does socioeconomic status predict course and outcome in patients with psychosis? *Social Psychiatry and Psychiatric Epidemiology* (2001) 36: 573–81.

29. S. Marwaha and S. Johnson, Schizophrenia and employment: A review. *Social Psychiatry and Psychiatric Epidemiology* (2004) 39: 337–49.

30. G. Leavey, K. Hollins, M. King et al., Psychological disorder amongst refugee and migrant schoolchildren in London. *Social Psychiatry and Psychiatric Epidemiology* (2004) 39: 191–5.

31. S. Pantelidou and T. Craig, Culture shock and social support. *Social Psychiatry and Psychiatric Epidemiology* (2006) 41: 777–781; R. Gater, B. Tomenson, C. Percival et al., Persistent depressive disorders and social stress in people of Pakistani origin and white Europeans in UK. *Social Psychiatry and Psychiatric Epidemiology* (2008) 44: 198–209.

32. E.g. M. King, J. Nazroo, J. S. Weich et al., Psychotic symptoms in the general population of England. *Social Psychiatry and Psychiatric Epidemiology* (2005) 40: 375–81.

33. D. Melzer, D.T. Fryers, R. Jenkins et al., Social position and the common mental disorders with disability. *Social Psychiatry and Psychiatric Epidemiology* (2003) 38: 238–43.

34. J. Todd, G. Green, M. Harrison et al., Social exclusion in clients with comorbid mental health and substance misuse problems. *Social Psychiatry and Psychiatric Epidemiology* (2004) 53: 519–87.

35. M. J. Maynard, S., Harding and H. Minnis, Psychological well-being in Black Caribbean, Black African, and White adolescents in the UK Medical Research Council DASH study. *Social Psychiatry and Psychiatric Epidemiology* (2007) 42: 759–69.

36. I. Collins and E. Paykel, Suicide amongst Cambridge University Students 1970–1996. *Social Psychiatry and Psychiatric Epidemiology* (2000) 35: 128–32.

37. D. J. Bartram, G. Yadegarfar and D. S. Baldwin, A cross-sectional study of mental health and well-being and their associations in the UK veterinary profession. *Social Psychiatry and Psychiatric Epidemiology* (2009) 44: 1075–85; P. Huxley, S. Reilly, E. Robinshaw et al., Interventions and outcomes of health and social care service provision for people with severe mental illness in England. *Social Psychiatry and Psychiatric Epidemiology* (2003) 38: 44–8.

38. Cf. Bifulco, Moran, Ball et al., Adult attachment style. I: Its relationship to clinical depression.

39. J. Nazroo, Y. Kamaldeep, S. Bhui et al., Where next for understanding race/ethnic inequalities in severe mental illness? Structural, interpersonal and institutional racism. *Sociology of Health and Illness* (2020) 42: 262–76.

40. A. Rogers and D. Pilgrim, *A Sociology of Mental Health and Illness* (6th ed.). Maidenhead: Open University Press, 2020.

Life, Change and Charisma: Memories of UK Psychiatric Hospitals in the Long 1960s

Thomas Stephenson and Claire Hilton

Introduction

Psychiatric hospitals across the UK were in various states of change during the long 1960s, influenced by legal, medical, ideological, social, psychological, financial and other factors. The Mental Health Act 1959 (MHA) created more liberal admission processes and encouraged community care. The Suicide Act 1961 decriminalised suicide and attempted suicide. New medications were available and multidisciplinary teamwork developed. Societal perspectives shifted concerning individuality, personal autonomy and human rights. In the face of a more educated, less class-deferent society, paternalistic 'doctor-knows-best' attitudes became less acceptable, although clinical styles which infringed on human dignity continued in many National Health Service (NHS) settings.[1] New organisations, such as the Patients Association, and older ones, such as the National Association for Mental Health (today, Mind), began to campaign for patients' health care rights (see also Chapter 14). Antiquated psychiatric hospitals were expensive to maintain and stimulated government policies to close them. Psychiatric hospital beds in England and Wales, which peaked at 148,000 in 1954, reduced to 136,000 in 1960 and to 94,000 in 1973 (see also Chapters 1 and 31).[2]

Decisions and actions within health care institutions, from central government down, impact on the lives of individual patients, their families, the staff and the wider community. However, too often, experiences of individuals are ignored in historical analyses. Recognising this for mental health care, oral history resources have been developed, such as the Mental Health Testimony Archive,[3] comprising patients' life stories and health service experiences. Some people wrote memoirs, such as psychiatrists William Sargant and Henry Rollin,[4] and community projects such as at the former Whittingham Hospital, Preston and Fairfield Hospital, Stotfold, are recording the lives of the people associated with them. To complement existing resources of personal experiences, we convened a witness seminar on psychiatric hospitals in the 1960s. A witness seminar allows invited witnesses to present their memories and to discuss them with each other and a participating audience. Challenge and comment are akin to open and immediate peer review. Seminars are recorded, transcribed, annotated and made available as a primary historical resource.[5]

Witness seminars are inevitably selective and subjective and include contributors' prejudices and personal agendas. These biases may be less evident in written archives, especially official or clinical documents, but they still exist and all sources need critical analysis. Our witness seminar aimed to be multidisciplinary, drawing on experiences from across the UK. Lifespan, health and competing commitments were factors limiting availability of witnesses. Unfortunately, we had only one patient witness and none from the civil service or black and Asian ethnic groups.

Table 6.1 Witness seminar participants quoted in this chapter

Name	Initials (used in text)	Role/context (1960s)	Affiliated hospital (1960s)
Dora Black	DB	Junior doctor	Napsbury, Hertfordshire
Bill Boyd	BB	Consultant psychiatrist and physician superintendent	Herdmanflat, East Lothian
John Bradley	JB	Consultant psychiatrist and medical director	Friern, London
Malcolm Campbell	MC	Junior doctor	Friern, London
Peter Campbell	PC	Patient	Addenbrookes, Cambridge; Royal Dundee Liff, Angus
Susanne Curran	SC	Mental welfare officer (psychiatric social worker)	Prestwich and Rossendale, Lancashire
John Hall	JH	Clinical psychologist	St Andrew's, Norwich
John Jenkins	JJ	Student nurse	Parc Gwyllt, Bridgend
David Jolley	DJ	Medical student	Severalls, Colchester
Jennifer Lowe	JL	Occupational therapist	Littlemore, Oxford
Peter Nolan	PN	Student nurse	Tooting Bec, London
Geraldine Pratten	GP	Lived with her family in a hospital staff house	Crichton Royal, Dumfries
Angela Rouncefield	AR	Junior doctor	Sefton General; Birkenhead General; North Wales, Denbigh
Peter Tyrer	PT	Junior doctor	St Thomas' and Maudsley, London
Harry Zeitlin	HZ	Junior doctor	Maudsley, London

In this chapter, we present some of the seminar themes, focusing on experiences in the hospitals and some of the clinicians and patients who inspired and influenced change. Discussion jogged memories onto other topics and anecdotes, such as ethics, leadership, gender and professional training, far more than can be explored in this chapter. The transcript, witnesses' biographies and a commentary on some of the more controversial themes are free to download.[6] In this chapter, references to the seminar are indicated by transcript page numbers and the speaker's initials (Table 6.1).

Onto the Wards

In the 1960s, most psychiatric hospitals were suburban or rural. Many were 'total institutions', as Erving Goffman described, places of residence and work where many like-situated individuals, cut off from wider society for an appreciable period of time, led an enclosed and formally administered way of life.[7] The public were often fearful of the hospitals (SC,20) and avoided them. Staff too could find them disconcerting, the 'foreboding experience of a very long, dimly lit corridor' (MC,25) could provoke panic (JB,50). MC (25) also remembered the 'overall pervading ... smell, a mixture of incontinence and disinfectant' and others recalled the foul odour of the sedative paraldehyde (JB,27), while written sources mentioned smells of vomit, faeces, cats, mothballs, cooking, ozone machines, flowers, talc and freshness.[8]

Psychiatric wards were gender segregated, but some hospitals were 'bringing the genders together for civilised activities' (DJ,12). Nevertheless, PC (16) recalled: 'men and women used to come down to mealtimes at slightly different times and sit at different tables. It was a brave person who made up a mixed table.' Whereas ward staff were usually of the same gender as their patients, doctors generally worked across several wards and were not. Women hospital doctors were few and far between,[9] and when they worked on the 'male side', there could be practical difficulties: 'no ladies [toilets] in the male units: a male nurse would stand outside the gents while I went in' (AR,47). Male and female wards also had different cultures. Since our nurse and patient witnesses (JJ; PN; PC) were all male, their descriptions might be less applicable to female wards. Male wards were more militaristic and arguably physically harsher than women's wards, which perpetuated different sorts of detrimental practices.[10]

Distressing mental symptoms could preoccupy a new patient:

> traumatised by my situation ... extremely anxious. I believed I'd been taken away to die ... I would wander around the ward. My concentration was extremely poor. I tried to watch the television but could make no sense of it. This distressed me greatly.   (PC,16)

Ward environments might add to distress:

> The day room always seemed crowded with constant movement. Although there were few comfortable places to sit, it was where patients smoked, had their meals, met visitors, listened to the radio, watched television, had cups of tea, sat alone or chatted in groups. No matter how often the ashtrays were emptied they were always full.   (PN,26)

Sometimes there were 'insufficient chairs. The only escape was to sit in the toilets smoking or just sleeping which often happened, thus blocking the use of some toilets' (PN,69). Some hospitals attempted to improve environments but patients might resist change:

> we got lovely comfortable chairs with coffee tables so that the patients could sit in nice little groups. Of course, when I came in the day after it was in action, the patients were all sitting around the wall .... backs to the wall and I said, 'What's happening?' And the nurses said, 'Well, that's what the patients wanted to do' so we just had to go along with it.   (BB,52)

Communal living arrangements, few personal possessions and the loss of usual social roles and relationships diminished patients' sense of individuality and promoted conformity with ward regimes.[11] Rigid regimes might ease life for staff but could be unhelpful to patients. PC (16) recalled:

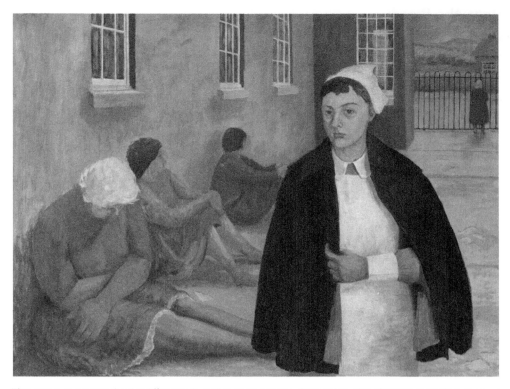

Figure 6.1 Institutionalised indifference: Russell Barton's painting, *Potential Murderers?* c.1960. © Bethlem Museum of the Mind.

> I found it very difficult to sleep. I remember lying in bed waiting for the right time to go and ask for chloral hydrate. Too soon, and I would be sent back to try again. Too late, and I would also be refused.

Some procedures, rules and inadequate facilities were also challenging to staff:

> I entered [the ward] briskly to prevent a possible key snatch or an escape attempt. The necessary rituals of saying good morning to the charge nurse and donning a white coat completed, the day started. Getting the patients up, dressed and washed before breakfast were priorities. Only having three wash basins and three toilets [for twenty-six patients] often delayed this process and frequently led to annoyances and confrontations. (PN,26)

Seminar participants spoke of interactions, between staff and patients, among patients and among staff. JJ (36) recalled an encounter with a senior nurse, who, because of his rank, was likely to influence staff attitudes and practices: 'I was given a very large key and taken ... to ward eight. [The nurse] only spoke a few words ... I will never forget ... "The key is the most important thing here and what it represents is your power over the lunatics."' The obsolete word 'lunatics' suggested outmoded attitudes towards patients, and 'power over' suggested a coercive culture, unlikely to foster kindness. Some staff showed 'institutionalised indifference' (Figure 6.1), walking past patients because 'being busy was preferable to being engaged' (PN,28), but there was also kindly interaction:

Assisting with [personal care] tasks, patients would sometimes confide to nurses such things as, 'It's my birthday today' or 'Today is the tenth anniversary of my leaving the army.' I often found myself captivated by observing the good-natured gentleness with which able bodied patients helped those less able. (PN,26)

PN's observation resonated with the 'kind of camaraderie' among patients which PC (17) experienced.

Medical staff as well as nurses could ignore patients' personal dignity. PC (17) described ward rounds:

We stood by our beds with our kit laid out neatly. The consultant and his retinue went from dormitory to dormitory and he interviewed us briefly where we stood and in front of all the other patients. It was nerve wracking, as ward rounds always are, but also lacking any confidentiality.

This style of ward round was unacceptable elsewhere, such as at Crichton Royal Hospital, Dumfries.[12]

Many staff, distressed by practices which they witnessed or experienced, lacked the confidence or know-how to challenge them. Juniors also feared that, in a culture of deference to seniors, antagonising those in authority might jeopardise their future careers. The NHS's first formal complaints guidance in 1966 had little effect and did not shift the defensive culture of NHS leadership.[13] However, NHS leaders began to acknowledge detrimental psychiatric hospital culture and practices in 1969, after inquiries into scandalously poor standards of psychiatric care.[14] Those reports echoed our witnesses' memories (JJ,36). The Ely Hospital, Cardiff, inquiry attributed bad practice to defective leadership in an inward-looking institution rather than to inherent malice.[15]

Some senior staff supported their distressed juniors in the event of a death by suicide (JH,28) but others did not. PN (27) recalled a recently discharged patient being found dead on Tooting Bec Common. The only acknowledgement from staff was that: 'I was asked to take his case-notes to the medical records office to be filed away.' Yet, for PN, 'His death profoundly affected me. There was no funeral, but I grieved for him.' Speaking about it fifty years later: 'I found myself back on that ward again. There was no emotional support, the term was never mentioned ... the way it was coped with was merely to ignore it' (PN,28). DB (40) also remembered a patient she had treated:

a seventeen-year-old epileptic girl ... she asked ... to go out into the grounds and she'd been very stable and I didn't see any reason why I shouldn't give her permission and I did. But there was a railway that ran on the north border of Napsbury Hospital ... And she was found dead on that railway track ... nobody was sure whether she'd deliberately gone and killed herself or whether she'd had an epileptic fit ... it was never really sorted out ... And I always wondered if I should have given her permission to go out ... I've remembered it for ... sixty years.

Historians have tended to see patients as victims and staff as perpetrators,[16] but the seminar pointed to a complex mix of experiences and emotions for both groups. Some staff had indelible painful memories and ongoing self-questioning about their own roles at the time (PT,30). Memories of unkindness haunted them, spurring them on to improve clinical practice over the course of their careers (JJ,37; PN,54).

Treatment

A daily routine, meaningful employment and social and leisure activities were all part of treatment, alongside medication and electroconvulsive therapy (ECT). New professions joined the hospitals, such as occupational therapists (OTs) and clinical psychologists, reflecting the challenges of accurate diagnosis, a broader range of treatments and a greater emphasis on discharging patients into the community. Psychologists, however, focused mainly on assessment (JH,42): 'Full psychometrics please' was often requested for a new inpatient, sometimes with its purpose difficult to ascertain (PC,19). JH (43) referred to routine psychometric testing as 'test bashing'.

Employment was considered to benefit self-esteem and well-being, through creativity and 'the involvement, fellowship, the jokes that would come from work' (DJ,16). At Severalls Hospital, 'the most damaged people' would 'turn cement', from which others would 'make slabs and they would sell the slabs in the town' (DJ,12). DJ (12) also pointed out 'what a tragedy at the moment, if you ask what people [with severe mental illness] are doing, there's no work' for them, referring to a report in 2013 which found UK employment rates of around 8 per cent for people with schizophrenia and stated that many more could work and wanted to do so.[17]

'Industrial therapy' (IT) fitted with the ethos of rehabilitation and discharge into the community. It was conceptualised as employing patients under clinical supervision in factory-type work appropriate to their individual needs, including providing psychological and economic satisfaction. If IT managers set up external business contracts, patients could be paid (JB,16). For patients engaged in non-IT hospital work, there were several material reward systems: cash; a 'token economy' based on psychological principles; and 'rewards in kind' which some senior psychiatrists criticised as 'out of keeping with modern views'.[18] Overcrowded wards lacking individual lockers for storing personal possessions put valued items at risk of theft and deterred hospitals from providing cash or tokens.[19]

Newly qualified OT JL (35) was deployed to a long-stay ward: 'I found it hard to feel that there was any good that I could do.' Bingo as an activity 'for heavily sedated patients, was very badly decided upon':

> Patients sat around tables with their bingo cards in front of them and one of us shouted out the numbers. We would then run around the tables moving the numbers for them and when a card was full, we would pick up a hand and shout, 'Come on Jan! Come on Alice!' or whoever it was, 'Shout Bingo! You've won!' It was impossible and exhausting.

JL (35) described her OT role as a 'cosmetic addition'. JH (42), another new hospital professional, commented: 'I was the first junior trained psychologist they had ever had, and to be honest I am not sure they knew what to do with me!' Hospital leaders developing multidisciplinary teams, with one eye on financial expenditure and uncertainty about what newcomers were able to do, could create impossible workloads.[20]

PC (19–20) described being treated with ECT, noting that it is given differently today:

> another patient [said] to me, 'Oh, you need ECT. You'll be given ECT. They'll do this and that to you in ECT.' And because ECT sounds awful, you start worrying about being given ECT . . . I remember being in a Nightingale ward and being lined up on a bed and the ECT machine worked its way down to you . . . You were just in the ward and the ECT machine came down to you and you could hear it getting nearer and nearer to you.

For many seminar participants, this disturbing description was a lasting memory of the day.

Medications, such as chlorpromazine, reserpine, imipramine and monoamine oxidase inhibitors which could modify the symptoms and course of 'functional' psychiatric disorders such as schizophrenia, were newly available.[21] DB (40) recalled their effect on her patients:

> In 1957 ... my senior registrar ... put everybody on reserpine ... it was like Oliver Sacks talked about with levodopa ... Many of them, just started walking and talking and being human again after having been doped for twenty years. It was really an amazing experience.

The outcome for one of these patients gives insights into rehabilitation processes and staff–patient dynamics:

> Dorothea had been on the ward for thirty years and she'd been cleaning the ward for thirty years, but she had been put on reserpine and she'd responded to it. I think she had been diagnosed originally as schizophrenic and she was really very well, and would we take her on [to clean our house]? ... I just gave her the keys ... and she went and cleaned my house ... And eventually she decided that she was well enough to leave the hospital and she got a job as a housekeeper for a local family who knew she was from Napsbury, so therefore they paid her hardly anything. And then she was successful at that job, so she got a better job and she used to come and visit ... bringing little presents for the children, she became a friend of the family. (DB,41)

The MHA, social expectations and policy ideas, along with new medications and a greater emphasis on rehabilitation, facilitated a move towards community care. The MHA allowed, but did not mandate, community care, with the result that local authorities were reluctant to fund it. Many hospitals built links with their local communities, but this was far from uniform, even between neighbouring hospitals (SC,21). It was dependent on the priorities of the local psychiatric leadership and staff creativity to nurture the links,[22] for instance by encouraging local people to volunteer to support patients with activities, such as knitting: 'Simple things but bringing people together to do things that they never did before' (DJ,13). At Herdmanflat Hospital, 'the Round Table, the young version of Rotary ... became very interested in the hospital, ran events, and visited' (BB,52). DJ (12) accompanied Dr Russell Barton to schools and colleges where 'Russell would be preaching the gospel and encouraging people not to be frightened of this place on the edge of the town'. From some hospitals, staff began to visit discharged patients at home and 'this ... blossomed into a full community nursing service' alongside improved liaison with local social services (JB,51). BB (52) described how bringing people together was 'quite a therapeutic thing', improving links with local clergy and with family doctors who had 'been a bit distant from the hospital'.

Evidence-Based Practice

Notions of clinical scientific evidence in the 1960s contrasted with those used today: PT (34) commented: 'When someone very important made a statement or made an observation about a clinical problem, that was evidence ... I suppose it was the only evidence we had to go on.' Seminar participants recalled working with, or being taught by, 'very important' charismatic people, such as William Sargant (1907–88), R. D. Laing (1927–89) and Russell Barton (1923–2002). Each had firmly held views. Sargant advocated biological treatments, including prolonged sleep, insulin coma, ECT and high doses of medication, often in combination. Diametrically opposed, R. D. Laing promoted 'anti-psychiatry' concepts with entirely psychosocial models of, and treatment for, mental illnesses such as schizophrenia. Barton was vociferous that psychiatric hospitals must provide humane, dignified and rehabilitative treatment, but in the 1960s his methods were considered almost as radical as those of Sargant and Laing. All three stood on the fringes of conventional psychiatry, generated enthusiasm and hostility and provoked public and professional debate. Their styles of communication were as contentious as their clinical methods: both could impact on patients and colleagues, with constructive and destructive outcomes.

Barton's humanity enthused DJ (12) and helped shape his life work. Like the nurses, junior doctors could be inspired to follow in the footsteps of their seniors or, if disturbed by their experiences, could become determined to do things better. PT (31) recalled:

> No one said anything about ethics. I first got my interest in randomised controlled trials by working for William Sargant . . . I learnt more from him by what he did to excess than from others who taught me more correctly . . . But . . . it really concerned me . . . was I complicit in this in my very first psychiatric post . . . ? The patient that got the insulin coma did get remarkably better (in the short term at least) and his parents were so pleased they gave a cheque to William Sargant, who gave it to me and said: 'Go and buy a couple of books.' The first one I bought was *Principles of Medical Statistics* by Austin Bradford Hill. [Working in Sargant's department] made me realise that doing things without any proper evidence was shocking.

Variable Standards

Many factors helped shape psychiatric hospital standards during the 1960s. No participants referred to poor standards in Scottish psychiatric hospitals. Scotland had similar mental health legislation to England and Wales but different policies on hospital closure, and new treatments and ideologies of deinstitutionalisation transformed care within them.[23] BB (53) noted that local people staffed Herdmanflat and the Royal Edinburgh Hospital, in contrast to the situation described south of the border. Staffing by local people (whose family and friends may also have been patients) may have facilitated communication and understanding between patients, staff and community, contrasting with hospitals which employed many staff recruited from further afield, who may have faced cultural and language challenges and lacked local social networks (PN,26; JH,46).

In England and Wales, government plans to close the psychiatric hospitals discouraged interest and expenditure on them.[24] The MHA abolished the supervisory body for the psychiatric hospitals, leaving them without external inspection or oversight for most of the decade, until a new inspectorate was established in 1969.[25] While historiographies about NHS psychiatric hospitals in the 1960s are overwhelmingly disparaging, oral history accounts suggest that standards were far from uniform. This is compatible with reports from independent inquiries into psychiatric hospital care which found 'wide contrasts' within hospitals, with grave concerns about some wards but not others.[26] SC (20) worked concurrently in a psychiatric hospital and a district general hospital and found better communication, team working and attitudes of the public to the psychiatric service and of the service towards the patients in the general hospital. John Wing and George Brown identified many differences between the three psychiatric hospitals they studied between 1960 and 1968.[27] They also highlighted the importance of idealistic leadership to improve standards, concurring with views of witnesses that leadership and vision were vital, such as to help overcome the tendency of staff to resist changing established practices previously regarded as safe and appropriate (JJ,38; HZ,38).

Conclusion

The 1960s were a decade of radical societal change, ideological battles within mental health services and a complex psychiatric hospital narrative.[28] New medication, the MHA, multi-disciplinary teams and ideals of community care provided opportunities to improve the lives of patients but not all hospitals grasped the nettle of implementation. Some in positions of responsibility endorsed neglect and old-fashioned methods, while others inspired improvements in patient care above and beyond expectations.

With the nature of medical 'evidence' ill-defined, and ethical frameworks unclear, clinical creativity by individual charismatic leaders entailed risks, particularly if associated with dogmatic inflexibility. Our witnesses' impressions, particularly about the extremes, from harshness and tragedies to humanity, were formative in their careers and persisted lifelong. Encounters with inhumane and disrespectful care and lack of autonomy for patients were unnerving for witnesses in the 1960s and for our seminar audience. It did not require an 'expert' to recognise the essence of 'good' and 'bad'. New or junior staff seemed more able to appreciate extremes than those accustomed to the local routines. Deference to seniority and a defensive leadership failed to enable the lower ranks to offer constructive criticism. However, people and practices perceived as 'good' provided role models and standards to emulate, whereas 'bad' spurred on others to achieve more humane and evidence-based care and treatment later in their careers.

Some witness seminar participants linked past to present. Why are there still scandals of care? How do we respond to practices we regard as unethical or harmful? Materially and scientifically psychiatric care has improved, but to what extent do unconstructive under-lying societal beliefs and expectations perpetuate? We can learn from the experiences of our forebears and use the themes raised in this seminar to help us reflect on our roles, obligations, practices and standards today.

Key Summary Points

- The witness seminar revealed perspectives on the past which are not readily available in written sources.
- The memory of a tragedy, such as the suicide of a patient, can haunt involved staff members lifelong.
- Individual senior staff were role models who had profound effects on the course of junior clinicians' future careers.
- Wide contrasts in clinical standards and practices existed within and between hospitals.
- Many aspects of psychiatric practice have improved since the 1960s but others have not. Supported employment has been lost in the era of community care, scandals of poor care recur and staff may still fear speaking up when they experience or witness substandard practices.

Notes

1.   G. Cohen, *What's Wrong with Hospitals?* Harmondsworth: Penguin, 1964.

2. For the 1960 figures, see E. Brooke, Factors affecting the demand for psychiatric beds. *Lancet* (1962) 2: 1211–13; for 1973, see Department of Health and Social Security (DHSS), *The Facilities and Services of Psychiatric Hospitals in England and Wales 1973*. London: HMSO, 1976, pp. 54–5.

3. British Library. Mental Health Testimony Archive, http://cadensa.bl.uk/uhtbin/cgisirsi/?ps=OlKuJBwhd1/ WORKS-FILE/0/49.

4. W. Sargant, *The Unquiet Mind: The Autobiography of a Physician in Psychological Medicine*. London: Heinemann, 1967; H. Rollin, *Festina Lente: A Psychiatric Odyssey*. London: BMJ, 1990.

5. T. Tansey, The History of Modern Biomedicine: What Is a Witness Seminar?, www.histmodbiomed.org/ar ticle/what-is-a-witness-seminar.html.

6. C. Hilton and T. Stephenson (eds.), *Psychiatric Hospitals in the UK in the 1960s*. London: Royal College of Psychiatrists, 2020, www.rcpsych.ac.uk/docs/default-source/about-us/library-archives/archives/witness-seminar-final-transcript-july-2020-small.pdf?sfvrsn=4bceec71_2.

7. E. Goffman, *Asylums: Essays on the Social Situation of Mental Patients and Other Inmates*. Harmondsworth: Penguin, 1980. The first edition was published in 1961.

8. R. Barton, *Institutional Neurosis*. Bristol: Wright, 1966, p. 25.

9. Royal College of Physicians (RCP), *Women and Medicine: The Future (Summary)*. London: RCP, 2009, www .rcr.ac.uk/sites/default/files/RCP_Women_%20in_%20Medicine_%20Report.pdf.

10. P. Nolan, The development of mental health nursing. In J. Carson, L. Fagin and S. Ritter, eds. *Stress and Coping in Mental Health Nursing*, 1–18. London: Chapman and Hall, 1995; B. Robb, *Sans Everything: A Case to Answer*. London: Nelson, 1967.

11. Barton, *Institutional Neurosis*.

12. R. Sneddon, Psychiatric geriatric assessment unit at Crichton Royal Hospital, *Nursing Mirror* (1967): x–xv.

13. Ministry of Health, *Methods of Dealing with Complaints of Patients*, HM (66)15. London: HMSO, 1966.

14. C. Hilton, A tale of two inquiries: *Sans Everything* and *Ely*. *Political Quarterly* (2019) 90: 185–93.

15. DHSS, *Report of the Committee of Inquiry into Allegations of Ill-Treatment of Patients and Other Irregularities at the Ely Hospital, Cardiff*, Cmnd. 3975. London: HMSO, 1969, pp. 115–16.

16. E.g. A. Scull. *Decarceration: Community Treatment and the Deviant – a Radical View*. Cambridge: Polity Press, 1984.

17. SANE, *Schizophrenia and Employment: Putting the Lived-Experience of Schizophrenia at the Heart of the Employment Agenda*. 2013, www.sane.org.uk/uploads/schizophrenia_employment_web.pdf (accessed 18 July 2020).

18. DHSS, *Report of the Committee of Inquiry into Allegations of Ill-Treatment of Patients*, p. 80.

19. Ibid., pp. 78–80, 123.

20. British Psychological Society (BPS), Psychology Special Interest Group in the Elderly (PSIGE) Newsletter 1981/82 (Typescript, BPS archives).

21. E. Shorter, *A History of Psychiatry: From the Era of the Asylum to the Age of Prozac*. New York: John Wiley, 1997, pp. 239–67.

22. DHSS, *Report of the Committee of Inquiry into Allegations of Ill-Treatment of Patients*, p. 115.

23. V. Long, 'Heading up a blind alley'? Scottish psychiatric hospitals in the era of deinstitutionalization. *History of Psychiatry* (2017) 28: 115–28.

24. E. Powell, Opening speech. In *Emerging Patterns for the Mental Health Services and the Public: Proceedings of a Conference at Church House Westminster, London on 9th and 10th March 1961*, 5–10. London: National Association for Mental Health, 1961. This speech was subsequently dubbed the 'Water Tower' speech. See also Ministry of Health, *A Hospital Plan for England and Wales*, Cmnd. 1604. London: HMSO, 1962.

25. A. Baker, Hospital Advisory Service. *BMJ* (1972) 15: 176–7.

26.   DHSS, *Report of the Committee of Inquiry into Whittingham Hospital*. Cmnd. 4861. London: HMSO, 1972, p. 40.

27.   J. Wing and G. Brown, *Institutionalisation and Schizophrenia: A Comparative Study of Three Mental Hospitals 1960-1968*. Cambridge: Cambridge University Press, 1970.

28.   J. Turner, R. Hayward, K. Angel et al. The history of mental health services in modern England: Practitioner memories and the direction of future research. *Medical History* (2015) 59: 599–624.

Mental Hospitals, Social Exclusion and Public Scandals

7

Louise Hide

Introduction

On 10 November 1965, a letter appeared in *The Times* newspaper drawing readers' attention to the ill treatment of geriatric patients in certain mental hospitals. The authors, who included members of the House of Lords, the eminent academic Brian Abel-Smith, two senior clerics and the campaigner Barbara Robb, asked readers to send in evidence that would help them to make a case for a national investigation that could give the Ministry of Health more 'effective and humane' control over such hospitals.[1] In response, hundreds of letters poured in. Many detailed appalling conditions and practices in 'geriatric' wards of psychiatric and general hospitals.

Two years later, towards the end of June 1967, a number of these accounts were published in *Sans Everything: A Case to Answer*.[2] In July, a group of student nurses convened at Whittingham Hospital near Preston in Lancashire to voice their concerns regarding inhumane treatment on some wards.[3] One month later, the *News of the World* newspaper exposed allegations of cruel practices and callous conditions which were subsequently revealed to have taken place at Ely Hospital in Cardiff. In late 1968, the police were called to investigate ill treatment of patients by male nurses at Farleigh Hospital in Somerset. While minor local inquiries were held into the allegations published in *Sans Everything*, broadly discrediting them, the inquiries into practices at Ely, Farleigh and Whittingham hospitals were the first in a long run of inquiries to be conducted into NHS psychiatric and 'mental handicap' hospitals, as they were then called, during the late 1960s and 1970s. They revealed a horrifying web of abuses, neglect, corruption and failures of care on certain wards – by no means all – and how they were facilitated by ingrained cultures that permeated socially, professionally and geographically isolated institutions.

This chapter provides an overview of the inquiries that took place into practices and conditions in some psychiatric and mental handicap hospitals, with a focus on the former. It describes the state of institutional care for people diagnosed with mental disorders in the post-war period and outlines the course this initial run of hospital 'scandals' took. It then examines why, when some ward cultures and hospital management practices had remained unchanged over decades, they were raised into public and political awareness at this particular point in time, bringing about changes in long-term care, particularly for older people in England and Wales.

Mental Hospitals in the Post-war Period

Following the Second World War, plans for the social reconstruction of the country, including a major reorganisation of health and social welfare systems, began to be implemented. Most hospitals were nationalised under the newly formed NHS and responsibility for them, including the large county mental and mental handicap hospitals, was passed from local governments to Regional Hospital Boards (RHBs) which were accountable to the Ministry of Health.

After the war, admissions into mental hospitals grew. By 1954, the rambling asylums of England and Wales contained around 154,000 people,[4] 46 per cent of whom had been resident for more than ten years,[5] often living on overcrowded and under-resourced wards. When the psychiatrist David H. Clark joined Fulbourn Hospital in Cambridge in 1953, he described his first visit to the 'back' wards:

> my conductor had to unlock every door; within the wards patients, grey-faced, clad in shapeless, ill-fitting clothes, stood still or moved about aimlessly . . . [In the men's dormitories] . . . chipped enamel chamber pots stood everywhere . . . the smell of urine was strong and there were no personal items of any kind to be seen in the cold rooms . . . there were no curtains on the windows . . . the furniture was massive, deep brown, dingy and battered.

By contrast, the Admission Villas were described as 'sunlit, pleasantly decorated one-storey buildings with an air of brisk purpose'.[6]

Interest in the symbiotic relationship between the environment, the body and the mind grew during the war. The 1946 Constitution of the World Health Organization (WHO) defined 'health' as 'a state of complete physical, mental and social well-being and not merely the absence of disease and infirmity'.[7] Theories around the psychosocial stirred the interest of sociologists and social psychiatrists into the effects of institutional environments on those who lived and worked inside them. Hospitals, including mental hospitals, were run along ingrained militaristic lines which were imposed on both staff and patients as a form of managing and controlling large numbers of people who might be mentally unwell. A strict routine was enforced from the moment patients got up in the morning until going to bed at night, which could be as early as 5 p.m. Personal possessions were often 'removed' on admission, clothing was shared, staff wore uniforms and doctors were referred to as medical 'officers'. Hierarchies were strict. Eric Pryor, who joined Claybury Hospital as a student nurse soon after the end of the war, explained how 'there was no fraternising, either with those above or below one's own rank . . . It was not etiquette for junior staff to speak to Medical Staff, Head Nurses or official visitors unless spoken to.'[8]

In Britain, the concept of 'institutionalisation' emerged into clinical discourse from the 1950s. The deputy physician superintendent at Claybury, Denis V. Martin, remarked in 1955 that terms such as 'becoming institutionalised' or 'well institutionalised' could often be found in clinical notes, meaning that a patient had 'more or less' surrendered to institutional life and was seen by nurses as 'resigned', 'cooperative' and not causing any trouble. The more institutionalised patients became, the more manageable and tractable their behaviour. In Martin's view, some doctors, who might be responsible for up to 300 patients, had a 'vested interest in maintaining the process of institutionalization' because it gave them more time to focus on the patients they found more therapeutically interesting. Yet it was nurses who managed the day-to-day lives of patients and 'ran' the wards. Martin argued that their training 'far more than the doctors' is destructive of individuality'.[9]

Russell Barton, a social psychiatrist and medical superintendent of Severalls Hospital in Essex, suggested that the institution was in itself pathogenic. Patients suffered from two conditions: one for which they were initially admitted and a second caused by the stultifying environment of the hospital resulting in a condition that was 'characterized by apathy, lack of initiative, loss of interest . . . [and] submissiveness'.[10] Perhaps the best-known indictment of the large institutions was *Asylums* (1961) by the Canadian sociologist Erving Goffman. Based on his study of a large mental hospital in Washington, DC, it was an excoriating critique of psychiatric hospitals and their effects on patients. Asylums were, according to Goffman, 'total institutions' which he defined as places of 'residence and work where a large number of like-situated individuals, cut off from the wider society for an appreciable period of time, together lead an enclosed, formally administered round of life'.[11]

Steps were taken to improve institutional life. During the war, a group of doctors, some of whom had been trained in psychotherapy, created more open and egalitarian therapeutic communities to help rehabilitate servicemen. Some of these approaches were subsequently adopted by social psychiatrists such as Clark and Martin to help patients regain a sense of independence and leave hospital. The large mental hospitals began to move away from the old custodial practices and follow guidance from the WHO which stated that the 'life within the hospital should, as far as possible, be modelled on life within the community in which it is set'.[12] Doors were unlocked and spaces were liberalised so that patients could move freely around the buildings and grounds. More therapeutic ward practices based on less rigid hierarchies and routines – nurses no longer wore uniforms and might be called by their first names – were introduced to help patients learn how to live more independently. These measures were bolstered from the mid-1950s by the introduction of new psychotropic drugs, such as chlorpromazine, which could alleviate severe psychotic symptoms. With the right medication and access to treatments such as electroconvulsive therapy (ECT) available in outpatient clinics, hospitalisation was no longer deemed necessary for many people experiencing serious mental health conditions.

New treatments, both biological and psychosocial, were matched by a strengthening political resolve to close the old asylums. In 1961, the Conservative minister of health, Enoch Powell, gave his 'water-tower' speech articulating the government's intention to reduce the number of psychiatric beds by half and to close the large isolated mental hospitals. The 1962 Hospital Plan mapped out how treatment would shift to psychiatric wards in district general hospitals.[13] It also signalled formally the beginning of the deinstitutionalisation process and the move towards care in the community (see also Chapter 31).

Two Standards of Care

Psychiatry's new therapeutic approach was not primarily intended for older, long-term patients who were believed to be suffering from incurable conditions, such as senile dementia, about which nothing could be done. When it came to distributing resources, services for younger people with acute conditions were prioritised over those for people with long-term chronic conditions, creating a two-tier system. Whittingham Hospital, which was the subject of a major inquiry in the early 1970s, is a good case in point. Located in an isolated spot some seven miles outside of Preston in Lancashire, it was a large sprawling institution that had been established in 1873. Some of the buildings had been modernised but the majority were described by the inquiry report as the old 'three-decker wards of 80 beds or more, with large cheerless day-rooms and grossly inadequate sanitary facilities'. In accordance with the government's plan to close the asylums, Whittingham was to be gradually run down until it could be closed. To that end, the number of occupied beds dropped from 3,200 in 1953 to slightly more than 2,000 in 1969.[14] This reduction was achieved through more 'active' psychiatry, when people with 'treatable' conditions were moved from Whittingham to acute psychiatric units. As a result, 86 per cent of inpatients who remained at Whittingham had been in the hospital for longer than two years and a high proportion were old.[15] The chairman of Whittingham's Hospital Management Committee – who was severely criticised in the inquiry – described this group of patients as 'the type who sit around all day just doing nothing but becoming cabbages'.[16]

The 'Scandals'

The depressing environment on some of Whittingham's long-stay wards was not uncommon. Early in 1965, Barbara Robb visited an acquaintance who had been admitted to Friern Hospital in North London. She was horrified by the dismal ward conditions and later described how older female patients in some hospitals were deprived of 'their spectacles, dentures, hearing aids and other civilized necessities' and left 'to vegetate in utter loneliness and idleness'.[17] Within months, Robb established the pressure group AEGIS (Aid for the Elderly in Government Institutions).[18]

Robb was a co-signatory of the letter to *The Times* mentioned in the Introduction to this chapter. In 1967, two years after its publication, she presented on behalf of AEGIS a book titled *Sans Everything: A Case to Answer* which included carefully chosen accounts that had been sent in by nurses and social workers describing heartbreaking cruelty, neglect and suffering on geriatric wards. The book caused a public outcry. The Labour minister of health, Kenneth Robinson, who had ignored Robb's earlier requests to investigate conditions at Friern, ordered the relevant RHBs to investigate the allegations relating to the hospitals in their region. The results of the inquiries were published in a single report.[19] Many of the original allegations were strenuously refuted and described as 'false', 'incomplete and distorted'; one informant was described as a 'highly emotional witness, prone to gross exaggeration'.[20]

Running simultaneously to the publication of *Sans Everything* was the exposure (without naming the hospital or individuals concerned) by the *News of the World* in August 1967 of allegations of patient mistreatment, failures of care and staff 'pilfering' at Ely Hospital in Cardiff, a former Poor Law institution primarily for 'sub-normal' or 'severely sub-normal' patients (see also Chapter 24). A delegation from the Ministry of Health had inspected Ely two years earlier when members had found appalling conditions yet done nothing to address them.[21] Worried about public criticism, the minister instructed the RHB to establish an inquiry into Ely, which was to be led by Geoffrey Howe QC.[22] The way in which the inquiry was set up – the structure of the committee and the terms of reference – was similar to the methods used to investigate the *Sans Everything* allegations. Howe did, however, extend the investigations beyond the events that took place to expose broader structural failings, including weak medical leadership, poor standards of nursing and an inadequate Hospital Management Committee.[23]

On 18 July 1967, just after the publication of *Sans Everything*, a meeting was convened at Whittingham Hospital by the Student Nurses Association which gathered to make a number of serious allegations of inhumane, cruel and even violent treatment of vulnerable older people on certain long-stay wards. Their complaints were consistently suppressed and ignored by the hospital. Two years later, a psychiatrist and a psychologist wrote directly to the Secretary of State alleging 'ill-treatment of patients, fraud and maladministration, including suppression of complaints from student nurses'. An inquiry was launched when allegations of ill treatment were concentrated on four long-stay wards, one of which had been run by the same Sister for forty-seven years.[24]

At Farleigh Hospital in Bristol, concerns about serious mistreatment and violence towards patients emerged at the end of 1968 when the police were called to investigate brutal treatment by male nurses of men with severe mental handicaps. Following judicial proceedings, when three of the nine nurses who had been charged received prison sentences, an inquiry was launched into the administrative systems and conditions of the hospital in order to understand the cultural and systemic mechanisms that had facilitated abuses of care over such a long period of time.

Claire Hilton has rightly argued that it was the publication of *Sans Everything* and the tireless work of Barbara Robb, among others, that triggered widespread revelations of abuses leading to Ely, which was the first inquiry into NHS care to be published in full.[25] The Whittingham Hospital Inquiry (1972) was also significant because, according to the sociologist John Martin, it 'dissected the organization which had allowed maltreatment and pilfering to occur, and which had stubbornly resisted all attempts to change old styles of care'. A socially and professionally isolated environment had been a major factor in allowing practices and customs to persist.[26] At least ten inquiries of national significance, and many other smaller ones, were conducted from the late 1960s and throughout the 1970s.[27]

Given that 'care' on long-term geriatric wards had often been so wretched for so long, and that so many knew about it, why did no one act before and how were such practices allowed to continue?[28] Sociologists Ian Butler and Mark Drakeford have argued that the 'everyday tragedies' that were revealed by the welfare scandals of the 1960s and 1970s are 'where meanings and historical significance become attached to acts and events that at other times might have passed almost unobserved'.[29] Widespread social change was in process, driven in part by human and civil rights campaigns, counterculture movements which challenged the prevailing establishment, including psychiatry (see Chapter 13 and 14), and service-user pressure groups like Mind which demanded greater rights for patients.[30] The isolated and dilapidated former asylums that housed ossified professional and social cultures were anachronistic and belonged to the past. They had to go.

The media played a crucial part in raising public awareness which, in turn, put pressure on the government to act. In addition to the *News of the World*, which had supported AEGIS and *Sans Everything*,[31] and broken the Ely story, *The Lancashire Evening Post* set up a 'press desk' in a local pub to gather information about malpractices at Whittingham Hospital before publishing 'A Big Probe into Allegations of Cruelty' in February 1970.[32] Television took the horrors of overcrowded wards and inhumane treatment into people's living rooms. In 1968, World in Action broadcast *Ward F13*, showing the harrowing conditions in which women were living on a female geriatric ward in Powick Hospital in Worcestershire, while younger patients with acute conditions were being treated in well-resourced facilities in the same hospital. In this case, it was the medical superintendent who had invited the cameras into the hospital so that viewers could see for themselves the inequities of the two-tier system.[33]

Change

As one inquiry after another was held during the 1970s, a pattern of underlying causes that could be attributed to such catastrophic failures of care began to emerge. They included geographical, social and professional isolation; patients with no one to advocate for them; an absence of formal complaints procedures; the privileging of task-centred nursing or other professional interests over the needs of patients; failures of leadership; poor administration and lay management; union intervention; inadequate training; and personal failings.[34] Threaded through these factors were deeply ingrained values and belief systems which had been passed on for years; these included ageism and the commonly held belief that older patients were suffering from inevitable and untreatable cognitive decline, which in many cases was erroneous (see also Chapter 22).

In 1969, the Labour MP Richard Crossman, who had replaced Kenneth Robinson and become the secretary of state for the newly formed Department of Health and Social Services, took over responsibility for hospitals providing long-term care. Crossman had a strong personal and professional interest in bringing about reform and quickly established an independent inspectorate, the Hospital Advisory Service, which was to evaluate and regulate long-stay hospitals.[35] An NHS ombudsman with a remit to introduce an effective complaints process was introduced in 1972.[36] While patient numbers fell, the government allocated more resources to long-stay hospitals. During the 1970s, medical and nursing staff levels rose in both psychiatric and mental handicap hospitals. Conditions were improved and there was some diversification into various sub-specialisms including psychogeriatric medicine.[37] Three important White Papers were produced by the DHSS: *Better Services for the Mentally Handicapped* (1971), *Services for Mental Illness Related to Old Age* (1972) and *Better Services for the Mentally Ill* (1975). The latter framed mental illness as a social as well as a medical issue and set out plans to improve the provision of community care through expanding local authority social services and to move away from institutional care.[38] This process took a decisive turn when a new Conservative government led by Margaret Thatcher came into power in 1979 and opened the provision of care to private, voluntary and independent sectors – often in large houses that were not fit for purpose. The old asylums began to close in the 1980s and valuable sites and buildings were sold, reducing the number of available hospital beds. When local authorities failed to provide suitable accommodation in the community, people who had left hospital were faced with the prospect of having nowhere to go.

Conclusion

This chapter has examined the ways in which 'exclusion' as a social mechanism allowed appalling conditions and practices to persist in mental hospitals over many years, leading to inquiries into the failures of long-term NHS care and subsequent scandals. Geographical remoteness led to professional exclusion as hospitals became increasingly inward-looking and medical and nursing staff lost touch with developments in their respective fields. The inquiries were an important catalyst that helped bring about the closure of the old asylums, many of which had played a central role in the segregation of people who were believed to be mentally unwell or socially 'undesirable' from society. The two-tier system had been active since the late nineteenth century. Embedding it into policy through deinstitutionalisation, from the early 1960s, imposed an additional layer of exclusion upon those who were left behind on the 'back' wards. Those who did leave the institutions could find themselves facing new forms of isolation as facilities in the community could fail to materialise or to provide adequate care.

While long-term care is now provided in smaller, usually privately owned, facilities, abuse, undignified treatment and neglect continue to be seen but unseen, known but unknown. Inquiries may be expensive and repetitive. They may need to be reimagined and reframed to engage with different questions and perspectives. Whatever their shortcomings, they remain vital mechanisms for uncovering harmful practices visited on vulnerable people. They can reassure the public and, crucially, highlight where changes need to be made by individuals and professional groups, as well as by management and policymakers.

Key Summary Points

- Between the late 1960s and early 1980s, at least ten major and many smaller inquiries were held into neglectful, abusive and violent practices in psychiatric and 'mental handicap' hospitals.
- Many institutions, or certain wards inside them, had become professionally isolated and severely under-resourced. Deeply ingrained cultures of harm and neglect had evolved over years.
- Growing interest in the effects of institutional environments on patients contributed to the post-war impetus to move care for acute conditions into the community, leaving long-stay wards more isolated than ever.
- The exposure of harmful practices by the press and campaigners compelled politicians to order inquiries which contributed to changes in the provision of long-term care and the widespread closure of the old Victorian asylums from the 1980s.
- While long-term care is now provided in smaller facilities, abuse, undignified treatment and neglect continue. Inquiries may need to be reimagined and reframed to engage with different questions and perspectives.

Acknowledgements

My thanks to Claire Hilton for her helpful comments.

Notes

1. Strabolgi et al., *The Times*, 10 November 1965; 13.

2. B. Robb, *Sans Everything: A Case to Answer*. London: Thomas Nelson, 1967. This was compiled on behalf of AEGIS.

3. NHS, *Report of the Committee of Inquiry into Whittingham Hospital*, Cmnd. 4861. London: HMSO, 1972.

4. H. Freeman, Psychiatry and the state in Britain. In M. Gijswijt-Hofstra, H. Oosterhuis, J. Vijselaar and H. Freeman, eds, *Psychiatric Cultures Compared: Psychiatric and Mental Health Care in the Twentieth Century: Comparisons and Approaches*, 116–40. Amsterdam: Amsterdam University Press, 2005.

5. J. Turner, R. Hayward, K. Angel et al., The history of mental health services in modern England: Practitioner memories and the direction of future research. *Medical History* (2015) 59(4): 599–624.

6. D. H. Clark, *The Story of a Mental Hospital: Fulbourn 1858–1983*. London: Process Press, 1996, pp. 1–2.

7. World Health Organization (WHO), *Constitution of the World Health Organization*. New York, 22 July 1946. https://apps.who.int/gb/bd/PDF/bd48/basic-documents-48th-edition-en.pdf.

8. E. H. Pryor, *Claybury 1893–1993: A Century of Caring*. London: The Mental Health Care Group, 1993, p. 106.

9. D. V. Martin, Institutionalisation. *The Lancet* (1955) 269: 1188–90.

10. R. Barton, *Institutional Neurosis* (3rd ed.). Bristol: John Wright & Sons, 1976, p. 2. (Originally published in 1959.)

11. E. Goffman, *Asylums: Essays on the Social Situation of Mental Patients and Other Inmates*. London: Penguin, 1991, p. 11. (Originally published in 1961.)

12. WHO, *The Community Mental Hospital: Third Report of the Expert Committee on Mental Health*. Geneva: WHO, 1953, p. 19.

13. Freeman, Psychiatry and the state in Britain.

14. NHS, *Report of the Committee of Inquiry into Whittingham Hospital*.

15. J. P. Martin and Debbie Evans, *Hospitals in Trouble*. Oxford: Basil Blackwell, 1984.

16. NHS, *Report of the Committee of Inquiry into Whittingham Hospital*; 5–6.

17. Robb, *Sans Everything*, p. xiii.

18. C. Hilton, *Improving Psychiatric Care for Older People: Barbara Robb's Campaign 1965–1976*. Cham: Palgrave Macmillan, 2017.

19. For a more detailed account of this process, see C. Hilton, A tale of two inquiries: *Sans Everything* and Ely. *The Political Quarterly* (2019) 90(2): 185–93.

20. NHS, *Findings and Recommendations Following Enquiries into Allegations Concerning the Care of Elderly Patients in Certain Hospitals*, Cmnd 3687. London: HMSO, 1968, pp. 23, 68, 36, 24, 82.

21. Hilton, A tale of two inquiries.

22. Howe later became Margaret Thatcher's longest-serving Cabinet minister, holding the posts of Chancellor of the Exchequer, Foreign Secretary and, finally, Leader of the House of Commons, Deputy Prime Minister and Lord President of the Council.

23. Martin, *Hospitals in Trouble*.

24. NHS, *Report of the Committee of Inquiry into Whittingham Hospital*, pp. 1, 11.

25. Hilton, A tale of two inquiries.

26. Martin, *Hospitals in Trouble*, pp. 9, 17.

27. Ibid., p. xi. In addition to Ely, Farleigh and Whittingham, similar major inquiries were held into Napsbury Hospital (1973), South Ockendon Hospital (1974) and Normansfield Hospital (1978). Dates relate to the publication of reports.

28. N. Stanley and J. Manthorpe, Introduction: The inquiry as Janus. In N. Stanley and J. Manthorpe, eds, *The Age of the Inquiry: Learning and Blaming in Health and Social Care*. London: Routledge, 2004.

29. I. Butler and M. Drakeford, *Scandal, Social Policy and Social Welfare*. Basingstoke: Palgrave Macmillan, 2005, p. 1.

30. Turner, Hayward, Angel et al., The history of mental health services in modern England.

31. Hilton, *Improving Psychiatric Care for Older People*.

32. Butler and Drakeford, *Scandal, Social Policy and Social Welfare*, p. 118.

33. Granada Television, Ward F13, *World in Action* broadcast, 1968.

34. Martin, *Hospitals in Trouble*, chap. 5.

35. P. Bridgen, Hospitals, geriatric medicine, and the long-term care of elderly people 1946–1976. *Social History of Medicine* (2001) 14(3): 507–23.

36. Hilton, *Improving Psychiatric Care for Older People*.

37. Turner, Hayward, Angel et al., The history of mental health services in modern England; Freeman, Psychiatry and the state in Britain.

38. The Health Foundation, '"Better services for the mentally ill" white paper'. The Health Foundation website, https://navigator.health.org.uk/theme/better-services-mentally-ill-white-paper.

Chapter 8

Mental Health Law: 'Legalism' and 'Medicalism' – 'Old' and 'New'

George Szmukler and Lawrence O. Gostin

Introduction

The 1959 Mental Health Act represented, by any standard, a 'paradigm shift' in the way in which mental illness was construed, not just in Britain but anywhere.

Its predecessor was the Lunacy Act of 1890. Kathleen Jones, in her influential *History of the Mental Health Services* characterised that Act thus:

> The Act itself is an extremely long and intricate document, which expresses few general principles and provides detail for almost every known contingency. Nothing was left to chance, and very little to future development.
>
> . . .
>
> From the legal point of view it was nearly perfect … From the medical and social viewpoint, it was to hamper the progress of the mental-health movement for nearly 70 years.[1]

Laws governing detention and treatment in the nineteenth century were developed in the setting of the expanding asylum system. The early enthusiasm for 'moral treatment' failed to live up to its promise. The numbers of those detained in the asylums grew far beyond what was originally envisaged.

Under the Lunacy Act 1890 admission to an asylum or licensed house depended on whether the case was *private* (involving a justice of the peace and two medical certificates) or *pauper* (involving a Poor Law receiving officer or the police, a medical certificate and a justice of the peace).[2]

Admission by inquisition, whose origins dated back to the fourteenth century applied to so-called Chancery lunatics – expensive and affordable only to those with large estates and great wealth. The alleged lunatic could request a trial of their sanity by jury.

There were detailed regimes of visitation by Lunacy Commissioners – unannounced, at an hour, day or night. A report book for instances of mechanical restraint was kept; a medical certificate was necessary for each instance.

Discharge arrangements were complex and could differ for private versus pauper patients. They might involve the person signing the petition for the reception, the authority responsible for the maintenance of the pauper patient, two Lunacy Commissioners – one legal and one medical – or three members of the visiting Local Authority committee.

The Mental Treatment Act 1930 followed a Royal Commission on Lunacy and Mental Disorder 1924–6.[3] It proposed that mental illness should be viewed like any other illness, and its recommendation that treatment should not necessarily be contingent upon certification was accepted. The Lunacy Act was amended but earlier legislation was not replaced. The Act introduced 'voluntary admission' by written application to the person in charge of the hospital. Non-objecting but non-volitional patients, called 'temporary', could be admitted under a non-judicial certificate. An essential condition in the application for reception of a 'temporary' patient was that the person 'is for the time being incapable of expressing (him)(her)self as willing or unwilling to receive such treatment'.[4] For many clinicians, the meaning of this provision lacked clarity, accounting for a huge variation in its use – from 34 per cent to 0 per cent.[5]

Magistrates continued to be involved in overseeing compulsory hospital admissions. The Act authorised local authorities to set up psychiatric outpatient clinics in general and mental hospitals, but the hospital remained the focal point for psychiatric provision.

The Mental Health Act 1959

The Mental Health Act 1959 followed the key recommendation of the Percy Royal Commission, established in 1954, 'that the law should be altered so that whenever possible suitable care may be provided for mentally disordered patients with no more restriction of liberty or legal formality than is applied to people who need care because of other types of illness'.[6]

The Act repealed all previous legislation.[7] Informal admission was now the usual method of admission. For the first time since 1774, there was no judicial authorisation for a compulsory admission. Patients could be admitted to any hospital or mental nursing home without any formalities. This replaced the 'voluntary admission' set down in the Mental Treatment Act of 1930 where the patient signed admission papers. Non-volitional patients could be admitted informally provided that they did not positively object to treatment.

Mental disorder was defined as '*mental illness*; or, *arrested or incomplete development of mind* (i.e. *subnormality or severe subnormality*); or, *psychopathic disorder*; or any other disorder or disability of mind'.

Psychopathic disorder was defined as a persistent disorder resulting in abnormally aggressive or seriously irresponsible conduct and susceptible to medical treatment. Persons were not to be regarded as suffering from a form of mental disorder by reason only of promiscuity or immoral conduct.

There were three kinds of compulsory admission:

Observation order: up to twenty-eight days' duration, made on the written recommendations of two medical practitioners stating that the patient either (1) is suffering from a mental disorder of a nature or degree which warrants his (*sic*) detention under observation for a limited period or (2) that he ought to be detained in the interests of his own health and safety, or with a view to the protection of other persons.

Treatment order: for up to a year, to be signed by two medical practitioners. The grounds were:

(a) The patient must be suffering *from* mental illness or severe subnormality; or from subnormality or psychopathic disorder if he is under the age of twenty-one.

(b) He must suffer from this disorder to an extent which, in the minds of the recommending doctors, warrants detention in hospital for medical treatment; and his detention must be necessary in the interests of his health and safety, or for the protection of other persons.

Emergency order: following an application made by the mental welfare officer or a relative of the patient and backed by one medical recommendation. The patient had to be discharged after three days unless a further medical recommendation had been given satisfying the conditions of a treatment order.

A *Mental Health Review Tribunal* (MHRT) alone took over the previous watchdog functions of the Lunacy Commission (which had later become the Board of Control). Detention could be reviewed at the request of patients or relatives or at the request of the minister of health. The tribunal consisted of an unspecified number of persons: legal members appointed by the Lord Chancellor; medical members appointed by the Lord Chancellor in consultation with the minister; lay members having such experience or knowledge considered suitable by the Lord Chancellor in consultation with the minister.

A patient was discharged by the Responsible Medical Officer (RMO), by the managers of the hospital, by an MHRT, by the patient's nearest relative – though with a possible RMO veto – or, in the case of *subnormality* or *psychopathy*, if the person had reached the age of twenty-five.

Guardianship, which had its origins in mental deficiency legislation and promised a degree of control in the community, could now be applied to those with a mental disorder.

Space does not allow us to discuss provisions for *mentally disordered offenders* in detail. In brief, courts could order admission to a specified hospital or guardianship for patients with a mental disorder of any kind, founded on two medical recommendations. Courts of Assize and Quarter Sessions could place special restrictions on the discharge of such patients. Power to grant leave of absence, to transfer the patient to another hospital or to cancel any restrictions placed on their discharge was reserved to the Home Secretary. Limitations were placed on the appeal of such patients to an MHRT. Those found 'Not guilty by Reason of Insanity' were detained during 'her Majesty's pleasure' by warrant from the Home Secretary. The Mental Health Act 1959 provisions by and large resemble those of today, with a significant change concerning the power of the MHRT in 1982, discussed later. The medical profession was united in its enthusiasm for the new provisions and the status of psychiatrists in the medical sphere was enhanced.

The Context of This Radical Change in Mental Health Law

A new optimism had emerged concerning the effectiveness of psychiatric treatment, with a new expectation that patients would return to their communities following a short admission. Jones talked in terms of 'three revolutions': pharmacological, administrative and legal.[8]

The 'Pharmacological Revolution'

The standing of psychiatry as a medical speciality, based on scientific principles, was boosted with the introduction in the early 1950s of the antipsychotic drug chlorpromazine. Admissions had become shorter and much more likely to be voluntary. The antidepressants, imipramine and iproniazid, were introduced later in the decade. New psychosocial interventions, such as the 'therapeutic community' and 'milieu therapy' looked promising. There was a sense of a 'therapeutic revolution'.

The 'Administrative Revolution'

A 1953 World Health Organization (WHO) report (*Third Report: The Community Mental Hospital*) described new models for mental health services. Combinations of a variety of services were proposed, including 'open door' inpatient units, outpatients, day care, domiciliary care and hostels. Earlier treatment, it claimed, meant fewer admissions; chronic patients could be satisfactorily cared for at home or boarded out. The report significantly influenced the Royal Commission's determinations.

There were other administrative considerations. In 1948, the new National Health Service (NHS) found itself responsible for the management of 100 asylums, each with its own regulations and practices. Their average population was around 1,500 patients. Patients with a 'mental illness or mental deficiency' occupied around 40 per cent of all hospital beds.[9]

The 'Legal Revolution'

Some legal matters were complicated by amendments introduced by the National Health Service (NHS) Act 1946. There was also a welfare state–influenced reimagining of law of this kind, now to be seen as an 'enabling' instrument as opposed to a coercive or constraining one.

Tackling the stigma of mental illness was another theme. There was agreement that stigma was heightened by what was called the 'heaviness of procedure' manifest in the magistrate's order, linking in the public's mind the deprivation of liberty for the purposes of treatment with that for the purposes of punishment.

Unsworth summarised the significance of the 1959 Act as a negation of the assumptions underlying the Lunacy Act:

> The [1959] act injected into mental health law a contrary set of assumptions drawing upon the logic of the view of insanity as analogous to physical disease and upon reorientation from the Victorian institution-centred system to 'community care'. . . . Expert discretion . . . was allowed much freer rein at the expense of formal mechanisms incorporating legal and lay control of decision-making procedures.[10]

A 'pendulum' thus had swung through almost its full trajectory, from what Fennell and others have termed 'legalism' to 'medicalism',[11] a form of paternalism.

A warning was sounded in parliament, however, by Baroness Wootton:

> Perhaps there is a tendency to endow the medical man with some of the attributes that are elsewhere supposed to inhere in the medicine man. The temptation to exalt the medical profession is entirely intelligible . . . but I think it does sometimes place doctors in an invidious position, and sometimes possibly lays them open to the exercise of powers which the public would regard as arbitrary in other connections.[12]

Mental Health Act 1983

Twenty-four years later, a new Mental Health Act was passed.[13] While the general outline of the 1959 Act was preserved, there was a significant swing of the 'pendulum' towards a new form of 'legalism'.

Among the changes introduced in the 1983 Act, the following were notable:

1. For the first time, the idea of consent to treatment, even if the patient was detained, made its appearance in mental health law. A requirement for consent was introduced for certain hazardous or irreversible treatments – psychosurgery and surgically implanted hormones. These now required the patient's consent and approval by a panel of three people, including a psychiatrist, appointed by the Mental Health Act Commission (see

item 4). Further, consultation with two persons professionally involved with the treatment (other than the patient's consultant) was needed. Electroconvulsive therapy (ECT) and the administration of medications for the mental disorder beyond three months required consent or a second opinion if the person could not or did not consent.

2. An expanded role and enhanced training was introduced for 'approved social workers' in respect of a social assessment.
3. Access to review of detention by the MHRT was expanded and now included patients under a 28-day 'assessment' order and automatic review with renewal of a treatment order. Patients became entitled to publicly funded legal representation
4. An oversight body concerning detained patients, the Mental Health Act Commission, was established. It will be recalled that there was no such body under the 1959 Mental Health Act.
5. Patients suffering from 'psychopathic disorder' or 'mental impairment' could only be detained if their behaviour was 'abnormally aggressive or seriously irresponsible' and if treatment was likely to alleviate or prevent a deterioration of their condition (i.e. a 'treatability' criterion').
6. A duty was placed on the District Health Authorities and local social services authorities to provide aftercare services for patients admitted on a treatment order or on some forensic orders.

In these domains, the rights of persons with a mental disorder were thus enhanced.

What Was the Context of These Changes?

In an extended history of mental health services, Jones began her analysis of the post-1959 period thus:

> After the passing of the 1959 Act, it would have been reasonable to expect a period of consolidation and cautious experimentation; but within two years, the whole scene changed. In 1961, a new Minister of Health, Enoch Powell, announced a policy of abolishing mental hospitals, and cutting psychiatric beds by half . . . Opposition to this draconian policy was muted by three new theoretical analyses . . . opposed to mental hospitals for very different reasons.[14]

She was referring to Szasz, Goffman and Foucault. We shall come to them later in this section (see also Chapter 20).

The Ministry of Health's *A Hospital Plan for England and Wales* followed Powell's 'Water Tower speech'. It proposed the restriction of hospital care mainly to the acute sector. Under a 'parity of esteem', this applied to psychiatry just as it did to the rest of medicine. Thus commenced a huge reduction in the number of hospital beds. At the same time, the Department of Health faced increasing fiscal pressures arising from the need to refurbish and maintain decaying public hospitals. The forces leading to the policy of deinstitutionalisation here overlapped with those acting to reduce admissions, including recourse to involuntary hospitalisation. Some noted an 'unnatural alliance' between civil rights advocates on the left, who distrusted the state and psychiatric expertise, and monetarist conservatives, who were concerned with the high institutional costs of mental health care (see also Chapter 31).

Highly publicised scandals involving mental hospitals continued – there were some twenty serious inquiries into maltreatment between 1959 and 1983. Faith in the effectiveness of medication – and in pharmaceutical companies, especially following the thalidomide inquiry – was faltering.

Proposals from some academic authorities that outcomes would improve if treatment were focused in the community rather than in hospitals were welcome to government. Evidence was offered that 'total institutions' like mental hospitals, in which almost every aspect of the resident's life is subservient to the institution's rules, far from being therapeutic, in fact contribute to a dehumanising erosion of personal identity, dependency and disability. Here Goffman's 1961 *Asylums* and Barton's 1959 *Institutional Neurosis* were influential.[15]

Joined to these criticisms was another set of voices denying the legitimacy of the psychiatric enterprise itself. Key figures in this loosely termed 'anti-psychiatry' movement included three psychiatrists – Thomas Szasz, R. D. Laing and David Cooper (see also Chapter 20). Szasz held that 'mental illness' was a 'myth' and had no kinship with 'real' illness; so-called mental illnesses were 'problems of living', not brain diseases.[16] From a rather different perspective, Laing and Cooper argued that insanity was an understandable reaction of some to impossible family pressures or, indeed, a society gone insane.[17] The experience of psychosis, they claimed, handled correctly – as opposed to conventional treatment – could be transformative.

In significant ways congruent with the 'anti-psychiatry' movement were the ideas of Michel Foucault. His *Histoire de la folie*, published in 1961, appeared in a much abridged form in English in 1965 (as *Madness and Civilization*) featuring a polemical introduction by David Cooper.[18] *Madness and Civilization* examined how the notion of 'mental illness' assumed the status of 'positive knowledge' or objectivity and its irreconcilability with society's growing valorisation of 'productive' citizenship. Foucault argued that psychiatrists' expertise lay in asylum-based governance and non-medical practices, such as techniques for the normalisation of certain sorts of socially transgressive behaviours.

Thus, while these figures differed significantly in their theories, they had in common a critique of psychiatry's basic tenets, its social role and the institutions in which these were realised. Their ideas found a place within a broader counterculture movement prominent in the 1960s and 1970s, which helped to bring them to the attention of a wider public.

A further significant influence was the civil rights movement in the United States, increasingly effective in the 1960s and 1970s. Civil rights were progressively asserted for groups subject to discrimination – African Americans, prisoners, women, persons with mental illness and persons with disabilities. An essential instrument was the law; a number of key legal decisions led to changes in institutional practices.

Increasingly publicised abuses of psychiatry in the Soviet Union during the 1970s and early 1980s seemed to point to the fact that, unless involuntary hospitalisation was the subject of special scrutiny, arbitrary detention could follow.

The key player in fostering reform of mental health legislation in the 1970s was the National Association for Mental Health (now Mind). Founded in 1946, it started as a traditional voluntary organisation, a partnership between professionals, relatives and volunteers, aimed at improving services and public understanding. Its character, described by Jones as 'duchesses and twin-set', changed in the 1970s (see also Chapter 14).

The organisation was shaken by a serious, though failed, attempt of a Scientology takeover. A 'consumer' orientation and a focus on human rights followed, marked by the appointment of Tony Smythe as director in 1974. He was previously secretary-general of the

National Council for Civil Liberties (NCCL, later named Liberty). Mind soon established a legal and welfare rights service.

Larry Gostin, co-author of this chapter, an American lawyer and recently a Fulbright Fellow at Oxford, was appointed first legal officer in 1975.[19] Both Gostin and Smythe had worked in the domain of civil liberties in the United States. While legal director for Mind, Gostin wrote *A Human Condition*, essentially Mind's proposals for reforming the Mental Health Act 1959.[20]

He stated:

> The [1959] Act is largely founded upon the judgment of doctors; legal examination has ceased at the barrier of medical expertise, and the liberty of prospective patients is left exclusively under the control of medical judgments which have often been shown in the literature to lack reliability and validity.[21]

Gostin challenged the assumption that compulsory detention automatically allowed for compulsory treatment. He proposed that all treatment to be given to an inpatient who cannot, or does not, give consent should be reviewed by an independent body. He argued for the concept of the 'least restrictive alternative' (which in turn required the provision of a range of alternative services). He also proposed an extended advocacy system.

Gostin took cases to the courts, ranging from the right to vote and consent to treatment to freedom of communication. A particularly successful example was the 1981 case, *X v The United Kingdom*, before the European Court of Human Rights, resulting in a new power for MHRTs to discharge restricted forensic patients. While at Mind, he formed a volunteer lawyers panel to represent patients at MHRT hearings.

Gostin subsequently received the Rosemary Delbridge Memorial Award from the National Consumer Council for the person 'who has most influenced Parliament and government to act for the welfare of society'.

The 1983 Mental Health Act thus marked a swing of the Act's 'pendulum', not especially dramatic, towards 'legalism' (or called by Gostin, 'new legalism'). It differed from Lunacy Act legalism by an accent on the rights of detained patients and their entitlements to mental health care, rather than ensuring that the sane were not mistakenly incarcerated as insane, or the detection of grossly irregular practices.

The newly established Mental Health Act Commission faced a daunting task. In addition to producing a Code of Practice, its oversight function involved up to 728 hospitals and units for mental illness and intellectual disabilities in England and Wales, together with 60 nursing homes which could come under its purview if they housed detained patients.

Mental Health Act 2007: An Amended Mental Health Act 1983

The next Mental Health Act followed thirty-four years later, in 2007.

The reduction in the number of mental health beds continued apace – England saw an 80 per cent reduction between 1959 and 2006. An argument grew in the 1980s that, as the locus of psychiatric treatment was increasingly in the community, so should be the option of involuntary treatment. Early moves in this direction were the 'long leash' – the creative use of 'extended leave' (ruled unlawful in 1985), the introduction of non-statutory Supervision Registers in 1994 and then the passing of the Mental Health (Patients in the Community) Act in 1995. This introduced Supervised Discharge, also known as 'aftercare under supervision'. This could require a patient to reside at a specified place and to attend places for medical treatment or training. Administration of treatment could not be forced in the community but the patient could be conveyed to hospital, by force if necessary, for persuasion or admission.

The 1990s saw a new turn – a growing public anxiety that mental health services were failing to control patients, now in the community and no longer apparently safely detained in hospitals, who presented a risk, especially to others (see also Chapter 28). The 1983 Act was labelled obsolete – as, for example, in a highly publicised publication, the *Falling Shadow* report, following the investigation of a homicide by a mental patient.[22]

A 'root and branch' review of the Mental Health Act 1983 was initiated by the government in 1998. Its purpose, as announced by the then Secretary of State for Health, Frank Dobson, was 'to ensure that patients who might otherwise be a danger to themselves and others are no longer allowed to refuse to comply with the treatment they need. We will also be changing the law to permit the detention of a small group of people who have not committed a crime but whose untreatable psychiatric disorder makes them dangerous.'

This led to what Rowena Daw, chair of the Mental Health Alliance, a coalition of more than seventy professional organisations and interest groups, called a seven-year 'tortured history' of 'ideological warfare' between the government and virtually all stakeholder groups.[23] The Mental Health Alliance was a unique development. Created in 1999, it incorporated key organisations representing psychiatrists, service users, social workers, nurses, psychologists, lawyers, voluntary associations, charities, religious organisations, research bodies and carers (see also Chapter 28).

Initially, a government-appointed Expert Committee chaired by Professor Genevra Richardson produced generally well-received recommendations founded on the principles of non-discrimination towards people with a mental illness, respect for their autonomy and their right to care and treatment. An impaired 'decision-making capacity' criterion was proposed, only to be overridden in cases of a 'substantial risk of serious harm to the health or safety of the patient or other persons', and there are 'positive clinical measures which are likely to prevent a deterioration or to secure an improvement in the patient's mental condition'.

However, as Daw notes:

> Government, on the other hand, had different priorities. It was driven by its wish to give flexibility in delivery of mental health services through compulsory treatment in the community; and its fear of 'loopholes' through which otherwise treatable patients might slip. In its general approach, the government followed a populist agenda fuelled by homicide inquiries into the deaths caused by mental health patients. Public concern and media frenzy went hand in hand to demand better public protection. ... The then Health Minister Rosie Winterton MP stated that 'every barrier that is put in the way of getting treatment to people with serious mental health problems puts both patients and public at risk'.[24]

A 'torrid passage' (Daw's words) of Bills through parliament involved two rejections, in 2002 and 2004, and finally, in 2007, an amending Act to the 1983 Mental Health Act was passed.[25]

Fanning has detailed the role of the containment of 'risk' in the generation of the 2007 Act.[26] He notes a swing back from 'legalism' to a new form of 'medicalism' – or 'new medicalism'. He explains:

The 1959 Act's medicalism . . . trusted mental health practitioners to take decisions for and on behalf of their patients according to clinical need. By contrast, the 2007 Act's 'New Medicalism' expands practitioners' discretion in order to enhance the mental health service's responsiveness to risk. This subtle shift in focus introduces a covert political dimension to mental health decision-making . . . the 2007 Act's brand of medicalism follows an inverted set of priorities to those pursued in the 1959 Act.[27]

Fanning examines a link to the characterisation of contemporary society, for example, by Beck and Giddens, as a 'risk society' – one preoccupied with anticipating and avoiding potentially catastrophic hazards that are a by-product of technological, scientific and cultural advances (see also Chapters 10 and 17). 'Risk' replaces 'need' as a core principle of social policy. It also leads to a culture of blame if adverse events should occur. Foucault's notion of 'governmentality' also enters Fanning's account – risk here offering an acceptable warrant for governmental disciplinary measures.

Another factor was the claim – disputed by a number of authorities – that risk assessment instruments had now achieved an acceptable degree of scientific precision as valid predictors of serious violent acts by persons with a mental disorder. The evidence is that risk assessment instruments for low frequency events, such as a homicide, result in a large preponderance of 'false positives' (see also Chapter 10).[28]

However, there is a problem with 'risk', Fanning argues. It is unclear what it really means. He claims:

Within reason, anything practitioners recast as evidence of a threat to the patient's health or safety or to others is enough to justify the deployment of the compulsory powers . . . Consequently, it undermines legal certainty and impairs the law's ability to defend patients' interests.[29]

The 2007 Act increased professional discretion on the role of risk by:

- simplifying and arguably broadening the definition of 'mental disorder';
- abolishing the 'treatability test' for psychopathy, requiring only that treatment be 'appropriate' – previously the treatment had to be 'likely' to be effective, now that must be its 'purpose';
- broadening the range of professionals able to engage the compulsory powers, by replacing the role of the 'approved social worker' with an 'approved mental health professional', who could be a psychologist, psychiatric nurse or occupational therapist. This reduced the separation of powers that existed between those with clinical and social perspectives; and
- introducing Supervised Community Treatment (or Community Treatment Orders, CTOs), effectively strengthening supervision after discharge by the imposition of a broad range of conditions. A failure to comply with the treatment plan may result in recall to hospital; and if treatment cannot be reinstituted successfully within seventy-two hours, the CTO may be revoked with reinstatement of the inpatient compulsory order. The patient may appeal against the CTO but not the conditions.

The reforms represented a substantial shift away from a focus on individual rights and towards public protection. An exception was a strengthening of the need for consent for ECT in a patient with decision-making capacity (except where it is immediately necessary either to save the person's life or to prevent a serious deterioration of their condition) and a right to advocacy (by an 'Independent Mental Health Advocate') for detained patients and those on a CTO.

Fanning goes on to claim that the 'new medicalism' maintains a 'residual legalism' in the amended Mental Health Act, which:

> arguably has a sanitising effect by conferring a veneer of legitimacy on 'sectioning' processes which may now be less certain, less predictable and primarily motivated by concern for public safety ... Far from being a minor statute which changes very little, the 2007 Act represents an entirely new moment in English mental health law and policy.[30]

At the same time as deliberations were in progress over reform to the Mental Health Act, parliament was passing the Mental Capacity Act 2005 in which the involuntary treatment of patients in general medicine and surgery was to be based on an entirely different set of principles – 'decision-making capacity' and 'best interests'.

Post-2007 Developments

Two drivers of reform garnered significant support during the first decade of the twenty-first century. The first was the proposal for capacity-based law or a more radical version, known as a 'fusion law'; the second was the adoption by the United Nations (UN) in 2006 of the Convention on the Rights of Persons with Disabilities (CRPD). Both aim at the elimination of unfair discrimination against people with a mental disorder.

A 'fusion law' refers to a single, generic law applicable to all persons who have an impairment in the ability to make treatment decisions, whether the cause be a 'mental disorder' or a 'physical disorder'.[31] It combines the strengths of the Mental Capacity Act 2005 – that is, a respect for autonomy, self-determination and the right to refuse treatment, almost entirely absent in the Mental Health Act – with the detailed regulation of involuntary detention and treatment – its authorisation, by whom, where, for how long, review and appeal mechanisms, all well specified in conventional mental health legislation but absent from the Mental Capacity Act. Involuntary treatment is restricted to those who lack 'decision-making capacity' and where it is in the person's 'best interests'. Northern Ireland passed such an Act in 2016 following the path-breaking Bamford Report of 2007.

The UN CRPD presents a huge challenge to conventional psychiatric practice. A number of authorities, including the UN CRPD Committee established by the UN to oversee the convention, holds that any 'substitute decision-making' (except perhaps by a proxy appointed by the person with a disability, and who will respect the person's 'will and preferences') is a violation of the CRPD. Thus, treatment against the objection of a patient is prohibited. It remains to be seen how the consequent debate with the many critics of this interpretation will play out.[32]

Scotland and Northern Ireland

Space permits only a brief account of the salient features of Scotland's legislation. Until 2003, Scottish mental health law was by and large similar to that of England and Wales (though it did retain in its 1960 Mental Health Act an oversight body – the Mental Welfare Commission and a role in compulsory admissions for a Sheriff). However, the Mental Health (Care and Treatment) (Scotland) Act 2003 marked a substantial departure:

- the principle of autonomy is prominent;
- it stipulates ten Guiding Principles (with no reference to risk or public safety);
- patients must be treatable if compulsion is to be used;
- while a criterion of risk to self or others is retained, an additional criterion must be met – a 'clinically significant impairment of treatment decision-making ability';
- compulsory treatment orders, inpatient or in the community, must be authorised by a Mental Health Tribunal;
- there is a right to independent advocacy;
- there is a special recognition of advance statements – a failure to respect the person's wishes needs written justification, which must be reported to the patient, a person named by the patient, a welfare attorney (if there is one) and the Mental Welfare Commission; and
- there is a choice of a named person rather than the nearest relative.

Few would deny that this law is far more rights-based than that in England and Wales. As mentioned in the section 'Post-2007 Developments', Northern Ireland has taken reform even further, having passed a 'fusion law'.

European Convention on Human Rights (Human Rights Act 1998)

It is beyond the scope of this chapter to give more than a brief reference to the influence on UK mental health law of the European Convention on Human Rights – later the Human Rights Act (1998). In 2007, Baroness Hale, then a member of the Appellate Committee of the House of Lords, summarised the impact as modest.[33] An exception was the 'Bournewood' case concerning a man (HL) with autism who was admitted to a hospital as an informal patient, and although he did not, or could not, object, it was apparent that he would not be allowed to leave if he were to wish to do so. His carers, denied access to him, initiated a legal action that he was being detained unlawfully. This progressed with appeals through the English court system up to the House of Lords in 1998, who decided HL's admission was lawful. His carers then took the case to the European Court of Human Rights, who, in 2004, ruled it was unlawful. This resulted in the Mental Health Act 2007 appending Schedules to the Mental Capacity Act establishing 'Deprivation of Liberty Safeguards' covering non-objecting hospital inpatients or care home residents who lacked decision-making capacity and, in their best interests, were not allowed to leave.[34]

Service User Movement

Similarly, limitations in scope only allow a brief consideration of the influence of service user organisations on changes in mental health law (see also Chapters 13 and 14). Service users had little direct involvement in the development of the 1983 Mental Health Act. While patient groups did form in the 1970s, the service user voice was not significantly heard until the mid-1980s.[35] It was reasonably prominent in the debate leading to the 2007 Act, and the major service user organisations joined the Mental Health Alliance. Within or outwith the Alliance, however, their voice was largely ignored by government.

Conclusion

We have traced the course of mental health legislation from 1959 to 2010. The broad sweep of the changes can be summarised schematically, allowing for a degree of simplification. We have adapted the idea from Fanning of locating each law within a space created by two orthogonal dimensions (Figure 8.1).[36] While Fanning finally did not support the schema, we propose that by reconceptualising the dimensions, it proves useful. The first dimension has at its poles 'legalism' versus 'clinical discretion' (or 'medicalism'). The second has a 'respect for autonomy' (or emphasis on decision-making capacity' and 'consent to treatment') versus 'protection from harm' (especially to others) dimension. The movements in this 'legal–clinical–social' space from the 1890 Act to the 1959 Act, then to the 1983 Act and the 2007 Act can be traced. The Richardson Committee's 1999 recommendations and the 2003 Scotland Act are also shown, as are the major directions taken in the first decade of the twenty-first century – the Northern Ireland 'fusion law' as well as the UN CRPD Committee's interpretation of the Convention (the claim that 'substitute decision-making' is to be abolished means that it is located at the top-right extreme or perhaps falls outside the space altogether).

It is pertinent to ask what has happened to the number of involuntary admissions over the period covered? In England, they declined steadily between 1966 and 1984, rose quite sharply and steadily until 2000 and then remained flat until 2010. The numbers then rose very sharply again (Figure 8.2). The contribution of changes in mental health legislation is difficult to determine. There were increases in involuntary admissions after both the 1983 and the 2007 Acts but other socio-political and administrative changes also occurred. Perhaps the most interesting observation is the stable rate between 2000 and 2008. This

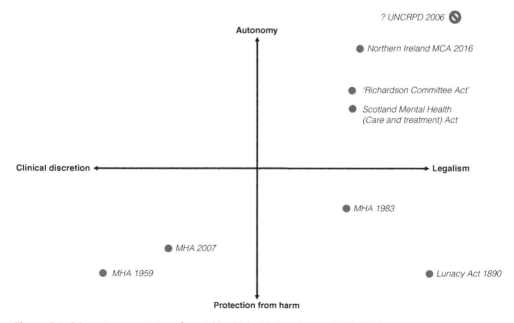

Figure 8.1 Schematic presentation of mental health legislation changes, 1890–2016

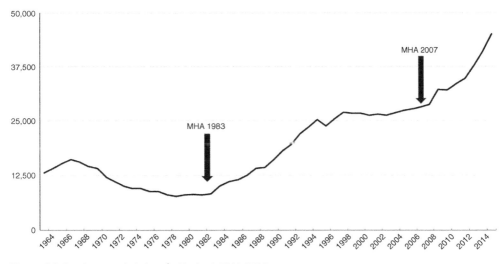

Figure 8.2 Involuntary admissions for England, 1964–2014

period was characterised by a substantial investment in community mental health services, suggesting that resources are a major determinant of the rate of involuntary admissions. Consistent with a resources contribution is the steep rise from 2009, a period of austerity.

Gostin observed that there is perhaps no other body of law which has undergone as many fundamental changes in approach and philosophy as mental health law.[37] We have seen that such law reflects shifts – in Jones's words, 'good, bad or merely muddled' – in social responses and values to an enduring and troubling set of human problems.[38] We agree with Fennell that, while such laws often may not obviously greatly affect substantive outcomes, they are important, if for no other reason, than they require professionals – and we would add the state and civil society – to reflect on, explain and justify what is being done.[39]

Key Summary Points

- The 1959 Mental Health Act represented, by any standard, a 'paradigm shift' in the way in which mental illness was construed, not just in Britain but anywhere. 'Legalism' of the 1890 Lunacy Act was replaced by 'medicalism'.
- While the general outline of the 1959 Act was preserved in the 1983 Mental Health Act, there was a significant swing of the 'pendulum' towards a new 'legalism'.
- Significant influences were the successes of the civil rights movement in the United States in the 1960s and 1970s that progressively asserted rights for groups subject to discrimination and the establishment of a legal and welfare rights service by the National Association for Mental Health (Mind).
- An argument grew in the 1980s that, as the locus of psychiatric treatment was increasingly in the community, so should be the option of involuntary treatment. The Mental Health Act 2007 represented a substantial shift away from a focus on individual rights and towards public protection.
- Two drivers of reform garnered significant support during the first decade of the twenty-first century. The first was the proposal for capacity-based law or a more radical version,

known as a 'fusion law'; the second was the adoption by the UN in 2006 of the Convention on the Rights of Persons with Disabilities (CRPD). Both aim at the elimination of unfair discrimination against people with a mental disorder.

- Changes in mental health law are traced within a space formed by two key dimensions: 'clinical discretion' versus 'legalism and 'autonomy' versus 'protection from harm'.

Notes

1. K. Jones, *A History of the Mental Health Services*. London: Routledge & Kegan Paul, 1972, pp. 176, 181.

2. Lunacy Act 1890, 53 Vict., c. 5.

3. Mental Treatment Act 1930, 20 and 21 Geo. V, c. 23.

4. Jones, *History of the Mental Health Services*.

5. S. Clarke, Mental Treatment Act 1930: Temporary patients. *British Medical Journal* (1933) 2(3793): 543.

6. *Report of the Royal Commission on the Law Relating to Mental Illness and Mental Deficiency 1954–1957*, HM Stationery Office, Cmnd 169, 1957.

7. Mental Health Act 1959, 7 & 8 Eliz. II, c. 72.

8. Jones, *History of the Mental Health Services*.

9. M. Gould, Mental health history: Taking over the asylum. *Health Services Journal* (May 2008) 1: 22–4.

10. C. Unsworth, *Mental Health Legislation*. Oxford: Oxford University Press, 1987, p. 231.

11. P. Fennell, Law and psychiatry: The legal constitution of the psychiatric system. *Journal of Law and Society* (1986) 13: 35–65.

12. Hansard, 217, June 1959.

13. Metal Health Act 1983, c. 20.

14. K. Jones, *Asylums and After: A Revised History of the Mental Health Services from the Early 18th Century to the 1990s*. London: Athlone Press, 1993, p. 159.

15. E. Goffman, *Asylums: Essays on the Social Situation of Mental Patients and Other Inmates*. New York: Doubleday, 1961; R. Barton, *Institutional Neurosis*. Bristol: John Wright & Sons, 1959.

16. T. S. Szasz, The myth of mental illness: Foundations of a theory of personal conduct. *American Psychologist* (1960) 15: 113–18.

17. R. D. Laing and A. Esterson, *Sanity, Madness and the Family*. London: Penguin, 1964; D. Cooper, *Psychiatry and Anti-Psychiatry*. London: Tavistock 1967. (Reprinted in 2001 by Routledge.)

18. M. Foucault, *Folie et déraison: Histoire de la folie à l'âge classique*. Paris: Plon, 1961. (Abridged and translated into English as *Madness and Civilization: A History of Insanity in the Age of Reason*, London: Tavistock, 1965.)

19. L. O. Gostin, From a civil libertarian to a sanitarian. *Journal of Law and Society* (2007) 34: 594–616.

20. L. O. Gostin, *A Human Condition: The Mental Health Act from 1959 to 1975: Observations, Analysis and Proposals for Reform*, Vol. 1. London: Mind, 1975.

21. Ibid., p. 35.

22. L. Blom-Cooper, *The Falling Shadow: One Patient's Mental Health Care, 1978–93*. London: Bloomsbury, 1995.

23. R. Daw, The Mental Health Act 2007: The defeat of an ideal. *Journal of Mental Health Law* (2007) 16: 131–48.

24. Ibid., p. 132.

25. Mental Health Act 2007, c. 12. An Act to amend the Mental Health Act 1983.

26. J. Fanning, Risk and the Mental Health Act 2007: Jeopardising liberty, facilitating control? PhD thesis, University of Liverpool, 2013; J. Fanning, *New Medicalism and the Mental Health Act*. Oxford: Hart Publishing, 2018.

27. Fanning, Risk and the Mental Health Act 2007, p. 61.

28. G. Szmukler, *Men in White Coats: Treatment under Coercion*. Oxford: Oxford University Press, 2018.

29. Fanning, Risk and the Mental Health Act 2007, p. 178.

30. Fanning, *New Medicalism*, p. 127.

31. J. Dawson and G. Szmukler, Fusion of mental health and incapacity legislation. *British Journal of Psychiatry* (2006) 188: 504–9; Szmukler, *Men in White Coats*.

32. G. Szmukler, 'Capacity', 'best interests', 'will and preferences' and the UN Convention on the Rights of Persons with Disabilities. *World Psychiatry* (2019) 18: 34–41.

33. B. Hale, The Human Rights Act and Mental Health Law: Has it helped? *Journal of Mental Health Law* (2007) 15: 7–18.

34. N. Allen, The Bournewood Gap (as amended?). *Medical Law Review* (2010) 18: 78–85.

35. P. Campbell, From little acorns: The mental health service user movement. In A. Bell and P. Lindley, eds, *Beyond the Water Towers*, 73–82. London: Sainsbury Centre for Mental Health, 2005.

36. Fanning, Risk and the Mental Health Act 2007.

37. L. O. Gostin, Contemporary social historical perspectives on mental health reform. *Journal of Law and Society* (1983) 10: 47–70.

38. Jones, *History of the Mental Health Services*, p. 352.

39. Fennell, Law and psychiatry.

Ken Clarke in Conversation with Peter Tyrer: My Role in Justice and Health

Peter Tyrer

Introduction

This interview was carried out with Ken Clarke on 24 September 2019 at the House of Commons. It was transcribed and subsequently edited by Ken and this text is placed in italics. The remainder of the text is written by Peter Tyrer.

Early Background

Ken Clarke and I were at the same Cambridge College, Gonville and Caius College, between 1959 and 1962. In the first year, we were in adjacent blocks in Tree Court, a square that is now deprived of trees but still has marvellous wisterias on the walls. Our paths hardly ever crossed. Ken soon became very involved in university politics and I was too preoccupied in organising a botanical expedition to Central Africa. Ken was attracted to Labour at first – his grandfather was a Communist – but then quickly changed to another party whose nature all now know. He was offered his place at Caius before being offered an Exhibition at Oxford University, which he turned down as he felt they were too pompous. Some jokers have suggested this was the reason Ken never became prime minister, as eleven of the last fourteen occupants of the position went to Oxford. The last to be educated at Cambridge was Stanley Baldwin.

The only other point of note that struck me when Ken was at Cambridge was his accent. He came from Langley Mill, a village that is in the middle of D. H. Lawrence country. Although he won a scholarship to Nottingham High School, very eminent in the Midlands, he must have had a fair dose of the typical and not unpleasant local accent and would have understood that 'silin' dahn in Stabbo' meant it was raining very hard in Stapleford (also near the Derbyshire border). He got on very well with the local miners, including those who had known D. H. Lawrence's father. Ken's father's associates did not think much of D. H. Lawrence, who they felt had got above himself by going away and 'writing mucky stories', so this gives you an idea of Ken's social milieu.

By the time he went to Cambridge, however, he was determined to become an MP and his accent had to change (remember this was 1959). He developed a Bertie Wooster-ish lad-di-dah accent with exaggerated rounded diphthongs, but this quickly changed into the voice everyone now knows. Ken is the only politician to be described as 'blokeish', a term impossible to define, but I think it really describes his voice. He doesn't talk down to people in any way and, even when disagreeing strongly, he retains the 'I'm just an ordinary chap trying to get my point over' that never sounds offensive. Mrs Thatcher had to have elocution lessons but from his early time in politics Ken never needed them.

The main point of describing this background is to show Ken is not your ordinary politician. He achieved almost all the top positions of state – failing to be elected leader of the Conservative Party on three occasions – and could be regarded overall as highly successful, through dint of great intelligence and very hard work. He was constantly amazed at how lazy and ill-informed so many of his colleagues were.

Consistency

The other thing that is important to emphasise in understanding Ken Clarke is his consistency. It is often said that politicians have to bend in the wind or be toppled, but Ken was an exception. Once he had come to a view, he held on to it unless there was compelling evidence otherwise. The main reason I suspect why he was not elected leader of the Conservative Party was his belief that the UK should be an intrinsic part of the European Community. Unlike many other politicians who changed their views greatly over the years, Ken stuck to his opinion and, if anything, has stressed it even more strongly in these Brexit years.

In his personal life, he has been equally consistent. He was married to Gillian, whom he met as an undergraduate when at Caius, for more than fifty years. She died in 2015 from cancer, and one of her last acts was to vote for her husband in the 2015 General Election. She was an absolute rock to him, especially in his early political years when he commuted between Nottingham and London almost daily.

He is even consistent in his support of football teams. He supports both Notts County and Nottingham Forest and tries to see one of them every Saturday (they play at home alternately); he has kept loyal to both. Even though Notts County has drifted down the leagues and is in danger of going into liquidation, while Nottingham Forest soared to great heights in the 1970s and won the European Cup twice, he has stuck with both teams.

Good Humour and Unflappability

In his memoir, *Kind of Blue*,[1] beautifully reflecting both his love of jazz and his semi-detached connection with the Conservative Party, Ken several times refers to the very true perception that 'I was so laid back I was almost horizontal'. He is not wounded by criticism – his wife was and tried to defend him – but he regards it as useful ammunition for his rejoinders, which are often very witty. His negotiations with the British Medical Association (BMA) over a new contract and negotiations for an internal market involved the chairman, Anthony Grabham,[2] and Ken used to point out his name repeatedly to illustrate that doctors were only interested in their wallets. Yet he also agreed that the BMA, in the end, had won the public relations battle over the new contract, and in my interview with him he conceded that the BMA was the union that he felt was more formidable than any other trade union because it could use the public as its main ally (see also Chapter 28).

Relevance of These Characteristics to Negotiations in Mental Health

I do not share the political views of Ken Clarke and it is equally possible to describe him as a highly intelligent but blinkered politician who has always seen the world through a kind of blue lens. Yet, in the interview, I conducted with him he was absolutely straight. 'Go ahead, start your recording, ask me anything you want.' I have to praise that in a politician. The changes he made to the transcript were very small, essentially typographical errors and improvement of clumsy expressions; and never once did he say 'I've changed my mind over that now' – consistency or stubbornness, you decide.

Ken was also highly regarded as a constituency MP. He represented the parliamentary constituency of Rushcliffe to the east of Nottingham for forty-nine years and improved the lot of his constituents greatly over that time. (I know, as I look over with envy from where I live in the adjacent constituency of Newark, which has been much less successful in gaining funding and new initiatives.) This constituency includes Saxondale Hospital, the former county mental hospital of Nottinghamshire, and Ken was aware of its assets and its failings. What he found most disturbing when Saxondale Hospital was destined to close was what he thought was sound evidence that some of the county dignitaries had managed to place their difficult and embarrassing relatives in the hospital for no good reason and that they had languished there for years.

My Interview

I was far from clear that I would be allowed to tape the interview with Ken when I saw him and only had a few notes jotted down. I was also limited by time. I saw him in Portcullis House, the new base for politicians opposite Big Ben, and he had to return to the House of Commons for a vote on the same evening. I apologise for any important omissions.

Q. Why did you introduce NHS Trusts?

One of the things I was concerned about when I became Secretary of State was to try and make the service much more accountable to its patients, and to stop it being so borne down by bureaucracy and dominated by industrial relations problems. The whole point of the purchaser/provider divide was to make sure what money was being spent on locally and to spend that money on the best outcomes for patients, the service and others in that locality. The service was for the locality, a strikingly novel idea that caused a lot of controversy. I had to reform the awful way in which the service was managed, with the responsibility diffusing out from the centre, not very effectively, saying how the service should be run in the rest of the country. We needed a better way of doing things. The idea of Trusts was to give more autonomy to the local users of services so they could answer for their perform-ances to their local public.

I intended to pass responsibility downwards from oversized headquarters in London and secure accountability upwards so the general public could see where decisions were made. This led to some interesting battles over the next three years but it generally went well.

Q. Was there ever a real risk that the John Moore proposal to have an insurance-based replacement for the NHS was likely to happen?[3]

There definitely was. If John Moore had not become unwell, the proposal would have gone ahead as Margaret Thatcher and John were quite agreed that this was precisely what they were going to do. She was convinced the American system was much superior to our own, with a system of personal insurance and the state paying the insurance premiums for those who could not afford it. When I became Secretary of State I quickly became aware that I was expected to take over the implementation of this policy.

But I quickly came round to the view that this was quite unacceptable. Nigel Lawson helped me by resisting Margaret Thatcher's urgings,[4] that those who paid these premiums could get tax relief on their private health insurance contributions. It took me many long meetings to persuade her (Margaret did listen to argument) to abandon her scheme, returning to mine that at least had a degree of market-related responsibility with a purchaser/provider split making sure that there was some fiscal discipline.

Before the purchaser/provider discussions nobody really knew that the NHS was spending its money on, and the idea that the money given might be linked to the outcomes was never contemplated. One trouble was that patients did not belong to any trade unions so their views about what was needed were never heard.

I never pretended I was introducing the final model for the National Health Service. I was wanting to change direction by putting in a framework that could be developed in the future. To some extent this has been achieved but now Simon Stevens of NHS England has developed the idea of integrating hospital and community care diluting the purchaser/ provider approach.[5]

Q. You mention in your memoirs that the BMA was the most difficult trade union you ever had to negotiate with. You were not very complimentary about the medical profession generally. Apart from Donald Acheson (then the Chief Medical Officer of Health), who you admired but who was not really part of the system, was there anyone in the BMA who you looked to for guidance and help?

Not really. Well the BMA was a trade union, even though at times they pretended not to be, with all sorts of high-minded statements for the general public, but basically, like all trade unions, they were always concerned about pay and conditions for their members. When I first arrived I was always advised I had to make concessions to the BMA. When I met Tony Grabham (muffled laughter about the significance of his surname) he tried to frighten me, telling me that all the previous Secretaries of State he had to deal with had all folded under the strain and that in the case of Barbara Castle he had reduced her to tears. But I wasn't going to buckle under this even when they got nasty and went public with advertisements pillorying me.[6]

Q. Do you think doctors were treated too generously in the pay decisions of 2004?

Yes it was generous. And the government at the time, like almost all governments, was trying to buy popularity. Of course, as you know, the doctors have always been regarded as a special case. When Aneurin Bevan said you had to stuff their mouths with gold he set the scene for the future. When the new contracts set reduced hours for much of their work for more pay most were rather surprised as they were going to be paid more for doing less.

Q. Was the Conservative government involved in any way with the introduction of the Dangerous and Severe Personality Disorder Programme (DSPD) introduced by the Labour Government in 1999?

I have no recollection that at any time we were considering such a programme. I think you have to give the responsibility to the Labour government. The trouble is with policies like this is that you now have this semi-presidential system where everyone listens to advisers and so when public opinion gets sufficiently animated new policies are introduced without ever having been thought through.[7]

Q. What are your views about the Private Finance Initiatives (PFIs)?

We introduced the idea of Private Finance Initiatives in the 1992–7 government but very few took them on as the Labour Party said they would abolish them if they came to power. When of course they were elected they immediately started to introduce them. They have unfairly been given a very bad name. This is mainly because of the appalling incompetence of the people who negotiated these contracts, with payments that extended far beyond completion of the project. In the end they turned out to be more expensive than public financing. At the time there was this obsession over keeping to targets for the public finances. Gordon Brown was saying continuously in the first two to three years about how prudent he was going to be as Chancellor.[8] *But the government was not bothered about anything that was not on the books, so the PFIs were not down anywhere amongst the figures, so the government's reputation for fiscal prudence could not be damaged in any way. My only explanation why the health authorities were allowed to go mad on PFI contracts was that the responsibility for the payments would pass on to a Minister appointed many years into the future.*

Q. Can I give you the example of one Trust close to me, Sherwood Forest Hospitals Foundation Trust, where the final bill for the new hospital is going to be more than thirty times the value of the initial cost. How could this happen?'

The problem was that the Trust people had no experience of any kind to negotiate the cost of such complex deals, so the people from these private organisations who negotiated these deals could not believe their luck, and took them to the cleaners. So the argument was quite simple. 'If you want your new hospital you can have it now. The payment for it will be made by someone else down the road, so don't worry.' So a sensible policy, well thought out and prudently applied at first, was quite discredited. Even in the early days when I was trying to get PFI going my approach was to say to each private financier that they could only get a return on their investment if they accepted a proportion of the risk.

The trouble was that the structure of these negotiations was quite unsuitable for the right contracts. People were appointed in the NHS with no experience, often on short-term contracts so they knew they would not have to pick up the flak down the line. So, in the Department of Health headquarters, we had some bright spark, hoping to make his way up the ladder, negotiating with British Oxygen's finest, knowing absolutely nothing about the oxygen market. So, as you can imagine, the results were very satisfactory for British Oxygen.

Q. Do you think there is a political solution to the imbalance in the funding of the NHS where a large proportion of the funding is going to elderly people like you and me, just to give them a few extra years of life, not always ideal ones, when it should be going to younger people with their lives ahead of them, including a large proportion with mental health problems?

The reason why we have not been able to reverse this trend is that the people in the mental health system do not have a voice. I recognised this when I became Secretary of State and had to close down these Victorian institutions like Saxondale Hospital in my constituency, where people had been kept for years with no voice and no influence. These old 'asylums' were absolutely shocking places so it was perfectly sensible to introduce this policy of care in the community, provided it was integrated with hospital care by psychiatrists and others in a coherent way.

The trouble is that care in the community was extremely unpopular. People noticed that suddenly there were strange people out in the street loitering by traffic lights and felt that they ought to be locked away somewhere like Mapperley or Saxondale (if they were in Nottingham),[9] and not being allowed to roam the streets.

The public believe that whenever there is extra money in the health service it ought to be spent on cancer patients or children, not on mental health, and populist Secretaries of State in populist governments accede to these requests, especially on cancer, a subject that terrifies the public so they feel if we spend more it might go away.

A more careful and balanced approach is possible but it does require a well-argued political defence. I separate that from the other problem you are touching on, which is the demographic one, the changing proportion of old and young people in society. The reason why there is an inexorable rising demand is the increasing age of the population that is creating a crisis in our health care system. We are going to have to find some way of meeting this demand. The burden of taxation is going to be spent increasingly on looking after the care of the elderly people and this is going to become unbalanced.

The big change is that so many people in their older years are going to need extra care. It is an extremely tricky political problem that has not been properly faced.

Q. But there has been an inter-Party group discussing this over some years. Is there any way in which this issue might be taken out of politics?

No, it can never be taken out of politics. The idea that it can be is quite wrong. Every time a bed-pan was dropped in South Wales there is a problem, which falls to the Secretary of State to deal with the consequences.

It will remain political while we have a totally free tax-paid health care system, even when it is linked to a social care system that is not comprehensively paid for at all by government.

Q. Should the NHS take over social care?

Well, we can't afford it. It's as simple as that. The debate about social care needs to be updated. It is perfectly obvious that if you provided the figures that would be necessary to pay for free care out of taxation it would be rejected out of hand. We need to introduce a more rational and fairer system. We need to come round to the idea that social care cannot be totally free and that we cannot avoid some financial burden. It may be possible to organise a national insurance system, but I'm not completely sure about that. We need to have something that takes account of the individual needs of patients and the responsibilities of society. The idea that somebody in a £2 m house should not be expected to pay for the costs of their care is ridiculous. Yet if this person did pay something, it should not mean that someone on a low income who has worked and struggled to pay for their needs over a working lifetime should also be required to pay. This would be clearly farcical.

The reason why we do not have a policy on social care is that no government has had the courage to produce one. Although there have been many attempts to resolve this all of them have proved to be deeply unpopular.

The trouble with our current populist system of government is that all decisions seem to be made by opinion polls. But opinion polls change, so they are no substitute for a properly organised policy. Anyone who suggests that social care should be paid for completely out of taxation would not be able to defend this at a time when there is rapidly increasing demand. So you then have to work out what means testing you are going to apply. A fairer, but not instantly unpopular solution for the twenty-first century, is to have some private insurance arrangements set up for social care.

We have to recognise where we are now. Both our education and health care systems are immeasurably better that when I was Secretary of State. Now we want someone with a well-thought-out plan for longer term reform, someone who can put their head down and not be worried about being unpopular. One of the big things about Margaret Thatcher was that she was not terribly interested in the reactions of the general public, she never looked at popular opinion, as she was a conviction politician.

There are two rules that need to be understood about reform. First, all change is resisted at first, and second, that anything that might cost more money is equally resisted. So you have to be aware of that from the beginning when you are making changes.

Q. Lastly, I want to turn to your time when you were at the Ministry of Justice when you were trying very hard to bring down the prison population. Why has this been so difficult when in other countries this aim has been more successful?

It is very disappointing. Even in America, in places where they have hard-line Republicans, they are beginning to reduce incarceration rates. We should be able to do better.

Q. In current forensic practice there are strong moves to improve the environments of people with significant mental health problems and to obtain early release, but there are many obstructions in the way. What can we do to help here?

There are good people in correctional institutions who recognise that getting people out of prison into good environments is the key to progress. There are far too many people in our prisons who are mentally ill and who require the proper treatment for their conditions. Of course this sometime requires secure accommodation. But we have to acknowledge that our current prisons do not allow adequate intervention for any of the mental health issues that they face.

At present we are having another of these populist drives to be tougher on law and order so we can bring more people into overcrowded institutions where it is almost impossible to do any worthwhile therapeutic work with them. There isn't the space, there aren't the personnel and almost all the effort is wasted. Currently we have Priti Patel who is waving this banner to be 'tough on crime'.[10] But it started long before her. Michael Howard, David Blunkett and others did quite a lot to raise the prison population dramatically.[11]

Priti is going to do her best to make her policy at the next general election a repeat of the old 'hang 'em and flog 'em' mantra. But there have been reactions against this. Michael Gove was on our side; [12] *he had sensible solutions.*

But, as for me, I have to say I failed to get a change in policy. I discussed it with David Cameron very frequently. [13] *He listened, but he was too nervous about the* Daily Telegraph *to do anything.*

When we had the Thatcher government it was different. When we had good policies that we believed were right we implemented them. But we had to get the timing right. We knew they would be unpopular at first but over time they would be accepted, so we had to bring them in early. Nowadays parliaments seem to be much shorter. It is also different as Prime Ministers now employ ranks of public relations specialists who seem to make all the decisions.

Q. Is there a place for conviction politics nowadays?

Of course. The time will come again. I regard myself as a conviction politician but at present we are in a small minority.

Conclusion

The interview finished and Ken popped across to the House of Commons for one of his final debates. In the chaotic last weeks of the 2017–19 government, there was doubt as to who was running the country and one proposition put forward was that he, as Father of the House, might be prime minister for at least a week or so. It did not come to pass, but it would have been a fitting end to a career, which, despite the gloomy words of Enoch Powell that he maintained applied to all politicians, certainly did not end in failure.

Notes

1.   K. Clarke, *Kind of Blue: A Political Memoir*. London: Pan Macmillan, 2016.

2.   Sir Anthony Grabham (b. 19 July 1930; d. 21 February 2015) was a surgeon and chairman of the BMA when Ken was minister of health.

3.   John Moore, Baron Moore of Lower Marsh (b. 26 November 1937; d. 20 May 2019) was secretary of state for health between 1987 and 1988. He was a great favourite of Mrs Thatcher and was often nicknamed 'Mr Privatisation', but this ended with his attempt to privatise the NHS.

4.   Nigel Lawson, now Baron Lawson of Blaby, was financial secretary to the Treasury when Ken was minister of health. He subsequently became chancellor of the exchequer.

5.   Sir Simon Stevens is chief executive of the NHS. He was health advisor to Tony Blair and Alan Milburn (former minister of health) for seven years and has been responsible for bringing independent organisations into the services of the NHS. This acknowledgement that John Moore may have abandoned the NHS as we know it was a revelation to me. Whatever one thinks of the internal market, and I for one feel it has failed and will need replacing in time, the possibility that the NHS principle of a service free at the point of need was so close to being lost is very alarming.

6.   Barbara Castle, Baroness Castle of Blackburn (b. 6 October 1910; d. 3 May 2002) was secretary of state for health between 1974 and 1976. She introduced the first legislation to expand community care in the White Paper *Better Care for the Mentally Ill* (1975).

7.   See Chapters 10 and 28.

8. Gordon Brown was shadow chief secretary to the Treasury at the time in Ken's account. He subsequently became chancellor of the exchequer in the Labour government of 1997 and prime minister between 2007 and 2010.

9. Mapperley and Saxondale Hospitals were, respectively, the mental hospitals for the city of Nottingham and the county of Nottinghamshire. Ken was MP for a constituency in the catchment area of Saxondale Hospital.

10. Priti Patel has been home secretary since 2019. She is well known for being tough on criminals.

11. Michael Howard and David Blunkett were former home secretaries.

12. Michael Gove is currently chancellor of the Duchy of Lancaster and former education secretary.

13. David Cameron, leader of the Conservative Party (2005–16) and prime minister from 2010 to 2016.

Chapter

10

UK Mental Health Policy and Practice

Jon Glasby, Jerry Tew and Sarah-Jane Fenton·

Introduction

Over five decades, we have seen major changes in mental health policy for adults and for young people, often influenced by shifts in the broader social, political and economic environment. This chapter summarises some of the main changes, drivers and issues, including the introduction of care in the community and the emergence of new discourses around recovery, marketisation and risk during the period 1960–2010.

From Asylum to Community Care

The Mental Health Act 1959 was a step change from previous legislation in foregrounding the provision of treatment, rather than mere confinement, as the core purpose of mental health services. This reflected wider changes in services, with informal treatment becoming available not only for inpatients but also for those outside hospital (with 144,000 outpatient clinic attendances in 1959 compared to virtually none in 1930). However, mental health was still very much a 'Cinderella service', with Mental Health and Mental Deficiency Hospitals containing 40 per cent of NHS inpatient beds but receiving only 20 per cent of the hospital budget.[1]

With a populist's ability to identify issues which chimed with the mood of the age, the Conservative health minister, Enoch Powell, saw the old Victorian asylums as being out of step with emerging expectations of a modern Britain. As well as being overcrowded and offering poor standards of care, their very architecture resonated as an uncomfortable symbol of a bygone age of Poor Law and Workhouse. In 1961, Powell captured this in his famous 'Water Tower speech' (for more details, see Chapters 1, 31).[2] He also recognised the attitudes, customs and practices (both social and professional) which were embodied in these buildings – the 'sheer inertia of mind and matter' – that would need to be overcome if services were to be transformed.

This landmark speech was followed by *A Hospital Plan for England and Wales*, which proposed the development of small-scale psychiatric units in District General Hospitals, with local authorities providing a full range of community services.[3] Much of this chimed with the aspirations of the more progressive elements within the mental health professions, who were keen to move out from the isolation (and perceived inferiority) of the old asylums and become part of mainstream health and social services provision. It suited both those with a more biological persuasion, with its emphasis on treatment rather than containment, and the emerging movement of social psychiatry with its emphasis on the social aspects of rehabilitation. However, despite the recognition of what was needed, and cross-party support for this agenda, financial pressures and institutional resistances continued to undermine any substantial implementation of community care. Although inpatient numbers were falling (from 160,000 in 1954 to 100,000 in 1974), there was inadequate investment in new community-based alternatives and concerns were starting to be expressed about the gap between rhetoric and reality.[4]

Recognising this, Barbara Castle, the Labour health minister, introduced the 1975 White Paper *Better Services for the Mentally Ill*.[5] This made explicit the level of community-based NHS and local authority provision that should be provided per 100,000 population, assuming a roughly equal commitment by the NHS and local authorities, with the latter taking on the main responsibility for those requiring longer-term support and reintegration into mainstream community living. It stated that 'joint planning of health and local authority services is essential' and that 'the policy can only be achieved if there is substantial capital investment in new facilities and if there is a significant shift in the balance of services between health and the local authority'.[6] What was less explicit were the mechanisms whereby this joint planning would be achieved; how 'bridge funding' could be provided for investment in new facilities before old hospitals could be closed and savings made; and how resources could be transferred from the NHS to local authorities to provide social care. These concerns were amplified by the unfortunate timing of the White Paper, coinciding with economic adversity following the oil crisis of 1973.[7]

Nevertheless, government funding was made available to pilot the proposed model of service provision in Worcestershire in an experiment known as the Worcester Development Project.[8] This allowed for comprehensive services to be established in the community without having to wait for any capital to be released and revenue saved from the closure of the old hospital. On the ground, progress was patchy, with teams in one part of the county moving quickly to relocate all their residents from the former asylum, while others were less committed to giving up previous ways of working – leading to a considerable delay in bringing about its final closure. Although GPs generally saw the new services as better for their patients, they also expressed concerns that they themselves were not properly trained for taking on a greater role in mental health.[9]

Although the intention was for this blueprint for a community service to be properly evaluated, this was not followed through. As a result, lessons were not learned as to what was actually needed, how much it would cost and how quickly the old hospitals could actually close – impeding further roll-out of the new service model. Whereas the Worcester Development Project had the benefit of bridging finance, this was not available elsewhere. Consequently, many people were discharged into lodgings or unsuitable accommodation with minimal support, arousing increasing public concern. During the hospital closure phase, more attention tended to be given to establishing psychiatric teams in new facilities in District General Hospitals than to integrating people back into mainstream community life. Crucially, there was no mechanism to transfer over funds to local authorities to create an appropriate infrastructure of community-based support.

A somewhat different story characterised developments in children's services. Here, there had been an established model of Child Guidance Clinics, located within local authority education services and having a strong psychosocial ethos. However, separate NHS hospital-based psychiatric services for young people were also now being developed alongside new adult provision. Early debates in the 1960s were about how to better integrate these service arms – but with little success.[10] Things came to a head (largely spurred on by all too familiar debates about a lack of adolescent inpatient beds and who should pay for what) in the 1986 report *Bridges Over Troubled Waters*.[11] This resulted in the advent of an integrated Child and Adolescent Mental Health Service (CAMHS) that was no longer split between the NHS and local authorities. However, there remained a lack of clarity as to how this should operate in practice, with the first national guidelines not arriving until the mid-1990s – and CAMHS remained hampered by lack of substantive financial investment.

Rights and Recovery

Although the 1959 Mental Health Act had been welcomed as a great advance, by the late 1970s the government and other stakeholders were suggesting that a review would be timely. Led by their legal director, Lawrence O. Gostin, Mind 'argued that many aspects of the treatment of those diagnosed as mental ill were an abuse or denial of their rights'.[12] Although the 1983 Mental Health Act retained much of the overall structure of the 1959 Act, a series of stronger safeguards were built in to enshrine the principle of the 'least restrictive alternative', including greater independence (and training) for Approved Social Workers; stronger (and quicker) rights of appeal for detained patients; and greater use of second medical opinions in relation to more controversial treatments such as psychosurgery and electroconvulsive therapy. Notably absent from the debates leading up to the new Act was any public or political concern as to the inherent dangerousness of people with mental health difficulties and hence any paramount necessity to protect the public against such people.

A little later in the decade, a new discourse emerged around the rights of young people to protection – which was reflected in the United Nations Convention on the Rights of the Child and the 1989 Children Act. This increased awareness of the need for more specific services to support children and young people with their mental health and well-being.[13] However, while this had more tangible impacts on local authority children's services (as in the provision of guardians ad litem to represent children's interests in court), it was less influential in relation to mental health where, for example, young people could still be sectioned and sent to adult psychiatric wards without any specific safeguards being put in place.

Linking in with wider movements around disability activism, people with lived experience of mental distress (often describing themselves as 'survivors' of the mental health system) started to assert their own voice through campaigning organisations such as Survivors Speak Out and the UK Advocacy Network and, to an increasing extent, voluntary organisations such as Mind. Particularly influential was the movement in the 1990s to claim and redefine the term 'recovery'.[14] Activists such as Pat Deegan in the United States and Ron Coleman in the UK promoted the idea of recovery as reclaiming a life worth living – where it would be for the person (and not professionals) to define what that life would look like. It offered a paradigm shift towards a more co-productive approach to practice – one that did not always sit easily with some of the established attitudes and practices of mental health professionals in its emphasis on areas such as empowerment, peer support and social inclusion.[15]

This user voice and the idea of recovery were influential in the development of the National Service Framework – although perhaps not as influential as many would have liked. Instead, it was articulated in documents that were less central to policy implementation: *The Journey to Recovery: The Government's Vision for Mental Health Care* and *A Common Purpose: Recovery in Future Mental Health Services* (the latter in collaboration with the Royal College of Psychiatrists).[16] Rather than transforming the mainstream of service provision, its influence tended to be in more circumscribed developments, such as the emergence of Recovery Colleges. Concerns started to be expressed that the idea of 'recovery' had lost its radical edge and had been appropriated by professional interests to support their agendas – for example, as a pretext for withdrawing services.[17] This marginalisation of user-defined recovery reflected a deep ambivalence within the system as to how (and whether) to move beyond rhetoric and situate people not as patients to be cured but as collaborators in their own recovery journeys.

Marketisation

This focus on rights was soon to be overtaken by a newly emerging discourse about management and efficiency in the delivery of public services – which came to dominate the policy agenda during Margaret Thatcher's premiership. Driven by the ideologies of neoliberalism and New Public Management that were taking hold in the United States, the priority was to make public services more efficient and 'business-like' using market mechanisms. A key proposal, based on the ideas of an American economist, Alain Enthoven, was that responsibility for purchasing care and providing services should be separated (the purchaser/provider split). NHS services would be bought from self-governing NHS Trusts which, in theory, would compete with one another, thereby encouraging greater responsiveness and cost-efficiency. A parallel (but different) marketisation of social care was introduced in the NHS and Community Care Act 1990, with local authorities as lead purchasers and the bulk of provision contracted out to the voluntary/private sectors (see also Chapter 3).

For mental health services, this fragmentation within and between different parts of the health and social care system simply exacerbated existing difficulties in ensuring strategic and operational collaboration. Partnership working was, in effect, part of government rhetoric rather than a practical possibility.[18] With no mechanism in place for enabling (or ring-fencing) a shift of funding from hospital beds to community care, many local authorities saw an opportunity, at a time of financial pressure, to cut back or abdicate many of their responsibilities in relation to mental health – apart from the statutory duty of providing Approved Practitioners to assess people under the Mental Health Act.

By contrast, relatively unaffected by marketisation, a more coherent approach was being taken forward in CAMHS. In *Together We Stand*,[19] a tiered model was proposed in which different levels of support and expertise were available in response to different levels of need. This was well received and described as a policy that 'captured the imagination of all and triggered a clear commitment to improve services'.[20] However, an unintended consequence was to compound existing problems around transitions (as most areas continued to only see children up to the age of sixteen, with adult services starting from the age of eighteen) – with no provision at all in some areas for sixteen-to-eighteen-year-olds who were either too old or too young for services.[21]

Risk and Public Safety

The primacy of economic efficiency as a policy driver came to be displaced by new discourses around risk and dangerousness that had become a key feature of 'late modernity' in the latter part of the twentieth century.[22] There emerged a widely held perception, aided and abetted by both politicians and professional interests, that risk and unpredictability could be eradicated across society by the appropriate application of management tools and technologies. While this had some positive impacts, for example in improving health and safety practices within industry, its impact on mental health services was less benign (see Chapter 23). By its very nature, mental distress challenges deeply embedded notions of rationality and predictability that underpin the organisation of civil society,[23] so it is perhaps not surprising that efforts to manage this perceived threat took on almost totemic significance for government. Despite the evidence that very few people with mental health problems commit homicides – and that the proportion of overall homicides committed by people with serious mental health problems has actually tended to decline during the transition to community care – certain incidents (in particular the death of Jonathan Zito on 17 December 1992) provided the focus for a widespread 'moral panic' fanned by the media (see also Chapters 23, 27, 28).[24]

While analysis of findings from homicide inquiries suggests that an investment in improving overall service quality and accessibility, rather than in devoting professional time to formal risk management procedures, is more likely to prevent potentially avoidable deaths,[25] this has not been reflected in policy or practice. Despite popular (and sometimes professional) misconceptions, research was demonstrating that, using the best available tools, practitioners working in the community cannot predict risk with an accuracy that is of any practical use.[26] This led to the unequivocal conclusion that:

> The stark reality is that however good our tools for risk assessment become . . . professionals will not be able to make a significant impact on public safety.[27]

Nevertheless, practices of risk assessment and management came to dominate both policy and practice in the 1990s and 2000s, often to the detriment of more progressive recovery-oriented practice. However, more recently, there have been some shifts towards more collaborative approaches to 'positive risk taking',[28] recognising that some degree of informed risk is part of normal life and that people cannot move towards recovery if they are overprotected (and potentially over-medicated).

One consistent finding from homicide inquiries was that people were often 'slipping through the net' because professionals and agencies were not working collaboratively or communicating well with one another. Unfortunately, this tendency was only exacerbated by the Thatcher government's market-led reforms. In the early 1990s, while one part of the Department of Health was drafting the NHS and Community Care Act and associated guidance, another part was introducing the Care Programme Approach (CPA) to promote better inter-agency working in managing the risks which were seen to be posed by people with mental illness.[29] While the former focused on assessment in relation to a concept of *need*, the latter was concerned with the assessment of *risk*. The former proposed that the key professional role was the *care manager* who had a limited role in terms of assessing need and purchasing services to meet that need. The latter prescribed a much more 'hands-on' role for the *key worker* (later renamed care co-ordinator) who would have an ongoing relationship with the service user, working with them to make sure that they were properly supported and services co-ordinated. In practice, the lack of integration between the two methods 'resulted in duplication of effort, excessive bureaucracy and construction of a barrier to effective joint working'.[30] This only started to be acknowledged by government in revised guidance, *Building Bridges*,[31] and, when this manifestly failed to resolve the splits and confusions, in a subsequent report entitled (with perhaps unconscious irony) *Still Building Bridges*.[32]

Modernisation of Mental Health Services

New Labour's approach to mental health policy from 1997 reflected somewhat contradictory drivers. On the one hand, there was a mounting concern in relation to the supposed dangerousness of people with mental health problems – as exemplified by the health secretary's assertion that 'care in the community has failed'.[33] On the other, there was a genuine concern to improve the effectiveness of services and take seriously issues such as stigma and discrimination.

Modernising Mental Health Services provided the first comprehensive government statement about the future direction of mental health policy since *Better Services for the Mentally Ill* in 1975. The following year, the *National Service Framework (NSF) for Mental Health in England* set out a ten-year plan for the development and delivery of mental health services for adults of working age,[34] with similar frameworks being produced by the devolved governments in Scotland and Wales. For the first time, there was a focus on mental health promotion – although mental health only came to be formally part of the public health agenda in England much later. For people with serious mental ill-health, the NSF encouraged implementation of functionalised mental health teams (Assertive Outreach and Crisis Resolution), putting greater organisational emphasis on services that could keep people out of hospital – but inadvertently taking the focus away from improving the effectiveness of hospital care itself (see also Chapters 11, 30). Probably the most influential innovation was the mainstreaming of Early Intervention in Psychosis teams, introducing an integrated psychosocial approach that was developed out of research in Australia and the UK.[35] Somewhat uniquely, these services spanned the divide between provision for adolescents and young adults – but only for young people with psychosis.

Following on from the NSF, there was a new stress on promoting social inclusion for people with mental illness and in ensuring that services benefited all sections of the population. A flurry of new policy documents emerged, including *Mainstreaming Gender and Women's Mental Health, Delivering Race Equality: A Framework for Action* and *Personality Disorder: No Longer a Diagnosis of Exclusion*.[36] Beyond this, there was a recognition that taking this agenda forward would require concerted action across government – work that was led by the Social Exclusion Unit within the Office of the Deputy Prime Minister.[37]

Set against the mainly progressive thrust of much of this policy agenda was a countervailing tendency driven by an overriding concern about managing risk. In framing his introduction to *Modernising Mental Health Services*, Frank Dobson, then secretary of state for health, promised that 'we are going to ensure that patients who might otherwise be a danger to themselves and others are no longer able to refuse to comply with the treatment they need'. This promise became translated into a political push, against concerted opposition from user and professional organisations (including the Royal College of Psychiatrists), to replace the 1983 Mental Health Act with more restrictive legislation. A first step was the appointment of an expert advisory committee under the chair of Professor Genevra Richardson in 1998. Unfortunately for the government's agenda, the committee decided to take a more balanced approach and recommended that the new legislation should foreground the principles of non-discrimination, consensual care and capacity – and that there should be a 'bargain' in which the state's right to take away people's liberty was to be balanced by a statutory duty to provide appropriate services (which, in many instances, might obviate the need to employ compulsion). In a somewhat cavalier way, the government chose to ignore the committee's recommendations and went ahead in setting out their agenda in the subsequent White Paper, *Reforming the Mental Health Act*.[38]

The most contentious aspect of the 2007 Mental Health Act was the introduction of Community Treatment Orders (CTOs). Under this provision, patients discharged from hospital could be required to accept medical treatment outside of hospital or face the sanction of a swift recall to hospital. Perhaps for fear of appearing 'soft' on public safety, CTOs came to be used much more widely than originally envisaged – despite the evidence from a randomised trial which showed that CTOs did not improve the effectiveness of community care as people on CTOs were just as likely to require readmission and did not experience any significant improvement in clinical or social functioning.[39]

From Illness to Well-being

The early 2000s saw an emerging political interest in the well-being of the general population alongside the need to better provide for those with more serious mental health problems difficulties. In 2006, Lord Layard, a health economist at the London School of Economics, published an influential report on the costs of failing to treat anxiety and depression.[40] The report stated that around 2.75 million people in England visited GP surgeries each year with mental health problems but were rarely offered effective psychological treatments. The central tenet of this argument was economic, based on the number of people unable to work due to mental health problems. Layard argued that 'someone on Incapacity Benefit costs £750 a month in extra benefit and lost taxes. If the person works just a month more as a result of the treatment (which is £750), the treatment pays for itself.'[41] In response, the government announced funding for a new Improving Access to Psychological Therapies (IAPT) programme, with a commitment to train 3,600 new therapists to offer a limited number of sessions of psychological treatment to more than 500,000 people. Whether or not this initiative delivered on its intended economic outcomes has not been evaluated, and the only comparative study to be conducted found that, while patients' well-being and mental health had improved over four- and eight-month intervals, outcomes were not significantly better than in comparator sites.[42]

Beyond the relatively narrow focus of the IAPT programme, the prioritising of mental well-being outcomes within wider social and economic policy initiatives came to achieve greater traction, particularly in Scotland. In England, a broader cross-governmental focus on mental well-being was taken forward in subsequent articulations of policy, *New Horizons* and *No Health without Mental Health*.[43] However, there was little ownership of these strategies within government (nationally or locally) and they were not accompanied by any funding or delivery mechanisms by which to translate such high level visions into reality. They did not link to any concerted investment in measures that might have ameliorated those adverse personal, social and economic circumstances that increase the likelihood of developing mental health problems – and, in particular, those adverse experiences affecting young people.[44]

Conclusion

As is usually the case with reviews of policy development, the picture that emerges is not one of consistent direction or continuous improvement. It is instead characterised by the influence of major competing discourses and pressures that both emerged internally within and more usually came to bear from outside of the immediate field of mental health (often influenced by broader economic, social and political changes). Overall, it is probably fair to judge that mental health services in 2010 were both substantially more effective and significantly more humane than those prevailing in 1960. However, were we to start with a blank sheet of paper and to design the most effective mental health service within the resources available, it might still bear relatively little resemblance to what has emerged over time. Of course, no generation starts with a blank sheet of paper, and there remains the challenge of how to think 'big' enough and engage co-productively with communities and those with experience of mental health difficulties, alongside professionals and other stakeholders, in envisioning and implementing a properly 'joined-up' strategy for delivering better mental health.

Key Summary Points

- The Mental Health Act 1959 and *A Hospital Plan for England and Wales* in 1962 set a direction for mental health services away from inpatient and towards outpatient and community care which enjoyed support across the political spectrum.
- There has been a shift of focus over time from rights and recovery to marketisation, risk and safety, modernisation and, finally, to well-being.
- There has been greater coherence in policy and consensus among staff in child and adolescent mental health than its adult counterpart, but service developments were hampered by chronic underfunding.
- Though, overall, it is probably fair to judge that mental health services in 2010 were both substantially more effective and significantly more humane than those prevailing in 1960, they have not fulfilled the aspirations held widely at the beginning of the period.

Acknowledgements

This chapter reproduces material from Glasby and Tew's (2015) *Mental Health Policy and Practice* (3rd ed., Basingstoke, Palgrave), with permission from Palgrave.

Notes

1. S. Goodwin, *Comparative Mental Health Policy: From Institutional to Community Care*. London: Sage, 1997.

2. E. Powell, Speech to the Annual Conference of the National Association of Mental Health (now Mind), 1961.

3. Ministry of Health, *A Hospital Plan for England and Wales*. London: HMSO, 1962.

4. R. M. Titmuss, *Commitment to Welfare*. London: George Allen & Unwin, 1968, pp. 106–7.

5. Department of Health and Social Security, *Better Services for the Mentally Ill*. London: HMSO, 1975.

6. Ibid., pp. 3, 86.

7. C. Webster, *The National Health Service: A Political History*. Oxford: Oxford University Press, 2002, p. 74.

8. R. Turner and G. Roberts, The Worcester Development Project. *British Journal of Psychiatry* (1992) 160: 103–7.

9. C. Bennett, The Worcester Development Project: General practitioner satisfaction with a new community psychiatry service. *Journal of the Royal College of General Practitioners* (1989) 39(320): 106–9.

10. D. Black, Are child guidance clinics an anachronism? *Archives of Disease in Childhood* (1983) 58: 644–5.

11. Health Advisory Service, Bridges Over Troubled Waters: A Report from the NHS Health Advisory Service on Services for Disturbed Adolescents. NHS Health Advisory Service, 1986.

12. N. Rose, Unreasonable rights: Mental illness and the limits of the law. *Journal of Law and Society* (1985) 12(2): 199–218, 199.

13. D. Cottrell and A. Kraam, Growing up? A history of CAMHS (1987–2005). Child and Adolescent Mental Health (2005) 10: 111–17, 112.

14. J. Tew, *Social Approaches to Mental Distress*. Basingstoke: Palgrave Macmillan, 2011.

15. J. Repper and R. Perkins, *Social Inclusion and Recovery*. London: Bailliere Tindal, 2003.

16. Department of Health, *The journey to recovery: the government's vision for mental health care*. London: Department of Health, 2001; Care Services Improvement Partnership (CSIP), Royal College of Psychiatrists (RCPsych) and Social Care Institute for Excellence (SCIE), *A Common Purpose: Recovery in Future Mental Health Services*. London: SCIE, 2007.

17. J. Tew, Towards a socially situated model of mental distress. In H. Spandler, J. Anderson and B. Sapey, eds, *Madness, Distress and the Politics of Disablement*, 69–81. Bristol: Policy Press, 2015. See also service user–led organisations such as Recovery in the Bin (https://recoveryinthebin.org/) who feel that 'the Recovery approach started with noble principles but has been co-opted by Neoliberal ideology and now mostly operates as cover for coercion, victim blaming, disability denial and removal of services'.

18. P. Bean and P. Mounser, *Discharged from Mental Hospitals*. Basingstoke: Macmillan, 1993.

19. Health Advisory Service, *Together We Stand: Commissioning, Role and Management of Child and Adolescent Mental Health Services*. London: HMSO, 1995.

20. Cottrell and Kraam, A history of CAMHS.

21. S.-J. Fenton, Mental health service delivery for adolescents and young people: A comparative study between Australia and the UK. PhD thesis, University of Birmingham and University of Melbourne, 2016.

22. U. Beck, *The Risk Society: Towards a New Modernity*. London: Sage, 1992.

23. M. Foucault, *Madness and Civilisation*. London: Tavistock, 1967; R. Porter, *Madness: A Brief History*. Oxford: Oxford University Press, 2002.

24. P. J. Taylor and J. Gunn, Homicides by people with mental illness: myth and reality. *British Journal of Psychiatry* (1999) 174: 9–14; A. Simpson, B. McKenna, A. Moskowitz et al., Homicide and mental illness in New Zealand, 1970–2000. *British Journal of Psychiatry* (2004) 185: 394–8; F. Holloway, Community psychiatric care: From libertarianism to coercion – 'moral panic' and mental health policy in Britain. *Health Care Analysis* (1996) 4: 235–43.

25. E. Munro and J. Rumgay, Role of risk assessment in reducing homicides by people with mental illness. *British Journal of Psychiatry* (2000) 176: 116–20.

26. S. Shergill and G. Szmukler, How predictable is violence and suicide in community psychiatric practice? *Journal of Mental Health* (1998) 7(4): 393–401.

27. E. Petch, Risk management in UK mental health services: An overvalued idea? *Psychiatric Bulletin* (2001) 25: 203–5, 203.

28. T. Stickley and A. Felton, Promoting recovery through therapeutic risk taking. *Mental Health Practice* (2006) 9(8): 26–30; R. Perkins and J. Repper, Recovery versus risk? From managing risk to the co-production of safety and opportunity. *Mental Health and Social* Inclusion (2016) 20(2): 101–9.

29. Department of Health, *The Care Programme Approach for People with a Mental Illness Referred to the Specialist Psychiatric Services*. London: Department of Health, 1995.

30. B. Hannigan, The policy and legal context. In B. Hannigan and M. Coffey, eds, *The Handbook of Community Mental Health Nursing*, 30–40. London: Routledge, 2003, p. 32.

31. Department of Health, *Building Bridges: A Guide to the Arrangements for Interagency Working for the Care and Protection of Severely Disabled People*. London: Department of Health, 1995.

32. Department of Health, *Still Building Bridges: The Report of a National Inspection of Arrangements for the Integration of Care Programme Approach with Care Management*. London: Social Services Inspectorate and Department of Health, 1999.

33. Department of Health, *Modernising Mental Health Services: Safe, Sound and Supportive*. London: Department of Health, 1998.

34. Department of Health, *National Service Framework for Mental Health: Modern Standards and Service Models*. London, Department of Health, 1999.

35. M. Birchwood, P. McGorry, H. Jackson et al., Early intervention in schizophrenia. *British Journal of Psychiatry* (1997) 170: 2–5; P. McGorry, Should youth mental health become a specialty in its own right? Yes. *British Medical Journal* (2009) 339: b3373; P. McGorry, E. Killackey and A. Yung, Early intervention in psychosis: Concepts, evidence and future directions. *World Psychiatry* (2008) 7: 148–56.

36. Department of Health, *Mainstreaming Gender and Women's Mental Health*. London: Department of Health, 2003; Department of Health, *Delivering Race Equality: A Framework for Action – Mental Health Services – Consultation Document*. London: Department of Health, 2003; National Institute for Mental Health in England (NIMHE), *Personality Disorder: No Longer a Diagnosis of Exclusion*. London: Department of Health, 2003.

37. Office of the Deputy Prime Minister, *Mental Health and Social Exclusion*. London: Office of the Deputy Prime Minister, 2004; Office of the Deputy Prime Minister, *Reaching Out: An Action Plan for Social Inclusion*. London: Office of the Deputy Prime Minister, 2006.

38. Department of Health. *Reforming the Mental Health Act – Part I: The New Legal Framework*. London: Department of Health, 2001; Department of Health. *Reforming the Mental Health Act – Part II: High Risk Patients*. London: Department of Health, 2001.

39. T. Burns, J. Rugkåsa, A. Molodynski et al., Community treatment orders for patients with psychosis (OCTET): A randomised controlled trial. *The Lancet* (2013) 381: 1627–33.

40. R. Layard and Centre for Economic Performance Mental Health Policy Group, *The Depression Report: A New Deal for Depression and Anxiety Disorders*. London: London School of Economics, 2006.

41. Ibid., p. 2.

42. G. Parry, M. Barkham, J. Brazier et al., *An Evaluation of a New Service Model: Improving Access to Psychological Therapies Demonstration Sites 2006–2009*. Final report. NIHR Service Delivery and Organisation programme, 2011.

43. Department of Health, *New Horizons: Towards a Shared Vision for Mental Health*. London: Department of Health, 2009; HM Government, *No Health without Mental Health: A Cross-government Mental Health Outcomes Strategy for People of All Ages*. London: Department of Health, 2011.

44. Mental Health Policy Commission, *Investing in a Resilient Generation: Keys to a Mentally Prosperous Nation*. Birmingham: University of Birmingham, 2018.

Chapter

11

Mental Health Policy and Economics in Britain

Paul McCrone

Introduction

Economics and health care are fundamentally linked. Financial arguments have been influential in the development of mental health services over the ages, from the establishment of asylums through to their demise and replacement with other forms of care. This chapter presents some of the economic arguments that have been used around the process of moving from a predominantly hospital-based form of care in 1960 to one in which community services were developed and expanded by 2010.

UK Economy and Health Spending, 1960–2010

The fifty-year period from 1960 to 2010 witnessed huge political and economic change in the UK. The post-war consensus whereby governments (Conservative and Labour) followed largely Keynesian economic policies (which were relatively interventionist) continued until the emergence of the Margaret Thatcher administration in 1979. 'Thatcherism' was characterised by a desire (whether achieved or not is debatable) to reduce the role of government and to promote the private sector. This was clearly relaxed to some extent during the Labour governments of 1997–2010, and the financial crisis towards the end of that period resulted in government once again accepting a heavily interventionist role in the economy.

The amount of funds that a society devotes to health care (whether through public or private spending) is fundamentally a decision made by society or individuals. According to the Organisation for Economic Co-operation and Development (OECD),[1] in 1960 gross domestic product (GDP) in the UK was £26.1 billion and by 2010 was £1.6 trillion. Adjusting for inflation gives an increase of some 336 per cent over this period. In 1960/1, the amount of GDP accounted for by health spending was 3.1 per cent and this had increased to 7.5 per cent by 2009/10.[2] This still leaves more than 90 per cent of GDP going on non-health activities and so there is room for increases albeit with proportional reductions elsewhere. Can this be achieved? Given that in other areas productivity gains can be achieved through technological advancements, products in these areas are prone to becoming cheaper in real terms. More labour-intensive sectors (health but also education) do not experience such productivity gains and so, as an economy develops, we should expect and even welcome a greater proportion of spending going on those areas. This is an argument put forward strongly by the influential American economist William Baumol.[3] However, governments around the world have appeared concerned about the rising costs of health care and cost-containment measures have been endorsed.

Unfortunately, it is not feasible to estimate how much funding has been allocated specifically to mental health care over the years. Different government agencies have had responsibility for this area and data have not been recorded consistently. In recent years, we do have such information for planned NHS spending. In 2007, for example, planned mental health expenditure amounted to £8.4 billion which was 12.4 per cent of all NHS spending.[4]

Economic Arguments around Deinstitutionalisation

Since the emergence of the large asylums in the Victorian period, there was an increase in the number of people detained in psychiatric hospitals, with stays frequently being long-term. The peak number of psychiatric beds in England was in 1955 (around 150,000 beds),[5] and this was followed by a gradual decline facilitated in part by the emergence of new antipsychotic medication such as chlorpromazine. However, the asylums remained and came in for substantial criticism. In 1961, Enoch Powell, who was a health minister in the ruling Conservative government, gave his famous 'Water Tower speech' which many consider to have paved the way for the ultimate demise of the asylums. In current times, the development of community services while still maintaining a huge stock of hospital beds might seem unfeasible (see also Chapters 1 and 2). However, it is clear from Powell's speech that the stated intention was not that finance would act as a barrier to developing alternative forms of care and indeed that around half of capital expenditure at the time was already taking place in the community rather than in hospitals. Importantly, whether there was professional acceptance of the need for this move is unclear.

Subsequent policy documents developed further the move to care outside of the long-stay institutions and economic factors clearly influenced these arguments. The report entitled *Hospital Services for the Mentally Ill*,[6] published in 1971, proposed integrating physical and mental health care within district general hospitals (interestingly, very different from what we have today). That report recognised the need for extra resources resulting from a desired high staff-to-patient ratio for care to be provided adequately. The realisation that community provision would require properly resourcing was shown in the 1975 report *Better Services for the Mentally Ill* (see also Chapter 10).[7] As well as emphasising that the running costs of community services would be high, the report also emphasised the imperative to upgrade the existing hospital services. Moving forward to 1989, the government published an official response to a seminal report led by Roy Griffiths (see also Chapter 12).[8] The *Caring for People* report set down the idea of a purchaser/provider split for health care, which has been revisited on a number of occasions up to the present day. It did not, though, ring-fence resources for community services (as had been called for) unless these were developed jointly between health and social care agencies.[9]

Financing Community Services

It is notable that, while many would have viewed the closure of asylums and the development of community services as a way of saving money, many in government and the policy world clearly were of the view that community services would not come cheaply. In her book *After the Asylums*, Elaine Murphy highlighted a number of financial issues relating to community care in the UK.[10] She noted the problem, which still applies today, that different agencies have different responsibilities in terms of provision and commissioning and this can lead to clashing priorities. When the asylums were established this was accompanied with a transfer of financial responsibility from local parishes to county councils who managed the asylums. With the emergence of the welfare state later in the twentieth century, housing benefit became available and this led to funds being transferred to the Department of Social Security. Jones pointed out that, while Joint Finance to encourage the development of community services became available from 1976, this represented just 1 per cent of NHS funds and discouraged the transfer of other funds from health authorities to local authorities. This, coupled with the immense pressure that local authorities came under in the early 1980s to contain spending (through rate capping, for example), meant that local services were poorly developed. The closure of long-stay hospitals should have released funds but unless whole wards or hospitals could be closed this would not materialise. In addition, the downsizing of hospitals meant that the costs per patient per day became very high. Jones was clear that to counter some of these problems there would need to be an effective system of bridging finance put in place (such as a dowry mechanism).

Rationale for Economic Evaluations

Any development in the way in which mental health care is provided has potential impacts on resources. New services usually require start-up costs and running costs can be quite different from those they are replacing. Clearly, there is a limit on funds available for health and social care. Economics is concerned with this issue of scarcity (hence it being dubbed the 'dismal science' by Thomas Carlyle in the nineteenth century) and whenever scarce resources are used in one particular way then there is an opportunity cost in that other potential uses for them are foregone.

The idea that resources are inherently scarce is a strong one – although it is important to bear in mind the arguments put forward by William Baumol described in the section 'UK Economy and Health Spending, 1960–2010'. This, coupled with the high demands for health care due in part to an ageing population but also demand for new ways of working, means that decisions are always being made about how best to use the resources we have available to us. This can be at a very specific level (e.g. what is the best form of care for someone with schizophrenia?) or at 'higher' levels (e.g. should we spend more on care for people with mental health problems or those with cancer?; should we be spending more on health or education or defence?). Such decisions have always been made and always will be. The methods of economic evaluation have been developed and operationalised to try and make this process better informed.

In establishing whether new forms of mental health provision represent value for money we need to combine information on the costs of care with evidence on outcomes. Simply focusing on costs is rarely sufficient – unless of course we are simply intent on identifying the least-cost option. Costs are, though, key to an economic evaluation and it is imperative that they are measured appropriately. In doing so, we must recognise that they can be borne by different agencies: the health service, social care departments, housing agencies, criminal justice services, education providers, social security systems, business, families and friends, and users of services themselves. Altering the way in which care is provided might have widespread impacts and capturing these is important. If one were to only focus on direct intervention costs, then key information might be missed. For example, some medications can be particularly expensive but if they result in savings elsewhere then such costs might well be offset if they prevent lengthy inpatient hospital stays or return patients more quickly to productive work.

Costs ultimately have to be either combined with or viewed alongside outcomes for those affected by changes in service delivery. In mental health care, this is of course primarily the user themselves, but families and wider society can also be affected. What outcomes should be included? Given that there is unlikely to be just one impact that is of interest, it may be that a range of outcomes are relevant. Policymakers in England (not the whole of the UK) generally favour the use of quality-adjusted life years (QALYs), which are a generic measure enabling, in theory, comparisons to be made across diverse health areas. QALYs have been used to evaluate mental health services but many would consider them to be too reductionist.

One outcome that has frequently been used in mental health evaluations has been the use of inpatient care. This has its merits. It is easily recorded and avoiding admission may be desirable. However, it has important limitations. It comes with an underlying assumption that inpatient care is 'bad' but for some it may be entirely necessary and good-quality care may be optimised in an inpatient setting. Furthermore, it is not a true outcome measure but rather a process measure. As such, it is more properly considered to be a cost rather than an outcome. Finally, use of inpatient care is directly associated with the provision of inpatient beds in the area. Reducing provision inevitably leads to reduced use.

Economics of Deinstitutionalisation

In the UK, the largest and most influential evaluation of a hospital closure programme was the Team for the Assessment Psychiatric Services (TAPS) study led by Julian Leff (see also Chapter 30).[11] This focused on the closure of the Friern and Claybury hospitals in North London in the 1980s and the health economic component was conducted by the Personal Social Services Research Unit (PSSRU) at the University of Kent, led by Martin Knapp and Jennifer Beecham.[12] The TAPS study followed cohorts of patients as they were discharged from the hospitals over several years, usually to long-stay residential facilities. Not surprisingly, the patients who were considered easier to place in the community were discharged first and they had noticeably lower average weekly costs of community services than those discharged later. These costs include the residential facility plus other services used while in the community and any subsequent hospital care. The authors of the TAPS study also looked at the comparative costs (in 1993/4 £s) of hospital- and community-based care.[13] This showed that the average weekly cost when still in the Friern Hospital and Claybury Hospital was £578 and £551 respectively. This compares to £539 during the first year following discharge for cohorts 1–7 and £562 in the fifth year following discharge for cohorts 1–3. What is clear from this is that the costs of community care were similar to hospital care and it was therefore not saving funds, even if that was desired by some.

Inpatient and Residential Care since Deinstitutionalisation

What can we say about inpatient care since the hospital closure programme has been largely completed? While the number of days spent in hospital for mental health reasons fell from when there was a peak number of 150,000 inpatients at any one time in 1955, in recent times the number of days has been fairly stable. Data from the Department of Health's Hospital Episode Statistics show that, in 1998/9, there were 7,029,445 days spent in hospital by people with a psychiatric diagnosis and, by 2009/10, the figure was 7,482,979.[14] This was also a time of comparatively high investment in community services and so probably indicates that this number of bed days (equivalent to around 20,000 beds) may be the minimum required.

Some patients do, though, remain as long-stay patients in hospital, and it is interesting to see what one year as an inpatient is equivalent to in terms of other forms of care. Box 11.1, where the numbers are based on unit costs produced by the University of Kent, shows that

> **Box 11.1** One Year in Hospital Is Equivalent to . . .
>
> 3,058 day care sessions
>
> 1,105 counselling sessions
>
> 1,095 staffed residential care days
>
> 577 outpatient appointments
>
> 969 psychologist contacts
>
> 2,803 community mental health nurse contacts
>
> 2,452 GP contacts

the amount of resources that could be provided is substantial.[15] Of course, it may be unfeasible for some to be discharged from hospital, but these figures do illustrate the alternatives that are available. Even though residential care is expensive, it is far less so than inpatient care. It is also worth pointing out that one day in prison has a cost of around £102 which is substantially lower than hospital costs.[16] It is well known that psychiatric morbidity in hospital is high, but the differences in costs between prisons and hospitals, especially secure units, can act as a disincentive to change location.

Inpatient stays remain a fundamental part of the care process within a mental health system and are also a highly expensive form of care. It is interesting therefore that there are relatively few studies that have investigated what actually takes place on inpatient wards and in particular there have been limited numbers of economic studies focusing on this. One major exception was the Patient Involvement in Improving the Evidence Base on Inpatient Care (PERCEIVE) study led by Til Wykes from King's College London and conducted in south London. This investigated care provided on seventeen inpatient wards and evaluated means of improving activities for patients. The economic analyses (described in depth by Sabes-Figuera and colleagues)[17] were a novel departure from usual studies that have examined inpatient costs in that the focus was on activities and staff contacts that patients considered to be meaningful to them. Study participants were asked what meaningful care they had received in the previous week and, from this information, costs were calculated. Further analyses attempted to identify which patient characteristics were predictive of variations on the costs across the sample.

The patients reflected those found on many inpatient wards in inner-city areas in the UK. Schizophrenia or bipolar disorder was the diagnosis of 65 per cent, compulsory detentions were experienced also by 65 per cent, and 53 per cent were from a minority ethnic group. Therapeutic activities, including ward meetings, had been experienced by 78 per cent of the sample which was relatively encouraging. Meaningful staff contacts were reported by 90 per cent of patients (including 59 per cent with nurses, 74 per cent with psychiatrists and between 20 and 33 per cent with other professionals). While this might seem reasonable, it does mean that some patients were reporting no meaningful contacts at all. When it comes to costs of meaningful care, the average for the week was £227. Psychiatrist contacts made up 48 per cent of this, nurse contacts were 13 per cent and other therapeutic activities were also 13 per cent. This figure of £227 per week is substantially below the cost *per day* on a ward if the conventional approach to estimating unit costs is used. The implication is that, although staff may have different views, patients perceive much care they receive to not be meaningful or therapeutic.

The abovementioned TAPS study investigated discharge from long-stay hospitals and usually this was to supported accommodation in the community. The Quality and Effectiveness of Supported Tenancies (QuEST) study more than twenty years later, led by Helen Killaspy from University College London, evaluated care delivered in different forms of supported accommodation.[18] A total of 619 residents were recruited for the study from residential care (which involved 24-hour staffing), supported housing (self-contained apartments with staffing up to 24 hours per day) and floating outreach arrangements (self-contained tenancies with staff support). Various clinical measures were taken as well as quality of life, and service use was recorded and costs calculated.

The QuEST study revealed that quality of life was similar in residential care and supported housing but was lower in floating outreach arrangements. Satisfaction with care was similar under all three models. Service use in the previous three months showed relatively high levels of care coordinator, psychiatrist and other doctor contacts. Inpatient care was received by relatively few participants. Total care costs were similar between residential care and supported housing, while care costs for those in floating outreach arrangements were around one-third lower. This was not surprising given that those in these forms of care would presumably have lower levels of need.

Economics of Specialist Services

Shortly after the election of the Labour government in 1997, the Department of Health published the *National Service Framework for Mental Health*.[19] This put forward the case for further developing specialist mental health services across the country. Three particular new models of teams and services were outlined: home treatment teams for people facing acute mental health crises; early intervention services for those with a first episode of psychosis; and assertive community treatment to improve contact with those who may be hard to engage with services. Though they had not been available across the whole country, such services had existed for many years in different settings. There was reasonably powerful evidence on the clinical benefits of the models but up-to-date evidence on their economic aspects was limited. A number of studies using similar methods were forthcoming though.

A randomised trial led by Sonia Johnson from University College London was conducted to compare a crisis intervention service with usual care in north London.[20] The main outcome in this study was inpatient use over a six-month follow-up period and this was shown to be substantially less for those receiving the crisis service. The costs of the two forms of care were calculated and, given the main outcome, it was not surprising that crisis intervention resulted in large cost savings (around 30 per cent) compared to usual care.[21]

The Lambeth Early Onset study led by Tom Craig and Philippa Garety at King's College London was another trial, this time comparing early intervention for first-episode psychosis with usual care.[22] The early intervention service resulted in reduced time in hospital. Costs for many services were higher for those receiving the service but total costs were lower due to the impact of reduced hospital time.[23]

The REACT study, led by Helen Killaspy, again at University College London, evaluated assertive community treatment in north London.[24] The randomised trial took inpatient days over an eighteen-month period as the primary outcome measure and found no significant difference between assertive community treatment and usual care. The economic evaluation measured a range of services and calculated costs of these. The average cost over the eighteen-month period was £34,572 for assertive community treatment and £30,541 for usual care. Most of this cost was accounted for by inpatient care.[25]

These three studies have demonstrated that early intervention and crisis services certainly appear to represent some value for money. Less clear is the assertive community treatment. One potential reason for the lack of a significant effect for that service model was that usual care by the time of the study was well developed – certainly compared to the comparator groups in some of the early studies of assertive community treatment.

Conclusion

Economic considerations were a key influence in the development of mental health care in the period between 1960 and 2010. While some initiatives might have been seen as cost-saving endeavours, it has been clear all along that good-quality mental health provision is not inexpensive. This, though, should not necessarily be seen as a problem – cost is only a monetary proxy for care provided and we would want care to be sufficient for those in need of it.

Key Summary Points

- Financial arguments have been influential in the development of mental health services over the ages, from the establishment of asylums through to their demise and replacement with other forms of care.
- In 1960, gross domestic product (GDP) in the UK was £26.1 billion and, by 2010, was £1.6 trillion. Adjusting for inflation gives an increase of some 336 per cent over this time period. In 1960/1, the amount of GDP accounted for by health spending was 3.1 per cent and this had increased to 7.5 per cent by 2009/10.
- Given that in other areas productivity gains can be achieved through technological advancements, products in these areas are prone to becoming cheaper in real terms. More labour-intensive sectors (health but also education) do not experience such productivity gains and so, as an economy develops, we should expect and even welcome a greater proportion of spending going on those areas.
- The TAPS study in north London in the 1980s showed that the average weekly cost when still in the Friern Hospital and Claybury Hospital was £578 and £551 respectively. This compares to £539 during the first year following discharge for cohorts 1–7 and £562 in the fifth year following discharge for cohorts 1–3. What is clear from this is that the costs of community care were similar to hospital care and it was therefore not saving funds, even if that was desired by some. However, prison costs are lower than hospital costs and this may discourage admission of mentally ill patients to appropriate clinical facilities.
- Health economic studies carried out in London and published between 1999 and 2009 suggest that, while home treatment teams for people in acute mental health crises and early intervention teams may save money, assertive outreach teams for difficult-to-engage patients may not. However, cost calculations do not address issues of quality of care and desired outcomes.

Notes

1. See OECD.Stat, https://stats.oecd.org/#.

2. R. Harker, *NHS Funding and Expenditure*. London: House of Commons Library, 2019.

3. W. J. Baumol, *The Cost Disease*. New Haven, CT: Yale University Press, 2012.

4. P. McCrone, S. Dhanasiri, A. Patel, M. Knapp and S. Lawton-Smith, *Paying the Price: The Cost of Mental Health Care in England to 2026*. London: King's Fund, 2008.

5. King's Fund, *Mental Health Under Pressure*. Briefing. www.kingsfund.org.uk/sites/default/files/field/field_publication_file/mental-health-under-pressure-nov15_0.pdf

6. Department of health and Social Security, *Hospital Services for the Mentally Ill*. London: HMSO, 1971.

7. Department of health and Social Security, *Better Services for the Mentally Ill*. London: HMSO, 1975.

8. R. Griffiths, *Community Care: Agenda for Action*. A Report to the Secretary of State for Social Services. London: HMSO, 1988.

9. Department of Health, *Caring for People: Community Care in the Next decade and Beyond*, Cm 849. London: HMSO, 1989.

10. E. Murphy, *After the Asylums: Community Care for People with Mental Illness*. London: Faber & Faber, 1991.

11. J. Leff, *Care in the Community: Illusion or Reality?* Chichester: John Wiley & Sons, 1997.

12. J. Beecham, A. Hallam, M. Knapp et al., Costing care in hospital and in the community. In Leff, *Care in the Community*, 93–108.

13. A. Hallam, Affording community care: Lessons from the Friern and Claybury psychiatric reprovision programme. *Mental Health Research Review* (1995) 2: 29–32.

14. Department of Health, Hospital Episode Statistics.

15. L. Curtis, *Unit Costs of Health and Social Care 2010*. Canterbury: University of Kent, 2010.

16. Ministry of Justice, *Costs per Place and Costs per Prisoner by Individual Prison*. https://assets.publishing.service.gov.uk/government/uploads/system/uploads/attachment_data/file/218347/prison-costs-summary-10-11.pdf

17. R. Sabes-Figuera, P. McCrone, E. Csipke et al., Predicting psychiatric inpatient costs. *Social Psychiatry and Psychiatric Epidemiology* (2016) 51: 303–8.

18. H. Killaspy, S. Priebe, S. Bremner et al., Quality of life, autonomy, satisfaction, and costs associated with mental health supported accommodation services in England: a national survey. *Lancet Psychiatry* (2016) 3: 1129–37.

19. Department of Health, *National Service Framework for Mental Health: Modern Standards and Service Models*. London: Department of Health, 1999.

20. S. Johnson, F. Nolan, S. Pilling et al., Randomised controlled trial of acute mental health care by a crisis resolution team: The north Islington crisis study. *British Medical Journal* (2005) 331: 599.

21. P. McCrone, S. Johnson, F. Nolan et al., Economic evaluation of a crisis resolution service: A randomised controlled trial. *Epidemiologia e Psichiatria Sociale* (2009) 18: 54–8.

22. T. K. J. Craig, P. Garety, P. Power et al., The Lambeth Early Onset (LEO) Team: Randomised controlled trial of the effectiveness of specialised care for early psychosis. *British Medical Journal* (2004) 329: 1067.

23. P. McCrone, T. K. J. Craig, P. Power and P. A. Garety, Cost-effectiveness of an early intervention service for people with psychosis. *British Journal of Psychiatry*. (2010) 196(5): 377–82.

24. H. Killaspy, P. Bebbington, R. Blizard et al., The REACT study: Randomised evaluation of assertive community treatment in north London. *British Medical Journal* (2006) 32: 815–20.

25. P. McCrone, H. Killaspy, P. Bebbington et al., The REACT study: Cost-effectiveness analysis of assertive community treatment in north London. *Psychiatric Services* (2009) 60: 908–13.

True Confessions of a New Managerialist

Elaine Murphy

Introduction

I became one of the new breed of medically qualified health service managers in the early 1980s and watched with fascination and some amazement at the upsurge in triumphs and disasters that accompanied the management revolution over the course of the following twenty years. In this chapter, I explore why the revolution happened, what went right and what went appallingly wrong for users of mental health services and for the professionals working in them. I end on a positive note; some aspects of mental health care improved over the forty years between 1970 and 2010 and quite a lot can be attributed to 'management'.

Three separate threads of causality in the changes in mental health services came together in the late 1970s: first, the oil crisis and its impact on global funding of health care; second, the drive to improve health care quality; and third, the global commitment to the deinstitutionalisation of people with serious mental disorders and profound learning/intellectual disabilities. Each one of these issues posed serious challenges; trying to cope with all three at once was bound to cause 'collateral damage' to the lives and careers of the cared-for and carers.

Health Care Funding

The 1973–4 oil crisis significantly raised prices and, shortly after, the Organization of the Petroleum Exporting Countries (OPEC) cut off supplies to several Western countries in retaliation for their support for Israel in its war with Egypt and Syria. Britain's ambassador to Saudi Arabia commented that the oil price rise represented 'perhaps the most rapid shift in economic power that the world has ever seen'.[1] The crisis underlined the importance of oil to the world economy in no uncertain terms. At that time, oil provided more than half of the world's energy needs – a situation that was not expected to change for the foreseeable future. Five of America's twelve leading firms were oil companies, as were Britain's top two: BP and Shell. 'The disappearance of cheap oil has transformed the world in which British foreign policy has to operate', noted the Foreign Office, with industrialised nations seeing their trading surpluses transformed into deficits almost overnight.

In the UK, this led to a stagnation in NHS funding through the years of the Labour administration. This was followed by an attempt to reduce and make more efficient the delivery of health care during the Thatcher years of 1979–90. The government then as now seemed not to understand that it is largely demographic change of an ever-ageing population that shifts demand once the parameters of provision have been established. The spending in real terms went up substantially from £9.2 billion in 1978/9 to £37.4 billion in 1991/2. Even adjusting for inflation, this rise is more than 50 per cent. However, the hyperinflationary effects of unionised NHS staff salary demands and an increase in pharmaceutical prices led to a real increase of only about 1.5 per cent. This, combined with real restrictions on acute hospital funding, contributed to the general perception of parsimonious funding for the NHS and subsequent raiding of conveniently 'underspent' mental health budgets by health authorities trying to balance their acute hospital budgets. Mental health underspends were largely caused by the poor recruitment of staff.[2] A quarter of all London general hospital beds closed during these years. Mental health suffered as a neglected poor relation.

The Drive to Improve the Quality of Health Care

These years also witnessed the advent of the systematic examination of health care quality, which perhaps began seriously with the work of Avedis Donabedian, who, in 1966, proposed a framework for a quality of care assessment that described quality along the dimensions of structure, process and outcomes of care. This galvanised the examination of quality in the US health system and prompted similar investigations in the UK.[3] Quality of care was defined as 'the degree to which health services for individuals and populations increase the likelihood of desired health outcomes and are consistent with current professional knowledge'. Health systems should seek to improve performance on six dimensions of quality of care: safety, effectiveness, patient-centredness, timeliness, efficiency and equity. It was clear that the current care systems could not do the job. Trying harder would not work. Changing systems of care, however, would, it was perhaps somewhat naively believed. It followed that what was true of acute hospital systems must also be true of mental health care systems. The desire to squeeze mental health services into a management framework designed for a different model of care, omitting the key role of social services, housing, employment and service users' own shifting perceptions of what they needed, was bound to lead to difficulties and the corrosion of trust among those who worked at the front line.

Received wisdom among health care pundits declared that health systems must be judged primarily on their impacts, including on better health and its equitable distribution; the confidence of people in their health system; and their economic benefit. Outcomes would depend on processes of competent care and positive user experience. The foundations of high-quality health systems were judged to include the population and their health needs and expectations; governance of the health sector and partnerships across sectors; platforms for care delivery; workforce numbers and skills; and tools and resources, from medicines to data. In addition to strong foundations, health systems would need to develop the capacity to measure and use data to learn. High-quality health systems should be informed by four values: they are for people and they are equitable, resilient and efficient.

The message was both seductive and impressive.[4] Mental health services, however, had no well-developed way of demonstrating outcomes for their patients; they were immediately at a disadvantage. Only process measures could be assessed; and what of the half of patients with serious psychotic illness who did not believe themselves to be ill and did not want to engage in services? Where did the model get us to there? Developing an outcomes framework in mental health was a challenge that would take years and still has not affected funding changes to better target effective services.

The Global Commitment to Deinstitutionalisation

The third major impact on services was the agenda driving deinstitutionalisation, one of public and moral necessity. This was based on a growing emphasis on human rights as well as advances in social science and philosophy attacking psychiatry and the boundaries of what constituted mental illness, which reached its height in the 1950s and 1960s. A series of scandals in the 1970s around the ill-treatment of mental health patients and a strong, vocal service user movement provided harrowing stories of people's experiences of care, which contributed to the opprobrium heaped on services. The timing, however, created the impression that somehow delivering mental health care 'in the community', wherever that was, would be cheaper than delivering care to long-stay patients in hospital.

This moral agenda, however, was supported by other developments that facilitated the possibility for transformation. Pharmaceutical advances demonstrated that people with severe mental illness could be treated and it became clear that institutionalisation itself was harmful. Politically, there was consensus among parties about the vision for mental health services. Gradually there emerged an economic impetus for deinstitutionalisation, which accelerated as large institutions became financially unsustainable and, in many cases, were occupying prime development land that finance directors perceived as capital asset money-spinners. Ostensibly the programme was geared towards achieving greater integration of health and social care provision with the development of alternative community services, to be delivered by local authorities, which, however, were never consulted and felt unreasonably put-upon.

New organisations were set up to manage the process of deinstitutionalisation and subsequently deliver services. Many of these were charities, including housing associations. With involvement from each stakeholder group (including the district health authority, local authority and voluntary sector), a key function of these new organisations was to broker relationships to ensure that no single organisation had sole ownership and to manage the power dynamics. They provided opportunities for people to connect around a new organisational form with its own identity and purpose, underpinned by a board and trustees who were accountable for the process and outcomes of transformation. These new organisations led on many aspects of the transformation, bringing new ideas. Subsequently, they received most of the funding, led on developing new services and created systems and structures to manage the transition, including workforce management and training. Yet the people who had previously managed the whole patient experience in hospitals were often left out in the cold, with doctors pigeonholed into 'drug prescribers' and senior nurses rejected as 'more institutionalised than the patients', an insulting and inaccurate phrase I heard often. The failure to engage with the traditional professional groups caused a serious waste of human resources in mental health services that is still not rectified.

There were in fact many excellent examples in existence before the closures. Psychiatric rehabilitation specialists had been quietly moving people out into group homes and community organisations since the late 1970s, demonstrating that this could be done well and improve patients' lives if well supported by clinicians. David Abrahamson had a successful programme running from Goodmayes Hospital in the London Boroughs of Newham and Redbridge from the mid-1970s that made a huge impact on my own philosophy of community practice.[5]

The deinstitutionalisation process involved a significant focus on managing the workforce. Where it resulted in the closure of individual wards, staff were absorbed into the wider organisation. Yet many mental health professionals who had been confident of their role as psychiatrists and nurses in an institution suddenly found themselves expected to take on different working patterns, leave the comfort of the professional silos that had hitherto dominated mental health services and take on completely alien tasks. Many resented it. An impatient senior management cadre, unable to perceive quite what the problem was, steamrollered through the closures, leaving resentful and uncomprehending consultant psychiatrists and senior nurses marooned in different locations from their patients and the staff teams they had previously worked alongside. Psychologists and occupational therapists, however, suddenly found their skills valued more highly and grasped the space left in the vacuum. In the 1980s, I visited a mental health service in Devon where the new community teams located in small dispersed market towns were struggling to provide a service without support from psychiatrists, since all the psychiatrists had remained recalcitrantly fixed to their offices in the old but much-loved Victorian mental hospital in Exeter. It took a new generation of appointments to solve a problem that should have been thought through at the outset.

Terrible mistakes were made as a result of an ideology of community care taking hold, in the face of obvious shortcomings for the most seriously ill and especially for those with profound learning/intellectual disabilities. Everyone had to be squeezed into the same model. Some saintly staff fought to bring common sense to a process that became the end rather than the means. In a devastating critique of the process he lived through in my own health district, Nick Bouras, one of the editors of this book, gave a personal account of the obstacles and challenges he faced in developing, researching and implementing services for people with intellectual disabilities.[6] In a very personal memoir of these years, he recorded the successes and frustrations of working in a system that does not always have a shared vision and the tenacity and enthusiasm that are necessary to reform an NHS service from the inside, in the teeth of every obstacle possible.

The cost of the deinstitutionalisation process, if done properly, was to prove much more expensive than originally forecast, and the most profoundly disabled were hugely expensive to care for satisfactorily in the community. I was a close observer of the closure of Darenth Park Hospital in Kent, a vast old mental handicap hospital in the South East Thames Regional Health Authority area, containing patients from all over Kent, East Sussex and inner and outer south-east London. Glennerster's economic analysis demonstrated that the final costs of care to the NHS, local authorities, the Department of Health and Social Security (DHSS) and Housing Corporation budgets were over a third more expensive than the old hospital. With modern buildings, a higher staff ratio and more personalised care plans, this is scarcely surprising. The extra costs fell on other public sector organisations that hitherto had borne few costs of care.[7] It took many years for the skills lost when the hospital closed to be learnt in the community, before a model of largely social care replaced the old nursing model. It is still not clear whether the very high costs of caring for the most disabled patients in this way is a good use of scarce resources. It is as possible to be institutionalised in a flat for two as it is in a ward for thirty.

Then Came Management

The creation of a large managerial stratum within the NHS in the 1980s and 1990s has been one of the most striking characteristics of reforms intended to develop a more efficient and 'business-like' service that was meant to address the problems of quality and efficiency. The majority of new managers had previously already been employed with clinical titles as senior nurses or belonging to other professional groups. As a result of the new job titles, the public's misperception was that an entirely new group of employees were draining resources from the clinical front line. The growth in managers was accompanied by a political rhetoric of decentralisation that cast local managerial autonomy to gauge and respond more easily to the needs and preferences expressed by local communities. In fact, the role of local populations in influencing decisions and determining priorities was considerably less than proclaimed by the sustained political rhetoric in favour of the local voices. That has remained the case. The NHS is done to people; it does not invite them to participate. Again the new purchaser/provider split, the creation of NHS Trusts and a general management structure within the NHS were never created to deal with mental health services but their implementation in mental health was inevitable as systems of financial and professional accountability were necessarily aligned with acute services.

One unforeseen problem was the sudden creation of a tier of managers, formerly labelled as 'administrators', with new power and authority beyond their wildest dreams. Trevor Robbins has suggested that one possible cost of this newfound authority is that its operation may be degraded under conditions of stress (e.g. resulting from exposure to a profusion of problems requiring difficult decisions). Speculatively, this may be manifest in part as the 'hubris syndrome', which he perceives as an acquired personality disorder that we see often afflicts politicians and others in leadership positions, with serious consequences for society.[8] The same phenomenon was witnessed in the NHS, generally, but I think especially in mental health services where passionately committed new-style managers felt that they could at last wage war on consultant psychiatrists who had had far too much power under the old regime to block developments and impose their own view of the world.[9]

In 1983, I was in a relatively recent appointment as Professor of Old Age Psychiatry at Guy's Hospital, my chair held at the United and Medical Dental Schools, part of the University of London. Crucially both chair and department were paid for by the NHS, so it was clear my job was going to be to develop a much-needed service for the locality as well as to engage in research and I was enthusiastic about the new community-based approach and anyone who would support my ideas. It was a time when Guy's Hospital, part of Lewisham and North Southwark Health Authority, was at the forefront of encouraging doctors into front-line management. One of my first tasks as a new professor, a request from the Department of Health, was to spend a day showing local services to Sir Roy Griffiths, a supermarket executive who had been commissioned to review the management of hospitals (see Chapter 3). I complained to him (this was a rare opportunity to get a hearing with a VIP) that the resources and beds were all in the wrong place; that the local authorities were much more important to my work than anyone recognised; and I had a long list of frustrations I could do nothing about. At the end of the day driving round Southwark and Lewisham, he said, 'So why aren't you and doctors who feel like you becoming managers?' It had never occurred to me. In his subsequent report, he concluded that the traditional NHS management had led to 'institutionalised stagnation'. The report's recommendations, including that hospitals and community services should be managed by general managers, were accepted and he promoted the idea that clinicians who spend the money in services must be responsible for managing it too. The changes introduced as a consequence of the Griffiths Report brought a large increase in general managers in the NHS, from 1,000 in 1986 to 26,000 in 1995, with spending on administration rising dramatically over the same period.[10]

I enthusiastically accepted an invitation to join the District Management Board, without any notion whatever of what 'management' might entail. There was no process of appointment, no one was consulted, but I vaguely thought it was something one could do on a Friday afternoon after everything important was wound up for the weekend. It did not occur to me then but rapidly became apparent that not only did other consultant and academic colleagues resent some female 'whipper-snapper' being appointed but several important men had been slowly waiting their term to be elected by their peers as consultant spokesman for the department. Furthermore, the district health authority was permeated by Labour Party political representatives from our inner-city boroughs who had a vehement revulsion of Thatcherite policies of any kind, whether it was competitive tendering of support services, performance management, devolved financial management or any kind of change in the configuration of even unsafe services. I developed an abiding respect for the NHS professional administrators who had over years learnt to bargain, negotiate, wheedle and cajole what they needed out of a heavy-handed NHS bureaucracy above them and a dismissive set of antipathetic local politicians around them. It was clear that my formerly successful strategy of steamrollering changes through sheer cussedness laced with charm would only go so far. I will admit to developing some hubristic self-confidence that was bound to fail as a long-term management strategy.

The tribal cultures in the NHS have never really been adequately tackled then or now. The problem is both educational and ideological. It is culture that separates medium-status managers and politicians who stay in a post for a relatively short time from high-status clinicians who consider themselves intellectually superior to the managers and who are in post far longer than the managers. Senior clinicians have professional support systems in the Royal Colleges and other institutions that monitor them. Loyalty to a professional specialism is far greater than to an individual employer. This is changing but only very slowly. Nurses felt as alienated from managers as doctors did. They felt that management was too theoretical and out of touch with the daily realities of providing care in a busy and harried environment. Managers were perceived by nurses as being too ready to redecorate their own offices when wards had crumbling paint. Managers saw nurses on the other hand as hopelessly traditional, having a very narrow perspective and largely concerned with making life tolerable for themselves rather than improving the patient's journey. These tribal stereotypes were wrong and fuelled by clinical resentments at what they saw as a misrepresentation of their commitment to their patients.

Conclusion

By 2010, many early managerial innovations had been accepted as normal. There was a far greater tolerance of the notion, hardly controversial, of operating within a budget for example. However, a distinctive feature of the early reforms was also a drive to co-opt professionals themselves into the management of mental health services and it seems that psychiatrists have been peculiarly unwilling to commit themselves away from patient and clinical work. Doctors and nurses rarely now become full-time managers, or even part-time 'hybrid' professional managers, although some are willing to take on temporary clinical director roles and participate in taking responsibility for budgets. One major mistake in the beginning was to emphasise management and downplay the role of personal leadership in inspiring and guiding clinical service change. Professional bodies are now actively supporting and even driving these changes. Clinical leadership has at last moved from 'the dark side' to centre stage at last. There is even a Royal College of Psychiatrists' textbook on how to be a psychiatrist manager.[11] That would have been unthinkable in 1970.

Key Summary Points

- Three key drivers that introduced the new managerialism into mental health services were funding constraints, the drive to measure health care quality and the move to deinstitutionalisation.
- A new cadre of managers, some of which were clinicians, but many of whom were not, often rode roughshod over traditional clinical administration and many psychiatrists and nurses felt ignored and undervalued.
- One major mistake in the beginning was to emphasise management and downplay the role of personal leadership in inspiring and guiding clinical service change.
- Managerialism brought a new understanding of budgets, human resources and objectives into mental health services that was largely positive but mental health services are still fashioned around systems that were established for the acute hospital sector and not readily adapted to mental health service provision.

Notes

1. M. Curtis, *Secret Affairs: Britain's Collusion with Radical Islam*. London: Serpents Tail, 2010.

2. K. Bloor and A. Maynard, Expenditure on the NHS during and after the Thatcher years: Its growth and utilisation. Working Paper No. 113, Centre for Health Economics, University of York 1993. www.york.ac.uk/media/che/documents/papers/discussionpapers/CHE%20Discussion%20Paper%20113.pdf.

3. A. Donabedian, Evaluating the quality of medical care. *Milbank Memorial Fund Quarterly* (1966) 44: 166–206.

4. T. Milewa, J. Valentine and M. Calnan, Managerialism and active citizenship in Britain's reformed health service: Power and community in an era of decentralization. *Social Science and Medicine* (1998) 47: 507–17.

5. D. Abrahamson, Shared housing and long-term mental illness. *Housing, Care and Support* (2014) 17: 41–7, https://doi.org/10.1108/HCS-12-2013-0026.

6. N. Bouras, *Reflections on the Challenges of Psychiatry in the UK and Beyond: A Psychiatrist's Chronicle from Deinstitutionalisation to Community Care*. Pavilion Publishing, 2017.

7. H. Glennerster, The costs of hospital closure: Reproviding services for the residents of Darenth Park Hospital. *Psychiatric Bulletin* (1990) 14: 140–3.

8. D. Owen, Hubris syndrome: An acquired personality disorder? A study of US Presidents and UK Prime Ministers over the last 100 years. *Brain: A Journal of Neurology* (2009) 132: 1396–1406, https://doi.org/10.1093/brain/awp008.

9. T. Robbins, Power, Neurobiology of decision making, gender and the exercise of power. 2017. Power, gender and hubris: Success and arrogance as risks to leadership in health care and beyond. Paper presented at the Royal Society of Medicine conference, London, 9 May 2017, www.daedalustrust.com/power-gender-hubris-conference-video-55-professor-trevor-robbins-neurobiology-of-decision-making-gender-and-the-exercise-of-power-2017.

10. C. Webster, *The National Health Service: A Political History*. Oxford: Oxford University Press, 2002, pp. 253–8.

11. D. Bhugra, S. Bell and A. Burns, eds, Management for Psychiatrists (4th ed.). London: RCPsych Publications, 2016.

Chapter 13

Subjectivity, Citizenship and Mental Health: UK Service User Perspectives

Peter Beresford and Liz Brosnan

In a viral 2009 TED Talk entitled 'The danger of a single story', Nigerian feminist author Chimamanda Ngozi Adichie said, 'How [stories] are told, who tells them, when they're told, how many stories are told, are really dependent on power . . . Power is the ability not just to tell the story of another person but to make it the definitive story of that person.'[1]

Introduction

The focus of this chapter is the impact that UK mental health service users/survivors have made on mental health policy and practice in the period covered by this book through their movement and survivor-led organisations. We write as part of this movement, which we believe probably represents the most significant development in this field and therefore one that demands careful and serious examination, particularly in its broader social, political, policy, cultural and economic contexts. It is our aim to develop that discussion and reflect on the ideas of subjectivity and citizenship as pertaining to this social history more broadly.

Training, Mental Health Services and Diversity

How can one chapter tell a story as diverse and multifaceted as our history? At the same time, it has been invisible to most educators of past generations of psychiatrists as we are aware from teaching students over the past decades. While painfully aware of our privilege as highly educated white, Jewish in the case of Peter, survivors of encounters with psychiatry, we have been participants and observers of the matters of which we write and seek to offer an overview of the history of the survivor movement in the UK up to the 2010. This signposts to other writers who can fill in the gaps for future scholarship and research.[2]

It is imperative that this narrative of our movement's struggles for subjectivity and citizenship is brought to the attention of future psychiatry students and trainees. They can get a foretaste for further encounters with the vibrant, dynamic and diverse layers of activism, resistance and collaboration by those activists and survivor/Mad scholars who demanded recognition for our rights, dignity and citizenship. We in our movements have variously been labelled mental patients and service users and claim our own designations as survivors and Mad scholars. Our narrative is necessarily partial, in that space will never permit a complete and definitive account of the diverse experiences, often glossed over in a homogenising simplification and omission of the underlying tensions, complexities and compromises evident over a period of rapid flourishing of activism and scholarship.

Another reason the opportunity to contribute this chapter is very welcome is because it allows us to point out an implementation gap in mental health services. As stated, we know generations of psychiatrists have not been educated about the activism and achievements within the user/survivor movements which left many practitioners ignorant of the autonomy and agency achieved over the past fifty years. The implementation gap arising from delays in research-based evidence filtering down to practice, plus systemic hurdles involved in changing academic course content, means that it may take years for new knowledge being developed within the user/survivor social movement activist and research endeavours to be accepted as legitimate perspectives. This is exemplified by experience delivering seminars to medical students during their psychiatric training, where my (LB) input on survivor research consisted of two-hour sessions on an elective module. When asked, the students could not speak about what the survivor-developed recovery concepts meant despite being two years into their medical studies already. These are the clinical leaders of the future. Hopefully, inclusion of a brief account of this activity in a significant social history of psychiatry will help future generations of psychiatrists be more aware of what survivor epistemology and tacit knowledge have contributed to our understandings of mental distress and madness.

We aim to introduce readers to the diversity of both activism and experiences within our heterogenous communities, including the silenced voices of BAME, LGBT and indeed women's specific experiences, particularly around motherhood. Very legitimate criticisms of both external and internal historical accounts highlight a homogenising narrative, which has presented accounts from a white, straight and able-bodied perspective. External academic accounts of the user movement have been challenged by the Survivor History Group as distorting and misrepresenting the agency of the service user movement.[3] Internally, the exclusion of the BAME communities' perspectives has been challenged recently by several writers, including Faulkner and Kalathil and Kalathil and Jones.[4] Carr has highlighted the heteronormativity of the user movement.[5] These are the internal reflections of a mature social movement which has developed historically across decades of struggles outlined in the section that follows. We aim also through this work to begin to introduce how the writers and activists in our movement have understood and addressed issues of subjectivity and citizenship.

Social History of the User/Survivor Movement

There is often talk in the UK about ensuring parity between physical and mental health services. This often relates to the funding of mental health services which has increasingly fallen behind that for physical health.[6] Perhaps more revealing are the differences in progress of these two branches of medicine within the National Health Service (NHS) made over this period. Thus, in physical medicine we have seen enormous innovation; the development of heart and other transplants, operations on foetuses, keyhole surgery, joint replacements, massively extended survival rates for many cancers, robotics used in surgery, greatly improved pain control, new diabetes treatments, drug drivers and so on – an almost endless list.

It looks like a very different story in mental health, where patients fifty years apart worryingly could expect little changed treatment. This includes a continuing emphasis on compulsion and restraint;[7] use of electroconvulsive therapy (ECT), despite its evidenced failings;[8] and the ongoing use of drugs like Largactil (chlorpromazine), with well-documented damaging effects like tardive dyskinesia.[9] The psychiatric system is still over-reliant on drug treatments. Psychiatric innovations like 'second-generation antipsychotics' have brought their own problems, including serious 'side' effects and their widespread and problematic use 'off-label' for groups they were not intended for, notably older people with dementia.[10] It has been estimated that a quarter of a million people are dependent on benzodiazepine and related minor tranquillisers, although it has long been known these should only be prescribed for very short periods of time.[11] The 'talking treatments' service users have long called for have been institutionalised to six sessions of cognitive behavioural therapy (CBT) through the IAPT (Improving Access to Psychological Therapy) programme; and such interventions have increasingly been directed at getting mental health service users into paid work, regardless of the nature and quality of such employment or of how helpful it is likely to be for their mental well-being.

Admittedly after massive delays, the grim Victorian 'lunatic asylums' are now largely gone, although some of their intimidating premises still serve as sites for 'treatment'. As other contributors in this book have pointed out, in 1961 Enoch Powell as health minister gave his famous 'Water Tower speech' promising to get rid of them. It was not until the Act of 1990 and the switch to 'community care' that this really happened and then, because the new policy was implemented so poorly, mental health service users, left without adequate help or support, were again stigmatised as 'dangerous' and a threat to 'the public' (see also Chapters 27 and 28).[12]

The lack of progression in the modern psychiatric system and its association with control, abuse and institutionalisation in the 1960s gave impetus to the development of a mental health service user/survivor movement in the UK.[13] While related 'mad person' protests and activism have been identified from the seventeenth century, Peter Campbell, a founding survivor activist, dated the modern UK survivor movement, which has grown on an unprecedented scale, to the mid-1980s, tracing its origins to earlier mental patient groups from the 1970s and acknowledging the help it received from progressive mental health professionals.[14]

The UK mental health service users/survivor movement can be seen as one of the 'new social movements' (NSMs) emerging globally in the second half of the twentieth century, largely based on shared identity and common experiences of oppression – thus the black civil rights, women's, LGBTQ and grey power movements. Certainly, welfare state user movements like those of survivors and disabled people highlighted their links and overlaps with these NSMs.[15] The UK disabled people's movement was in some ways a separatist one, arguing for different kinds of support to that which had been provided and developing its own underpinning model or theory – the social model of disability and related philosophy for change of 'independent living'.[16] The same separatist drive and radically different philosophy does not seem to have been true of the mental health/survivors' movement. The many groups and user organisations that emerged often operated *within* the psychiatric system, its services and related voluntary organisations and were sometimes directly linked with and funded by the services. While the movement did not have the same kind of distinct philosophical basis or perhaps independence as the disabled people's movement, nonetheless it has highlighted a number of common principles that have endured:

- The lives of mental health service users are of equal value to those of others.
- Mental health service users have a right to speak for themselves.
- There is a need to provide non-medicalised services and support.
- Service users' first-hand experience should be valued.

- Discrimination against people with experience of using mental health services must end.[17]

The emergence of the survivor movement, like other service user movements, was also facilitated by the political shift to the right from the late 1970s which was associated with both a renewed emphasis on the market and devaluing of the state and a growing government rhetoric for consumer rights in public services. While this did not necessarily chime with service users' calls for more say and empowerment, it opened doors to them and heralded a new stage in the broader interest in democratisation and public/user participation. Key stages in this history vary from country to country but include the following:

- Working for universal suffrage in representative democracy and the achievement of social rights, like the right to decent housing, education and health, from the late nineteenth to mid-twentieth century.
- Provisions for participatory democracy and community development, associated with the 1960s and 1970s.
- Specific provisions for participation in health and social care, from the1980s through to the first decade of the twenty-first century.
- State reaction and service user–led renewal as conflicts and competing agendas become more explicit, from 2010 onwards.[18]

While mental health service users/survivors were organising and campaigning before the 1980s, from then onwards their activities mushroomed in scale, visibility, impact and effectiveness.[19] Local and national survivor-led organisations were established. International links were developed. There were organisations that focused on particular issues, like the Hearing Voices Network, as well as some that linked with and included other groups of service users, beyond mental health service users/survivors. These included, for example, the Wiltshire and Swindon Users Network as well as Shaping Our Lives, organisations which engaged with a broad range of disabled people and service users, including people with learning difficulties and long-term conditions. There was an emphasis on organising and offering mutual support to mental health service users/survivors who faced particular barriers – for example, if they had difficulty being in public spaces or whose distress might be particularly difficult for them to deal with at particular times – as well as on working together for change.[20]

Much was achieved in many different areas, not least a major challenge to conventional assumptions that service users could not contribute and be effectively involved.[21] Some local groups made arrangements with local hospitals and service providers, enabling members to be on wards to offer information, advice and advocacy. Schemes for collective as well as self-advocacy developed. Service users began to establish user-run services, providing crisis, out-of-hours, advocacy, advice, support and telephone services based on shared experience and first-hand knowledge. Some service users gained skills as survivor/user trainers and took part in academic and in-service training for professional and other mental health workers, offering insights from their lived experience. In social work, this was extended with the new social work degree introduced in 2001, leading to service users and carers being required to be part of all aspects and stages of qualifying training, with a budget from central government to facilitate this.[22]

Survivors and their organisations became involved in processes of service monitoring, quality control, audit, evaluation and review. Perhaps most significantly, the mental health service user movement has developed its own survivor research and research initiatives. Not only have these offered fresh insights on mental health policy and practice, as well as distress from the perspectives and lived experience of survivors, and producing a growing cannon of both qualitative and quantitative research, but they have also resulted in the establishment of a major Service User Research Enterprise (SURE) unit at the internationally feted Institute of Psychiatry, Psychology and Neuroscience in London and also led to a growing number of survivors gaining doctorates and other research qualifications, sourcing research funding, publishing in peer-reviewed journals and securing mainstream research posts.[23] There were some early examples of user-researchers controlling their own research projects, most notably the work in the Sainsbury Centre for Mental Health and the Strategies for Living project in the 1990s;[24] but most of the efforts of user researchers have been occurring within academic spaces that have constrained the parameters of what was possible working within mainstream and services-led research projects. Nevertheless, there has been a flourishing of writing by user-researchers since the initial publication by Beresford and Wallcraft.[25]

However, while survivors and their organisations made significant progress from the 1980s onwards, it often felt from within like two steps forward and one step back. They were unable to achieve any level of funding parity in relation to traditional charitable organisations, and their significant reliance on funding from within the psychiatric system limited their independence.[26] Despite their innovative thinking about new kinds of support, few user-led services were supported or sustained in practice. Increasingly their ideas, from peer support and self-advocacy to recovery and self-management, were taken over and subverted by traditional power holders and service providers. The psychiatric system showed an enormous capacity to resist change while incorporating it at a rhetorical level.[27]

Two convincing arguments have been offered to explain mental health service users' frequent reluctance to distance themselves from conventional psychiatry even though their movement offers a clear philosophical challenge to its medical model, confirmed by research.[28] First seems to have been the fear that, if they challenge the underpinning medical model, then they will be dismissed as in denial about their own pathology and lack of rationality.[29] Second, there seems to be a more generalised reluctance to sign up to any monolithic theories about themselves for fear that these again might dominate and damage them in the same way that they feel psychiatric thinking long has done.[30] However, this has changed with the emergence of Mad studies.[31] While its flowering in the UK and internationally takes us beyond the period covered by this book, its origins and emergence can be traced to that time and therefore it has clear relevance to this discussion.

Subjectivity and Research

The narrative recounting of the user/survivor movement in the UK would be incomplete without considering the direction towards academic participation which flourished over two decades and initiated a new positioning of user-researchers into academic spaces. This generation of user-researchers took us into the struggles for legitimacy as knowers of our own experiences, holders of our own subjectivity.

Often derided by clinician researchers as of lesser credibility than its binary opposite objectivity, subjectivity designates the experience under investigation as a valid source of knowledge. Within the social sciences, decades of healthy debate and controversy surround the standing of knowledge embodied by marginalised peoples excluded from the academy and elite spaces where knowledge about their communities has been generated without their participation. The epistemological bias has been called out by scholars from the marginalised communities, leading to critical new scholarship in, for example, feminist and women's studies, working-class scholarship and Marxist studies, critical race studies and decolonial and disability studies, all of which informed the early mental health user-researchers, and latterly the emergence of Mad studies. Disability studies, for example, fostered a reaction to able-bodied researchers describing the position of disabled people, without any benefits returning to the people studied in terms of material changes to their living situation in congregated institutionalised settings. The work of Oliver, who pioneered the idea of emancipatory disability research, inspired the early user-researchers who railed against their exclusion from knowledge generation about them by detached and objective researchers.[32]

A core element of these critical intellectual and activist endeavours is that they give value and priority to the situated knowledge of those who live with their mental health 'conditions' and under oppressive societal structures, for example physically disabled or racialised people. In the mental health field, user/survivor researchers have equally put forward the arguments that those closest to the experiences under investigation have greater tacit knowledge and insights into the phenomena being studied. This privileging of subjectivity has led to greater insights into, for instance, the experiences of hearing voices, those who self-harm, survivors of suicide attempts and those who undergo ECT.[33]

Later scholarship has illuminated the accumulated experiences of structural oppressions which have greater impact on people with other marginalised identities: racialised people, queer people and other minorities in society. The concept of intersectionality – developed by Kimberle Crenshaw– describes how black women's experiences cannot be understood by solely examining patriarchal oppressions as their racialised experiences were often ignored or silenced by white feminists and their experiences as women not understood within anti-racist movements.[34] Likewise, Kalathil has pointed out how racialised mental health service users experience intersectional oppressions due to the white majorities in the user movement spaces and sanism (prejudice and discrimination against mental health) within anti-racist movements.[35]

There is now increasing recognition of the significance of subjective experience and this has led to demands that survivors be heard and listened to as individuals and not just treated as a statistic or diagnosis. Survivors' claims for validating our subjective knowledge are core to the demands to have our stories listened to. Recent scholarship has dealt with these struggles for justice as knowers of our own experience deploying theoretical concepts such as epistemological justice.[36] Additionally, narrative therapy has led to innovations in how to recognise and address the many oppressions which induce trauma.[37] The significance of the growing evidence on the prevalence of earlier adverse experiences in people who later present to mental health services validates the movement's historical demands for listening to those who use services.[38] This has resulted in a growing demand for trauma-informed mental health services which give people space to tell their stories before arriving at any treatment decisions.

A narrative justice framework has emerged from narrative therapy and trauma work, which highlights the 'storytelling rights' of survivors of injustice and oppression. Narrative justice approaches defend people's rights to 'name their own experiences; to define their own problems, and to honour how their skills, abilities, relationships, history and culture can contribute to reclaiming their lives from the effects of trauma'; and the framework centres on an ethical question: 'When meeting with people whose problems are the result of human rights abuses and injustices, how can we ensure we do not separate healing from justice?' The Dulwich Centre, an Australian-based narrative therapy organisation, has created a Charter of Story-Telling Rights,[39] which include the right of survivors 'to define their experiences and problems in their own words and terms' and 'to be free from having problems caused by trauma and injustice located inside them, internally, as if there is some deficit in them. The person is not the problem, the problem is the problem.' These narrative justice aims are consistent with many of the rights claimed by service users over the decades.

Citizenship

We are not isolated individuals but live in families and in societies. How people treat us once it becomes known that we have experienced distress or acquired a psychiatric diagnosis leads to the final part of our considerations, that is, struggles for citizenship. Citizenship is a concept embedded within political theory and participatory democracy, which asserts the rights of everyone to participate in a society even though not all have equal access to citizenship privileges.[40] Citizenship is linked to the notion of belonging to a society, of having rights and associated duties. In human rights legal scholarship and disability rights, disabled people are rights holders, for which the state is the duty bearer; that is, the state has obligations towards its citizens. Of course, many reject the notion of citizenship as an inclusive concept because many people around the world are denied citizenship and it is applied unequally based on difference.[41] Nevertheless, when understood in the context of second-class citizenship, it can be a useful way to examine the experiences of people with mental health diagnoses.

There is pervasive stigma and discrimination against people using mental health services (for a fuller discussion, see also Chapter 27). However, we draw attention to a specific aspect of discrimination against psychiatrised people and the way it denies them full citizenship and most essentially epistemic justice as knowers of our own realities. Sanism, a term coined by Perlin, is expanded on in greater depth by Mad scholars.[42] Sanism, they argue, operates to deny us credibility and citizenship, positioning us as lesser citizens. Indeed, sanism is used to justify separate laws to treat people against their will, as mental health legislation is drawn up by governments to address this anomaly in citizenship and human rights.[43]

The legal basis for state violence, as identified by early advocates against forced removal to psychiatric establishments and treatment imposed by medical experts against one's will,[44] has been described as akin to kidnapping. Lindow has argued that any other people undergoing forced removal and interventions experienced as traumatic would receive post-traumatic counselling and support.[45] It is this practice along with the institutionalisation of many people, preventing full participation in society, which were the primary concerns of the many psychiatric survivors who participated in the negotiation of the UN Convention on the Rights of Persons with Disabilities (CRPD) (see Chapter 8). Detailed discussion of the UN CRPD is beyond the scope of this chapter, but there is a wide and growing body of literature and activism considering the rights of people to live lives where they are fully encouraged to be active in their communities and it warrants serious attention from all areas of psychiatry and all mental health professionals.[46]

Conclusion

Our account concludes at the point where new knowledges have blossomed due to international collaborations enabled by developments in internet access and the arrival of survivor researchers and Mad scholars into academic spaces. It is necessarily short and incomplete, as a full narrative would itself fill volumes. It is offered in an attempt to introduce readers to work that is usually ignored, undervalued and struggling for adequate funding which would allow the work to blossom further and demonstrate its potential to contribute to practice both inside and independently of mental health services.

Key Summary Points

- The user/survivor movement represents a most significant development in mental health and therefore demands careful and serious examination, particularly in its broader social, political, policy, cultural and economic contexts.
- Generations of psychiatrists have not been educated about the activism and achievements within the user/survivor movements, which left many practitioners ignorant of the autonomy and agency achieved over the past fifty years.
- The UK mental health service users/survivor movement is one of the 'new social movements' (NSMs), including black civil rights, women's, LGBTQ and grey power, emerging globally in the second half of the twentieth century, largely based on shared identity and common experiences of oppression.
- The survivor movement, like other service user movements, was facilitated by the political shift to the right from the late 1970s which was associated with a renewed emphasis on the market, devaluing of the state and growing government rhetoric for consumer rights in public services. While this did not necessarily chime with service users' calls for more say and empowerment, it opened doors to them and heralded a new stage in the broader interest in democratisation and public/user participation.
- In the mental health field, user/survivor researchers have put forward the arguments that those closest to the experiences under investigation have greater tacit knowledge and insights into the phenomena being studied.

Notes

1. C. N. Adichie, The danger of a single story, Ted Talks [Online], July 2009, www.ted.com/talks/chimaman da_ngozi_adichie_the_danger_of_a_single_story?language=en.

2. EURIKHA and Still we Rise at www.eurikha.org.

3. N. Crossley, *Contesting Psychiatry: Social Movements in Mental Health*. Abingdon: Routledge, 2006; Survivor History Group. The Survivor History Group takes a critical look at historians. In M. Barnes and P. Cotterell, eds, *Critical Perspectives on User Involvement*, 7–18. Bristol: Policy Press, 2012.

4. A. Faulkner and J. Kalathil, *The Freedom to Be, the Chance to Dream: Preserving User-led Peer Support in Mental Health*. London: Together, 2012; J. Kalathil and N. Jones, Unsettling disciplines: Madness, identity, research, knowledge. *Philosophy, Psychiatry, and Psychology* (2016) 23: 183–8.

5. S. Carr, Seldom heard or frequently ignored? Lesbian, gay and bisexual (LGB) perspectives on mental health services. *International Journal of Human Rights in Healthcare* (2010) 3: 14.

6. D. Campbell, Mental health still losing out in NHS funding report finds. *The Guardian*, 16 January 2018, www .theguardian.com/society/2018/jan/16/mental-health-still-losing-out-in-nhs-funding-report-finds.

7. A. Molodynski, J. Rugkåsa and T. Burns, Coercion and compulsion in community mental health care. *British Medical Bulletin* (2010) 95: 105–19.

8. D. Rose, P. Fleischmann and T. Wykes, Consumers' views of electroconvulsive therapy: A qualitative analysis. *Journal of Mental Health* (2004) 13: 285–93.

9. J. R. Scarff and D. A. Casey, Newer oral atypical antipsychotic agents: A review. *Pharmacy and Therapeutics* (2011) 36: 832.

10. Ibid.

11. J. Davies, T. C. Rae and L. Montagu, Long-term benzodiazepine and Z-drugs use in England: A survey of general practice. *British Journal of General Practice* (2017) 67: e609–13, https://bjgp.org/content/67/662/e609.

12. A. Rogers and D. Pilgrim, *Mental Health Policy In Britain: A Critical Introduction* (2nd ed.). Basingstoke: Palgrave Macmillan, 2001.

13. L. O. Gostin, From a civil libertarian to a sanitarian: 'A life of learning'. Presidential address to the Faculty Convocation, Georgetown University Law Center, Washington, October 2010.

14. P. Campbell, The service user/survivor movement. In J. Reynolds, R. Muston and T. Heller et al., eds, *Mental Health Still Matters*, 46–52. Basingstoke: Palgrave, 2009.

15. A. Lent, *British Social Movements since 1945: Sex, Colour, Peace and Power*. Basingstoke: Palgrave Macmillan, 2002.

16. J. Campbell and M. Oliver, *Disability Politics: Understanding Our Past, Changing Our Future*. London: Routledge, 1996.

17. Survivors Speak Out. Charter of needs and demands (Edale Conference Charter), agreed and presented at the Survivors Speak Out conference, London, 18–20 September 1987.

18. P. Beresford, Public participation in health and social care: Exploring the co-production of knowledge. *Frontiers in Sociology* (2019) 4: 41.

19. J. Reynolds, R. Muston, T. Heller et al., eds, *Mental Health Still Matters*. Basingstoke: Palgrave, 2009.

20. F. Branfield, P. Beresford, E. J. Andrews et al., *Making User Involvement Work: Supporting Service User Networking and Knowledge*. York: Joseph Rowntree Foundation and York Publishing Services, 2006.

21. P. Beresford and P. Campbell, Participation and protest: Mental health service users/survivors. In M. J. Todd and G. Taylor, eds, *Democracy and Participation: Popular Protest and New Social Movements*, 326–42. London: Merlin Press, 2004.

22. Ibid.

23. A. Sweeney, P. Beresford, A. Faulkner, M. Nettle and D. Rose, eds, *This Is Survivor Research*. Ross-on-Wye: PCSS Books, 2009.

24. N. Kotecha, C. Fowler, A. Donskoy et al., *A Guide to User-focused Monitoring*. London: Sainsbury Centre for Mental Health, 2007; A. Faulkner and S. Layzell, *Strategies for Living: A Summary Report of User-led Research into People's Strategies for Living with Mental Distress*. London: Mental Health Foundation, 2000, www.mentalhealth.org.uk/sites/default/files/strategies_for_living_update.pdf.

25. P. Beresford and J. Wallcraft, Psychiatric system survivors and emancipatory research: issues, overlaps and differences. In C. Barnes and G. Mercer, eds, *Doing Disability Research*, 66–87. Leeds: The Disability Press, 1997.

26. B. I. Field and K. Reed, The rise and fall of the Mental Health Recovery model. *International Journal of Psychosocial Rehabilitation* (2016) 20.

27. Ibid.

28. P. Beresford, R. Perring, M. Nettle and J. Wallcraft, *From Mental Illness to a Social Model of Madness and Distress? Exploring What Service Users Say*. London: Shaping Our Lives and National Survivor User Network (NSUN), 2016.

29. P. Campbell, The history of the user movement in the United Kingdom. In T. Heller, J. Reynolds, R. Gomm, R. Muston and S. Patterson, eds, *Mental Health Matters: A Reader*, Basingstoke, Macmillan and Open University, 1996.

30. A. Plumb, *Distress or Disability? A Discussion Document*. Manchester: Greater Manchester Coalition of Disabled People, 1994.

31. B. A. LeFrançois, R. Menzies, G. Reaume, eds, *Mad Matters: A Critical Reader in Canadian Mad Studies.* Toronto: Canadian Scholars' Press, 2013.

32. Campbell and M. Oliver, Disability politics. In M. Oliver and C. Barnes, eds, *Social Policy and Disabled People: From Exclusion to Inclusion.* London: Longman, 1998.

33. P. Bullimore, Altering the balance of power: Working with voices. *International Journal of Narrative Therapy & Community Work* (2003) 2003: 22, https://search.informit.com.au/documentSummary;d n=634012147835668;res=IELIND; D. Corstens, E. Longden and R. May, Talking with voices: Exploring what is expressed by the voices people hear. *Psychosis* (2012) 4(2): 95–104; R. Waddingham, Me and the meds: A personal story of a dysfunctional relationship. *Mental Health Nursing (Online)* (2014) 34: 16. https://search .proquest.com/openview/b3dba5224a627611ac441c0e99cdc31b/1?pq-origsite=gscholar&cbl=135348; L. R. Pembroke, *Self Harm.* Brentwood: Chipmunka Publishing, 2005; D. Webb, A role for spiritual self-enquiry in suicidology? Thinking about suicide. PhD thesis, Victoria University, 2006; Rose, Fleischmann and Wykes, Consumers' views of electroconvulsive therapy.

34. K. Crenshaw, Mapping the margins: Intersectionality, identity politics, and violence against women of color. *Stanford Law Review* (1990) 43: 1241.

35. J. Kalathil, *Dancing to Our Own Tunes: Reassessing Black and Minority Ethnic Mental Health Service User Involvement.* London: National Survivor User Network in collaboration with Catch-a-Fiya, https://survivor-research.com/publications/dancing-to-our-own-tunes-reassessing-black-and-minority-ethnic-mental-health-service-user-involvement/.

36. S. Leblanc and E. A. Kinsella, Toward epistemic justice: A critically reflexive examination of 'sanism' and implications for knowledge generation. *Studies in Social Justice* (2016) 10: 59–78.

37. S. Madigan, *Narrative Therapy.* Washington, DC: American Psychological Association, 2011.

38. A. Sweeney, B. Filson, A. Kennedy, L. Collinson and S. Gillard, A paradigm shift: Relationships in trauma-informed mental health services. *BJPsych Advances* (2018) 24: 319–33.

39. D. Denborough, Recent developments in narrative responses to social suffering (n.d.), http://therapeutic conversations.com/wp-content/uploads/2012/05/David-Denborough-handout.pdf.

40. I. M. Young, *Inclusion and Democracy.* Oxford: Oxford University Press, 2000.

41. Ibid.; R. Lister, *Citizenship: Feminist Perspectives* (2nd ed.). Basingstoke: Palgrave Macmillan, 2003.

42. L. Brosnan, 'The lion's den': The epistemic dimensions of invisible emotional labour in service-user involvement spaces. *Journal of Ethics in Mental Health* (2019) 10: 1–6.

43. F. Beaupert, Freedom of opinion and expression: From the perspective of psychosocial disability and madness. *Laws* (2018) 7: 3.

44. V. Lindow, *Self Help and Alternatives.* London: Mental Health Foundation.

45. V. Lindow, Power and rights: The psychiatric system survivor movement. In R. Jack, ed., *Empowerment in Community Care*, 203–21. Boston, MA: Springer, 1995.

46. F. Beaupert and L. Brosnan, The CRPD and weaponizing absent knowledges: Countering the violence of mental health law. In J. Russo, P. Beresford and K. Boxall, eds, *Routledge Handbook of Mad Studies.* Abingdon: Routledge, 2020.

14

How the Voice of People with Mental Health Problems, Families and the Voluntary Sector Changed the Landscape

Paul Farmer and Emily Blackshaw

Introduction

The years 1960–2010 mark a period of radical transformation for mental health in Britain. Like all social change, there were many actors in enabling the transformation to take place. This chapter focuses on the role of people with 'lived experience', their families and voluntary organisations in acting as catalysts, enablers and, in some cases, architects for change. The move from institutionalised care to care in the community was partly caused by, and in turn further strengthened, the voices of people with mental health problems. People with mental health problems and the friends and family who supported them, alongside other stakeholders and practitioners, formed, influenced and supported voluntary mental health organisations. The voluntary sector has since been a prominent and vocal force in mental health, supporting the rights of those with mental health problems and filling gaps in service provision, where community care has sometimes fallen short. Charities are in a unique position, sitting outside of statutory care and clinic-based spaces, allowing them to build reciprocal and trust-based relationships with the communities that they serve. The voluntary sector must continue to push for the voice of people with mental health problems to be front and centre of mental health service delivery and policymaking.

Deinstitutionalisation: From Asylums to Care in the Community

Going back as far as the Middle Ages, asylums were the main route of care for those with mental health problems.[1] Asylums existed in an unregulated and inconsistent form across England in the eighteenth century, and it was not until the 1808 Country Asylums Act that 'Lunatic Asylums' were officially established for the poor and 'criminally insane'. These were further regulated with the 1845 Lunacy Act, which importantly changed the status of those it served from 'people' to 'patients'.[2] Up until the establishment of the National Health Service (NHS), mental health services were subject to the 1890 Lunacy Act and the 1930 Mental Treatment Act, which set the terms for compulsory detention and treatment without certification.[3] As one patient described their experience of being committed to Ticehurst Asylum in 1875, 'my liberty, and my very existence as an individual being, had been signed away behind my back'.[4] People had no voice, they were 'out of sight and out of mind', locked away by a society which simply could not cope with mental ill health and consequentially stigmatised those who had mental health problems.

The First World War threw mental health problems into sharp relief. Approximately 80,000 British soldiers were treated for a range of war neuroses, generally known as 'shell shock', presenting with symptoms including tics, obsessive thoughts, fatigue and paralysis.[5] Military medical professionals acknowledged the need to act on mental health, in order to preserve the morale and manpower of their troops, but this was far from the era of 'psychological modernity' that some argued enlightened post-war Britain.[6] Psychotherapy remained the exception to the rule in terms of treatments for shell shock, which included medicinal remedies of iron, arsenic and Ovaltine as well as electrotherapy.[7] Some doctors, such as W. H. R. Rivers (who famously treated the poet Siegfried Sassoon at Craiglockhart War Hospital) explored the psychological causes of shell shock, prescribing the 'talking cure' alongside creative activities.[8] The collective trauma experienced by the British public during the First and Second World Wars may also have softened attitudes towards mental health and its treatment.

After the Second World War, society in Britain became increasingly concerned with social fairness, reflecting the wider political consensus for universal human rights (UN/ European declarations on human rights, later extended to the rights of disabled people),[9] as well as marked changes in social order and structures, including the provision of universal health care. Two key changes started to emerge: the formation and gathering of voluntary organisations and the increasing opportunity for people with mental health problems to have a voice. These were not always easy encounters, with deep-seated stigma and resistance to the idea that 'the mad' could possibly have a view. Equally, family voices were often marginalised, caught between the clinician and the service user. In Alan Bennett's *Untold Stories*, he refers to his mother's history of depression and his grandfather's suicide and bemoans the lack of support available for families without unusual symptoms, 'mistake your wife for a hat and the doctor will never be away from your bedside'.[10]

A Series of Scandals: Increased Service User Voice and Pressure from the Voluntary Sector

In the 1950s and 1960s, several mental health hospital scandals broke, supported by accounts from people who were treated there, including Farleigh, South Ockendon and Normansfield (see also Chapter 7). The investigation into long-stay wards at Ely Hospital in Cardiff took place between 1967 and 1968 and is often cited as the start of 'an avalanche of scandal in mental health,'[11] although an earlier exposé *Sans Everything: A Case to Answer* foreshadowed many of the revelations.[12] The Ely Committee reported evidence of rough and cruel treatment, inhumane and threatening behaviour towards patients and the pilfering of patients' belongings and food.[13] Despite the best attempts of the government (the Ministry of Health sought to keep the Ely inquiry private, limiting a public appeal for witnesses and keeping the scope of the inquiry narrow),[14] the allegations were supported and the story broke, shocking a concerned public and leading to increased governmental pressure. Other prominent scandals were featured heavily in the media, including the Shelton Hospital fire and overcrowding at Warwick Central Hospital, and calls for action were demanded by voluntary organisations. Mind (then known as the National Association for Mental Health, NAMH) condemned the handling of the inquiries in the *Observer* and worked in solidarity with service user groups such as the Patients' Association calling for more independent inquiries and support for the Post-Ely Working Party.[15] Calls for changes to the 1959 Mental Health Act were also supported by the combined voices of people with mental health problems and pressure from groups such as NAMH.[16]

The voluntary sector remained at the forefront of the ongoing call for deinstitutional-isation. The then minister of health, Enoch Powell, made his remarkable 'Water Tower speech' at NAMH's annual conference in March 1961, where he called for the closure of large psychiatric hospitals, menacingly describing them as 'isolated, majestic, imperious, brooked over by the gigantic water-tower and chimney combined, rising unmistakeable and daunting out of the countryside'.[17] This was promptly followed by supportive legislation, including the 1962 A Hospital Plan for England and Wales, calling for the closure of all mental health beds by 1975, and the 1971 Hospital Services for the Mentally Ill White Paper, proposing the complete abolition of the hospital system for mental health care (see also Chapter 1).

The movement towards deinstitutionalisation in the 1960s and 1970s was considered a 'public and moral necessity'.[18] This shift in approach from institutionalised care to care in the community has been attributed to many causes, including the rise of psychopharma-cology, a desire to cut public expenditure, an increased emphasis on human rights and advances in social science and philosophy (see also Chapter 31).[19] Bolstering the call for the closure of asylums was a strong service user voice, providing harrowing accounts of experiences of care and calling for patient emancipation. The Mental Patients' Union was one such group established in 1973 to demand civil and economic rights for patients, including the abolition of compulsory treatment, increased communication of treatment options and risks and the abolition of isolation as treatment.[20] NAMH was also centring the voices of people with mental health problems in its work, with a 1969 article in Hospital World emphasising that the charity had 'developed from a polite, reassuring body, uttering words of comfort to all those involved with mental health, to an organisation which is now firmly on the side of the patient and not at all scared of speaking its mind when the need arises'.[21]

The journey from institutionalised to community care dominated NAMH annual conference agendas over this period – from 'Rehabilitation and Resettlement of Mentally Disordered People' in 1977 to 'Breakthrough: Making Community Care Work' in 1994. These events were often characterised by outpourings of frustration and anger about the poor state of services, the coercive nature of poor-quality treatment and the lack of support or recognition for people with their own experiences of mental health problems. These events acted as a convening point for many people who had struggled to find a voice.

Were Communities Ready for Care in the Community?

Deinstitutionalisation in mental health care involved three core strategies: discharging patients from hospital wards; decreasing or halting hospital admissions; and implementing alternative community-based interventions (see also Chapter 30).[22] Discharging patients and reducing admissions was largely successful, with a sharp reduction from 143,700 mental health inpatients in England in 1950 to 49,000 in 1990; the length of stays also reduced dramatically from an average stay of 863 days in 1950 to just 83 days in 1990.[23] The success of implementing community-based interventions, however, was less certain. As part of the reconfiguration of mental health services under the 1962 Hospital Plan for England and Wales, acute psychiatric inpatient services were developed at general hospitals, outpatient capacity was increased and local authorities developed community mental health teams.

The voluntary sector played a crucial role alongside local and district health authorities in managing and delivering community-based services.[24] Throughout the gradual closure of psychiatric hospitals, it became increasingly clear that community statutory services could not meet all the needs of people who were experiencing mental distress or had learning/intellectual disabilities. This placed a greater responsibility on the families of those with mental health problems in terms of providing care.[25] It also coincided with an increase in voluntary sector organisations supporting people with mental health problems. Groups of psychiatrists, people experiencing mental health problems and other stakeholders organised themselves into voluntary sector organisations. There was an established legacy in this. Samaritans had been founded by vicar Chad Varah in 1953. The origins of the Mental Health Foundation were established as the Mental Health Research Fund in 1949. The oldest mental health charity in the UK had been Together for Mental Wellbeing, which was originally established in 1879 and had worked to find housing for female patients discharged from asylums.

Mind had been founded as the National Association for Mental Health in 1946. In 1971, NAMH launched its twenty-fifth anniversary Mind campaign, which was so successful that, in 1972, the organisation adopted Mind as its new name. The campaign sought to clarify the organisation's aims, raise funds, increase public awareness of mental health and improve hospital and community services. Under the influence of the organisation's new director, Tony Smythe, it took on a social model of care and sought to support those also receiving care in the community, as well as in hospital. As part of the 1974 strategy, Mind worked to establish more regional offices, in order to support local Mind associations across England and Wales. It also strengthened its campaign for improvements to services at a local level, as it became increasingly evident that statutory services could not meet the needs of all people experiencing mental health problems. From the 1970s through to the 1990s, concern around community care dominated the charity's public education and fundraising campaigns: 'Home from Hospital' in 1976 emphasised the housing problems faced by people discharged from hospital wards; 'A Better Life' in 1986 called for increased resources in order to develop an effective local network of care; and 'Breakthrough! Community Care' in 1994 attempted to advance a service user–centred and holistic approach to mental health care in the community.[26]

Local associations for mental health were newly established throughout this period in response to the needs of the community. Often formed by family members or local community leaders following the closure of an asylum, local Minds and other voluntary organisations provided hope and help in communities where people with mental health problems were often feared and stigmatised. Since this point, local Minds grew in number up to more than 200 by the start of the next century and had grown in scope too. Today, local Minds offer a variety of services to the public, including counselling and psychological therapies, housing schemes, social clubs and day centres. Arguably, voluntary and community organisations can go beyond what is offered by statutory services delivered in clinical settings; they become rooted in the communities in which they are situated, work alongside people with mental health problems to provide user-led interventions and become trusted by those people they serve.[27]

While support for people was an important role for the voluntary sector, it was not sufficient. As seen in the section 'A Series of Scandals: Increased Service User Voice and Pressure from the Voluntary Sector', there was a wider need for people to be regarded as equal citizens, receiving respect in society. This required mobilisation on a societal level, with campaigning, legal work and policy influencing a part of this new agenda for change. The 1970s marked a decided change in Mind's positioning in the voluntary sector. In 1975, the first legal officer was appointed and Mind began promoting itself as a lobbying group. In a 1981 issue of *Mind Out*,[28] Mind's then medical advisor, Anthony Clare, noted that 'Mind has developed a lusty appetite for legal reform and the issue of patients' civil rights'. Prominent campaigners who worked at Mind included civil rights lawyer Larry Gostin, Labour MP Tessa Jowell and disability and mental health campaigner Liz Sayce. In 1979, the legal and welfare rights service became a fully fledged legal department (see also Chapter 8). Mind's subsequent campaigns again demonstrated the preoccupation with deinstitutionalisation – from the 'Home from Hospital' 1976 campaign, highlighting the housing problems faced by people with mental health problems, to the 1986 'A Better Life' campaign, raising public awareness of the lack of resources for the development of a local network of care. Gostin's 1975 publication with Mind, *A Human Condition*, is said to have largely influenced the 1982 Mental Health (Amendment) Act, including increased opportunities for tribunal review, as well as detailed regulations for consent and treatment.[29] The 'Breakthrough! Community Care' campaign in 1994 demanded 'proper care in the community'. In January 1995, Tessa Jowell MP presented the Community Care Bill to the House of Commons alongside Mind, which highlighted the failures of the government to properly implement the Community Care Act, meaning that care in the community was 'far from an effective reality'.

The Role of Family, Friends and Carers

Mental health care in the community meant shared care of people with mental health problems, from both mental health professionals and family members. The Schizophrenia Fellowship (now Rethink Mental Illness) was founded in 1972, after a father, John Pringle, shared his son's experience of schizophrenia in the *Times*. In 1973, Rethink launched its first support groups for carers and three years later received its first government funding to expand this work.[30] Then, in 1995, Rethink published its ground-breaking *Silent Partners* report commissioned by the Department of Health, which was the largest survey at that time of those caring for people with mental health problems. Many of the issues highlighted in that survey still resonate today. The C4C (Caring for Carers) survey reported on seventy-one UK respondents who were caring for a family member with a severe mental illness in 2015.[31] It found that family caregivers had typically cared for their relative for sixteen years and spend approximately twenty-nine hours per week caregiving. The report also highlighted that support for these carers was lacking and they often felt unheard. Worryingly, the UK ranks the highest internationally in terms of perceived stigma felt by family caregivers in seeking professional help.

More recently, the efforts of carers, in the form of family and friends, have been better recognised in mental health service provision and research. As highlighted in a 2017 paper on carer involvement in mental health inpatient units,[32] engaging carers in mental health treatment can help to improve patient symptoms and quality of life as well as reduce inpatient admissions.[33] Consequently, more and more mental health policies recommend the involvement of carers in the treatment of people with mental health problems. For instance, the 2010 UK publication *Recognised, Valued and Supported: Next Steps for the Carers Strategy* focused on how best to support both carers and those they care for.[34] The 2014 Care Act built on these intentions by enabling carers to complete a carer's assessment to obtain support from their local authority.

Despite these positive steps, many barriers still exist that prevent carers from becoming fully involved in their family member's or friend's mental health care, with perspectives of people with mental health problems and carers still sorely lacking in services and research literature.[35] Carers of people receiving mental health care in the UK have experienced difficulties in navigating these services, with communication gaps and discontinuities in treatment. In a qualitative exploration of these experiences, a carer of her son with schizophrenia expressed her frustration with repeated staff changes in services: 'as soon as I get to know one, then they've gone. It used to be very upsetting, very disruptive, because every time there was a new doctor or a new key worker or a new social worker, or whoever, you've got to start right from scratch.' Another woman caring for her husband with schizophrenia expressed the difficulties when carers have to work with mental health professionals with whom they have no established contact: 'it's an absolutely vital lifeline to have somebody that knows you, that listens to you, that responds to you, at the other end of the phone.' Voluntary organisations such as Rethink and the Carer's Trust are still fighting to support these individuals in carer roles and to ensure their voices are at the centre of conversations around mental health support in the UK.

Tackling Stigma

Stigmatising attitudes towards mental health problems have existed in various forms since before the establishment of asylums in Britain. For a long time, stigma meant that people experiencing mental health problems were kept out of sight. As segregated care moved to care in the community, the conversation shifted from concern for the welfare of those patients discharged into the community to fears of dangerousness and a desire to protect the public. The murder of Jonathan Zito ignited public fear and popular 'mad axeman' and 'psychopathic murderer' myths dominated debate around community care.[36] People were keen to protect themselves and the communities in which they lived; a survey carried out in 1994 by the Department of Health showed that 22 per cent of people in the UK felt that locating mental health facilities in a residential area would downgrade the area.[37] Fears of dangerousness still exist today and are perpetuated in the media. For instance, a study in 2019 of tweets about mental health generated by the UK national press revealed that 24 per cent of tweets presented mental illness as 'bad news' stories, as opposed to 'understanding' stories.[38] The global director of Time to Change, Sue Baker OBE, stressed that 'we are still picking up the pieces from terrible headlines of "mad psycho killers" mid to late 90s'.[39]

The voluntary sector and government increased their efforts to tackle these stigmatising attitudes towards mental health. In 1997, the Health Education Authority launched their making headlines initiative, pushing for less sensationalised portrayals of mental illness in the national press. A study at the time showed that nearly half of articles in the news media referencing mental health presented it negatively and associated mental illness with criminality and violence.[40] The SHiFT anti-stigma campaign was launched to promote a disability-inclusion model of mental health and involved cross-departmental governmental input. In more recent times, Rethink and Mind jointly launched the Time to Change campaign in 2007 to tackle stigma, which has reported a 9.6 per cent positive change in attitudes towards mental health between 2008 and 2016. While stigmatising attitudes towards mental health still exist today, these are slowly starting to change for the better.

These campaigns were centred around the voices of people with mental health problems. Time to Change established a community of thousands of champions, people with lived experience, who could tell their own story.[41] These champions challenge stigma around mental health by sharing their experiences, talking about their mental health, forming campaigning groups and influencing the work of the Time to Change campaign. One champion, Sophie, feels that 'involving yourself in open and non-judgemental conversations regarding mental health is an absolutely crucial first step towards fighting stigma and ending discrimination'.[42] This work has helped to put the voices of people with mental health problems at the forefront of mental health campaigning. As one champion, Sian, puts it, 'the way society views mental health is changing. We are talking more and more, showing people that it is OK not to be OK, that it can happen to any of us.'[43] By the time the period 1960–2010 was coming to an end, the same voices were back on the streets campaigning for better mental health legislation.

Mind's approach to tackling stigma has long been focused on creating space for the voices of those experiencing mental health problems. For instance, the October 1974 edition of *Mind Out* was devoted entirely to the experiences and views of people with experience of mental health problems, and in 1987 Mind launched the service user advisory group Mindlink.[44] Mind continues to ensure that lived experience is at the centre of its work, with people with mental health problems involved in strategy planning, service development as well as governance, with a commitment that at least half of Mind's board have lived experience of mental health problems.

Conclusion

The voluntary sector has been an adaptive but constant source of support for individuals with mental health problems throughout this period of dramatic transformation in mental health services between 1960 and 2010. Charities sought to assist in providing local-level support when the vast majority of care moved from hospital wards to care in the community. The voluntary sector also fought to tackle the stigmatising attitudes towards mental health that negatively impacted communities as mental health patients were discharged. Ensuring that people with lived experience of mental health problems were heard and respected has been at the core of this work. Charities, such as Mind, continue to fight against stigmatising attitudes and to develop and deliver user-led community-based interventions to support all those people in need of help.

Key Summary Points

- The move from institutionalised care to care in the community was partly caused by, and in turn further strengthened, the voices of people with mental health problems.
- Charities are in a unique position, sitting outside of statutory care and clinic-based spaces, allowing them to build reciprocal and trust-based relationships with the communities that they serve.
- Mind (then known as the National Association for Mental Health, NAMH) condemned the handling of the 1970s inquiries into psychiatric hospitals in the *Observer* and worked in solidarity with service user groups such as the Patients' Association calling for more independent inquiries. Mind's approach to tackling stigma has long been focused on creating space for the voices of those experiencing mental health problems.

- Worryingly, the UK ranks the highest internationally in terms of perceived stigma felt by family caregivers in seeking professional help. The Schizophrenia Fellowship (now Rethink Mental Illness), founded in 1972 after a father, John Pringle, shared his son's experience of schizophrenia in the *Times*, launched its first support groups for carers and three years later received its first government funding to expand this work.
- Time to Change established a community of thousands of champions, people with lived experience, who could tell their own story. These champions challenge stigma around mental health by sharing their experiences, talking about their mental health, forming campaigning groups and influencing the work of the Time to Change campaign.

Notes

1. S. Lawton-Smith and A. McCulloch, *A Brief History of Specialist Mental Health Services*. London: Mental Health Foundation, 2013.

2. A. Rogers and D. Pilgrim, *Mental Health Policy in Britain*. London: Palgrave Macmillan, 2001.

3. J. Turner, R. Hayward, K. Angel et al., The history of mental health services in modern England: Practitioner memories and the direction of future research. *Medical History* (2015) 59: 599–624.

4. H. C. Merivale, *My Experiences in a Lunatic Asylum: By a Sane Patient*. Glasgow: Good Press, 2019.

5. F. Reid, 'His nerves gave way': Shell shock, history and the memory of the First World War in Britain. *Endeavour* (2014) 38: 91–100.

6. T. Loughran, Shell-shock and psychological medicine in First World War Britain. *Social History of Medicine* (2009) 22: 79–95.

7. Loughran, Shell-shock and psychological medicine; Reid, 'His nerves gave way'.

8. T. E. Webb, 'Dottyville': Craiglockhart War Hospital and shell-shock treatment in the First World War. *Journal of the Royal Society of Medicine* (2006) 99: 342–6.

9. N. Bouras, Historical and international perspectives of services. In C. Hemmings and N. Bouras, eds, *Psychiatric and Behavioural Disorders in Intellectual and Developmental Disabilities*, 3rd ed., 1–14. Cambridge: Cambridge University Press, 2016.

10. A. Bennett, Untold *Stories*. London: Faber & Faber, 2008.

11. I. Butler, M. Drakeford and J. Campling, *Scandal, Social Policy and Social Welfare*. Bristol: Policy Press, 2005; C. A. Hilton, A tale of two inquiries: *Sans Everything* and Ely. *The Political Quarterly* (2019) 90: 185–93.

12. B. Robb, *Sans Everything: A Case to Answer*. London: Thomas Nelson, 1967.

13. C. Hilton, Whitewash and after: 'Most good is done by stealth.' In C. Hilton, *Improving Psychiatric Care for Older People*, 201–49. London: Palgrave Macmillan, 2017.

14. Ibid.

15. Ibid.

16. Turner, Hayward, Angel et al., The history of mental health services in modern England.

17. Enoch Powell's Water Tower Speech 1961. High Royds Hospital website (n.d.), www.highroydshospital.com /resource/enoch-powells-water-tower-speech-1961/.

18. A. Charlesworth, R. Murray, L. Bennett et al., *Making Change Possible: A Transformation Fund for the NHS*. London: Health Foundation and the King's Fund, 2015.

19. Lawton-Smith and McCulloch, Brief History of Specialist Mental Health Services; Turner, Hayward, Angel et al., The history of mental health services in modern England; Charlesworth, Murray, Bennett et al., Making change possible.

20. Unknown [S.], The Mental Patients Union, 1973. libcom.org website, 21 March 2017, https://libcom.org/history/mental-patients-union-1973.

21. Mind, A history of Mind. Mind website (n.d.), www.mind.org.uk/about-us/what-we-do/our-mission/a-history-of-mind/.

22. Charlesworth, Murray, Bennett et al., Making change possible.

23. Turner, Hayward, Angel et al., The history of mental health services in modern England.

24. Charlesworth, Murray, Bennett et al., Making change possible.

25. A. J. Shah, O. Wadoo and J. Latoo, Psychological distress in carers of people with mental disorders. *British Journal of Medical Practitioners* (2010) 3: 18–25.

26. Mind, A history of Mind.

27. L. Weeks, Mental health charities can help people where the NHS cannot. *The Guardian*, 30 April 2015.

28. Cited in Shah, Wadoo and Latoo, Psychological distress in carers of people with mental disorders.

29. C. Ford, *Mind the Gap: A History of Mind and the Impact of the 1960s Civil Rights Movement on Its Development*. Bristol: University of Bristol, 2016.

30. Rethink, Our history. Rethink website (n.d.), www.rethink.org/aboutus/who-we-are/our-history/.

31. B. Vermeulen, H. Lauwers, N. Spruytte et al., *Experiences of Family Caregivers for Persons with Severe Mental Illness: An International Exploration*. Leuven: LUCAS KU Leuven/EUFAMI.

32. D. Giacco, A. Dirik, J. Kaselionyte and S. Priebe, How to make carer involvement in mental health inpatient units happen: A focus group study with patients, carers and clinicians. *BMC Psychiatry* (2017) 17: 1–13.

33. E.g. R. M. Norman, A. K. Malla, R. Manchanda, R. Harricharan, J. Takhar and S. Northcott, Social support and three-year symptom and admission outcomes for first episode psychosis. *Schizophrenia Research* (2005) 80: 227–34.

34. Department of Health, *Recognised, Valued and Supported: Next Steps for the Carers Strategy*. London: HMSO, 2010.

35. L. E. Rose, R. K. Mallinson and B. Walton-Moss, Barriers to family care in psychiatric settings. *Journal of Nursing Scholarship* (2004) 36: 39–47.

36. See the published lecture J. Laurance, *Pure Madness: How Fear Drives the Mental Health System*. London: Faculty of Public Health, 2002, https://www.kingsfund.org.uk/sites/default/files/puremadness.pdf.

37. Time to Change, Attitudes to Mental Illness 2013 Research Report, February 2015.

38. M. Bowen and A. Lovell, Stigma: The representation of mental health in UK newspaper Twitter feeds. *Journal of Mental Health* (2019): 1–7.

39. F. Morse, The Sun newspaper's '1,200 killed by mental patients' headline labelled 'irresponsible and wrong.' *The Independent*, 7 October 2013.

40. G. Ward, *Making Headlines: Mental Health and the National Press*. London: Health Education Authority, 1997.

41. Time to Change, Personal stories. Time to Change website (n.d.), www.time-to-change.org.uk/personal-stories.

42. Time to Change, We can build a society that cares about people with mental health problems. Time to Change (Personal Stories 2016) website, 17 August 2016, www.time-to-change.org.uk/blog/we-can-build-society-cares-about-people-mental-health-problems. This is in the public domain and not to be used for marketing/campaign materials.

43. Time to Change, 'Self-stigma' is real and we need to talk about it. Time to Change (Personal Stories 2019) website, 2 December 2019, www.time-to-change.org.uk/blog/self-stigma-real-and-we-need-to-talk-about-it. This is in the public domain and not to be used for marketing/campaign materials.

44. Ford, *Mind the Gap*.

Chapter 15

Women in UK Psychiatry and Mental Health

Gianetta Rands

Introduction

Throughout this chapter, it is accepted that women's mental and emotional health are affected by their roles in society, their relationships with other people, their own health and welfare and their financial independence. Some relevant laws enacted between 1960 and 2010 are described. Some experiences of women as mental health professionals and as patients during this time period are considered.

Women's Lives in 1960

One source of insight into the lives of women at the end of the 1950s and during the 1960s is Jennifer Worth's book *Call the Midwife* (2002),[1] later turned into a BBC series portraying people's lives in London's docklands. Many women stopped working when they married. Sex before marriage was frowned upon. Women often had ten or more children. Maternal death rates were high, usually due to postpartum haemorrhage or sepsis. Contraception was the rhythm method or condoms. Illegal terminations could be procured as 'back street abortions' that too often resulted in fatal sepsis or painful pelvic scarring and infertility. Large extended families lived in small tenements with outdoor toilets and no hot water. Domestic violence was brushed off by police and others as 'just a domestic'.

In 1960, most psychiatric treatment took place in large mental hospitals, the old lunatic asylums, that were among the first employers to provide equal pay to men and women, thanks to Henry Fawcett.[2] These were also some of the first medical institutions to employ women doctors, some of whom progressed to careers as psychiatrists, such as Eleanora Fleury and Helen Boyle.

By the early 1960s, conditions in the asylums were miserable for patients and staff, as described by Bradley.[3] Barbara Robb, a psychoanalyst working in north London, was horrified by conditions in her local asylum. Her book *Sans Everything* shook the establishment and the long process of closing asylums began (see also Chapters 1 and 7).[4]

Mother's Little Helper

'The problem that has no name' slowly emerged in the consciousness of Betty Friedan as she analysed replies to a questionnaire sent to her cohort of 1942 graduates from Smith College, a women-only university in Massachusetts, United States. Women in the late 1950s and early 1960s were not happy. When they consulted their doctors there was 'nothing wrong' with them. Their problem had no name. Friedan's analysis evolved into her book *The Feminine Mystique* described by the *New York Times* as 'one of the most influential non-fiction books of the twentieth century'.

Table 15.1 Timeline of laws and events significant for women and mental health, 1960–2010

Date	Legislation	Professional Landmarks	Key People
1841		The Association of Medical Officers of Asylums and Hospitals for the Insane founded in the UK; became Medico-Psychological Association (MPA) in 1865	
1894		MPA admitted first woman member	Eleanora Fleury (1867–1960)
1926		MPA became the Royal Medico-Psychological Association (RMPA)	
1939			Helen Boyle (1869–1957) first woman president, RMPA
1960s		Medical training; 30% women	
1961	Suicide Act		
1963		The oral contraceptive pill available to women in the UK	
1965/9	Murder (Abolition of Death Penalty) Act		
1967	The Abortion Act		
1967	Sexual Offences Act		
1968		The Ford sewing machinists strike; women employees demanded equal pay to men in equivalent jobs	Barbara Castle; as first secretary of state and secretary of state for employment (1968–70)
1970	Equal Pay Act		Barbara Castle
1971		RMPA became the Royal College of Psychiatrists	

Year	Event	Names
1971	First refuge for victims of domestic abuse opened in London. In 1993, renamed Refuge, offering advice and refuge to victims of domestic abuse	Erin Pizzey Jack Ashley, Labour MP, House of Commons address (1973) coined the term 'Domestic Violence'
1975	Sex Discrimination Act	
1976	Women's Psychotherapy Centre, London	Susie Orbach Luise Eichenbaum
1983	The Mental Health Act	
1984	First clinic for benzodiazepine withdrawal	Heather Ashtor
1985	The Gillick Decision, House of Lords	
1985	Prohibition of Female Circumcision Act	
1990	Human Fertilisation and Embryology Act	Amended legal abortions from 28 to 24 weeks, except if extreme risk to mother
1993	Women presidents elected by RCPsychiatrists	Fiona Caldicott (1993–6); Sheila Hollins (2005–8); Susan Bailey (2011–14); Wendy Burn (2017–20)
1996	Women in Psychiatry Special Interest Group (WIPSIG) created	Jane Mounty Anne Cremona Rosalind Ramsay

Table 15.1 (cont.)

Date	Legislation	Professional Landmarks	Key People
1998	The Human Rights Act		
2003	Sexual Offences Act	Marital or spousal rape was now illegal	
2003		In psychiatry, 36% of consultants and 22% of fellows were women	
		1 in 5 higher trainees were in flexible or part-time posts	
2004	Domestic Violence, Crime and Victims Act		
2005	The Mental Capacity Act, enacted 2007		
2006	Safeguarding Vulnerable Groups Act		
2010	The Equality Act		

One of many republications of this book is a Penguin Modern Classic edition, 2010, with an introduction by Lionel Shriver.[5] Shriver refers to the award-winning television series *Mad Men*, in particular the character Mrs Betty Draper as the embodiment of the feminine mystique. She has everything a woman could want – handsome high-earning husband, beautiful suburban house filled with modern domestic gadgets, two healthy children, time for self-pampering and money for pretty clothes. She had married young and rejoiced that she wasn't a frumpy 'career-girl'. Why was she unhappy?

Although Friedan's research has been criticised for focusing on a few hundred, middle-class, highly educated, white women in the United States, her findings showed insights into a massive, international problem. *The Feminine Mystique* has been credited with sparking the second wave of feminism in which equality was the main issue.

Other Smith College alumna are Nancy Reagan, Barbara Bush, Gloria Steinem and Sylvia Plath (Class of 1955). Plath, in her writings and her tragic short life, embodied something of the problem that has no name. As a talented poet and writer, the restrictions and drudgery of being a housewife overwhelmed her mental health. She was diagnosed as clinically depressed, received electroconvulsive therapy (ECT) and tragically killed herself in 1963.

Sylvia Plath died in London. A few miles away, Mick Jagger and Keith Richards were creating their legendary rock and roll genre. In 1966, they released this song:

Mother's Little Helper

Kids are different today, I hear every mother say
Mother needs something today to calm her down
And though she's not really ill, there's a little yellow pill
She goes running for the shelter of a mother's little helper
And it helps her on her way, gets her through her busy day

It goes on:

And if you take more of those, you will get an overdose
No more running for the shelter of a mother's little helper
They just helped you on your way, to your busy dying day

These lyrics were seen as a response to public criticism of the younger generation's use of recreational drugs at a time when married women were being prescribed increasing amounts of calming medications such as meprobamate and diazepam (Mother's Little Helper). Both these drugs are prescribed sedatives and are now known to be addictive. Meprobamate (Miltown or Equanil) can be lethal in overdose. Valium (diazepam), one of the first benzodiazepine group of drugs, was launched in 1963, and in 1978 more than 2 billion tablets were prescribed in the United States alone.

In 1984, in her practice in Newcastle, Heather Ashton noticed the difficulties people had in withdrawing from benzodiazepines and set up the first clinic to help with this. Her manual *Benzodiazepines: How They Work and How to Withdraw* has guided millions around the world in this difficult task.[6]

Sedation was an easy way to manage women presenting with 'the problem that had no name'. As in the case of Betty Draper, alcohol was another sedative increasingly resorted to by unhappy housewives.

As the 1960s progressed towards the 'Summer of Love' (1969), addiction to sedatives, alcohol and other recreational drugs all spiralled (see also Chapter 25). Another group of medications that had a massive effect on the mental and physical health of women was the pill: oral contraception for women.

The Pill: Women Control Family Planning

The oral contraceptive (OC) pill is a tablet taken every day, or twenty-one per twenty-eight day cycle, by women wanting to avoid pregnancy. Interest in combining a progesterone-type drug with an oestrogen-type drug for this purpose started in the 1930s. It wasn't until synthetic versions of these hormones were available that they could be tested in women. In the UK, the first OCs were made available via Family Planning Clinics (FPCs) from 1963.

By 2010, thirty-three varieties of combined OC, five varieties of progesterone-only OC and other hormonal contraception such as subcutaneous implants, intrauterine devices and vaginal rings were available in the UK. The pill could be prescribed to girls under sixteen provided they were 'Gillick competent' in which case 'parental rights' do not exist.[7]

The impact on women's lives and health was huge. Not only could they control their fertility but these drugs were used for other inconvenient and incapacitating conditions such as menorrhagia (heavy bleeding), dysmenorrhoea (painful periods), endometriosis, premenstrual tension and acne.

Women's health improved because they were not constantly having babies. The risks associated with pregnancy, such as death, septicaemia, anaemia, urinary tract infections, incontinence and deep-vein thrombosis, reduced as the number of pregnancies reduced. The age that women married increased, the number of children they had decreased and more women succeeded in higher education and professional careers. There were concerns that decoupling sex and pregnancy caused an increase in promiscuity and pressure on young women to have sex before they were fully consenting.

With effective contraception available, women with serious illnesses, be they mental, physical or genetic predispositions, could choose whether or not to have babies. For instance, a woman with bipolar affective disorder needing lithium to stay well could choose to avoid pregnancy as lithium is toxic to the foetus (teratogenic).

Mental Illnesses Associated with the Menstrual Cycle and Pregnancy

The three main psychiatric diagnoses associated with the menstrual cycle and pregnancy are premenstrual dysphoric disorder, postnatal depression and postpartum psychosis.

Premenstrual tension refers to a collection of mood and somatic symptoms experienced by many women in the luteal phase of their cycles, that is, after ovulation and before menstruation. Some 3–8 per cent of women experience severe symptoms that constitute a diagnosis of premenstrual dysphoric disorder. These women have a higher risk of postnatal depression and mood disorders during their menopause.

Postnatal depression affects 10–15 per cent of new mothers within the first two months of giving birth and sometimes starts in the last few months of pregnancy. Postpartum psychosis affects about 1 in 1,000 women who give birth and usually comes on very quickly in the first few weeks after having a baby. It has a high risk of suicide and infanticide and needs urgent treatment, usually in hospital and preferably in a mother and baby unit.

These conditions are treatable once they are diagnosed. Research and collaborations between psychiatrists, obstetricians, gynaecologists, general practitioners and scientists led to criteria for diagnoses and improvements in services and training. By the end of the 2010s, these mental illnesses were taken seriously in the UK.[8]

Laws Affecting Women in UK Psychiatry and Mental Health, 1960–2010

In 1961, the Suicide Act was passed. Before this, anyone found trying to kill themselves could be prosecuted and imprisoned. This law applied to England and Wales. In Scotland, suicide was never an offence. In Northern Ireland, text from the Suicide Act was incorporated into their Criminal Justice Act 1966.

The Abortion Act, passed in October 1967 and effective from April 1968, made medical termination of pregnancy (abortion) legal up to twenty-eight weeks in England, Wales and Scotland. A pregnant woman could obtain termination of her pregnancy if two medical practitioners agreed that continuing with that pregnancy would risk her life, mental or physical health, or put any of her existing children at risk. Northern Ireland decriminalised abortion in October 2019, effective from 31 March 2020. To quote Bradley 'unwanted pregnancy, whether due to contraceptive failure, rape or incest was often a precursor of severe depression or suicide'.[9]

The Sexual Offences Act 1967 legalised homosexuality between consenting men aged twenty-one years and over, reduced to eighteen years and over in 1994. Before then, women, knowingly or unknowingly, willingly or unwillingly, in sham marriages would have experienced collateral damage, suffering confusion, deceit, emotional distress and mental illnesses.

Barbara Castle, in her roles as first secretary of state and secretary of state for employment (1968–70) intervened in the Ford machinists strike of 1968 in which women employees demanded pay equal to their men colleagues in equivalent jobs. The awareness of widespread pay inequality precipitated the Equal Pay Act 1970 which gained royal assent in May 1970 but was, curiously, not commenced until 1975. It made discrimination between men and women, in their terms and conditions of employment, illegal. It applied to the whole of the UK except Northern Ireland. Castle, in her role as minister of transport (1965–8), also introduced breathalysers, seat belts and speed limits, all of which have benefited the lives of women.

The Sex Discrimination Act 1975 gained royal assent in November 1975. It specifically covered discrimination and harassment on the grounds of sex or marital status in employment, training and education. It was one of a clutch of equality and discrimination laws that were repealed and incorporated into the Equality Act in 2010.

The current version of the Equality Act 2010 lists protected characteristics as age, disability, gender reassignment, marriage and civil partnership, race, religion or belief, sex and sexual orientation.[10] Discrimination, harassment and victimisation are prohibited in employment and private and public services. The Act applies in England, Wales and Scotland but has limited application in Northern Ireland.

Other legislation passed in the UK during this time period and relevant to the mental health of women includes the Prohibition of Female Circumcision Act 1985 and the Domestic Violence, Crime and Victims Act 2004 which gave legal protection to victims of crime, particularly domestic violence. The first refuge for women victims of domestic violence opened in London in 1971. The Sexual Offences Act 2003 made marital, or spousal, rape illegal. Before that, a husband could force 'conjugal rights' on his wife claiming ongoing consent through their marriage contract. The 2003 Act reinforced the importance of consent and that, if someone is unable to consent or their consent is obtained by force or intimidation, the sex act is not consensual.

The Human Rights Act was passed in the UK in 1998. It legislated that public organisations, including government, police and local councils, must treat every person resident in the UK equally, with fairness, dignity and respect. It is based on articles of the European Convention on Human Rights (ECHR). Another important law incorporating ECHR articles as principles is the Mental Capacity Act 2005, commenced in 2007. This Act enshrines a person's right to make their own decisions based on informed consent and defines a process for making decisions when a person lacks mental capacity.

The Feminist Movement

Women's movements have a long history, at least 500 years, and international representation. Friedan describes progress made as 'two steps forward, one step back'.[11] Since then feminism has been documented as 'waves', which inevitably implies troughs.

Feminism as an ideology is based on equality of men and women in all aspects of society, education, employment, politics, economics and human rights. It is about equality of value, opportunity and reward. The principles of feminism have been incorporated into many areas, such as feminist philosophy, psychology and sociology, and into specific groups, such as black and intersectional feminism.

First-wave feminism covers women's rights movements' demand for, and gain of, suffrage. Many also demanded equality of educational opportunities. This aim continued into the second wave of feminism, in the 1960s and 1970s, that primarily focused on equality and non-discrimination. As these ideals were enshrined in laws, there was the reasonable assumption that they would soon be achieved. It slowly became evident that this was not so, igniting the third wave of feminism in the early 1990s. This was more multiracial than previous waves, and the concept that social conditioning was the cause of gender inequalities and discriminations was key. The phrase 'a matrix of domination' incorporates the idea that gender inequality interacts with homophobia, classism, colonisation and capitalism across the globe, in a way that holds back progress in all those areas.[12] The use of social media around 2010 sparked new interest in feminism which started ripples of the fourth wave.

Feminists of the 1970s reinstated the title 'Ms' as a formal way to address women without specifying their marital status. It had previously been used in the seventeenth and eighteenth centuries when, like 'Miss' and 'Mrs', it was a derivation of Mistress. Doctors in the 1920s rejected the title 'Doctress' and many women doctors use Dr or Professor not only because they indicate training and academic achievements but also because they are non-gendered titles.

Aspects of Mental Health Services, 1960–2010

With mental health services in the 1960s under-resourced and neglected, the anti-psychiatry movement was an attractive alternative (see also Chapter 20). In the 1970s, there was a flurry of reports about sexual and violent crimes on psychiatry wards and inappropriate behaviour of professionals. The Kerr/Haslam Inquiry (2005) investigated two psychiatrists, William Kerr and Michael Haslam, working in York in the 1970s and 1980s, both of whom had been found guilty of indecent assaults against women psychiatric patients.[13] The report found that numerous complaints had not been taken seriously; professionals raising concerns (whistle-blowing) were not heard; whistle-blowing was detrimental to careers, and there was a culture of loyalty to colleagues, tolerance of sexualised behaviours and a predominantly male hierarchy of doctors and female nurses that reinforced gender power dynamics.

Several good recommendations were made. All Mental Health Trusts were to display information leaflets about assessments and treatments. Complaints procedures needed to be clear, and Independent Mental Health Advocates (IMHAs) and Patient Advice and Liaison Services (PALS) were to be provided. The report's recommendations about protecting vulnerable adults were incorporated into the Safeguarding Vulnerable Groups Act 2006.[14]

In the 1980s, the psychiatric paradox was described. Women go to psychiatry services for help but instead get blamed for their own illnesses and those of others. Penfold and Walker write that

> 'Blame the victim' models lead to the scapegoating of mothers, blaming the rape victim and battered wife, dismissing the prostitute as primitive or deviant, accusing the alcoholic's wife of causing her husband's downfall, pointing the finger at the little girl who is assumed to have seduced her innocent father, and attributing women's addiction to tranquillisers to neuroticism and inadequacy.[15]

They describe protection of perpetrators with reference to psychiatry's function as a social regulator.

Perusal of standard psychiatry textbooks from the 1980s provides evidence for some of these allegations. Their indexes contain few references to women, abuse or perinatal illnesses. A short paragraph about the mental effects of the menopause concludes 'psychiatric symptoms at this time of life could equally well reflect changes in the woman's role as her children leave home, her relationship with her husband alters, and her own parents become ill or die'. The recommendations of the Kerr/Haslam report were needed and eventually implemented throughout the UK.

The Women's Therapy Centre, London, opened in 1976 to offer individual and group psychotherapy to women who, for many reasons, were not able to access other mental health services. It was a social enterprise started by psychotherapists Susie Orbach and Luise Eichenbaum based on their principles of social feminism and their skills in psychotherapy and psychoanalysis. Some of its successes have been to increase the understanding of what it means to grow up as a girl in patriarchal societies, to expand their developmental theory and feminist relational practice and to write books and lectures that are used internationally.

Developments in Mental Health Services since 1960 that have specifically benefited women include Perinatal Psychiatry, Child and Adolescent Mental Health Services, Intellectual Disability and Old Age Psychiatry, the latter because women live longer than men. There have been extensive debates about women-only wards that usually conclude that what matters is good, well resourced, multi-professional teams providing assessment and treatment in a co-operative, collegiate way, with sufficient resources to do their jobs well. With these in place, the demands for single-sex wards diminish.

Private psychoanalysis and psychotherapy thrived in many areas of the UK from 1960 to 2010. A list of women psychoanalysts in Great Britain in the twentieth century includes Enid Balint and Clare Winnicott.[16] Enid Balint (1903–94) was a social worker and psychoanalyst. She married Michael Balint in 1953 and introduced him to casework techniques she used to train social workers. These formed the basis for Balint groups in which transference and countertransference are used to analyse clinical cases and the doctor–patient relationship. Balint methodology is usually attributed to Michael but evidence indicates that Enid needs attribution.

Clare Winnicott (1906–84) also trained as a social worker and psychoanalyst and taught at the London School of Economics (LSE) throughout her career. She was interested in the psychic life of children who had suffered loss and separation, how to communicate with them and the role of social workers as 'transitional participants'. She described ideas such as 'transitional objects' before she married Donald Winnicott in 1951. Whose idea was 'the good-enough mother'?

Attribution for the ideas and work of women therapists, doctors and scientists has been skewed for years, their contributions being invisible and/or claimed by male colleagues. Famous examples include Rosalind Franklin's work on DNA crystallography and June Almeida's discovery in 1964 of coronaviruses.

In addition to statutory and private mental health service developments, since 1960 there has been an expansion in voluntary organisations and self-help information for people in emotional distress and managing mental illnesses (see also Chapter 14).[17]

Women Psychiatrists

When training as a medical student and psychiatrist in the 1970s and 1980s it was not unusual for a lecturer to announce 'I will refer to the doctor as He and the patient as She, whatever their sex, just for clarity'.

In 1894, after a year debating whether 'man/men' could include woman/women the Medico-Psychological Association (MPA, predecessor of the Royal College of Psychiatrists) rewrote its rules and admitted its first woman psychiatrist Eleanora Fleury (1867–1960). Helen Boyle (1869–1957) became a member of the MPA in 1898 and, in 1939, became its first woman president.[18]

A 1960s analysis of medical staffing predicted that, in 1964, 1,730 medical students would qualify as doctors, 1,330 men and 400 women. They assumed two-thirds 'wastage' of women to marriage, leaving 1,464 'working doctors'.[19] In 1967, 30 per cent of the UK medical school intake were women. Two surveys of qualified women doctors, by the Medical Practitioners Union and the Medical Women's Federation, found that 80 per cent of respondents actively worked as doctors and nearly half were in full-time work. The researchers concluded that 'the overall wastage of women doctors is not as alarming as is suggested'.

In 1974, the then health secretary Barbara Castle expressed her intention to improve opportunities for women working part-time in the NHS. Part-time and flexible jobs and training posts now offered options for different work–life balance choices for women and men professionals working in mental health services.

Psychiatrists Jane Mounty, Anne Cremona and Rosalind Ramsay describe the Women in Psychiatry Special Interest Group (WIPSIG) within the Royal College of Psychiatrists. Its initial objectives were to improve both the working lives of women psychiatrists and the provision of care to women using mental health services. The need for part-time jobs and job-shares had been acknowledged, but employers preferred full-time doctors who, at that time, worked up to eighty hours per week.[20]

They note that 'by November 2003, 47% of core trainees, 53% of higher trainees, 55% of staff grade and associate specialists, and 36% of consultants in psychiatry, were women. Twenty-two per cent of College Fellows were women, and there were 21 women professors of psychiatry. One in five higher trainees was training flexibly.'

The second aim of this group was to highlight the service provisions for women patients. Professor Dora Kohen is quoted thus:

> Half the patients in mental health services are women, although in Old Age services women outnumber men by 2:1 (women live longer). Anxiety, depression and eating disorders are all more common in women. Socio-economic and psychological factors associated with poverty, unemployment and social isolation play a considerable part in female mental illness. Other disorders such as puerperal psychosis, postnatal depression and premenstrual dysphoric disorder are specific to women.[21]

Gender inequality continues in clinical and academic medicine. In a recent review of the evidence for inequalities in pay, career progression, citations and authorships of academic papers, clinical awards and senior leadership roles, the authors conclude that 'equality is not just about having a level playing field, it is about unleashing talent'. They challenge science journals to improve the gender balance of their editorial boards.[22]

Conclusion

In 1988, *Punch* magazine published the Miss Triggs cartoon, now guaranteed immortality by its reproduction in Mary Beard's book *Women and Power: A Manifesto*.[23] It is a line drawing of an unspecified board meeting of five men and one woman, with the caption 'That's an excellent suggestion, Miss Triggs. Perhaps one of the men here would like to make it.'

Most women immediately recognise this situation. It's a common experience of everyday sexism which includes silencing, misattribution of skills, talents and contributions, and gender inequality.

Add to this social and institutional structures that perpetuate inequality and discrimination and the toll on women's mental health seems obvious. In 2010, social media had not yet become ubiquitous and its effect on young people's mental health, particularly that of young women, was not known. However, it was known that one in four women experienced domestic abuse, only 6 per cent of rape cases resulted in prosecution and that the prevalence of mental illnesses in young women and teenage girls was increasing. Unforeseen events such as economic collapse and new disease outbreaks seem to affect women disproportionately in their 'double shift' responsibilities (career and domestic) and a world that remains, predominantly, designed for men.[24]

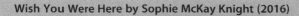

Wish You Were Here by Sophie McKay Knight (2016)

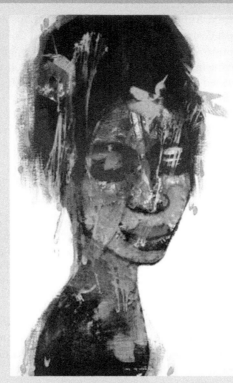

Wish You Were Here is part of the Chrysalis project at the University of St Andrews, in which conversations of women at all stages of their careers in science research were interpreted by the artist Sophie McKay Knight. The images she created were displayed in the Byre Gallery in St Andrews as part of the Women in Science Festival 2016. Sophie McKay Knight has said of this artwork,

> Throughout it all I was thinking about what people had told me about being apart from loved ones in order to pursue their careers & the instability of contracts and not really having any permanence. The single figure in 'Wish you were here' represents that dual positive/negative sense of being alone and yet deeply connected to 'work' – which both does and does not make up for any associated loss.[25]

Key Summary Points

- Women's lives changed profoundly between 1960 and 2010. The main contribution to this was hormonal contraception and its impact on women's mental and physical health.
- Mental health services changed from asylum-based inpatient facilities to community-based services and from male doctor–dominated organisations towards multidisciplinary collegiate teamwork.

- By 2010, discrimination and inequality persisted despite forty years of laws making these illegal.
- While many organisations now monitor gender equality data, research is needed to discover why inequality and discrimination are so resistant to change and what factors perpetuate this status quo.
- The effects of social stresses, economic or pandemic, seem to disproportionately burden women who work 'double shifts' to balance work and home commitments with predictably adverse effects on their mental and physical health.

Notes

1. J. Worth, *Call the Midwife*. London: Merton Books, 2002.

2. Henry Fawcett. Wikipedia entry, https://en.wikipedia.org/wiki/Henry_Fawcett.

3. J. J. Bradley, Sixty years in psychiatry. *Medico-Legal Journal* (2017) 85(4): 210–14, https://doi.org/10.1177/0025817217721381.

4. C. Hilton, A woman the government feared: Barbara Robb (1912–1976). In G. Rands, ed., *Women's Voices in Psychiatry*, 205–14. Oxford: Oxford University Press, 2018.

5. B. Friedan, *The Feminine Mystique*. London: Penguin, 2010. (Originally published in 1963.)

6. G. Ferry, Heather Ashton obituary. *The Guardian*, 18 November 2019. H. Ashton, *Benzodiazepines: How They Work and How to Withdraw [The Ashton Manual]*, online publication, www.benzo.org.uk/bzmono.htm.

7. NSPCC Learning, Gillick competency and Fraser guidelines, NSPCC Learning website, June 2020, https://learning.nspcc.org.uk/child-protection-system/gillick-competence-fraser-guidelines; see also Gillick v West Norfolk and Wisbech AHA [1985] UKHL 7 (17 October 1985), House of Lords, www.bailii.org/uk/cases/UKHL/1985/7.html) (HL).

8. K. Abel and R. Ramsay, *The Female Mind: A User's Guide*. London: RCPsych Publications, 2017.

9. Bradley, Sixty years in psychiatry.

10. The Equality Act 2010, www.legislation.gov.uk/ukpga/2010/15/pdfs/ukpga_20100015_en.pdf.

11. Friedan, *The Feminine Mystique*.

12. Patricia Hill Collins. Wikipedia entry, https://en.wikipedia.org.wiki/Patricia_Hill_Collins.

13. HM Government, *The Kerr/Haslam Inquiry [report]*. Cm. 6640. www.gov.uk/government/publications/the-kerrhaslam-inquiry-report.

14. Safeguarding Vulnerable Groups Act 2006. Wikipedia entry, https://en.wikipedia.org.wiki/Safeguarding_Vulnerable_Groups_Act_2006.

15. P. S. Penfold and G. A. Walker, *Women and the Psychiatric Paradox*. Montreal: Eden Press, 1983, p. 245.

16. Women psychoanalysts in Great Britain. *Psychoanalytikerinnen: Biografisches Lexikon*, www.psychoanalytikerinnen.de/greatbritain_biographies.html.

17. Abel and Ramsay, *The Female Mind*.

18. F. Subotsky, The entry of women into psychiatry. In Rands, *Women's Voices in Psychiatry*, 39–49.

19. A. Rimmer, A history of women in British medicine. In Rands, *Women's Voices in Psychiatry*, 25–38.

20. J. Mounty, A. Cremona and R. Ramsay, History of the Royal College of Psychiatrists' Women's Mental Health Special Interest Group. In Rands, *Women's Voices in Psychiatry*, 57–72.

21. Ibid., p. 66.

22. J. F. Breedvelt, S. Rowe, H. Bowden-Jones et al., Unleashing talent in mental health sciences: Gender equality at the top. *British Journal of Psychiatry* (2018) 213(6): 679–81, https://doi.org/10.1192/bjp.2018.249.

23. M. Beard, *Women and Power: A Manifesto.* London: Profile Books, 2017.

24. C. Criado Perez, *Invisible Women: Exposing Data Bias in a World Designed for Men.* London: Chatto & Windus, 2019.

25. The project artwork is available under the Creative Commons Attribution (CC BY 4.0) terms and conditions: https://creativecommons.org/licenses/by/4.0. Credit: Chrysalis, paintings exploring women in science. Credit: Original painting (acrylic on canvas) by Sophie McKay Knight, with imagery contributed by women scientists from the University of St. Andrews, as part of the Chrysalis Project coordinated by Dr Mhairi Stewart. Attribution 4.0 International (CC BY 4.0).

Biological Psychiatry in the UK and Beyond

Stephen Lawrie

Introduction

What is 'biological psychiatry'? With biology being the scientific study of life, if one took the word literally, one could legitimately question whether there is any other kind of psychiatry.[1] By this definition, psychology is part of biology. As taught in schools and universities, however, biology is the more constrained study of living organisms and includes anatomy, physiology and behaviour; human biology includes all those aspects as well as genetics, anthropology and nutrition and so on. That is still quite broad.

What biological psychiatry is usually taken to mean is the search for neurobiological underpinnings of mental illness and application of drug and other physical treatments for them. This, of course, assumes that the brain–mind are sufficiently interlinked to justify that approach – something that is taken as read by most doctors and should be self-evident to anyone who has ever consumed any psychoactive drug, including caffeine and alcohol. What biological psychiatry does not (overtly) include are those key elements of human understanding that are the essential tools in the trade of the effective clinician: the application of insights from experience, perhaps informed by the arts and humanities, to the clinical encounter. There are, of course, those members of our broad church of psychiatry that prioritise psychosocial approaches to understanding and psychotherapy as treatment. To some of them, and many outside psychiatry, biological psychiatry is or at least can be reductionistic – reducing or ignoring the mind to little or nothing more than the brain. Anything so 'mindless' would be just as bad as dualism or mentalistic 'brainlessness'.[2] One would, however, be hard-pressed to find any so-called or self-declared biological psychiatrist who does not pay heed to the importance of our mental lives.

The Rise of Psychopharmacology

In the 1940s, the therapeutic armamentarium available to psychiatrists included barbiturates and not much else. During the 1950s, cutting-edge neuroscience demonstrated the existence of neurotransmitters in the brain. Coincidentally, several new drugs were discovered, including tricyclic antidepressants, monoamine oxidase inhibitors (MAOIs), antipsychotics and lithium. One of the eminent pharmacologists of the age, John Henry Gaddum, was interested in LSD and proposed a role for serotonin (5-hydroxytryptamine, 5HT) in mood regulation. Gaddum was Professor of Pharmacology at the University of Edinburgh from 1942 to 1958 and in Cambridge from 1958 to 1965.

Two young psychiatrists working in Gaddum's departments, George Ashcroft and Donald Eccleston, proposed the monoamine theory of depression. The theory received initial support from a study that showed patients with depression had lower levels of the main 5HT metabolite 5-hydroxy indole acetic acid (5HIAA) in cerebrospinal fluid (CSF) than neurology patient 'controls' undergoing lumbar air encephalography.[3] Strong support came from a study conducted in what was by then the Medical Research Council (MRC) Brain Metabolism Research Unit, in which CSF was sampled under standardised conditions – 5HIAA not only correlated with the severity of depression but normalised on remission.[4] Less appealingly, levels were also low in those with schizophrenia (but not in mania). This apparent early success was further reinforced when Alec Coppen and colleagues at the MRC Neuropsychiatric Research Unit in Epsom, Surrey, showed that adding tryptophan (TRP, a 5HT precursor) to the antidepressant tranylcypromine helped get patients dramatically better, almost as effectively as electroconvulsive therapy (ECT).[5]

Decreased free and/or total TRP levels in the plasma and CSF in depressed patients were replicated in several labs,[6] but Coppen was always concerned that it all could be a secondary change to depression and subsequent work by Ashcroft led him to the same conclusion.[7] The weight loss and elevated cortisol of depression were just two of many possible confounders.[8] On the other hand, several studies showed that rapid TRP and 5HT depletion – through, for example, ingesting a TRP-free amino acid drink – reduces mood in healthy volunteers and in those who are depressed or have recovered. This realisation led to extensive work on neuroendocrine disruptions in depression – particularly in Oxford – including demonstrations that hormonal responses were blunted in depression and normalised by some antidepressants and lithium, including ECT in patients and electroconvulsive stimulation in animals.

There is, of course, an analogous story to be told about the role of the adrenergic system in depression but the UK contribution to this was less central. Although there is no question that many treatments for depression act on the serotoninergic and other monoamine systems, it has not been established whether there is an abnormality of serotonin metabolism or that treatments correct it. It is more complicated than that. The 5HT system is probably modulating other processes critical to the development and maintenance of depression, such as adaptive responses to aversive events.[9] Low 5HTIAA levels in CSF may mark severity and are associated with, and maybe even predictive of, impulsive, violent suicidal behaviour. This also seems to be true, however, of schizophrenia.[10]

Nevertheless, subsequent work employing functional neuroimaging as a window on the brain has shown that single and repeated doses of various antidepressants increase the recognition of happy facial expressions, and amygdala responses to them, while decreasing amygdala response to negative affect faces, in healthy people and in those with depression.[11] These effects are also seen after seven days' administration in healthy participants and are maintained during longer-term treatment. Further, long-term administration of selective serotonin reuptake inhibitor (SSRI) or norepinephrine reuptake inhibitor antidepressants can enhance synaptic plasticity and block the synaptic and dendritic deficits caused by stress.[12]

Landmark Clinical Trials

The advent of rigorous randomised controlled trials (RCTs) also coincided with the availability of many new drug treatments for depression, bipolar disorder and schizophrenia. Even if a simple monoamine theory of depression was not to survive, a series of landmark clinical trials carried out by psychopharmacologists and psychiatrists of various persuasions in the 1960s and 1970s established that antidepressants and other biological approaches to major psychiatric disorders worked.

The Clinical Psychiatry Committee of the MRC, which included epidemiologists like Archie Cochrane and Austin Bradford Hill, published its clinical trial of the treatment of depressive illness in the *British Medical Journal* in 1965.[13] No fewer than 250 patients in London, Leeds and Newcastle aged 40–69 years with an untreated primary depressive illness (characterised by persistent low mood, with at least one of the following: morbid or delusional guilt, insomnia, hypochondriasis and psychomotor retardation or agitation) were randomised to ECT (4–8 treatments), 150 mg imipramine, 45 mg phenelzine or placebo over 4 weeks. About one-third of those on placebo improved notably but this was almost doubled in those on imipramine and more than doubled in those given ECT – and these differences were maintained at six months. Moreover, in those who had responded to imipramine, continuation with 75–150 mg over a further six-month period meant that only 22 per cent relapsed as compared to 50 per cent randomised to placebo.[14]

During the 1960s, Baastrup and Schou working independently and then together in Denmark, conducting studies that suggested lithium was effective in acute mania and had prophylactic properties. However, to Aubrey Lewis and Michael Shepherd in the MRC Social Psychiatry Unit at the Institute of Psychiatry (IOP) in London, lithium was 'dangerous nonsense' and 'a therapeutic myth', which, in their opinion, was based on 'serious methodological shortcomings' and 'spurious claims' (see also Chapters 2 and 17).[15] Schou and Baastrup undertook a double-blind discontinuation trial with patients with 'manic-depressive illness' successfully treated with lithium who were then randomly allocated to continue on lithium or placebo. Lithium was superior in preventing relapse – but only in typical cases.[16] Coppen and colleagues randomised sixty-five patients with recurrent affective disorders to lithium or identical-looking placebo in four centres for up to two years – 86 per cent of those on lithium (0.73–1.23 meq per litre) were judged by independent psychiatrists and psychiatric social workers to have had no further episodes over that time, as compared to 8 per cent of the placebo group.[17] What is more, lithium seemed to be equally effective in unipolar and bipolar patients.

Following observations that the turnover of 5HT was greatly increased by the administration of the amino acid TRP, Donald Eccleston (having moved to Newcastle) led the introduction of a new '5HT cocktail' or 'Newcastle cocktail' therapy for severe depression. Using l-tryptophan alone or combined with other drugs, such as phenelzine (or clomipramine) and lithium, frequently produced dramatic improvement in otherwise chronically treatment-resistant depressed patients.[18]

The landmark study of the use of antipsychotic drugs in acute schizophrenia was carried out with more than 400 patients admitted to 9 centres around the United States, about a half of whom were in their first episodes.[19] By the end of the trial, 75 per cent of the patients receiving antipsychotic showed moderate or marked improvement, whereas only about 23 per cent did on placebo. It was left, however, to British social and biological psychiatrists to robustly demonstrate that these drugs also reduced the risk of relapse in the longer term – whether with oral medication or depot long-acting intramuscular injection.[20]

Innovative British Neuroimaging

The independent realisation that X-ray intensity reduction by the brain could be accurately measured and reconstructed into a brain image earned Allan Cormack (Tufts University) and Godfrey Hounsfield (Electric & Musical Industries (EMI), Middlesex) the Nobel Prize for Physiology/Medicine in 1979 for the development of computer assisted tomography. This was all the more remarkable as Hounsfield had gone to work for EMI immediately after school, making him the first person to win a Nobel Prize without going to university since Albert Einstein. Computerised tomography (CT), as it came to be known, became available for clinical use in 1971. Demonstration systems for CT of the head were installed in Glasgow, London and Manchester and the first body scanner (the CT5000) was installed for research at the Northwick Park Hospital (NPH) MRC Clinical Research Centre (CRC) on the outskirts of London in 1975.

Tim Crow was Head of the CRC Division of Psychiatry and intrigued that many patients with schizophrenia had cognitive impairment. He gave the young Glaswegian émigré Eve Johnstone the task of using CT to see if this might have an organic basis. Mid-axial brain slice photographs were traced three times each to calculate an average lateral ventricle-to-brain ratio (VBR), which was markedly increased in the patients.[21] One can imagine how the finding that schizophrenia – a 'functional' psychosis – might have an organic basis was greeted by social psychiatrists, psychotherapists and neurologists at the time. Indeed, the copy of the paper in the *Lancet* in the IOP library reputedly had 'Rubbish' scrawled across it. Regardless, the finding was widely replicated, as was the association with cognitive impairment.[22]

Important work contributing to the development of magnetic resonance imaging (MRI) as a non-invasive means of imaging brain and body in greater detail was done in Aberdeen by John Mallard and in Nottingham by Peter Mansfield (for which he was to share the 2003 Nobel Prize with Paul Lauterbur of Illinois, United States). US business and researchers capitalised upon this and the landmark MRI studies in schizophrenia were done there.[23] It was clear by the turn of the millennium that people with schizophrenia had reduced whole brain volumes and additional decrements in parts of the prefrontal and temporal lobes.[24] Further, there is a consistent association between these reductions and negative and positive symptoms respectively.

This work stimulated a resurgence of interest in the neuropathology of mental illness, especially schizophrenia, which provides independent confirmation of the findings and suggests they derive from the reduced density of neurons and glia, and lesser dendritic arborisation.[25] These could, of course, partly derive from antipsychotic medication, as well as the other effects of long-term illness and alcohol excess. However, the demonstration of similar but lesser changes in relatives and first episode cases,[26] and in those at elevated clinical risk,[27] with further reductions as some develop schizophrenia, has opened the way to potentially using neuroimaging to predict schizophrenia – which remains a very active global research effort.

Functional Neuroimaging

The first robust evidence that patients with schizophrenia had 'hypofrontality' – underactive prefrontal lobes – came from Ingvar and Franzén at the Karolinksa Institute in Sweden.[28] The British contribution was to rather undermine confidence in this finding. Researchers in Edinburgh and London demonstrated that hypofrontality was more anatomically constrained, that it could also be found in depression and even that 'hyperfrontality' could be found in unmedicated first episode patients.[29] Consequently, a *Lancet* editorial could pronounce 'Hypofrontality RIP' in 1995.

Following Chris Frith's lead, several important positron emission tomography (PET) studies at the MRC Cyclotron Unit at the Hammersmith Hospital in London showed a complex but compelling picture of neurofunctional correlates of symptoms, especially of auditory–verbal hallucinations. These findings suggested that such hallucinations are associated with under-activation of language areas in the brain concerned with the monitoring of inner speech.[30] These insights depended upon a technique that could analyse whole-brain tracer data. Karl Friston not only invented a Statistical Parametric Mapping procedure to do this but also would apparently stay up all night adding functions if one was needed for a particular analysis.

The Functional Imaging Laboratory (FIL) was founded in 1994, within the Institute of Neurology, following a major grant award from the Wellcome Trust. It pioneered new neuroimaging techniques such as functional MRI (fMRI) for understanding human cognition. Generously and wisely, Friston made his 'SPM' programme for analysing these data freely available and supported from the FIL and it remains the industry standard worldwide. The combination of fMRI and SPM facilitated more sophisticated studies to map auditory hallucinations, to relate them to dysconnectivity between language regions in the brain and to integrate these findings with dopamine signalling.

Dopamine

Two independent North American groups demonstrated in the early 1970s that the clinical potencies of antipsychotic drugs very strongly correlated with their ability to inhibit tritiated (3 H) dopamine binding to postsynaptic receptors in mammalian brain samples. Clinical trials at NPH reinforced a dopaminergic theory of schizophrenia but also showed that it applied to other psychotic disorders.[31] Some post-mortem studies also showed that the binding of 3 H–labelled spiroperidol was increased in parts of the basal ganglia and amygdala, but other studies suggested it was secondary to drug treatment. An early PET study with spiroperidol 77Br-brominated to emit gamma rays found an increase in activity in drug-free patients, but this too was disputed – with sometimes heated exchanges between the labs leading this work at Johns Hopkins and the Karolinksa.

It was only with the development of another tracer – fluorodopa – which is incorporated into dopamine and therefore measures dopamine synthesis and turnover that the dopamine story in schizophrenia has been clarified. Using fluorodopa PET, researchers at Imperial and Kings Colleges in London have shown that young people at high clinical risk of psychosis have elevated dopamine turnover in the striatum, which correlates with psychotic (but not other) symptoms, is highest in those most likely to become ill and increases as they develop a psychotic disorder.[32] (It should be noted, however, that there is a similarly strong strand of evidence that glutamatergic neurotransmission is also disrupted in schizophrenia.)

A Note on Dementia Imaging

Psychiatrists of many persuasions were among the vanguard of researchers using early neuroimaging techniques to study morphological and perfusion pattern changes in the brain in Alzheimer's disease and to distinguish them from those in multi-infarct dementia and from normal controls. Indeed, a generation of Old Age psychiatrists – inspired by Martin Roth in Newcastle and then Cambridge – did much to develop wider scientific and clinical interest in these conditions. As neurologists became more interested, they established that brain atrophy can be visualised by CT or MRI and that serial imaging and quantifying the degree of atrophy could aid diagnosis. Indeed, CT or MRI is now routinely recommended in many clinical guidelines in the evaluation of possible dementia and is now included in some diagnostic criteria. Further, Ian McKeith and John O'Brien have led the application of the accurate and reliable measure of low dopamine transporter activity in the brain in making a diagnosis of Lewy body dementia as distinct from others.[33]

The Cochrane Collaboration and Evidence-Based Medicine

The Cochrane Collaboration was founded in 1993 in response to Archie Cochrane's earlier call for up-to-date, systematic reviews of all relevant RCTs across health care (see also Chapter 17). Many academic and clinical psychiatrists from different specialties were early and enthusiastic contributors, and dedicated groups for schizophrenia and dementia were among the first to get established and publish reviews.

It quickly became evident that the RCT literature in psychiatry was about as good or bad as it was in most of medicine – with the notable exceptions of neurology and cardiology – in that there were far too many small, short and poorly reported trials. Nonetheless, systematic reviews and meta-analyses of the best available evidence showed that antidepressants and antipsychotics successfully treated acute depression or schizophrenia and that continuing effective treatment for a year compared with treatment discontinuation reduced relapse rates from around 41 per cent to 18 per cent for depression (31 RCTs, 4,410 participants)[34] and from 64 per cent to 27 per cent for schizophrenia (65 RCTs, 6,493 patients).[35] These differences of 23 per cent and 37 per cent mean that, on average, about one in three or four patients will benefit from taking these drugs over a year – and these are some of the largest treatment effects in the whole of medicine. There was even RCT evidence (32 RCTs, 3,458 patients) that lithium reduced suicide and overall mortality, although these were based on (fortunately) small numbers of deaths.[36] The UK ECT review group included service users and established that real ECT was significantly and substantially more effective than simulated or sham ECT (6 RCTs, 256 patients, all done in the UK in the 1970s) and more effective than pharmacotherapy (18 trials, 1,144 participants).[37]

Cochrane, as it has become known, and the wider rise of what might be called the evidence-based medicine movement came at roughly the same time as the development and aggressive marketing of the new 'atypical' antipsychotics (and valproate and various antidepressants) as more effective and/or better tolerated than the old drugs. Varying definitions of atypicality, study populations, outcomes and the reporting of these meant that well-conducted RCTs could show that 'olanzapine beats risperidone, risperidone beats quetiapine, and quetiapine beats olanzapine' and that all were, of course, better than the standard comparator drug haloperidol (as was required for FDA approval). Even if some or all of the apparent benefits were down to these new antipsychotics being used at lower doses than psychiatrists had got into the bad habit of using when prescribing older drugs,[38] Big Pharma had realised this. There was a clear need for independently funded and conducted RCTs.

This realisation led to the Clinical Antipsychotic Trials in Intervention Effectiveness (CATIE) study, which is probably the largest and most expensive clinical trial ever done in schizophrenia. It cost the US taxpayer the best part of $100 million. Lieberman and colleagues randomised 1,493 patients at 57 US sites to one of five treatments.[39] The primary outcome measure of continuing medication was only achieved in 26 per cent of people at eighteen months but this was about 10 per cent higher in patients allocated to take olanzapine – even if they also tended to put on weight and suffer metabolic derangements.

In the UK, the CUtLASS trial showed similarly slight, if any, advantages of the newer antipsychotics,[40] while the BALANCE trial showed that lithium was superior to valproate in preventing relapse in bipolar disorder.[41] Systematic reviews showed that the new anti-depressant, mood stabilising and antipsychotic drugs did not have simple class effects and each drug had subtle differences in terms of reducing certain symptoms and causing various adverse effects.

Laying the Groundwork and Going Global for Genetic Advances

It has long been known that major psychiatric disorders aggregate in families. This was conclusively demonstrated for schizophrenia by Gottesman and Shields in 1966,[42] while working at MRC Psychiatric Genetics Unit at the IOP, with the assistance of Elliot Slater. He had kept records of twins of whom at least one had a diagnosis of schizophrenia. Taken together with data from eleven earlier major twin studies, an identical twin was at least forty times more likely to have schizophrenia than a person from the general population and a fraternal twin of the same sex around nine to ten times as likely. These data strongly suggested a strong genetic basis for schizophrenia and adoption studies outside the UK proved it.

Ongoing twin studies at the IOP established beyond doubt that the heritability of schizophrenia, schizoaffective disorder and mania were substantial and similar (82–85 per cent). What was controversial was the mode of inheritance – whether it was due to a small number of rare but highly penetrant mutations or more attributable to polygenic liability in a diathesis stress-model. The identification of a chromosomal translocation from t1:11 in a large Scottish family in 1990 led to the identification of the 'DISC1' (Disrupted in Schizophrenia 1) gene.[43] The association was, however, strongest when the mental disorders in the phenotype included recurrent major depression and adolescent conduct and emotional disorders. Even though this family may be unique and common variants in DISC1 are not (at least as yet) identified as risk factors for any specific disorder, this discovery kept the field going during the long lean years of non-replicated linkage and association studies.

What was to transform psychiatric genetics was the Human Genetics Project (HGP). This started in 1990, funded by the US Department of Energy and the US National Institutes of Health and supported by the Wellcome Trust through the Sanger Centre in Cambridge. The first draft of the complete sequence of nucleotides in the human genome was published in 2001 and launched modern human genetics. The identification of rare, penetrant genetic variants causing monogenic diseases boomed in the following years and paved the way for the systematic screening of disease genes in diagnostic services – including those with severe learning disability. The HGP also brought about advances in technology, particularly 'next-generation sequencing', which led to the first available arrays for genome-wide association studies (GWAS).

The early psychiatric GWAS did not lead to significant findings, which led to some losing faith in the approach. Others persisted, and in one of the first and best examples of collaboration science the Wellcome Trust Case Control Consortium published (in 2007) the then largest GWAS to date and set the scene for the spate of gene discovery that was to follow. They examined approximately 2,000 individuals for each of seven major diseases and a shared set of approximately 3,000 controls and identified 24 independent association signals including one in bipolar disorder (and 1–9 in coronary artery disease, rheumatoid arthritis, type 1 and type 2 diabetes and Crohn's disease).[44]

The Psychiatric Genomics Consortium was also formed in 2007, which allowed thousands of samples from all over the world to be shared. This collaboration quickly delivered the first significant findings from GWAS for schizophrenia, as well as evidence that major psychiatric disorder was very highly polygenic.[45] Nevertheless, some rare mutations of large effect were clearly implicated in neurodevelopmental disorders such as autism, attention deficit hyperactivity disorder (ADHD) and schizophrenia.[46]

It has become increasingly clear in the past decade that GWAS is a numbers game. Pooling 100,000 cases of schizophrenia and controls led to no fewer than 108 schizophrenia-associated genetic loci becoming evident.[47] Adding another 35,000 people identified another 37 'hits' and more are on the way. Indeed, the success of GWAS in schizophrenia has led to it being called the poster child of the GWAS generation. Bipolar disorder and depression are now yielding their genetic secrets too.

It is, however, equally clear that the genes identified are pleiotropic – that is, they have multiple effects and so do not map neatly on to specific disorders. Just as the rare mutations increase the risk for a variety of conditions, the risk variants for common psychiatric disorders overlap to a large extent. Nonetheless, there are likely to be some specific genes and biological pathways as well as others cutting across disorders. Although such insights have yet to lead to innovations in the clinical management of patients, they certainly have promise for diagnostics and therapeutics.

The Decade of the Brain and the Next Ten Years

While the psychiatric geneticists have been trailblazing, the neuroimaging research community have organised themselves into large global consortia employing common and increasingly innovative methods. Most notably, the Enhancing Imaging Genetics through Meta-Analysis (ENIGMA) consortium have combined data from thousands of scans which have confirmed and strengthened the results from previous studies and meta-analyses and delivered novel insights into the genetics of neuroimaging measures. The application of mathematical graph theory tools to neuroimaging data provides a way of studying neural systems efficiency at a whole-brain (connectome) level.

Most excitingly, contemporary neuroscience and philosophy see the brain–mind (after Reverend Thomas Bayes) as testing hypotheses about the world, from previous experience, against ongoing experience and updating the inner model of the world as required.[48] In essence, structural and functional disturbances of fronto-temporal brain systems could reduce their reliable co-ordinated input, disrupt reality testing and impair the use of memories to guide perception and action. Most of the research thus far has been done on schizophrenia – with some replicated findings if not yet a true consensus – but this and other forms of 'computational psychiatry' offer objective measures of otherwise subjective impressions that promise to be revealing across psychiatry and indeed neuroscience as a whole.[49]

It has also become clear in the last ten years that the structural and functional neuroimaging findings in various disorders overlap to a large degree. To some extent, this is hardly surprising given the overlap in genetic and environmental risk factors and the comorbidities of mental disorders. The increasing incorporation of psychosocial risk markers – such as the role of personality, childhood adversity and stress and their biological correlates – into multivariate risk models of mental illness alongside polygenic risk scores and machine learning approaches to data analysis will advance progress towards clinical applications. Despite these complexities, there has been notable progress in developing neuroimaging biomarkers of depression and schizophrenia in the 2010s.[50]

Conclusion

This has, of necessity, been a relatively brief and focused review of fifty years and more of research endeavour. It has also been positive in stressing replicated advances and ignoring less profitable research streams, such as the red herring of the 'pink spot' in schizophrenia. Equally, however, British psychiatrists have made major contributions to understanding and treating many conditions – including autism, ADHD, anxiety and alcohol and drug dependence – which we have not had the space to do justice to.

Overall, it is difficult to avoid the conclusion that 'biological psychiatry' has been a success. Indeed, the historian Edward Shorter said as much as far back as 1999.[51] However, it makes little sense to talk of a biological psychiatry pursued by biological psychiatrists. It is simply medicine done by doctors who specialise in the diagnosis and management of mental illness.

Disquietingly, far too many psychiatrists seem unaware that drug treatments in psychiatry are about as good as in the rest of medicine.[52] As for the research, we should redouble our efforts to find biomarkers of diagnosis and in particular of treatment response. This is within our grasp if the field receives the research funding that reflects the societal costs of the conditions we deal with. This is also what the patients with these conditions and their carers want, as the James Lind Alliance (JLA) has demonstrated. The JLA, whose infrastructure is funded by the UK National Institute for Health Research (NIHR), brings patients, carers and clinicians together, in Priority Setting Partnerships, to identify and prioritise unanswered questions. There is a remarkable convergence of interests in, for example, determining causes, better diagnosis, early interventions, personalised approaches and better treatments with fewer adverse effects.

Key Summary Points

- Many scientists, academic and clinical psychiatrists have contributed to the search for the biological basis of mental illness, leading to many notable discoveries and particular advances in understanding schizophrenia.
- RCTs have established beyond reasonable doubt the efficacy of antidepressants, ECT, antipsychotics and mood stabilisers.
- The most striking diagnostic advances have been made in identifying the genetics of learning disability and in developing neuroimaging and blood-based biomarkers of dementia.
- Polygenic risk scores and machine learning of neuroimaging and other data have real potential to impact upon clinical practice and improve patient care.
- Psychiatrists should join those affected by mental illness in calling for increased funding to identify biomarkers, develop new treatments and improve services.

Notes

1.   S. B. Guze, Biological psychiatry: Is there any other kind? *Psychological Medicine* (1989) 19: 315–23.

2.   L. Eisenberg, Mindlessness and brainlessness in psychiatry. *British Journal of Psychiatry* (1986) 148: 497–508.

3.   G. W. Ashcroft and D. F. Sharman, 5-Hydroxyindoles in human cerebrospinal fluids. *Nature* (1960) 186: 1050–1.

4. G. W. Ashcroft, T. B. Crawford, D. Eccleston et al., 5-hydroxyindole compounds in the cerebrospinal fluid of patients with psychiatric or neurological diseases. *The Lancet* (1966) 2: 1049–52.

5. A. Coppen, D. M. Shaw and J. P. Farrell, Potentiation of the antidepressive effect of a monoamine-oxidase inhibitor by tryptophan. *The Lancet* (1963) 1: 79–81.

6. A. Coppen, E. G. Eccleston and M. Peet, Total and free tryptophan concentration in the plasma of depressive patients. *The Lancet* (1973) 2: 60–3.

7. E. Shorter, *How Everyone Became Depressed.* Oxford: Oxford University Press: 2013.

8. B. J. Carroll, M. Feinberg, J. F. Greden et al., A specific laboratory test for the diagnosis of melancholia: Standardization, validation, and clinical utility. *Archives of General Psychiatry* (1981) 38: 15–22.

9. J. F. W. Deakin and F. G. Graeff, 5-HT and mechanisms of defence. *Journal of Psychopharmacology* (1991) 5: 305–15.

10. S. J. Cooper, C. B. Kelly and D. J. King, 5-Hydroxyindoleacetic acid in cerebrospinal fluid and prediction of suicidal behaviour in schizophrenia. *The Lancet* (1992) 340: 940–1.

11. C. J. Harmer, R. S. Duman and P. J. Cowen, How do antidepressants work? New perspectives for refining future treatment approaches. *Lancet Psychiatry* (2017) 4: 409–18.

12. Ibid.

13. British Medical Research Council, Clinical trial of the treatment of depressive illness. *British Medical Journal* (1965) 1: 881–6.

14. R. H. Mindham, C. Howland and M. Shepherd, Continuation therapy with tricyclic antidepressants in depressive illness. *The Lancet* (1972) 2: 854–5.

15. E. Shorter, The history of lithium therapy. *Bipolar Disorders* (2009) 11(Suppl 2): 4–9.

16. P. C. Baastrup, J. C. Poulsen, M. Schou, K. Thomsen and A. Amdisen, Prophylactic lithium: Double blind discontinuation in manic-depressive and recurrent-depressive disorders. *The Lancet* (1970) 2: 326–30.

17. A. Coppen, R. Noguera and J. Bailey, Prophylactic lithium in affective disorders: Controlled trial. *The Lancet* (1971) 2: 275–9.

18. W. A. Barker, J. Scott and D. Eccleston, The Newcastle chronic depression study: Results of a treatment regime. *International Clinical Psychopharmacology* (1987) 2: 261–72.

19. National Institute of Mental Health Psychopharmacology Service Center Collaborative Study Group, Phenothiazine treatment of acute schizophrenia: Effectiveness. *Archives of General Psychiatry* (1964) 10: 246–61.

20. J. P. Leff and J. K. Wing, Trial of maintenance therapy in schizophrenia. *British Medical Journal* (1971) 3: 599–604; S. R. Hirsch, R. Gaind, P. D. Rohde, B. C. Stevens and J. K. Wing, Outpatient maintenance of chronic schizophrenic patients with long-acting fluphenazine: Double-blind placebo trial. Report to the Medical Research Council Committee on Clinical Trials in Psychiatry. *British Medical Journal* (1973) 1: 633–7.

21. E. C. Johnstone, T. J. Crow, C. D. Frith, J. Husband and L. Kreel, Cerebral ventricular size and cognitive impairment in chronic schizophrenia. *The Lancet* (1976) 2: 924–6.

22. S. W. Lewis, Computerised tomography in schizophrenia 15 years on. *British Journal of Psychiatry* (1990) 157 (Suppl 9): 16–24.

23. R. L. Suddath, G. W. Christison, E. F. Torrey, M. F. Casanova and D. R. Weinberger. Anatomical abnormalities in the brains of monozygotic twins discordant for schizophrenia. *New England Journal of Medicine* (1990) 322: 789–94.

24. S. M. Lawrie and S. S. Abukmeil, Brain abnormality in schizophrenia: A systematic and quantitative review of volumetric magnetic resonance imaging studies. *British Journal of Psychiatry* (1998) 172: 110–20.

25. P. J. Harrison, N. Freemantle and J. R. Geddes, Meta-analysis of brain weight in schizophrenia. *Schizophrenia Research* (2003) 64: 25–34.

26. S. M. Lawrie, H. Whalley, J. N. Kestelman et al., Magnetic resonance imaging of brain in people at high risk of developing schizophrenia. *The Lancet* (1999) 353: 30–3.

27. C. Pantelis, D. Velakoulis, P. D. McGorry et al., Neuroanatomical abnormalities before and after onset of psychosis: A cross-sectional and longitudinal MRI comparison. *The Lancet* (2003) 361: 281–8.

28. D. H. Ingvar and G. Franzén, Distribution of cerebral activity in chronic schizophrenia. *The Lancet* (1974) 2: 1484–6.

29. K. P. Ebmeier, S. M. Lawrie, D. H. Blackwood, E. C. Johnstone and G. M. Goodwin, Hypofrontality revisited: A high resolution single photon emission computed tomography study in schizophrenia. *Journal of Neurology, Neurosurgery, and Psychiatry* (1995) 58: 452–6.

30. P. K. McGuire, D. A. Silbersweig, I. Wright et al., Abnormal monitoring of inner speech: A physiological basis for auditory hallucinations. *The Lancet* (1995) 346: 596–600.

31. E. C. Johnstone, T. J. Crow, C. D. Frith, M. W. Carney and J. S. Price, Mechanism of the antipsychotic effect in the treatment of acute schizophrenia. *The Lancet* (1978) 1: 848–51.

32. O. D. Howes, S. K. Bose, F. Turkheimer et al., Dopamine synthesis capacity before onset of psychosis: A prospective [18 F]-DOPA PET imaging study. *American Journal of Psychiatry* (2011) 168: 1311–17.

33. I. McKeith, J. O'Brien, Z. Walker et al., Sensitivity and specificity of dopamine transporter imaging with 123I-FP-CIT SPECT in dementia with Lewy bodies: A phase III, multicentre study. *Lancet Neurology* (2007) 6: 305–13.

34. J. R. Geddes, S. M. Carney, C. Davies et al., Relapse prevention with antidepressant drug treatment in depressive disorders: a systematic review. *The Lancet* (2003) 361: 653–61.

35. S. Leucht, M. Tardy, K. Komossa et al., Antipsychotic drugs versus placebo for relapse prevention in schizophrenia: A systematic review and meta-analysis. *The Lancet* (2012) 379: 2063–71.

36. A. Cipriani, H. Pretty, K. Hawton and J. R. Geddes, Lithium in the prevention of suicidal behavior and all-cause mortality in patients with mood disorders: A systematic review of randomized trials. *American Journal of Psychiatry* (2005) 162: 1805–19.

37. UK ECT Review Group, Efficacy and safety of electroconvulsive therapy in depressive disorders: A systematic review and meta-analysis. *The Lancet* (2003) 361: 799–808.

38. J. Geddes, N. Freemantle, P. Harrison and P. Bebbington, Atypical antipsychotics in the treatment of schizophrenia: Systematic overview and meta-regression analysis. *British Medical Journal* (2000) 321(7273): 1371–6.

39. J. A. Lieberman, T. S. Stroup, J. P. McEvoy et al., Effectiveness of antipsychotic drugs in patients with chronic schizophrenia. *New England Journal of Medicine* (2005) 353: 1209–23.

40. P. B. Jones, T. R. Barnes, L. Davies et al., Randomized controlled trial of the effect on Quality of Life of second- vs first-generation antipsychotic drugs in schizophrenia: Cost Utility of the Latest Antipsychotic Drugs in Schizophrenia Study (CUtLASS 1). *Archives of General Psychiatry* (2006) 63: 1079–87.

41. BALANCE investigators and collaborators, J. R. Geddes, G. M. Goodwin et al., Lithium plus valproate combination therapy versus monotherapy for relapse prevention in bipolar I disorder (BALANCE): A randomised open-label trial. *The Lancet* (2010) 375: 385–95.

42. I. I. Gottesman and J. Shields, Schizophrenia in twins: 16 years' consecutive admissions to a psychiatric clinic. *British Journal of Psychiatry* (1996) 112: 809–18.

43. D. St Clair, D. Blackwood, W. Muir et al., Association within a family of a balanced autosomal translocation with major mental illness. *The Lancet* (1990) 336: 13–16.

44. Wellcome Trust Case Control Consortium, Genome-wide association study of 14,000 cases of seven common diseases and 3,000 shared controls. *Nature* (2007) 447: 661–78.

45. International Schizophrenia Consortium, S. M. Purcell, N. R. Wray et al., Common polygenic variation contributes to risk of schizophrenia and bipolar disorder. *Nature* (2009) 460: 748–52.

46. N. M. Williams, I. Zaharieva, A. Martin et al., Rare chromosomal deletions and duplications in attention-deficit hyperactivity disorder: A genome-wide analysis. *The Lancet* (2010) 376: 1401–8.

47. Schizophrenia Working Group of the Psychiatric Genomics Consortium, Biological insights from 108 schizophrenia-associated genetic loci. *Nature* (2014) 511: 421–7.

48. P. C. Fletcher and C. D. Frith, Perceiving is believing: A Bayesian approach to explaining the positive symptoms of schizophrenia. *Nature Reviews Neuroscience* (2009) 10: 48–58.

49. K. J. Friston, K. E. Stephan, R. Montague and R. J. Dolan, Computational psychiatry: The brain as a phantastic organ. *Lancet Psychiatry* (2014) 1: 148–58.

50. A. T. Drysdale, L. Grosenick, J. Downar et al., Resting-state connectivity biomarkers define neurophysiological subtypes of depression. *Nature Medicine* (2017) 23: 28–38; A. Li, A. Zalesky, W. Yue et al., A neuroimaging biomarker for striatal dysfunction in schizophrenia. *Nature Medicine* (2020) 26: 558–65.

51. E. Shorter, *A History of Psychiatry: From the Era of the Asylum to the Age of Prozac.* New York: Wiley and sons, 1997, p. vii.

52. S. Leucht, S. Hierl, W. Kissling, M. Dold and J. M. Davis, Putting the efficacy of psychiatric and general medicine medication into perspective: Review of meta-analyses. *British Journal of Psychiatry* (2012) 200: 97–106.

Chapter

17

The Pharmaceutical Industry and the Standardisation of Psychiatric Practice

David Healy

Introduction

The 1950s saw the largely serendipitous discovery in clinical settings of a series of psycho-tropic drugs, produced primarily in the pharmaceutical divisions of European chemical companies. This accompanied the discovery of antibiotics and medicines for other clinical conditions. While there were large chemical companies and a proprietary medicines industry, there was then no pharmaceutical industry as we know it. The nascent companies producing psychotropics, however, were quick to set up international meetings that brought basic scientists and clinical delegates together from all continents.

1960–80

In the wake of the Second World War, German psychiatry and medicine lost ground, opening a door for English to become the lingua franca of the medical world. This and the detour American psychiatry took into psychoanalysis fostered the reputations of British psychiatrists.

As of 1960, British academic psychiatry was 'social'. Social meant epidemiological rather than committed to the idea that mental illness was social rather than biological in origin. Social psychiatrists began thinking in terms of the operational criteria and other procedures that would enable research on the incidence and prevalence of nervous problems. Among the leading figures were Michael Shepherd, John Wing and others from the Institute of Psychiatry, who worked to establish methods which laid the basis for an international pilot study of schizophrenia on the one hand to studies on the incidence of primary care nervous disorders, not then part of psychiatry, on the other. These latter studies provided a template for other studies undertaken since then that, perhaps even more in mental health than in any other branch of medicine, created markets for pharmaceuticals.[1]

This group of psychiatrists played a central role in incorporating mental disorders into the *International Classification of Diseases*, which influenced the third edition of the American *Diagnostic and Statistical Manual of Mental Disorders* (DSM) that, published in 1980, laid a basis, along with controlled trials, for an industrialisation of psychiatry.

Randomised controlled trials (RCTs) originated in Britain. The first RCT had been done by Tony Hill on streptomycin in 1948. Michael Shepherd at the Institute of Psychiatry became a coordinator of the Medical Research Council (MRC) clinical trials committee soon after and, working with Hill, fostered the development of RCTs within mental health. Shepherd also ran the first placebo-controlled parallel group RCT comparing reserpine to placebo in anxious depression, which reported in 1955.

RCTs have since invaded medicine. This was not because they are a good way to evaluate a drug but because of the thalidomide crisis. The birth defects thalidomide caused led, in 1962, to a set of amendments to the US Food and Drugs Act that made RCTs the primary method to evaluate treatment. It was not clear then that the necessary focus on a primary end point RCTs require made them, almost by definition, a poor method to evaluate a treatment. Food and Drug Administration (FDA) regulations made RCTs the standard through which industry made gold, and trials done across medicine ever since have been industry-related.[2]

Before 1945, there were few academic psychiatry posts outside of Germany. After the war, university posts were created in the United States, the UK and elsewhere. Through the 1960s, however, there were comparatively few academic psychiatrists globally and this scarcity along with the involvement of British academics in early epidemiological research, the development of protocols for RCTs and their facility at English gave them a magisterial status at international meetings.

Among the notable figures were Martin Roth, whose concepts of endogenous and neurotic depression were influential. Linford Rees was a prolific clinical trialist. Michael Shepherd brought a scepticism of the enthusiasm for new drugs, most clearly demonstrated in high-profile arguments about the role of lithium (see also Chapters 2 and 16). Max Hamilton is perhaps the best-known figure now, by virtue of having his name on the standard scale for assessing the efficacy of antidepressant drugs – the Hamilton Rating Scale for Depression.

Hamilton's 1974 view about this scale seems prescient:

> It may be that we are witnessing a change as revolutionary as was the introduction of standardization and mass production in manufacture. Both have their positive and negative sides.[3]

Rating scales, along with operational criteria and RCTs, have made for a standardisation of clinical practice and a development of managed services that have latterly left US and UK psychiatry, and health services more generally, increasingly similar – where, in 1960, they could not have been more different.

In the years between 1960 and 1980, clinicians like George Ashcroft, Alex Coppen, Michael Pare, Donald Eccleston and others played a part in formulating monoamine,[4] especially serotonergic, hypotheses for mood disorders and in bringing the notion of a receptor into psychopharmacology, along with researchers in pharmacology like Merton Sandler, Gerald Curzon, Geoff Watkins, John Hughes and others.[5] These hypotheses were discarded by the 1970s but in the 1990s in the hands of pharmaceutical marketing departments they provided a basis for a bio-babble that has profoundly shaped public culture.[6]

In 1974, the British Association for Psychopharmacology (BAP) formed. The BAP became a forum for lively interdisciplinary exchanges for twenty years after which, as in other forums, the divide between clinicians and neuroscientists became increasingly hard to bridge.[7] The BAP provided a template for a European College of Psychopharmacology and at the same time a European Psychiatric Association was forming, which along with a World Psychiatric Association was largely underpinned by industry funding.

In addition to new tricyclic antidepressants and neuroleptics for traditional illnesses, LSD, benzodiazepines and contraceptives were at the centre of vigorous debates in the 1960s, playing a key role in stimulating revolutionary ferment in 1968. Did these drugs enhance or diminish us? In the case of the deinstitutionalisation that followed the introduction of the psychotropic drugs, who was being deinstitutionalised – patients or mental health staff?[8]

As a symbol of the role of medicine and psychiatry in particular, at this time, in 1968, revolting students occupied and ransacked the Paris office of Jean Delay, the discoverer of chlorpromazine, and occupied the Tokyo Department of Psychiatry for ten years, protesting against the biological experiments being undertaken. The biochemical psychopharmacology being undertaken by clinicians like Coppen in England and Van Praag in Holland appeared dehumanising.[9]

While psychotropic drugs were a focus for concern, it was the prospect of Big Medicine and medical arrogance rather than Big Pharma that was alarming at the time. Physicians working in industry such as Alan Broadhurst at Geigy did a great deal to 'market' depression, along with the tricyclic antidepressants and the Hamilton Rating Scale. This was considered respectable medical education then rather than disease mongering as it might be seen now.[10] George Beaumont, also at Geigy, took a lead in the promotion of clomipramine as a treatment for obsessive-compulsive disorder (OCD).[11]

1980–2000

While anti-psychiatry seemed largely contained in the 1970s, from 1980 mainstream figures in Britain like Peter Tyrer, Malcolm Lader and Heather Ashton raised concerns about the risks of dependence on benzodiazepines that seemed continuous with anti-psychiatric concerns about psychotropic drugs in general.[12] It was at this point that the pharmaceutical industry slipped into the line of fire,[13] symbolised by a set-piece engagement when Ian Oswald accused Upjohn of fraud in clinical trials of their hypnotic Halcion.[14]

Benzodiazepine dependence fed into a growing public debate about both mental health and health issues since, from 1980 onwards, more people were encountering psychiatrists and physicians than ever before, as both psychiatry and medicine deinstitutionalised from acute inpatient care into chronic disease management in outpatient and outpatient care (i.e. hypertension, osteoporosis, Type 2 diabetes, etc.).

Prior to 1980, other than for major events such as heart transplants, health rarely featured in the media but, in the 1980s, routine stories about benzodiazepine dependence in TV programmes like *That's Life* marked a change and health stories now figure in every issue of almost every newspaper and regularly on the headlines of news bulletins.

The media focus then was on breakthroughs and risks. As of 1970, the word risk had featured in the headlines and abstracts of medical articles on 200 occasions.[15] By 1990, prior to any mention of *Risk Societies*, this figure was more than 20,000 articles. Within health, a new numbers-based operationalism pitched medicines as a way to manage risks.

The benzodiazepine controversies opened a door for the Royal College of Psychiatrists to promote a Defeat Depression Campaign in 1990, whose message was that, rather than treat the superficial symptoms of anxiety, it would be better to diagnose and treat underlying depressions with non-dependence–inducing antidepressants.

This campaign coincided with the development and launch of selective serotonin reuptake inhibiting drugs (SSRIs). Eli Lilly and other companies ensured the Defeat Depression message was heard. The campaign helped make Prozac and later SSRIs into blockbuster drugs – drugs which earned a billion or more dollars per year – something unheard of before 1990, even though within three years of its launch there were more reports to regulators of dependence on another SSRI paroxetine than on all benzodiazepines over a twenty-year period.

The triumph of Prozac with its message of becoming Better than Well in books like *Listening to Prozac*, accompanied by a race to complete the Human Genome Project, seemed around 1990 to be ushering in a new biomedical era that left historians from Roy Porter to Roger Cooter wondering if it was possible any longer to write history of medicine. The term Biological Psychiatry was coined at this time.[16]

The years around 1990 also saw the emergence of evidence-based medicine (EBM). EBM pitched RCTs as offering gold standard knowledge of what medical drugs did and argued that this kind of knowledge should replace the knowledge born from clinical experience. The supposed validity of the RCT process meant that even trials funded by pharmaceutical companies would offer valid knowledge, although physicians needed to remain alert to tricks companies might get up to on the margins of trials.

As with RCTs, EBM largely began and took shape in Britain, symbolised by the establishment of the Cochrane Collaboration in 1992 (see also Chapter 16). Cochrane's mission was to review trials systematically, whittle out duplicate publications and take a critical view of efficacy. Around 1990, the pharmaceutical industry seemed increasingly powerful, leading to the establishment of organisations like No Free Lunch that encouraged physicians to beware of Pharma-bearing gifts. For many, Cochrane and EBM seemed the best tool with which to rein in the pharmaceutical industry, given its focus on scientific procedures rather than morality.

Until 1980, clinical trials had been run in single universities or hospitals by academics who knew their patients. By 1990, they were multicentred and run by clinical research companies who collected the trial data in a central repository to which no academics or physicians had access. The reporting of trial results was contracted out to medical writing agencies so that the articles were mostly ghostwritten with academic names chosen for the authorship lines primarily for their value to marketing rather than their knowledge of the issues. British psychiatrists were no longer magisterial figures, who could make or break a drug; they had become ciphers in an industrial process, taking second place to Americans who had now discovered biological psychiatry. The appearances of scientific process remained the same, so few physicians or psychiatrists and no one outside the profession had any sense of the changes.

The first medical guidelines appeared in the mid-1980s aimed at stopping clearly unhelpful practices like stripping varicose veins. As of the early 1990s, a series of bodies like the BAP began to develop guidelines based on RCTs that made recommendations about what to do rather than what not to do. Industry also began to support guidelines but stopped when companies realised their control of publications meant they controlled the guidelines others created.

Industry control of the evidence became almost complete with the establishment by a Labour government of the National Institute for Clinical Excellence (NICE; now the National Institute for Health and Care Excellence) guideline apparatus in 1997. We appeared to have an independent body sifting the evidence without anyone realising that the evidence being sifted had been mostly ghostwritten and there was no access to the underlying data.

Events following a 1990 paper in the *American Journal of Psychiatry* brought home the change. This paper carried accounts of six cases of patients becoming suicidal on Prozac that offered compelling evidence of causality as traditionally established in medicine.[17] Eli Lilly, the makers of Prozac, claimed their trials did not show that Prozac caused suicidality and that, while individual cases might be harrowing, the plural of anecdote was not data.[18] Lilly's defence ran in the *British Medical Journal* (*BMJ*), whose editor, Richard Smith, was a proponent of EBM. Lilly's defence, hinged on a meta-analysis, seeming to show industry playing by EBM rules.

Prozac survived. The *BMJ* missed the fact that the small print of the meta-analysis showed a significant excess of suicidal acts on Prozac compared to placebo. The tie-up between *BMJ* and Lilly fuelled support for EBM and transformed medical journals and clinical practice. Up till then, clinicians had received regular drugs bulletins outlining the hazards of treatments, but these were replaced by guidelines which only mentioned benefits. Journals preferentially published RCTs and meta-analyses, which companies paid for, and it became close to impossible to publish case reports or anything on the hazards of treatment.[19] Few clinicians noted that the party most consistently exhorting them to practice EBM was the pharmaceutical industry. Industry profits, meanwhile, grew twentyfold in the thirty years from 1980 to 2010. EBM did not rein in industry.

Through to the 1990s, many significant problems on treatment, such as the acute sexual effects on antidepressants or tardive dyskinesia on antipsychotics, were recognised within a year or two of a drug's launch. After 1990, significant treatment hazards such as impulsivity disorders on dopamine agonists, enduring sexual dysfunction following finasteride, isotretinoin and antidepressants, and the mental state changes linked to asthma drugs like montelukast might wait twenty to thirty years, the expiration of a patent, or company efforts to market new drugs, to come to light.[20] If treatment hazards cannot be formally recognised, they are unlikely to be registered in clinical practice. As a result, an increasing part of patients' experience no longer registered on the eyes or ears of clinicians.

2000–2010 and Beyond

In 2002, a Labour government made NICE guidelines central to a new National Health Service (NHS) plan, which aimed at levelling up health provision supposedly in accordance with best practice. Guidelines would also enable managers to ensure clinicians delivered services rather than exercised discretion and allow nurses and other staff to replace doctors to carry out defined tasks. Health services began to replace health care, and in the new services the exercise of medical discretion was a problem rather than something to be celebrated.

The transition from care to services became clear in 2004, when NICE began drawing up guidelines for the treatment of childhood depression, just as a crisis developed about the efficacy and safety of antidepressants given to children. Investigative journalists rather than scientists, academics or clinicians scrutinised what was happening and found that the clinical trial literature was entirely ghostwritten or company-written and that publications claiming treatments were effective and safe were at odds with what RCT data showed. A *Lancet* article and editorial 'Depressing Research' suggested no guidelines should be written unless there was access to the data.[21]

The crisis was raised in a House of Commons Health Select Committee meeting later that year, but in response both the editor of the *Lancet* and a founder of the Cochrane Collaboration assured the committee that the ghostwriting of clinical trials and the lack of access to trial data were not a significant problem.[22]

There was a brief stay in the increasing rate of antidepressant prescriptions to children in Britain just after this, but antidepressants are now the second most commonly prescribed drugs to teenage girls after contraceptives, in the face of thirty RCTs of antidepressants given to depressed minors – all negative.[23]

In 1960, RCTs were expected to temper the enthusiasm for new treatments generated by open studies claiming astonishing benefits. A negative RCT would stop therapeutic bandwagons – as with the demise of the monoamine oxidase inhibitor (MAOI) antidepressants following a negative MRC trial in 1965. Now psychiatry leads the world in having the greatest concentration of negative trials ever done for any indication in any age group, but this has had no effect, other than a paradoxical one, on rates of treatment utilisation.

When concerns first arose around 2004 about the use of antidepressants in children the problem could be seen as a rotten apple in a barrel problem that could be put right by professional and media attention. There was some professional attention to the problem of children and antidepressants around 2004 with the then president of the Royal College, Mike Shooter, instituting a review of conflict of interest policies. Industry warned the College to back off.[24]

We now appear to have a rotten barrel with politicians, health bureaucrats, academics and the media unable to grapple with a problem that extends to both the efficacy and the safety of all drugs across medicine. There are limp discussions about the need to rein in conflicts of interest – transparency – predicated on the idea that we are still dealing with rotten apples. At a time when it would be helpful to have some magisterial clinicians, it is difficult to see any psychiatrist the industry might be worried about.

Almost all industries have an interest in standardising methods and processes. This standardisation and operationalism is at the heart of what is called neoliberalism but has arguably been more apparent in medicine (neo-medicalism) than in any other domain of life since 1980.[25] Just as in 1976, according to the then prevalent dogmas of the Chicago School of Economics, the money supply in Chile became a thermostat function that dictated how the Chilean economy would operate, so in medicine *numbers*, such as those for blood pressure, peak flow rates, bone densities, rating scale scores or the five of nine criteria needed to make a diagnosis of depression in DSM, now dictate what happens.

The room for discretion vanished with the development of guidelines which were embraced by governments of both right and left and in particular the Labour government in the UK, who saw a means to level up care. Instead, guidelines provided a vehicle to expand the role of management in clinical practice, transforming what had been health care into health services and making health part of the wider service sector.

Qualitative assessments of a patient, which had been judicial in nature, best exemplified in the effort to establish whether a treatment is causing an adverse effect or not, were replaced by quantitative processes against which clinical practice would be evaluated.[26]

In 2016, the pharmaceutical industry declared they were pulling out of mental health because they could make more money elsewhere. There was no apparent fiduciary duty to physicians or patients; their primary fiduciary duty to their shareholders required a maximising of revenues.

Industry's intention was to turn to anti-inflammatory drugs, among others. This turn did not mean that mental health would be neglected completely but that anti-inflammatory drugs would be developed which would come at a high cost and could then be sold for a variety of indications such as mental health disorders. It is no surprise that in the last decade we have heard a lot more about a possible inflammatory basis to mood disorders – an inflammo-babble. It is unlikely this move will lead to cures of nervous problems in that, as Goldman Sachs recently noted, curing patients is not a good business model.[27]

Conclusion

In the 1960s, after an astonishing flood of new drugs, a nascent pharmaceutical industry, previously run by chemists and clinicians, brought in management consultants to ensure the breakthroughs continued. The consultants installed professional managers and recommended process changes involving an outsourcing of clinical trials and medical writing initially, followed by drug discovery as drug pipelines dried up. Latterly, public relations have been outsourced so that pharmaceutical industry personnel rarely defend industry in public. Debate about the role of drugs or hazards linked to drugs has been silenced, as media organisations adopt policies to avoid False Balances – a strategy introduced by industry think tanks, the mirror image of Doubt Is Our Product. If drugs are approved by regulators and endorsed in guidelines, dissenting viewpoints should not be aired in order to avoid alarming the public.

The standardisation of processes extended to clinical services in the 1990s and to professional bodies like the Royal College of Psychiatrists from around 2010. An installation of managers is one of the headline features of these changes, but these are not managers in the sense of people who manage conflict or who are entrepreneurial. They are rather bureaucrats ticking operational boxes. This is bad for drug discovery, inimical to health care and may toll a death knell for psychiatry as a profession. Psychiatrists, on current trends, are more likely to end up as middle-grade managers, ensuring nurses and others meeting with patients adhere to guidelines and minimise risks to the organisation, than as clinicians who might exercise discretion or academics who might follow a serendipitous observation.

Key Summary Points

- As of 1960, British academic psychiatry was 'social'. Social meant epidemiological rather than committed to the idea that mental illness was social rather than biological in origin. The designation 'biological psychiatry' became current in the 1990s.
- In the 1960s, after an astonishing flood of new drugs, a nascent pharmaceutical industry, previously run by chemists and clinicians, brought in management consultants to ensure the breakthroughs continued but drug discovery in psychiatry has dried up.
- The pharmaceutical industry has colonised medical research, education and clinical practice. EBM and clinical guidelines have served to extend rather than contain the influence of the industry.
- Antidepressants are now the second most prescribed drugs to teenage girls after contraceptives, in the face of thirty RCTs of antidepressants given to depressed minors – all negative.
- While they came with drawbacks, through to 1990 the psychotropic drugs introduced from the late 1950s onwards extended the range of clinical capabilities and likely did more good than harm. It is difficult to make the same claims about developments since 1990.

Notes

1. M. Shepherd, Psychopharmacotherapy: Specific and non-specific. In D. Healy, ed., *The Psychopharmacologists*, Vol. 2, 237–58. London: Arnold, 1998.

2. D. Healy, *Pharmageddon*. Berkeley: California University Press, 2012.

3. M. Hamilton. In P. Kielholz, ed., *Depressive Illness, Diagnosis, Assessment, Treatment*. Berne: Hanns Huber Publishers, 1972.

4. G. Ashcroft, The receptor enters psychiatry. In D. Healy, ed., *The Psychopharmacologists*, Vol. 3, 180–200. London: Arnold, 2000; A. Coppen, Biological psychiatry in Britain. In D. Healy, ed., *The Psychopharmacologists*, Vol. 1, 265–86. London: Chapman and Hall, 1996.

5. M. Sandler, The place of chemical pathology in psychopharmacology. In Healy, *The Psychopharmacologists*, Vol. 1, 381–400; G. Curzon, From neurochemistry to neuroscience. In Healy, *The Psychopharmacologists*, Vol. 2, 307–24.

6. D. Healy, Trouble in the Freudian gulf. *British Medical Journal* (1999) 318: 949; D. Healy, Serotonin and depression: The marketing of a myth. *British Medical Journal* (2015) 350: h1771.

7. D. Healy, The history of British Psychopharmacology. In H. Freeman and G. E. Berrios, eds, *150 Years of British Psychiatry, Volume 2: The Aftermath*, 61–88. London: Athlone Press, 1996.

8. Healy, *Pharmageddon*.

9. Ibid.

10. A. Broadhurst, Before and after imipramine. In Healy, *The Psychopharmacologists*, Vol. 1, 111–34.

11. G. Beaumont, The place of clomipramine in psychopharmacology. In Healy, *The Psychopharmacologists*, Vol. 1, 309–28.

12. M. Lader, Psychopharmacology: Clinical and social. In Healy, *The Psychopharmacologists*, Vol. 1, 463–82.

13. M. Bury and J. Gabe, A sociological view of tranquilliser dependence: Challenges and responses. In I. Hindmarch, G. Beaumont and S. Brandon, eds, *Benzodiazepines: Current Concepts*, 211–26. Chichester: John Wiley, 1990.

14. I. Oswald, The hypnotic business. In Healy, *The Psychopharmacologists*, Vol. 3, 459–78.

15. J. A. Skolbekken, The risk epidemic in medical journals. *Social Science and Medicine* (1995) 40: 291–305.

16. S. Guze, Biological psychiatry: Is there any other kind? *Psychological Medicine* (1989) 19: 315–23.

17. M. H. Teicher, C. Glod and J. O. Cole, Emergence of intense suicidal preoccupation during fluoxetine treatment. *American Journal of Psychiatry* (1990) 47: 207–10.

18. C. M. Beasley, B. E. Dornseif, J. C. Bosomworth, M. E. Sayler, A. H. Rampey and J. H. Heiligenstein, Fluoxetine and suicide: A meta-analysis of controlled trials of treatment for depression. *British Medical Journal* (1991) 303, 685–92.

19. Healy, *Pharmageddon*.

20. Ibid.

21. Editorial, Depressing research. *The Lancet* (2004) 363: 1335; C. Whittington, T. Kendall, P. Fonaghy, D. Cottrell, A. Cotgrove and E. Boddington, Selective serotonin reuptake inhibitors in childhood depression: Systematic review of published versus unpublished data. *The Lancet* (2004) 363: 1341–1345.

22. House of Commons Health Select Committee, *The Influence of the Pharmaceutical Industry*. Fourth report of session 2004–2005. HC 42-1. London: The Stationery Office, p. 56 et seq.

23. D. Healy, J. Le Noury and J. Jureidini, Paediatric antidepressants: Benefits and risks. *International Journal of Risk and Safety in Medicine* (2019) 30: 1–7.

24. Healy, *Pharmageddon*, chap. 7, pp. 220–1.

25. D. Healy, *Shipwreck of the Singular. Healthcare's Castaways*. Toronto: Samizdat Health, 2021.

26. D. Healy and D. Mangin, Clinical judgments, not algorithms, are key to patient safety. *British Medical Journal* (2019) 367: l5777.

27. T. Kim, Goldman Sachs ask in biotech report: Is curing patients a sustainable business model. *CNBC*, 11 April 2018, www.cnbc.com/2018/04/11/goldman-asks-is-curing-patients-a-sustainable-business-model.html.

Chapter

18 The Evolution of Psychiatric Practice in Britain

Allan Beveridge

Introduction

In 1960, the typical psychiatrist was male, white and British-born. He would spend most of his working day in a mental hospital. The majority of his patients would be compulsorily detained and many would have spent long periods incarcerated.[1] He would not be a member of the Royal College of Psychiatrists as this organisation was not created until 1971. Instead, he would probably have attained a Diploma in Psychological Medicine (DPM) but would not have participated in a formal training scheme, as these did not exist either.[2] In assessing his patients, he would have had a limited number of diagnoses at his disposal. Homosexuality was one of the diagnoses and he might use aversion therapy to treat the 'condition'.[3] He could prescribe antipsychotic medication, such as chlorpromazine and haloperidol, and antidepressants, such as imipramine, amitriptyline and phenelzine. He could also prescribe electroconvulsive therapy (ECT), though he might have to administer the anaesthetic himself. He could employ phenobarbitone and intramuscular paraldehyde for sedation, and he might resort to the use of the padded cell and the straitjacket, which were still available in some mental hospitals. He might have some expertise in psychodynamic psychotherapy, but this would depend on where he was working and whether the local psychiatric culture favoured such an approach. There was little in the way of specialisation, so he would be expected to deal with all the patients referred to him, the referrals coming almost exclusively from the general practitioner. At this time, the number of psychiatrists was small, and his contact with other colleagues outside his work would be at meetings of the Medico-Psychological Association (MPA) or in the pages of the *Journal of Mental Science*, the forerunner of the *British Journal of Psychiatry*, which was established in 1962.

By 2010, the typical psychiatrist was quite likely to be female and non-white, as, by this stage, many doctors had emigrated to Britain from the Indian subcontinent, Africa, the Caribbean and the Middle East. She would be working in a community resource centre or in a psychiatric unit in a district general hospital and most of her patients would be voluntary. She would receive referrals from not only general practitioners but also psychologists, social workers, occupational therapists, the police and other agencies. The range of problems she encountered was much larger than in 1960 and the expectation of cure or relief of symptoms was much higher.[4] She would be a member of the Royal College of Psychiatrists, having passed her exams and participated in a training scheme, which involved rotating around the different psychiatric specialties. She would have access to many more diagnoses, some of them contentious, such as attention deficit hyperactivity disorder (ADHD), though homosexuality would no longer be considered a psychiatric condition. She would have a greater range of medications from which to choose, such as lithium and other mood stabilisers, though there had been no major breakthrough in psychopharmacology since the 1950s. She would be versed in psychodynamic psychotherapy, which was now a mandatory part of her training, and she would also be familiar with cognitive behavioural therapy and, perhaps, dialectical behavioural therapy and interpersonal therapy. The number of psychiatrists in Britain in 2010 was considerably larger than it had been in 1960, and there were now many specialties, such as addictions, psychotherapy, old age psychiatry, forensic psychiatry, liaison psychiatry, community psychiatry, intellectual disability psychiatry and rehabilitation. There were more conferences at which to meet colleagues, and the *British Journal of Psychiatry* had expanded to include other publications, such as the *Psychiatric Bulletin*, which focused on everyday clinical matters.

What sources are available to understand the day-to-day clinical experience of British psychiatrists during this period? As well as the secondary literature, there are witness seminars,[5] where clinicians discuss past events. There are also various interviews with psychiatrists, but these tend to be focused on white men and on those who trained in London, more particularly at the Maudsley.[6] It is difficult to discover what clinical life was like for women, though Angela Rouncefield, who worked in Liverpool in the 1960s, remembers that psychiatry, like the rest of medicine then, was very male-dominated and that she felt she was constantly having to prove herself.[7] It is also difficult to find the testimonies of people from ethnic minorities and those working in the so-called periphery. There tends to be much more written about England than other parts of Britain. Andrew Scull has criticised this exclusively Anglocentric approach, which, although he was referring to Scotland, could equally apply to Wales and Northern Ireland:

> With few exceptions, English-centred historiography . . . largely neglected the very different Scottish approaches to the containment and treatment of the mad . . . the scholarship of the time embodied the presumption (infuriating for the Scots, and typical of the English) that either the only thing that mattered was what occurred south of the border; or alternatively and without giving the matter much thought, what happened in England was also what occurred in politically subordinate Scotland.[8]

Within the limitations of the archival record, this chapter will attempt to examine the evolution of psychiatry between 1960 and 2010, as it was experienced by psychiatrists of the era.

The Beginning of the Era

In 2019, the social psychiatrist Tom Burns remembered the 1960s thus (see also Chapter 20):

> in the late 60s, when I was doing this, psychiatry was . . . quite prestigious. I mean nowadays it's all looked down on, psychiatry, it's a job that people who can't get proper medical jobs do. It wasn't like that then. It was the year of Ronnie Laing, and all that stuff, and but it was quite an exciting thing to do. And it did have its own glamour and prestige, you know, it wasn't seen as something that people who couldn't get other jobs did.[9]

The Mental Hospital

The old mental hospitals were still standing in 1960 but not all were the repressive institutions of folklore. Bill Boyd, who worked at Rosslynlee Hospital outside Edinburgh, remembers:

It was very comforting and comfortable because Rosslynlee was still traditional under a very excellent and benign Physician Superintendent, Dr Andy Hegarty, I found I was accepted there very easily. There was a very informal, warm atmosphere amongst doctors, nurses and all the staff and there was a lot going on there too – out patient clinics in the local towns, patients coming up as day-patients, looking back now the services were remarkably advanced.[10]

In contrast, Hugh Freeman had more unpleasant memories:

My first experience of it, though, was as a locum at Wakefield, immediately before the Army. The neuroleptic era was just beginning then, but this mental hospital was quite Hogarthian in many ways, and some of the staff seemed to me as peculiar as the patients. When I first arrived there, on a misty January night, it was like the opening of a Hammer film.[11]

Malcolm Campbell, a neurologist, remembers his shock in the early 1960s when he started work at Friern Hospital, in London with its quarter-of-a-mile-long corridor providing the entrance to more than thirty wards, crammed with patients.[12] A recent witness seminar demonstrated that the quality of mental hospitals varied greatly throughout the country, and there was a suggestion that the standard of care was higher in Scotland.[13]

Changes were afoot, however. The 1957 Report of the Royal Commission on the Law Relating to Mental Illness and Mental Deficiency (Percy Commission, 1957) was a crucial turning point in mental health policy in the UK.[14] It urged relocating mental health care from hospital to community settings and inspired the 1959 Mental Health Act, which empowered local authorities in England and Wales to establish community mental health provision.

Psychiatrists tended to see the 1959 Act as benign in its impact on services and patient experience, partly because it allowed them, through the procedure of voluntary admission to mental hospitals, to implement improvements in treatment and care which had been foreshadowed in the 1950s. Services were dominated institutionally and intellectually by psychiatrists.[15] Although the 1959 (England and Wales) and 1960 (Scotland) Acts differed in some respects, there were enough similarities between the two to anticipate that the drive in England and Wales to close down psychiatric hospitals would be mirrored north of the border. However, as Victoria Long has pointed out, the Scots were not as convinced as their English counterparts that psychiatric hospitals could be rapidly emptied of their patients.[16]

Bill Boyd remembers:

I was Chairman of the Scottish Division, we were accused in Scotland of not being as advanced as the south in terms of cutting back on beds and putting people into the community. I remember very clearly writing to the *Scotsman* on behalf of the Division pointing out that psychiatrists were at the forefront of developing Care in the Community but that we as a group were not prepared to put our patients out of hospital until we were confident that community facilities and indeed public attitudes had matured to a level where it was reasonable to move our patients into Community Care.[17]

Rehabilitation

During the 1970s, the numbers of patients in psychiatric hospitals fell. This was the era of 'deinstitutionalisation'. In 1970, Wing and Brown's classic *Institutionalism and Schizophrenia* was published.[18] The authors compared three psychiatric hospitals and found that the social environment had a considerable effect on the mental state of the patients. The more deprived the environment, the worse the outcome. However, too much stimulation could also have adverse effects on the patients as well. The London social psychiatrist, Jim Birley, maintained that the goal of rehabilitation was to find the appropriate level for each patient.[19] Diagnosis was not so important in predicting outcome for these patients. Developing living skills was more important, and here clinical psychologists and occupational therapists played a crucial part, while Industrial Rehabilitation Units helped patients get back into the way of work. However, Birley conceded that the early optimistic belief that patients could become independent was not borne out by experience. There was the danger of what he termed 'transinstitutionalisation', whereby patients were merely transferred from hospital to other deprived environments, such as boarding houses, nursing homes or the street. In addition, after the 1960s employment fell and it was less easy for the mentally ill to find jobs.

Birley also felt that many psychiatrists were not particularly interested in looking after the long-term mentally ill. By 1970, many acute psychiatric units had been built in general hospitals, and these proved more attractive to psychiatrists. Birley observed:

> Psychiatrists, like most doctors, prefer to look after patients who get better . . . Psychiatric departments of medical schools, where most psychiatrists were trained, felt that they required a regular supply of acute and preferably 'new' cases for teaching.[20]

As a result, many psychiatrists had not been trained in the management of the chronically mentally ill, whom, Birley maintained, they often perceived as unattractive in appearance, behaviour and level of hygiene. In addition, many psychiatrists felt vulnerable outside the hospital, working with different staff with different approaches, though some greatly enjoyed it.

As well as the efforts to move the long-term psychiatric residents outside asylum walls, there was the movement to treat patients in the community, known as social or community psychiatry. As Tom Burns recalled, the flagship of social psychiatry was the therapeutic community movement, which encompassed Fulbourn, Napsbury, Dingleton and Henderson Hospitals.[21] Although a pioneer and an enthusiast, he recognised some of the difficulties:

> You're stripped of the normal paraphernalia of status. You know, you've got an outpatient clinic in medicine, there are receptionists and nurses and medical students and being a consultant is good for your ego, you know, you're the expert that everything circles around. If you do social psychiatry, it's you and perhaps one of your colleagues, a nurse or social worker, plus the patient and their family on their territory.
> . . . when I look back on it, the, particularly when social psychiatry started to move out more and more into sort of community-based work and stripping away all these structures that we normally relied on, I, I think we probably underestimated how important they are to sustain people in difficult jobs . . . So, I think one thing that we've gotten wrong a bit was that we turned our back a little bit too much on the benefits of institutional care. I mean, not for the patients, but for us.[22]

The lack of sufficient resources for community care of the mentally ill was already causing frustration to clinicians.[23]

Other Developments

Hugh Freeman recalled: 'there was no tradition of multidisciplinary team working; that was one of the achievements of our efforts in the '60s',[24] a sentiment which David

Goldberg also expressed.[25] Tom Burns felt that the sectorisation of psychiatric services into geographical 'catchment areas' which began in the 1960s was a major and valuable development.[26]

Further, as Turner (see also Chapter 23) and colleagues observed:

> The 1970s also saw significant innovations in treatment and service delivery, led by clinicians responding to these challenges. There was increasing use of psychological treatments with an evidence base and widespread acceptance that the services needed to acknowledge and counteract the social devaluation of their users.[27]

With the rundown of the old mental hospitals, came the setting up of psychiatric units in general hospitals. The advocates claimed they would lead to a reduction of stigma, greater accessibility for patients and a closer alliance between psychiatry and general medicine, leading to improvements in the patients' physical health.[28] For many psychiatrists, it was a great step forward. Maurice Silverman, working at Blackburn commented:

> I think the basic difference is that in the DGH [district general hospital] unit, as a psychiatrist, you have a very much more intimate relationship with other personnel and with the surrounding community. Under 'other personnel', I'm including other consultants in every specialty, the GPs in the area, and community social workers.[29]

Others, though, were less keen. Thomas Freeman, who worked at Gartnavel Royal in Glasgow, commented:

> I was perhaps going to swim against the tide as by 1963–1964 there was already talk of the mental hospital becoming superfluous. Hope was now pinned on the new medications and on the psychiatric unit of the general hospital. I strenuously opposed this, pointing to the fact that as yet we were without aetiologically based treatments. Chronically ill patients would remain with us; where else were they to go? Today we have the legacy of these optimistic forecasts and the actions which were based on them.[30]

Professor Elaine Murphy (see also Chapter 12) also complained:

> Psychiatrists pressed for more convenient and congenial facilities in DGHs – the time spent with the long-term patients decreased in asylums and in the community. By the time the Royal College of Psychiatrists was established in 1971, training was focused on short term and emergencies.[31]

Murphy contended that there had emerged a two-tier system in England, with the new DGHs and the old, less well-funded asylums. Goldberg objected to the practice at the Maudsley of sending their seriously mentally ill patients, who had relapsed, to local mental hospitals.[32]

There were significant differences, however, between England and Scotland in their attitude towards psychiatric units sited in general hospitals. According to Long:

> [Health] Departmental officials in Scotland believed that general hospitals lacked a number of resources specially designed to assist psychiatric patients, and favoured upgrading mental hospital care by using the small drop in inpatient numbers to relieve overcrowding and close down wards in old, obsolete buildings. Psychiatric units in general hospitals, they believed, should not be developed at the expense of existing mental hospitals, and efforts

should be made to integrate the two forms of provision to stop a two-tier service developing.[33]

The Royal College of Psychiatrists and the Development of Specialties

The Royal College of Psychiatrists was founded in 1971. As Bewley shows, the path to its establishment was tortuous and many psychiatrists as well as doctors from other disciplines opposed it.[34] Trainee psychiatrists, who were worried about the entrance requirement of a formal examination, campaigned successfully for the provision of adequate ongoing education before they were expected to sit such an exam. Hugh Freeman discussed the lack of formal training before the advent of the College:

> At that time, the psychiatric profession here was very small, compared with today, and the greater part of it consisted of doctors who had grown-up in mental hospitals under the apprenticeship tradition. There was very little alternative to that, as the Universities and teaching hospitals provided only very few places indeed for those who wanted to train in psychiatry.[35]

The period witnessed the growth of a rapidly ageing population – by 1990, half of all long-stay beds were occupied by old people with dementia.[36] The response was the development of the psychiatric care of the elderly, which had its origins in the late 1960s (see also Chapter 22).[37] R. A. Robinson at the Crichton Royal Hospital in Dumfries was an early pioneer. In 1970, the government urged that psychogeriatric assessment units should be set up in general hospitals. According to Arie and Jolley,[38] the main progress was in the development of services and they contended that the emphasis on bringing treatment to the patient's home led the way for the rest of psychiatry. Further, the links with medicine contributed to the reintegration of psychiatry into medicine, at least to some extent.

Following the 1959 Mental Health Act in England and Wales, there was a reduction in the number of locked wards in psychiatric hospitals.[39] In the early 1970s, there were only eight forensic psychiatrists in England (see also Chapter 29). Following the Butler Report in 1975, there were more than 150 consultants. When he was interviewed in 1990, the Edinburgh forensic psychiatrist Derek Chiswick said:

> Forty years ago a handful of forensic psychiatrists spent their time giving evidence in the various 'hanging' trials . . . which decided whether a murderer was to live or die. Today the picture has changed. Forensic psychiatrists are fully involved in both assessment and treatment (the latter very important) of a wide range of mentally abnormal offenders . . . You will find forensic psychiatrists in various clinical settings including the maximum security or special hospitals (of which there are five in Britain), in the new regional secure units which have developed in England (though not in Scotland), in ordinary psychiatric hospitals and clinics, and also visiting psychiatrists to prisons.[40]

However, in the 1980s, following the killing of a social worker by a mentally ill individual, it became mandatory in England to set up a homicide inquiry if a mentally ill person committed a murder. As a result, all English psychiatrists, and, indeed, all mental health workers, practised within a 'blame culture' setting, and this culture was also apparent, albeit to a lesser degree, in Scotland, though it did not have the same mechanism of automatic inquiries (see also Chapters 8 and 28).

Dr Max Glatt inaugurated the first unit for alcoholism at a mental hospital in Britain in 1951; between then and 1973, more than twenty such units were established by the NHS (see also Chapter 25).[41] However, research in the 1970s cast doubt on this approach, demonstrating that many could be improved by outpatient treatment alone or brief interventions.

Bruce Ritson describes how the approach to alcohol problems evolved during this period:

> A strongly held view at that time was that people who were alcoholic had become so because of some underlying psychological problem. The emphasis – and this is what attracted me in the first place – was on finding out what the psychodynamics of their particular addiction were and then trying to help, usually with group psychotherapy and sometimes with individual psychotherapy or couple therapy. The focus was on finding an underlying psychic cause, which I do not think I would really go along with now. Sometimes there is an underlying cause, but often it is the outcome of chronic exposure to excessive drinking and the psychological harm is secondary.[42]

There was a long-running campaign to persuade the College to accept that training in psychotherapy should be an integral part of the training of general psychiatrists. Heinz Wolff, a psychotherapist at University College London, observed:

> I recall how hard we had to fight to have the first Guidelines for the Training in Psychotherapy accepted by the Council and other committees in 1971. For me it was less important exactly what the guidelines said but rather that the College should acknowledge the importance of training of psychiatric trainees in dynamic psychotherapy.[43]

In 1993, the College published guidelines making training in psychotherapy a mandatory requirement for qualification as a psychiatrist.[44]

Until the 1970s, dedicated liaison services were virtually unknown in Britain. A special interest group in liaison psychiatry was set up in the early 1980s.[45] The specialties of intellectual disability, child psychiatry and others also evolved during this period.

Crisis of Confidence among Psychiatrists

The advent of the Conservative government in 1979 saw the rapid development of the New Right, which explicitly encouraged both privatisation and competition. The first service user movements appeared in the early 1970s, demanding civil and economic rights for patients in the community, and, in parallel, pressure groups such as Mind began to agitate for changes to the 1959 Act (see also Chapters 13 and 14).[46] In *Psychiatry in Dissent*, published in 1980, Clare judged that contemporary psychiatry was in an unhealthy state, with problems of recruitment, lack of resources and its lowly status in the medical hierarchy.[47] Writing in 1983, Sedgwick delineated many of the circumstances that undermined the authority of psychiatrists.[48] He noted the failure to accept psychiatric expertise in the legal courts following the Peter Sutcliffe trial, the popularity of anti-psychiatric arguments and the collusion of this attitude with the political 'New Right'. An editorial in 1985 in the *Lancet* claimed that psychiatry was a 'discipline that had lost its way'.[49] In 1986, Bhugra reported on the largely negative public perception of psychiatry.[50]

Writing in 1989, Tom Harrison, a psychiatrist from Birmingham, reported on the concerns of his consultant colleagues:[51]

First is the declining morale of the psychiatrist and second are the rising expectations of other mental health workers . . . Other professions in mental health have been influenced by a number of factors. These include: a broadening knowledge base and range of skills, increasing specialisation, more graduate nursing recruits, less acceptance of authoritarian management, often accompanied by idealistic enthusiasm, and increasing independence of operation with less direct supervision.

More generally, Hugh Freeman lamented:

The NHS was one of the best things that ever happened in Britain. I find that the shift in the philosophy of the service is, with a widespread loss of idealism and commitment, the most disturbing change of all. It derives mainly from the domination by managers and account-ants, who seem to have no personal concern with the objectives of a Health Service, but of course, it's also part of a general cultural shift away from the liberalism and sense of community of the post-war period.[52]

Psychiatry found itself criticised by patients, relatives, anti-psychiatrists and other mental health professionals. Birley observed:

Psychiatrists responded to these criticisms . . . in various ways. A positive approach was to view critics as potential allies . . . Another reaction was to strive to make psychiatry more scientific . . . but turning to medical science was liable to omit the social and behavioural disciplines.[53]

According to Rogers and Pilgrim, these opposing attitudes have continued into the twenty-first century (see also Chapters 5 and 20).[54] In a paper in the *British Journal of Psychiatry* in 2008, Craddock and his colleagues warned:

British psychiatry faces an identity crisis. A major contributory factor has been the recent trend to downgrade the importance of the core aspects of medical care . . . Our contention is that this creeping devaluation of medicine is damaging our ability to deliver excellent psychiatric care. It is imperative that we specify clearly the key role of psychiatrists in the management of people with mental illnesses.[55]

In response, Bracken and his colleagues countered by arguing that a rigid adherence to the medical model was inappropriate in treating mental illness, and, instead, they favoured an approach which focused on an understanding of the social and existential aspects of the patient.[56]

Conclusion

At the beginning of this chapter, the clinical world of the psychiatrist in 1960 was contrasted with that of his counterpart in 2010. It would be facile to view the changes in psychiatry during this period as one of straightforward progress. Certainly, there were many improvements. The old asylums, many of which were overcrowded and untherapeutic, were largely closed or had their bed numbers reduced and more patients were now cared for in the community. The patient's voice was more likely to be heard and attended to than in the past. A witness seminar for English mental health workers concluded: 'that one of the most important and striking changes in the history of post-war British mental health care has been the rise of the service user perspective'.[57] There were now more psychiatrists and they came from more diverse backgrounds than before, with many more women in the profession. However, morale had declined, though personal experience and anecdotal evidence suggest that this was less so in Scotland. There was disagreement as to whether psychiatry should be seen primarily as a branch of medicine or whether it should be more concerned with the psychological and social aspects of patients' distress. Roy Porter noted a paradox: while psychiatry had reformed its old institutions and now offered a wider range of therapies, the general public had responded with a resurgence of suspicion and lack of confidence in psychiatrists.[58]

Key Summary Points

- The era saw the gradual closure of the mental hospitals and the development of care in the community – a process known as 'deinstitutionalisation'.
- Community care revealed its own problems: some patients were merely transferred to different kinds of institution; there was a lack of funding; and there was an unease among some psychiatrists at working outside the hospital.
- There was the innovative development of multidisciplinary teams; sectorisation; and district general hospitals (DGHs).
- The Royal College of Psychiatrists was founded in 1971, leading to formal education schemes for trainees and the creation of psychiatric specialties.
- The psychiatric profession underwent a crisis of confidence as a result of several factors: the increasing privatisation of the health service; the challenge to its authority from both other mental health professionals and the emerging service user movement; and problems with recruitment.

Acknowledgements

Thanks to Nicol Ferrier, Femi Oyebode and Bruce Ritson for their helpful comments and advice with this chapter.

Notes

1.   J. Turner, R. Hayward, K. Angel et al., The history of mental health services in modern England: Practitioner memories and the direction of future research. *Medical History* (2015) 59(4): 599–624.

2.   M. Shepherd and D. Watt, In M. Shepherd, ed., *Psychiatrists on Psychiatry*, 185–203. Cambridge: Cambridge University Press, 1982.

3.   R. Davidson, Psychiatry and homosexuality in mid-twentieth century Edinburgh: The view from Jordanburn Nerve Hospital. *History of Psychiatry* (2009) 29(4): 403–24.

4.   Turner, Hayward, Angel et al., The history of mental health services in modern England.

5.   C. Hilton and T. Stephenson, eds, *Psychiatric Hospitals in the UK in the 1960s [Witness Seminar]*. London: RCPsych Publications, 2020.

6.   G. Wilkinson, ed., *Talking about Psychiatry*. London: Gaskell, 1993.

7.   Hilton and Stephenson, *Psychiatric Hospitals*.

8.   A. Scull, The peculiarities of the Scots? Scottish influences on the development of English psychiatry, 1700–1980. *History of Psychiatry* (2011) 22(4): 403–15.

9.   M. Smith (Creator) (8 August 2019). Social Psychiatry Oral History Interviews. University of Strathclyde. Transcripts (zip).10.15129/7ada.0b9e-98eb-429d-98ac-486413ecf36a. Tom Burns. Interviewed by Linsey Robb. 11 May 2015.

10. B. Boyd. In conversation with David Tait. *Psychological Bulletin* (1997) 21: 769–74.

11. G. Wilkinson, In conversation with Hugh Freeman. *Psychological Bulletin* (1993) 17: 388–404.

12. Hilton and Stephenson, *Psychiatric Hospitals.*

13. Ibid.

14. V. Long, 'Heading up a blind alley'? Scottish psychiatric hospitals in the era of deinstitutionalization. *History of Psychology* (2017) 28(1): 115–28.

15. Turner, Hayward, Angel et al., The history of mental health services in modern England.

16. Long, 'Heading up a blind alley?'.

17. Boyd, In conversation with David Tait.

18. J. K. Wing and G. W. Brown, *Institutionalism and Schizophrenia.* Cambridge: Cambridge University Press, 1970.

19. J. Birley. Rehabilitation. In H. Freeman, ed., *A Century of Psychiatry*, 253–6. London: Mosby, 1999.

20. Ibid.

21. Smith, Social Psychiatry Oral History Interviews.

22. Ibid.

23. Turner, Hayward, Angel et al., The history of mental health services in modern England.

24. Wilkinson, In conversation with Hugh Freeman.

25. Hilton and Stephenson, *Psychiatric Hospitals.*

26. T. Burns, *Our Necessary Shadow: The Nature and Meaning of Psychiatry.* London: Allen Lane, 2013.

27. Turner, Hayward, Angel et al., The history of mental health services in modern England.

28. A. Clare, *Psychiatry in Dissent: Controversial Issues in Thought and Practice* (2nd ed.). London: Routledge, 1980.

29. H. Freeman, In conversation with Maurice Silverman. *Psychological Bulletin* (1992) 16: 385–90.

30. Perspective. Thomas Freeman. *Psychological Bulletin* (1988) 12: 306–9.

31. E. Murphy, *After the Asylums: Community Care for People with Mental Illness.* London: Faber & Faber, 1991.

32. Hilton and Stephenson, *Psychiatric Hospitals.*

33. Long, 'Heading up a blind alley?'.

34. T. Bewley, *Madness to Mental Illness: A History of the Royal College of Psychiatrists.* London: RCPsych Publications, 2008.

35. Wilkinson, In conversation with Hugh Freeman.

36. Murphy, *After the Asylums.*

37. T. Arie and D. Jolley, Psychogeriatrics. In Freeman, *A Century of Psychiatry*, 260–4.

38. Ibid.

39. P. Snowden and H. Freeman, Forensic Psychiatry. In Freeman, *A Century of Psychiatry*, 265–9.

40. D. Chiswick, Conversation piece: The forensic psychiatrist. *Postgraduate Medical Journal* (1990) 66: 68–9.

41. B. Ritson, Alcoholism. In Freeman, *A Century of Psychiatry*, 218–22.

42. Conversation with Bruce Ritson. *Addiction* (2010) 105: 1346–54.

43. S. Bloch, In conversation with Heinz Wolff: Part 2. *Psychological Bulletin* (1989) 13, 337–42.

44. J. Holmes, The integration of psychiatry and psychotherapy. *Psychological Bulletin* (1995) 19: 465–6.

45. P. Aitken, G. Lloyd, R. Mayou et al., A history of liaison psychiatry in the UK. *Psychological Bulletin* (2016) 40 (4): 199–203.

46. Turner, Hayward, Angel et al., The history of mental health services in modern England.

47. Clare, *Psychiatry in Dissent*.

48. P. Sedgwick, The fate of psychiatry in the new populism. *Psychological Bulletin* (1983) 7: 22–5.

49. Anon. Psychiatry: A discipline that has lost its way. *The Lancet* (1985) 325: 731–2.

50. D. Bhugra, The public image of psychiatry. *Psychological Bulletin* (1987) 11: 105.

51. T. Harrison, The role of the consultant psychiatrist in the clinical team. *Psychological Bulletin* (1989) 13: 347–50.

52. Wilkinson, In conversation with Hugh Freeman.

53. Birley, Rehabilitation.

54. A. Rogers and D. Pilgrim, *A Sociology of Mental Health and Illness* (5th ed.). Maidenhead: Open University Press, 2014.

55. N. Craddock, D. Antebi, M.-J. Attenburrow et al., Wake up call for British psychiatry. *British Journal of Psychiatry* (2008) 193: 6–9.

56. P. Bracken, P. Thomas, S. Timimi et al., Psychiatry beyond the current paradigm. *British Journal of Psychiatry* (2012) 201: 430–4.

57. Turner, Hayward, Angel et al., The history of mental health services in modern England.

58. R. Porter, Two cheers for psychiatry! The social history of mental disorder in twentieth century Britain. In H. Freeman and G. E. Berrios, eds, *150 Years of British Psychiatry, Volume 2: The Aftermath*, 383–406. London: Athlone Press, 1996.

19

The Changing Roles of the Professions in Psychiatry and Mental Health: Psychiatric (Mental Health) Nursing

Kevin Gournay and Peter Carter

Introduction

To begin – a word about the term psychiatric (mental health) nursing. In this chapter, we use the term 'mental health nursing' as this is the legal term to describe the profession. A UK Department of Health review in 1994 recommended: 'the title of mental health nurse be used both for nurses who work in the community and for those who work in hospital and day services'.[1] Indeed, both authors who were once 'registered mental nurses' became 'registered mental health nurses'. Nevertheless, the terms 'psychiatric nurse' and 'community psychiatric nurse' (CPN) are still in common usage. The 1994 change in terminology was but part of a move to change the more general language used in psychiatry, leaving us with a somewhat oxymoronic term to describe what we do for people with psychiatric problems. In some parts of the chapter (particularly in describing the pre-1994 period), we refer to psychiatric nursing rather than mental health nursing.

This chapter describes some of the changes and key events that have taken place in this fifty-year period so as to illustrate the nature of the history. We therefore describe:

- Psychiatric nursing in the 1960s.
- The development of community mental health nursing.
- A profession characterised by an increase in skills and knowledge: nurses as therapists, prescribers, researchers.
- Inpatient care.
- Nurses and other psychiatric professionals.

Psychiatric Nursing in the 1960s

Both authors commenced their career in psychiatric nursing in the late 1960s and are therefore able to offer their observations and commentary on the changes in their profession over this fifty-year period. For readers interested in a complete history of the profession from the sixteenth century to the 1990s, there is perhaps no more authoritative account than that of Professor Peter Nolan.[2]

When we began our careers in the large asylums, in one sense it was like stepping back in time (see also Chapter 6). We were vaguely aware that the care and treatment of the mentally ill was undergoing what, with the benefit of hindsight, were enormous changes – such changes being so well described in Anthony Clare's landmark book *Psychiatry in Dissent*.[3] However, as mere student nurses at the bottom of a hierarchy, we were largely unaware of the detail of these changes, particularly because the wards where we began our careers were characterised by the use of rigid routines and a uniformity of approach. The medical superintendent still reigned, with doctors most certainly seen as a different species to nurses. The wards where we worked were dormitory-style, often overcrowded, with little space for personal possessions and certainly – for most patients – little privacy. Some hospitals had wards of up to 100 patients; many had central dining rooms and in some cases central bathing facilities, where patients would troupe up once or twice a week for a bath or a shower. One of us recollects a charge nurse appointed to do nothing else but supervise bed-making – this task then being delegated to several long-stay patients. Charge nurses (and ward sisters on the female side of the hospital – the integration of male and female patients only beginning slowly at the end of the 1960s) supervised the cleaning and other domestic duties carried out by patients. Ward domestic staff only began to appear in the late 1960s; in some hospitals, later. As this was the era just after National Service, many of the male charge nurses had served in the military, and thus an ethos of authority pervaded the atmosphere of the wards. Ward sisters were similarly figures of authority. Our female counterparts were chastised for any incorrect wearing of their uniform, starched aprons still being the order of the day. It took many years more for uniforms to disappear from psychiatric inpatient care settings – the revolution to the wearing of 'mufti' not really beginning until the mid-1970s.

Many of the patients that we looked after were totally institutionalised, and in some of the 'long-stay wards' where we worked, we had little or no conversations with many of our patients. They were often over-medicated with chlorpromazine, haloperidol and similar drugs; many incapacitated by Parkinsonian symptoms. Some of the locked wards had 'airing courts' where patients would either stand and stare at nothing in particular or stride around apace with what, on reflection, was akathisia, the interminable restlessness caused by phenothiazine tranquillisers.

Patients were provided with a range of social and recreational outlets, including the hospital cinema and once-a-week dances, where the male and female patients could mix under supervision. Most hospitals had a patient football and cricket team, with games organised between hospitals. Musical patients joined the hospital band and many hospitals put on pantomimes (one for staff and one for patients). All of these activities came within the responsibility of a member of nursing staff who was often given the title 'activities coordinator'. Such was the importance of this role that these nurses were employed at ward sister/charge nurse grade or above.

On the wards, within a few short weeks, we witnessed many patients receiving electro-convulsive therapy (ECT) for their depression or acute psychosis, and some patients who were deemed to require 'building up' were given morning courses of modified insulin therapy, with the 1960s seeing the era of insulin coma therapy falling into disuse. Those of us who began nursing in the 1960s also remember patients being treated with modified narcosis, that is, being medicated with barbiturates so that sleep prevailed for much of the 24-hour period. Any sense of patient empowerment or 'user involvement' was years away.

Some of our experiences in the three years of training to become registered nurses involved placements in industrial therapy units within the hospital, where patients often worked thirty hours a week or more, for derisory levels of pay. It was here that one might find a 'technical instructor'. Through the 1960s, hospitals began to employ occupational therapists; they were few in number but not as rare as clinical psychologists (179 in 1960; that number rising to 399 in 1970 and nearly 9,000 in 2010).[4] In the 1960s, the value of work became formally recognised as a method of rehabilitating the seriously mentally ill – inspired by a number of psychiatrist pioneers, notably Dr Douglas Early,[5] who developed one of the first industrial therapy units in Bristol. All patients who could work did so. Hospitals were often relatively self-sufficient with various workshops. In 1960, some hospitals ran thriving farms; indeed, until the 1970s, the NHS employed shepherds and farm hands to work alongside 'farm nurses' to oversee the work of the patients. These farms fell into disuse and were sold off, with proceeds going to the Exchequer rather than back into the NHS.

The 1960s were a time of full employment and some of the more able long-stay patients, whose only home was the hospital where they had resided for many years, began 'working out' in local factories and other industries. Their employers were very pleased to see workers who would do exactly what they were told and work without complaint. One of the ironies of this 'working out' population was the fact that some of these long-stay patients began to earn more money in factories than some members of the nursing staff. However, while pay for nurses was low, student and newly qualified nurses were able to aspire to being able to move into a hospital house at subsidised rent and to a full pension at fifty-five. In the late 1960s, many nurses were institutionalised themselves, with their only social outlet being the use of a staff social club in the grounds of the hospital. The 'Club' (which served alcohol at much lower prices than in pubs) was the focus of not only staff social activity but often also the social activity of their families because many hospitals were at some distance from the local town. Male staff were encouraged to join the hospital's football and cricket teams. In the London area, the London Mental Hospitals Sports Association ran a football league of teams formed from the staff of the many mental hospitals that ringed the London area. Some hospitals recruited nursing staff on the basis of their sporting prowess rather than any other attribute, such was the importance of the hospital team.

Nursing staff recruits, who trained in the schools of nursing that were situated in hospital grounds, came from the local area, often as part of a family tradition. Recruits also came from the Republic of Ireland and, increasingly, from a number of more distant countries, notably Mauritius, Malaysia and the Caribbean islands. At this time, nurses did not need to demonstrate the, then, marker of a good general education, that is, five GCE O levels. Nurses without GCEs would pass a General Nursing Council test that examined general literacy, numeracy and general knowledge.

In our six-week introduction to our education and training as registered mental nurses in our respective schools of nursing, we learned a great deal about the 1959 Mental Health Act and came to understand the importance of the principle of treatment as an informal patient. In the hospital, we came across doctors and nurses who were trying to effect change, but these were in a minority. Some of our nurse tutors told us about Laing, Szasz, Cooper and Goffman. However, most qualified staff had never heard about such figures and were highly disparaging about the changes that were so clearly afoot following Enoch Powell's 1961 'Water Towers speech' (see also Chapter 1).[6] By then, most hospitals had smaller short-stay units, often located away from the main hospital. The late 1960s saw the first drug addiction units and the start of units where medication was not the central approach. Day hospitals were beginning to appear. Nevertheless, most nurses were still largely engaged on 'long-stay' wards with their time spent in supervising activities of daily living and ensuring that good order prevailed. The growth of district general hospital psychiatric units was to follow from the mid-1970s onwards.

The idea that psychiatric nursing would one day become an all-graduate profession, or, indeed, a profession in its true sense at all, never crossed anyone's mind. In the 1960s, none of us envisaged a future where we could become 'responsible clinicians' under the Mental

Health Act, independent prescribers of medicine or leaders of multidisciplinary teams that included consultant psychiatrists. Neither did we envisage a future when psychiatric nurses rose to other positions of influence and importance – for example, becoming chief executives of sprawling mental health trusts, responsible for managing budgets of many millions of pounds, leading national initiatives or chairing the development of NICE guidelines.

The Development of Community Psychiatric Nursing

In 1954, two psychiatric nurses who were working in a large psychiatric hospital, Warlingham Park in Surrey, were seconded to provide outpatient care and to assist patients discharged from the hospital to establish themselves in the community. This initiative was followed by the development of a service from Moorhaven Hospital in Devon in 1957. As White has described,[7] community psychiatric nursing slowly developed and, by 1973, formal training for CPNs was established, with a first course at Chiswick College in London. The development of long-acting (depot) injections of antipsychotic medications led to an increase in the number of CPNs.[8] To begin with, the role of the CPN was simply to administer the injection. However, it quickly became apparent that extrapyramidal side effects were a problem and the role of the CPN expanded to the monitoring of side effects, alongside taking more responsibility for the assessment of mental state and risk. On a more negative note, CPNs were delegated to running depot clinics, where literally dozens of patients would attend at a time for their fortnightly injection and spend only a brief period with the nurse. While these patients were in receipt of medications that would be of some benefit, the brief interactions with the CPNs did little to provide the patient and, importantly, the family with any meaningful input to address social or psychological needs.

CPN practice began to change in the 1970s, and by the 1980s many CPNs began to base themselves in primary care settings with GPs and work largely with people with common mental disorders, such as general anxiety, relationship difficulties and 'stress'. A survey of CPNs in England in 1989 showed that one-quarter of CPNs did not have a single client with a diagnosis of schizophrenia on their caseload.[9] The CPN interventions used could be described as counselling rather than any specific evidence-based approach. From the early 1990s, the practice of CPNs took another turn, with CPNs returning to a focus on people with serious and enduring mental illness, such as schizophrenia. This renewed focus was prompted by the results of two research trials. One randomised controlled trial of CPNs in primary health care in North London showed that CPN intervention produced little or no benefit.[10] An economic analysis, based on that trial, demonstrated that, per unit of health gain, CPN interventions yielded far fewer benefits than interventions with patients with schizophrenia.[11] At the same time, another trial, in Manchester, demonstrated that training CPNs to undertake psychosocial interventions with families caring for a relative with schizophrenia provided benefits to families. This CPN intervention also led to an improvement in both positive and negative symptoms in patients, with some evidence that CPN intervention reduced inpatient episodes.[12] Thus began an era that extends to the present, where a large majority of CPN work is focused on people with serious and enduring illnesses. The scope of training for CPNs widened to include mental state and risk assessments and a range of psychosocial interventions, including cognitive behaviour therapy and family interventions. Thus, by the early 2000s, CPNs had become a central resource in delivering high-quality community care, with important roles in crisis intervention and early intervention teams.

The wide dissemination of this work owes a great deal to the Sir Jules Thorn Trust, a charity that, in or around 1990, provided substantial funds to develop training in psychosocial interventions for CPNs at the Institute of Psychiatry, Psychology and Neuroscience, King's College London and the University of Manchester; this being originally known as the 'Thorn Nurse Programme'.[13] The programme was disseminated across the UK and then increasingly opened up to all mental health professionals. Thorn has evolved into the multidisciplinary training provided to community mental health teams in 2020. From its beginnings in 1990, Thorn nurse training was led by a multidisciplinary group that included one of the pre-eminent figures in psychiatry at the time, Dr Jim Birley, who had been Dean of the Institute of Psychiatry. Jim Birley was generous with his time and took a great interest in not only the programme but all those involved. As this chapter reflects throughout, many of the very positive developments in psychiatric nursing owe much to the contribution of a number of psychiatrists who have recognised the importance of the nursing profession in the care of the mentally ill.

A Profession Characterised by an Increase in Skills, Knowledge and Responsibility

Between 1960 and 2010, there were significant developments in the education and training of mental health nurses. The syllabus for mental health nurse training was updated in 1964 to include psychology and sociology for the first time. It also suggested that student nurses should spend some time outside their hospital on community placements. This represented a major break with traditional training, which had been geared solely towards preparing nurses for work within institutions. By the turn of the century, all preregistration training was located in universities – the hospital training schools having closed in the early 1990s. By 2000, the syllabus covered a wide range of topics, both theoretical and practical, with an emphasis on evidence-based approaches.[14] By 2010, degree-level education required students to acquire a breadth and depth of knowledge that was in great contrast to their counterparts in 1960. While their time in clinical placements was more limited, they were expected to critically analyse and reflect on the clinical practice that they observed. There was also a growing expectation that a significant number of the student body would go on to further study, with growing numbers expected to complete further training to equip them with specialist skills and some to continue on to master's level.

Arguably, one of the most influential figures in the development of specialist nurse roles was Professor Isaac Marks, a distinguished psychiatrist rather than a nurse. Marks's career has been devoted to three central topics: first, the adherence to an evidence-based approach for all that we do in psychiatry; second, the development of methods for treating common mental disorders (particularly those that cause considerable handicap, e.g. obsessive-compulsive disorder (OCD) and severe agoraphobia); and, finally, innovations that could extend treatment to wider populations. Marks was one of the first to develop computer assisted treatments for common mental disorders.[15] As a young psychiatrist, not long in the UK from South Africa and then at the Maudsley Hospital/Institute of Psychiatry, he identified the core elements of effective behavioural treatment for anxiety disorders, notably phobias and OCD. These core elements were exposure and, in the case of OCD, response prevention.[16] Marks also realised that these therapies were, in one sense, the domain of practice of clinical psychologists. However, on the other hand, psychologists were few in number and it was clear that this workforce would be unable to deliver treatment to the tens, or hundreds, of thousands of patients who might be responsive to these new psychological treatments. He realised that psychiatric nurses might be suitable for training in these methods, particularly because of their background general experience of dealing with people with a wide variety of mental health problems in various settings. Thus, in 1972, Marks began the Nurse Therapy training programme. Over a pilot programme lasting three years, he developed a rigorous training for nurses to become autonomous therapists. The results of this study and subsequent research demonstrated very clearly that, both clinically and economically, nurses could be effective autonomous therapists.[17] From 1975 onwards, Nurse Therapy Training (a full-time course of eighteen months) led to the graduation of literally hundreds of nurses from sites in the UK and the Republic of Ireland. Arguably, this programme seeded the developments for more widespread training in psychological methods, culminating in the Improving Access to Psychological Therapies programme that began in 2006, in which nurses have played leading roles in development, education, evaluation and dissemination.[18]

In another enormous change in the responsibilities of psychiatric nurses, the year 1992 saw changes in legislation which meant that nurses were able to prescribe from an extended formulary. Following a number of policy reviews and with a change in the NHS landscape,[19] the law was changed so that, following an approved and comprehensive training programme, independent nurse prescribers would be able to prescribe any licensed medicine for any medical condition, providing it was within their expertise. Thus, towards the end of the period covered by this chapter, psychiatric nurses across the country were beginning to receive such training and the requisite legal authority. In practice, this meant, for example, that an independent nurse prescriber could make changes to the patient's medication, thus enabling psychiatrists to spend more time with patients whose needs were complex and who might have significant physical comorbidities. Overall, nurse prescribing was welcomed by the psychiatric profession. However, some opposition has come from nursing academics, who objected to nurses being enveloped by the 'medical model'.[20] By 2010, it became clear that, while mental health nurse prescribing was growing slowly, the way in which nurse prescribing was used across the NHS varied considerably and there was still some disagreement regarding the most appropriate settings for this work.[21]

In 2007, the Mental Health Act was amended so that nurses could become a 'responsible clinician' or an 'approved mental health professional', important roles in the supervision and safeguarding of the rights of patients subject to the involuntary provisions of the Act. These legal changes were prompted by the fact that CPNs had, since 1991, become 'care coordinators', with a wide range of responsibilities under the Care Programme approach.[22]

In another development that followed improvements in the education and training of psychiatric nurses, they acquired sufficient skills to be able to lead and conduct research trials that would meet the standard required of high-impact psychiatric journals. Thus, in the same edition of the British Journal of Psychiatry in 1994, the results of two research trials involving CPNs were published, both led by graduates of Marks's Nurse Therapy Programme.[23] By the year 2000, the Medical Research Council had begun the funding of postdoctoral fellowships for mental health nurses. This enabled nurses who already had a PhD and some research training to go on to complete postdoctoral courses in subjects such as epidemiology, statistics and trial design. Towards the end of the first decade of the present century, psychiatric nurses began to figure in the range of research studies funded by the National Institute of Health Research (NIHR). By this time, nurses had also begun to take leading parts in the National Institute for Health and Care Excellence (NICE) and the

Cochrane Collaboration. The year 1995 saw the inauguration of the first chair in psychiatric nursing at the Institute of Psychiatry/Maudsley Hospital. This development was due to the efforts of Sir David Goldberg, at that time Professor of Psychiatry, who had become a great friend to nursing some years before in Manchester as a collaborator on the aforementioned trial of training nurses in psychosocial interventions.[24]

Changes in the Nursing of Inpatients

In 1960, there were around 150,000 patients in the large mental hospitals; by 2010, there were 23,000.[25] The reduction in bed numbers over the years resulted in nurses needing to provide care for a population with acute episodes of illness that posed significant challenges for nursing staff. Many patients had the additional problem of drug and alcohol use. Two important problems had become the source of great concern: patient suicide and violence. The National Confidential Inquiry into Suicide and Homicide by People with Mental Illness (established in 1996) published its first report, *Safety First*, in 2001.[26] This reported that 16 per cent of all inquiry cases of suicide in England were psychiatric inpatients. These tragic events were most likely to be by hanging, most commonly from a curtain rail and using a belt as a ligature. Wards were also seeing higher levels of violence.[27]

The NHS responded to the matter of inpatient suicide by spending vast sums on making wards safer, resulting in a great reduction in suicide rates.[28] At the same time, three nursing bodies, the United Kingdom Council for Nursing Midwifery and Health Visiting (the predecessor body to the Nursing and Midwifery Council); the Royal College of Nursing and the Standing Nursing Midwifery Advisory Committee for the UK responded to the challenge with a number of surveys, literature reviews, visits to services and consultations with all interested parties to begin developing recommendations for changing nursing practice. Eventually NICE guidelines on the management of disturbed and violent behaviour in mental health and emergency settings were published in 2005,[29] with the guidelines leading to much-improved standards for the observation of patients at risk and improved training in the prevention and management of violence.

Nursing and Other Professions in Psychiatric Settings

As noted, and for a range of reasons, in 1960 nurses were at the very bottom of a hierarchy. In 2010, most newly qualified nurses were graduates and could go on to develop a wide range of specialist skills. Importantly, the remuneration for nurses was, in relative terms, much improved. A nurse qualifying in 2010 could aspire to become a nurse consultant, a director of nursing or an NHS Trust chief executive. While pay is still a contentious issue, senior nurses earn salaries that are within the same range as social workers, occupational therapists and psychologists.

In clinical settings, by 2010 many clinical services and multidisciplinary teams were led by nurses. By this time, nurses were performing roles that had, only a few years before, belonged to other disciplines – for example, providing high-quality psychological treatments, prescribing medication or making recommendations in respect of detention in hospital. Arguably, this blurring of roles made for a more harmonious approach to patient care, with nurses, by 2010, being highly skilled and much-respected members of the professional psychiatric community.

Conclusion

It would not be an exaggeration to say that, in comparison with all other professions in psychiatry, nursing changed beyond recognition between 1960 and 2010. Nurses became members of an established profession. Over the years, the profession saw the acquisition of a wide range of knowledge and skills that in most ways have reflected the changing landscape in psychiatry, notably following the closure of the large hospitals. The question now posed is, what changes will take place in our profession in years to come?

Key Summary Points

- Psychiatric (mental health) nursing is a relatively young profession that developed with great speed over this fifty-year period. In 1960, nearly all nurses were employed in large mental hospitals.
- While education and training were improving, nurses' roles in the 1960s largely involved the care and supervision of institutionalised patients. The pay and status of nurses were low, with nursing at the bottom of a medically led hierarchy.
- The 1970s saw a great expansion in community psychiatric nursing; the development of Nurse Therapy training; and the gradual emergence of multidisciplinary teams.
- The education and training of nurses improved, as did pay conditions and status; and by 2010, nursing was becoming an all-graduate profession.
- The end of the era saw nurses becoming independent prescribers and skilled clinicians. Changes in the Mental Health Act meant that nurses could assume additional roles by becoming 'responsible clinicians' or 'approved mental health professionals'.

Notes

1. Department of Health, *Working in Partnership*. London: HMSO, 1994.

2. P. Nolan, *A History of Mental Health Nursing*. London: Stanley Thornes, 1993.

3. A. Clare, *Psychiatry in Dissent: Controversial Issues in Thought and Practice*. London: Tavistock, 1976.

4. J. Turner, R. Hayward, K. Angel et al., The history of mental health services in modern England: Practitioner memories and the direction of future research. *Medical History* (2015) 59: 599–624.

5. D. Early, The Industrial Therapy Organisation (Bristol): A development of work in hospital. *The Lancet* (1960) 2: 754–7.

6. J. E. Powell, Speech by Rt hon Enoch Powell; Report of the National Association for Mental Health Conference, 1961.

7. E. White, Community mental health nursing: An interpretation of history as a context for contemporary research. In J. Macintosh, eds, *Research Issues in Community Nursing* (Community Healthcare Series). London: Palgrave, 1999.

8. J. Bennett, J. Done, P. Harrison-Reed and B. Hunt, Development of a rating scale/checklist to assess the side effects of antipsychotics by community psychiatric nurses. In C. Brooker and E. White, eds, *Community Psychiatric Nursing: A Research Perspective*, Vol. 2. London: Chapman & Hall, 1995.

9. White, Community mental health nursing.

10. K. Gournay and J. Brooking, The CPN in primary health care: An outcome study. *British Journal of Psychiatry* (1994) 165: 231–8.

11. K. Gournay and J. Brooking, An economic analysis of the work of mental health nurses in primary care. *Journal of Advanced Nursing* (1995) 22: 769–78.

12. C. Brooker, I. Falloon, A. Butterworth, D. Goldberg, V. Graham-Hole and R. Hillier, The outcome of training community psychiatric nurses to deliver psychosocial interventions. *British Journal of Psychiatry* (1994) 165: 222–30.

13. C. Gamble, The Thorn Nurse training initiative. *Nursing Standard* (1995) 9: 31–4.

14. R. Newell and K. J. M. Gournay, *Mental Health Nursing: An Evidence-Based Approach* (2nd ed.). Edinburgh: Churchill Livingstone, 2009.

15. I. Marks, K. Cavanagh and L. Gega, *Hands-on-Help: Computer Aided Psychotherapy*. New York: Psychology Press, 2007.

16. I. M. Marks, *Fears Phobias and Rituals*. Oxford: Oxford University Press, 1987.

17. I. Marks, *Nurses As Therapists in Primary Care*. London: RCN Publications, 1985.

18. D. M. Clark, R. Layard, R. Smithies, D. A. Richards, R. Suckling and B. Wright, Improving access to psychological therapy: Initial evaluation of two UK demonstration sites. *Behaviour Research and Therapy* (2009) 47: 910–20.

19. K. J. M. Gournay and R. Gray, Should mental health nurses prescribe? Maudsley Discussion Paper No. 11, Institute of Psychiatry, London, 2001.

20. P. Barker and P. Buchanan-Barker, First, do no harm: Confronting the myths of psychiatric drugs. *Nursing Ethics* (2012) 19: 45–63.

21. D. Dobel-Ober, N. Brinblecombe and E. Bradley, Nurse prescribing in mental health: A national survey. *Journal of Psychiatric and Mental Health Nursing* (2010).

22. Department of Health. *The Care Programme Approach for People with a Mental Illness*. London: Department of Health, 1990.

23. Gournay and Brooking, The CPN in primary health care; Brooker, Falloon, Butterworth et al., The outcome of training community psychiatric nurses to deliver psychosocial interventions.

24. Brooker, Falloon, Butterworth et al., The outcome of training community psychiatric nurses to deliver psychosocial interventions.

25. Turner, Hayward, Angel et al., The history of mental health services in modern England.

26. *Safety First: Report of the National Confidential Inquiry into Suicides and Homicides by People with a Mental illness*. University of Manchester, 2001.

27. S. Wright, R. Gray, J. Parkes and K. J. M. Gournay, The prevention and therapeutic management of violence in acute in patient psychiatry: A literature review and evidence based recommendations for good practice. *Review for United Kingdom Council for Nursing Midwifery and Health Visiting*. London: NMC Library, 2002.

28. K. J. M. Gournay, Patient safety: Reducing harm and saving lives. *British Journal of Mental Health Nursing* (2014) 3: 96–7.

29. NICE, *Violence: The Short-Term Management of Disturbed/Violent Behaviour in Psychiatric In-patient Settings and Emergency Departments*. Clinical Guideline 25. London: NICE, 2005.

Critical Friends: Anti-psychiatry and Clinical Psychology

Tom Burns and John Hall

The immediate post-war period in the UK was focused on the establishment of the welfare state. There was a broad consensus that the old order had failed and that those who had served and sacrificed should be heard. Mental health services had been absorbed into the NHS from the local authorities, although this had not been a foregone conclusion.[1] This aligning with NHS practice threw the disparities in care into stark relief. The Percy Commission was established in 1957 to enquire into the care of mentally ill and learning disabled patients. This resulted in the 1959 Mental Health Act and also mandated social services spending on discharged patients. As well as tightening up the supervision of compulsory care, it brought health and social care together, enabling the development of geographical catchment area services and the growth of British community and social psychiatry.

These developments were accelerated by the discovery of antipsychotics in 1954 and the first tricyclic antidepressants in 1958 and 1960. Confidence in psychiatry's future outside the asylum was high. This is nowhere more evident than in the health secretary Enoch Powell's much-quoted 'Water Tower' speech to the Mind conference in 1961 and in legislation with the 1962 *Hospital Plan*.[2]

Despite its unprecedented progress (or perhaps because of it), the 1960s onwards found psychiatry's legitimacy challenged on two fronts. In the 1960s and 1970s, a dramatic onslaught came from the celebrity 'anti-psychiatrists' (a term coined by David Cooper in 1967). Also, alongside this, a relative newcomer to mental health services – clinical psychology – was rapidly growing in power and influence.

The Anti-psychiatrists

The anti-psychiatry movement can be understood as one front in the baby boomers' assault on the old order. Social turmoil and rebellion characterised the next two decades, from the civil rights movement in the United States, through the Vietnam protests and the student revolts that erupted in Paris in May 1968. The established order was challenged and in many aspects upended. Psychiatry's prominence in this counterculture owes much to the anti-psychiatrists and, in particular, to four iconic books. These all appeared within eighteen months of each other in 1960–1.

Each of these very different books was entirely independent – their authors had no connection with each other before or after their publication. They came to be seen as the four seminal texts of the anti-psychiatry movement. This term was never accepted by the authors themselves but it has endured. All four spoke powerfully to psychiatry's relationship with society, with an unflinching demand that both must change.

Laing

The first to appear was R. D. (Ronnie) Laing's *The Divided Self* (1960),[3] which went on to become an international campus bible. Laing was a Scottish psychiatrist who trained in psychoanalysis in London. He was heavily influenced by existentialism, particularly by Jean-Paul Sartre. He saw the struggle of the 'psychotic patient' through the existentialists' lens of becoming rather than being. As agents of our own identity and destiny, we create ourselves by the choices we must constantly make (as Sartre wrote in 1946, 'Man is condemned to be free').[4]

Laing believed that psychotic patients were struggling against confusing and contradictory messages to make sense of their experiences. Their confusion communicates itself to us as a threat to our ontological security (our confidence in our own stable identity). We then contain this anxiety through diagnosis. Laing proposed an approach of 'existential phenomenology', which seeks to understand the patient's struggle for identity rather than clarifying signs and symptoms as in classical phenomenology. This existential phenomenology requires full engagement rather than traditional professional distance.

Such direct engagement was to avoid 'objectifying' the patient. Sartre insisted that humans simply cannot be understood as objects because identity inheres in active agency (choices). A 'snapshot' diagnosis would miss the individual's most important quality – their agency.

Laing was a wonderful writer. He had an ability to engage fully with very disturbed patients and conveyed these experiences vividly and humanely. A striking and charismatic speaker, his message was taken up enthusiastically by a youthful readership. His second book (*Sanity Madness and the Family*, with Aaron Esterson 1964) became an iconic film, *Family Life*, in 1971, spreading the message even wider.[5]

Laing was a restless individual in both his intellectual and his personal life. His later writing became increasingly obscure, partly coloured by his alcohol and drug abuse. His impact on psychiatry began to fade as he shifted his focus to the emerging global counterculture.

Foucault

Madness and Civilization is the English translation of Foucault's abridged PhD thesis published in 1961.[6] Foucault's approach was historical and he argued that 'madness' was timeless but 'the madman' was a recent construction. Foucault ascribed this new identity to the 'great confinement', which occurred in France in the mid-seventeenth century. The enormous 'grands hôpitaux' had been established in Paris to contain the poor, the mad and the socially disruptive. They were a response to France's rapid economic and social development and new categories were required to facilitate this extrajudicial incarceration.

Foucault's writings continue to have enormous influence in the social sciences and wider cultural circles. 'Mental illness' as a convenient label to remove uncomfortable and supposedly deviant individuals, who are unable to contribute economically, remains a pervasive trope. Franco Basaglia, responsible for Italy's radical reforms in the 1970s, repeatedly insisted that psychiatric diagnoses were based on economic inutility and resulted in social exclusion. Current thinking around stigma derives much from these ideas and those of labelling theory – that an imposed identity, once accepted, becomes a self-fulfilling prophecy and an impediment to recovery and social reintegration.

Goffman

The Canadian-American sociologist Erving Goffman spent 1955–6 in participant observation (effectively 'undercover') in a large Washington mental hospital. *Asylums: Essays on the Social Situations of Mental Patients and Other Inmates* (1961) was the result and had an enormous impact on psychiatry.[7] Unlike Russell Barton's 1959 book *Institutional Neurosis*,[8] explaining the apathy of psychotic inpatients as a side effect of institutional care, Goffman believed it resulted from deliberate policy.

Goffman coined the term 'total institutions' to include mental hospitals, prisons, monasteries and even the military. Such all-embracing organisations needed to 'manage' large numbers of people efficiently. Goffman described a range of initiation rituals, rigid rules, hierarchies and roles that stripped away individual identity. The result was predictable and pliable individuals. Monotonous routines and the absence of personal choice generated dependency and apathy. This process of 'institutionalisation' served the institution's needs, not the individual's.

Goffman's also observed that real power within the institution often originated low down the organisational hierarchy. Rather than the doctors and senior nurses controlling the wards, the nursing aides, cleaners and even more-established patients made the day-to-day decisions. They ran the ward on simple moral concepts of good and bad behaviour and punishment and reward rather than on notions of symptoms and treatment.

Like Laing, Goffman could write striking prose and captivate his reader. He, however, presented evidence, not just a theoretical revision. Despite its highly critical message, *Asylums* was readily taken up by the profession. Underscored by regularly occurring scandals, it became a central text in the deinstitutionalisation movement. His observations of hospital power structures fed into the development of modern multidisciplinary working.

Szasz

Thomas Szasz escaped Soviet-dominated Hungary at age eighteen and trained in medicine and psychiatry in the United States. He remained active as a psychiatrist in both private and university practice for the rest of his life. He wrote more than thirty books, of which *The Myth of Mental Illness* (1961) is the most famous.[9] He makes two basic points (reiterated throughout his subsequent books). The first is that mental illnesses are not 'real' illnesses because they have no physical markers (such as glucose levels in diabetes). The second, following on from this but clearly reflecting experiences of oppression under Soviet occupation, is that there is absolutely no justification for treating 'mental patients' against their will. As any special treatment is an abuse of power, no allowance can be made for any criminal or deviant behaviour. There is no 'insanity clause'. So the murderer with psychosis goes to prison and can there receive treatment but even then only if they consent.

Szasz had, and continues to have, a powerful influence outside the profession. His message is immediate and simple and resonates with liberalism and anti-authoritarianism. He was also an effective communicator and used vivid (albeit questionable) examples to make his points: 'If I speak to God I am a Christian, if God speaks to me I am schizophrenic.' Szasz became a figurehead for anti-psychiatry groups such as the Scientologists, and his ideas find a home with civil libertarians. However, because their message is essentially so simplistic, with no striking insights or reinterpretations of established assumptions, they rarely figure in professional discourses about psychiatry.

Anti-psychiatry's Impact

Although often perceived as infuriating and superficial by many clinicians, anti-psychiatry certainly raised public interest in the profession. In the late 1960s and early 1970s, it was 'cool' to be a psychiatrist. Recruitment, ironically, improved. By this time, the British anti-psychiatrists were moving away into the broader worldwide counterculture. In 1967, they staged the Dialectics of Liberation Congress at the Roundhouse in London with keynote speeches from anti-psychiatrists, beat poets, black activists and more. By 1970, Kingsley Hall (the most high-profile manifestation of UK anti-psychiatry) had collapsed amidst acrimony and discord. The caravan had moved on.

British Psychiatry's Response to the Anti-psychiatrists

The mainstream psychiatric response to the anti-psychiatrists was essentially to ignore or dismiss them.[10] Some brave individuals engaged publicly with the argument but it was rarely constructive or successful. The sight of the eminent Michael Shepherd spluttering with incredulity on TV at proposals from a young enthusiast that psychiatry really had nothing to offer a psychotic young mother left most reluctant to engage in what seemed a dialogue of the deaf. Responses based on pragmatism and experience simply had no impact on ideology. In their article about Basaglia's reforms, Kathleen Jones and Alison Poletti record this impotence:

> [we] remained mystified by the insistence of Psichiatria Democratica on 'closing the mental hospital' when it was patently obvious that mental hospitals were not being closed. ... When the Trieste team say 'We closed the mental hospital' they do not mean 'We closed the mental hospital'. They mean 'We broke the power of the mental hospital over the patients'.[11]

In his 1970 book *Psychiatry in Dissent*, Anthony Clare tried to engage with the debate, particularly in his chapters 'Concepts of mental illness' and 'What is schizophrenia?'[12] He forensically examined Laing's proposals and Joseph Berke's portrayal of Mary Barnes's 'journey' through psychosis. Experience is impotent, however, against what Andrew Scull calls 'word-magic'.[13] In addition, Clare is preaching to the converted – few who bought *The Divided Self* also bought *Psychiatry in Dissent*.

Radical (Critical) Psychiatry and Post-psychiatry

In understanding the impact of the anti-psychiatrists in the 1960s and 1970s, it is important to remember that psychiatry has never been without vociferous critics. In the following decades up to 2010, there have constantly been groups of dissident voices, both within and outside the profession. The most prominent of these critical groups are the radical psychiatry group and the post-psychiatry movement.

The radical psychiatrists include senior and respected figures, several with academic appointments. Joanna Moncrieff at University College London (UCL) has persistently challenged the claims for efficacy of prophylactic drug treatments such as lithium and maintenance antipsychotics.[14] Derek Summerfield at the Institute of Psychiatry has written prolifically about the imposition of diagnoses such as post-traumatic stress disorder (PTSD) and depression on more diffuse human problems (and in particular the export of these 'Western' concepts).[15]

The post-psychiatry movement draws on the ideas of postmodernism.[16] It emphasises the loss of faith in science as an effective solution for current problems and questions its status as a privileged discourse among others. It emphasises social and cultural contexts and places ethics before technology.

Both the radical psychiatry group and the post-psychiatrists differ fundamentally from the earlier anti-psychiatrists in that they are focused on 'improving' psychiatry and limiting its poor (damaging) practice. This is fundamentally more a technological than an ideological attack despite some of the language. Both have been fuelled by the one-sidedness of the evolving biomedical model within psychiatry and the disquieting growth in power of 'Big Pharma'. The muted response of orthodox psychiatry to these critics undoubtedly stems from similar shared concerns (albeit less extreme) being widespread throughout the profession. Psychiatry has learnt to coexist with its internal critical friends. This may reflect its need to pay urgent attention to a more cogent threat to its status growing alongside it in the multidisciplinary team.

Psychiatry and Psychology

Psychology and psychiatry relate to each other at three different levels. They are distinct conceptual and methodological disciplines, with border territories of abnormal and medical psychology. Psychologists and psychiatrists relate to each other as immediate clinical colleagues in day-to-day practice; and their professional bodies relate to each other in the context of their own competition for political influence and funding. The British Psychological Society (BPS) was founded in 1901, gained its Royal Charter in 1965 and represents all psychologists, both academic and applied. In most of these areas, there has been co-operation and mutual acknowledgement of each other's knowledge and skills – and there have been differences and mutual criticisms.

It is no surprise that the strongest advocates for psychological input to the new NHS were psychiatrists in the asylums and mental handicap hospitals. This built on pre-existing joint practice between psychiatrists and educational psychologists (and social workers) in the Child Guidance Clinics that were set up from the late 1920s and on the less well-known joint working in military settings during the Second World War, as colleagues in both military selection and training.

Psychiatrists initially wanted psychologists to bolster their search for a more measurable and scientific psychiatry. Consequently, the two main functions of the early psychologists were as psychometricians ('test-bashers') – mainly with ability, personality and projective tests – and to contribute to doctor-led research projects. Yet growth in numbers before 1960 was very slow; in that year, there were only around 180 clinical psychologists in England and Wales, with a few in Scotland.

Changes in Clinical Psychology, 1960–2010

The scope and nature of the work of clinical psychologists in Britain, and their numbers, have changed almost beyond recognition from that early period.[17] Many of those early clinical psychologists were former educational psychologists who had moved into the NHS. In 1957, there were only three formal training courses in Britain, and it was also possible to qualify simply by a three-year apprenticeship.

Involvement in anything that could be called treatment was forbidden – not least by Aubrey Lewis at the Maudsley – but if it could be called education or training that might be permitted. In the mental handicap field, clinical psychologists had an early innovative role, as shown by the work of Jack Tizard and Neil O'Connor at the Medical Research Council's Social Psychiatry Research Unit and of the Clarkes at the Manor Hospital at Epsom.[18]

The Todd Report on medical education led to the establishment of both new medical schools and new university departments of psychiatry from the 1960s. The new professors of psychiatry – many of them trained at the Maudsley – were keen to appoint clinical psychologists, and they were strong supporters of the new regional clinical psychology training courses that developed from that period.

Two factors then conspired to broaden the fields of activity of psychologists beyond psychiatry and so to loosen the control of psychiatrists over their work. In 1974, the creation of area health authorities meant that the management of clinical psychologists was often transferred to an area officer, and clinical psychologists began to be seen as a resource for other areas of clinical work, such as neurology and paediatrics. In 1977, the DHSS-sponsored report on the role of psychologists in the health services,[19] chaired by William Trethowan (then professor of psychiatry at Birmingham), recommended that clinical psychologists 'should have full professional status' in the NHS and should develop specialist services beyond psychiatry. Some psychiatrists resented and vehemently opposed these proposals; others felt the recommendations did not go far enough.

A third factor was the explosive growth of behaviour therapy, soon expanded to cognitive behavioural therapy (CBT) and which changed the core role of clinical psychologists in all clinical fields.[20] From the early 1960s, the increasing evidence for the effectiveness of behaviour therapy, initially for anxiety-related conditions, led to high levels of demand for psychological services – not least from GPs. From the 1980s, the major expectation of clinical psychologists was a contribution to psychologically informed treatments and to psychiatric rehabilitation, with increasing demand in outpatient and Community Mental Health Team (CMHT) settings and significant developments in work with older adults, for example.

Hans Eysenck, the deliberately provocative and now controversial professor of psychology at the Institute of Psychiatry up to 1983, has often been seen as the representative leading clinical psychologist in Britain. While he was a prodigiously productive researcher, he did not himself see patients and his influence on clinical and professional practice has been overstated,[21] with Monte Shapiro and Jack Rachman instead having been central to developments in training and CBT at the Maudsley during the early part of this period.

Away from the London and the Maudsley, David Smail in Nottinghamshire and Dorothy Rowe in Lincolnshire, for example, promoted more reflective and critical stances,[22] with other firebrands such as Don Bannister at Bexley Hospital. Other centres developed their own highly productive research programmes, such as at Birmingham, Edinburgh, Manchester and Oxford.

A number of effective professional and academic leaders worked closely with the Department of Health, and with the Royal College, to influence policy and improve practice. These included the three clinical psychologist members of the Trethowan Committee – Alan Clarke, Gwynne Jones and May Davidson. In a later generation, psychologists such as Glenys Parry and Anne Richardson worked very effectively within the Department of Health.

Fifty years on, in 2010, this led to there being 8,800 clinical psychologists in England and Wales who had trained at one of the thirty-five 3-year highly selective university doctoral programmes throughout the UK that adopted a 'scientist-practitioner' model of training. In

2010, the lead psychologist within a service was likely to be as experienced as the consultant psychiatrist. Psychologist-led research programmes mushroomed, and the BPS is now an equal partner with the Royal College in contributing to mental health–related NICE guidelines. With the advent of general management, clinical psychologists can be clinical directors or Trust CEOs and, with the 2007 Mental Health Act, could be responsible clinicians (RCs) in their own right.

In 1960, there would typically be one relatively inexperienced psychologist in a mental hospital, working essentially as a subordinate scientific technician, when psychiatric services were emerging from the hierarchical systems that existed before the 1959 Mental health Act. So the crucial underlying factor in the changing relationships between the two professions over the period is the shift from a marked imbalance in power and experience to a position of equivalence in expertise within their own fields and of equality in experience and numbers.

So What *Is* Distinctive about Clinical Psychologists?

The distinctive characteristic of psychologists is their felt primary identity as psychologists, acquired during their initial education and training and sustained by their ongoing professional relationships and exercise of distinctive skills and perspective. First degrees in psychology are not vocational. Although the curriculum has to cover core issues required by the BPS, degrees vary significantly in their content and orientation. Many potential clinical psychologists choose to take courses in abnormal psychology that often adopt a critical approach to psychiatry.

Psychology has become one of the most popular undergraduate subjects in Britain, so entry to clinical psychology is highly competitive, with trainees already high academic achievers. They are in effect required to have several years' 'relevant' experience before beginning their clinical training. One significant consequence of this is that most trainees are several years older than most medical students when they begin medical school.

Simon Sinclair, himself a psychiatrist, explored from a social anthropological perspective the socialisation process which medical students undergo, forming what he considered a distinctive 'embodied disposition' or 'medical habitus'.[23] Clinical psychologists are undoubtedly socialised into their roles, but they have gone through a different intellectual and social journey to doctors. They have much in common with other psychological colleagues also working in mental health – health, child, counselling and forensic psychologists as well as clinical neuropsychologists.

Psychologists are, however, now also entering the mental health field in other guises. Completely unexpectedly, the Labour government elected in 1997 gave priority to mental health. The 1999 Adult Mental Health National Service Framework (NSF) identified the need to improve staffing and uncovered serious difficulties in recruitment.[24] In 2000, a commitment was made to train a thousand 'graduate primary care mental health workers' – in practice, nearly all psychology graduates – to administer brief psychological therapy techniques in GP settings, and the 2007 Improving Access to Psychological Therapies (IAPT) programme brought in even more psychologists to NHS mental health services. Add in the psychology graduates who are now training as mental health nurses and occupational therapists, for example, and psychologists are now embedded in the NHS mental health services at every level.

Inter-professional Co-operation, Competition and Criticism

What psychologists in health care and psychiatrists share is their concern for their patients – or clients or service users, as you will – and their families. When working well as a team, or as immediate colleagues, their concerns lead to a fuller understanding of the needs of their patient and to a wider range of available interventions. With experience, the assumption by mental health workers from all professions of origin of key worker roles and with the cross-professional take-up of post-basic training in new therapeutic modalities, there has been a softening of professional differences. When workers from different disciplinary backgrounds have worked together for thirty years or more, coping with very demanding and distressing circumstances, mutual confidence and trust deepen.

The professional bodies collaborate in a number of areas: the 1995 joint Royal College and BPS policy on psychological therapies in the NHS is an early example.[25] Yet there remain tensions within the BPS, earlier primarily a learned society with an open membership, with it recognising only in 1966 that it needed to also become a professional body and it now fighting to represent academic and research psychologists in a highly competitive funding environment.

There is competition between differing biomedical, psychological and social perspectives: applied psychologists do not privilege biomedical explanations for the myriad range of distress, disability and dysfunction they encounter. R. E. Kendell, in his 2000 Royal College presidential lecture,[26] explicitly saw clinical psychologists as direct professional competitors; he could 'visualise a scenario in which clinical psychology might seem ... to both general practitioners and to the Health Departments ... to be both the most important source of therapeutic skills and professional advice in the mental health field'. An important example of such challenges to conventional psychiatric thinking is Richard Bentall's book on the nature of psychosis.[27]

There is direct financial competition in the mental health private practice marketplace with the increased numbers of psychologists and other psychological therapists and counsellors. More psychologists engage in the lucrative business of court work and in the sound bite media comments that influence public attitudes to mental health.

There can still be strains to relationships, usually when one or another person plays power games or holds rigidly to a particular position and is unwilling to compromise; but for every rigid controlling psychiatrist encountering bumptious young psychologists, there have been supportive psychiatrists mentoring their new colleagues.

Just as there is critical and radical psychiatry, so there is critical and radical psychology. There has been no shortage of clinical psychologists challenging their own profession, with David Pilgrim, for example, being a trenchant critic for thirty years.[28] The sociologist Nikolas Rose has similarly been a trenchant critique of the 'psy' professions.[29]

Conclusion

The world of mental health has changed markedly over the past sixty years. Boundaries between normality and abnormality, sickness and health, are complicated by different ideas of distress and dysfunction. The voice of patients (experts by experience) now challenges our authority and mental health policy is firmly in the public and political arena.

To pretend that all is now well in the world of professional mental health practice is dangerous. Psychiatrists and clinical psychologists can be good clinical colleagues and conceptual sparring partners; however, both psychiatrists and clinical psychologists must be open to criticism, whether friendly or unfriendly.

Key Summary Points

- Psychiatry has never been without vociferous critics.
- Anti-psychiatry raised legitimate, albeit irritating, concerns about psychiatric practice.
- Clinical psychologists in Britain now outnumber psychiatrists, with an enormously expanded clinical remit.
- Lead psychologists are now as experienced as consultant psychiatrists and vie for leadership.
- To pretend that all is well in the world of professional mental health practice and relationship is dangerous.

Acknowledgements

Parts of this chapter were published in *Lancet Psychiatry* in 2020 to mark sixty years since the publication of Laing's *The Divided Self*.[30]

Notes

1. C. Webster, *The National Health Service: A Political History* (2nd ed.). Oxford: Oxford University Press, 2002.

2. E. Powell, Enoch Powell's 'Water Tower' speech, 1961; Ministry of Health, *A Hospital Plan for England and Wales*. London: HMSO, 1962.

3. R. D. Laing, *The Divided Self*. London: Tavistock, 1960.

4. J.-P. Sartre, *L'existentialisme est un humanisme* [Existentialism and Humanism]. Paris: Les Editions Nagel, 1946.

5. R. D. Laing and A. Esterson, *Sanity, Madness and the Family*. London: Tavistock Publications, 1964.

6. M. Foucault, *Madness and Civilisation: A History of Insanity in the Age of Reason*. New York: Random House, 1965.

7. E. Goffman, *Asylums: Essays on the Social Situation of Mental Patients and Other Inmates*. Harmondsworth: Penguin Books, 1960.

8. R. Barton, *Institutional Neurosis*. Bristol: John Wright, 1959.

9. T. S. Szasz, *The Myth of Mental Illness: Foundations of a Theory of Personal Conduct*. London: Paladin, 1972.

10. M. Roth, Presidential address: Psychiatry and its critics. *Canadian Psychiatric Association Journal* (1972) 17: 343–50.

11. K. Jones and A. Poletti, The 'Italian experience' reconsidered. *British Journal of Psychiatry* (1986) 148: 144–50.

12. A. Clare, *Psychiatry in Dissent*. London: Tavistock Publications, 1976.

13. A. Scull, *Psychiatry and Its Discontents* (1st ed.). Berkley: University of California Press, 2019.

14. J. Moncrieff, *The Myth of the Chemical Cure: A Critique of Psychiatric Drugs*. London: Palgrave Macmillan, 2007.

15. D. Summerfield, The invention of post-traumatic stress disorder and the social usefulness of a psychiatric category. *British Medical Journal* (2001) 322: 95–8.

16. P. Bracken and P. Thomas, Postpsychiatry: A new direction for mental health. *British Medical Journal* (2001) 322: 724–7.

17. J. Hall, D. Pilgrim and G. Turpin, eds, *Clinical Psychology in Britain: Historical Perspectives* (History of Psychology Centre Monograph No 2). Leicester: British Psychological Society, 2015.

18. A. M. Clarke and A. D. B. Clarke, *Mental Deficiency: The Changing Outlook*. London: Methuen, 1958.

19. Department of Health and Social Security (DHSS), *The Role of Psychologists in the Health Services* (The Trethowan Report). London: HMSO, 1977.

20. S. Marks, Psychologists as therapists: The development of behavioural traditions in clinical psychology. In Hall, Pilgrim and Turpin, eds, *Clinical Psychology in Britain: Historical Perspectives*, 194–207.

21. R. D. Buchanan, *Playing with Fire: The Controversial Career of Hans J. Eysenck*. New York: Oxford University Press, 2011.

22. D. Smail, *Taking Care: An Alternative to Therapy*. London: Dent, 1987; D. Rowe, *Depression: The Way Out of Your Prison* (3rd ed.). London: Routledge, 2003.

23. S. Sinclair, *Making Doctors: An Institutional Apprenticeship*. London: Bloomsbury, 1997.

24. Department of Health, *National Service Framework for Adult Mental Health*. London: Department of Health, 1999.

25. Royal College of Psychiatrists and the British Psychological Society, *Psychological Therapies for Adults in the NHS: A Joint Statement*. Report No. CR37. London, 1995.

26. R. E. Kendell, The next 25 years (RCPsych presidential valedictory lecture). *British Journal of Psychiatry* (2000) 176: 6–9.

27. R. Bentall, *Madness Explained: Psychosis and Human Nature*. London: Allen Lane, 2003.

28. J. Pilgrim and A. Treacher, *Clinical Psychology Observed*. London: Routledge, 1992.

29. N. Rose, *Governing the Soul: The Shaping of Private Self* (2nd ed.). London: Free Association Books, 1990.

30. T. Burns, A history of antipsychiatry in four books. *Lancet Psychiatry* (2020) 7: 312–14.

Changing Generations I: Children, Adolescents and Young People

Arnon Bentovim

Introduction

This chapter will review the societal and political context in which there was an evolution of approaches to address the mental health needs of children and young people.[1] In the 1960s and 1970s, stimulated by socio-cultural changes, new innovations in therapeutic approaches were introduced, including family therapy and cognitive behavioural therapy (CBT). The first major longitudinal and epidemiological research studies were carried out. In the 1970s and 1980s, there were challenges to the state's capacity to deal with a variety of social problems and various forms of child maltreatment were identified. A national multidisciplinary assessment and management framework was introduced aimed at protecting the child, supporting families and developing appropriate treatment initiatives. In the 1990s and 2000s, further interventions were developed to reverse the impact of social exclusion – for example, Sure Start. There was a consolidation of practice, including both general and highly specialised services, and further development in research and training.

The Societal Context: 1960s and 1970s

During the post-war years, the promotion of national growth and well-being had been a priority with the establishment of the National Health Service (NHS) and the welfare state.[2] Then, as a result of post-war fertility and the baby boom, demographics tilted towards youth; by the 1960s and 1970s, fuelled by the 'youth culture', there was a marked change towards an anti-establishment cultural phenomenon in the Western world. Disaffected young people rebelled against the Vietnam War. Socially progressive values grew, encompassing feminism, women in leadership roles, environmentalism, civil rights, a sexual revolution relaxing social taboos, easier birth control, repeal of sexist laws and gay liberation. There were also increasing stresses, family break-ups, divorce and single parenthood.

Traditions: Child and Adolescent Psychiatry in the 1960s and 1970s

The Child Guidance Movement

The child guidance clinic model was established in the 1930s: the 'trinity' of a psychiatrist seeing the referred child, a social worker engaging with the mother and an educational psychologist testing the child and liaising with the school.[3] Many child and adolescent psychiatrists underwent psychoanalytic training. Psychiatric social workers trained in casework skills and educational psychologists had a background in teaching.

Regular sessions were offered to the child or young person, promoting an attachment through a child-centred approach, using play and artistic materials to encourage the expression of feelings. The approach gave the child the experience of an adult creating a warm, positive attachment and facilitated reflecting on their lives, sharing traumatic and stressful events and trying to make sense of their anxieties and depressed mood as well as managing behaviours, solving problems and finding solutions. Casework with mothers to support them in the challenging task of parenting provided an opportunity for mothers to reflect on their own experiences, current and historical stresses, and relationships, which were influencing their parenting. They were helped in managing their children's challenging behaviour as well as being emotionally responsive and understanding. The psychologist supported the child or young person in the educational context. By 1970, there were 367 clinics in the UK.

Child Psychotherapy

There was significant controversy in working therapeutically with children and young people.[4] Anna Freud's approach at the Hampstead Clinic emphasised the supportive 'ego-strengthening' role of the therapist and the use of play materials, games and activities to promote growth and resilience. Kleinian approaches at the Tavistock Clinic centred on the object-relations, transference and counter-transference interpretation of children's play and responses to the therapist in order to resolve early sources of anxiety and promote maturation.

Winnicott, a paediatrician and psychoanalyst who gained renown from his wartime broadcasts, supported an independent/'middle' group approach – illustrated through his demonstrations of 'squiggle' drawing encounters with children. The child and the therapist challenged each other to turn a shape into an image, thus reflecting experiences which could be built on as part of a creative encounter. Winnicott built on the notion of transitional space underpinning play and creativity (see also Chapter 15).[5]

The Association of Child Psychotherapists, established in 1949, fostered different approaches and maintained a continuity of traditions of training in working intensively with children, adolescents and young people. Work developed with special populations of children – in residential and care contexts and with autistic spectrum disorders and learning/intellectual disability. Related creative forms of therapeutic work have developed – play therapy, art and music therapy and educational therapies.

Innovations: 1960s and 1970s

Developments of Family Therapy and Multidisciplinary Practice

Although effective, the child guidance clinic model proved static and unresponsive to the changing societal dynamics. A striking development was the growth of family therapy.[6] Bowlby introduced family meetings to reinforce individual therapy; Skynner, a group analyst, worked with the family as a group. A seminal paper by Bateson, 'The Double-Bind Theory of Schizophrenia', in 1962, asserted that disordered communication led to pathological outcomes. Children's mental health difficulties were triggered and maintained by pathological family interactions. Minuchin developed 'structural' approaches, working with family communications, boundaries and alliances aiming to alter interactions between family members and improve the functioning of the child. The model was transmitted widely by videos of therapeutic work, large-scale dramatic demonstrations and public media forums, an approach which contrasted vividly with traditional more private and reflective approaches.

Therapists were trained in experiential approaches such as 'moving family sculptures' and 'role play' to facilitate the development of skills and understanding. Live supervision of clinical work took place through one-way screens and electronic bugs in the ear. Despite reservations, there was an enthusiastic take-up of the approach. Child and adolescent psychiatrists, psychologists and social workers started working with families and collaborated to establish training, which led to the founding of the Association of Family Therapy in 1976, rebalancing the dynamics between the different professionals. Therapeutic skills could be developed and effective therapy delivered to children and their families by a range of professionals across health and social care as well as education.

Developments in Cognitive Behavioural Therapy (CBT)

CBT emerged as an amalgam of behavioural and cognitive theories of human behaviour.[7] Behavioural therapy had been developed in the 1960s and included Patterson's parent-training model, introducing consistent approaches to managing challenging disruptive behaviour. An increased awareness of the role of cognition led to the transition to CBT in the 1970s. Internal thought processes (e.g. self-talk) began to be viewed as both targets and mechanisms of change, with an emphasis on improving cognitive skills linked with modifying behaviour. Self-instruction emerged to teach impulsive children how to control their behaviour.

Psychological disorders were attributed to maladaptive cognitive processes, with psychological vulnerabilities developing as a result of early socialisation experiences within the family. Specific CBT approaches for children and young people incorporated parent training and the development of children's mastery over their own environment. Specific protocols emerged for the treatment of anxiety and depression, trauma-focused CBT and parent training. The Triple P and Incredible Years programmes have been widely adopted. CBT has become a well-established, online, self-guided approach, which is as effective as face-to-face treatments in appropriate circumstances.

Developments in Research and Practice in Child and Adolescent Mental Health

Attachment

Bowlby's 1951 review of maternal deprivation in *Maternal Care and Mental Health* had a significant influence on the development of research in the field.[8] He highlighted the core role of maternal attachment for the secure development of the child. Psychoanalytic colleagues criticised his emphasising the role of real-life experiences rather than the inner world. Rutter praised positive consequences, for example parents staying with their children in hospital but echoed feminist criticisms that even brief daily maternal separations were assumed to be harmful.[9] He observed that the controversy generated empirical research about children's development, family relationships and the importance of good-quality alternative care. The 'attachment' concept has played a key role in professional and public awareness about the care of children and the security and organisation of attachment and mental health and as a target for therapeutic work.

Research Methodologies, Assessment and Measurement

Assessing and measuring the nature, extent and severity of mental health difficulties is an essential component of research and practice.[10] Questionnaires, interviews and observational approaches help to identify the presence of disorders, including depressed mood, anxiety, traumatic responses, anti-social behavioural symptoms and concentration difficulties.

Longitudinal research identified cohorts of children at birth followed through to adulthood, establishing continuities of mental health disorders between childhood, adolescent and adult life, identifying harmful and protective influences on development. Following the development of children through to adulthood has also been a popular theme in TV documentaries.

The 1970 Isle of Wight Study, led by Rutter,[11] was a key development in *epidemiological research*, demonstrating the value in screening whole populations and interviewing children, adolescents, young people and families. The epidemiological model has examined many influences on children and young people's development, including prenatal factors, smoking and alcohol misuse; family factors – parental mental health, neglect and abuse, separation and divorce; and community and school influences. This knowledge has influenced public health, preventative approaches, support for parenting and clinical practice.

Measures of family and parenting relationships include attachment quality and parenting capacity. *The Multiaxial Approach to Diagnosis*, introduced in 1975, provided a way to describe complexity – the nature of the presenting disorder, the level of intellectual functioning, medical factors and the psychosocial factors, including family characteristics. Assessing the effectiveness of therapeutic approaches in research and practice enhances professional and public awareness of the value of treatments.

Specific Disorders of Emerging Public Interest

Self-harming suicidal behaviour, anorexia nervosa, and other eating disorders are the main mental health conditions in young people which can lead to death.[12] Widely publicised tragic cases of young people with talent and promise self-harming – cutting, over-dosing, killing themselves – led to demands for improved and accessible mental health services. Increasing numbers of young people were presenting with self-starvation, distorted body image and a fear of fatness, associated with obsessive self-control of eating and calorie counting. There is continuing debate about societal aspirations for an idealised slim body shape and young people identifying with models or dancers.

Autistic disorders and attention deficit hyperactivity disorder (ADHD) are key neurodevelopmental disorders. Rutter delineated autism as a separate, specific disorder with deficits in social skills, empathy, problems of speech and non-verbal behaviours as well as repetitive stereotyped behaviours.[13] High-functioning individuals were identified with Asperger's syndrome and sometimes showed areas of abilities, talents and exceptional skills – for example, mathematical, musical and artistic, an interest fostered by films and TV series.

ADHD is a neurodevelopmental disorder with a classic pattern of short attention span, inattentiveness, hyperactivity, and impulsiveness, and is recognised in schools and families.[14] Treatment with psychostimulants improved concentration and educational attainment and demands for treatment followed, evoking controversy about the potentially harmful effects of medication in general and on children's growth and development.

The Recognition of Child Maltreatment: 1970s and 1980s

The Battered Child

A key to recognising child maltreatment was the publication in 1962 of Kempe and colleagues' highly influential paper 'The Battered-Child Syndrome'.[15] Images of bruising and broken bones focused the thinking of child health practitioners worldwide. The sequence of identification in society of different forms of maltreatment followed:

- *Physical abuse* – burns, fractures and bruises; a child 'deserving punishment'
- *Neglect and failure to thrive* – unawareness of the needs of the child
- *Emotional abuse* – rejection and scapegoating
- *Exposure to violence* – domestic violence and abuse
- *Sexual abuse* – sexual interest and exploitation of the child and young person.

There was also the recognition that a rare unintended consequence of mothers staying with children in hospital was that, despite appearing loving and close, some came to be understood as seeking support through having a sick child. Symptoms could be falsified or exaggerated, resulting in factitious illness states – Munchausen's syndrome by proxy or non-accidental poisoning.[16]

Epidemiological research revealed the extent of maltreatment, its under-reporting and the long-term impact on physical and mental health.[17] Finkelhor described 'polyvictimisation', the exposure to multiple forms of maltreatment over childhood.[18] As maltreatment can be defined as a criminal action, a social problem or a health disorder, a multidisciplinary response was advocated, led by social services. Practitioners from the police, health and social care and education were encouraged to 'Work Together' to recognise the signs of child maltreatment, carry out the necessary assessments, ensure the child or young person is protected though legal processes if necessary and provide intervention to help the child and family. This included appropriate treatment for complex parental mental health issues, including alcohol and substance abuse. Prosecution was reserved for the most serious injuries. There was increasing awareness of the intergenerational traumatic impact on children's health and development and the need to provide a range of therapeutic interventions.

Recognition of Sexual Abuse

Our survey of professionals working with children in 1981 revealed that the sexual abuse of children was recognised as a crime not a focus of child protection,[19] an attitude which has persisted. Following wider publication on the issue, many individuals who had suffered sexual abuse and exploitation in silence came forward to speak about their persisting traumatic experiences. There is continuing evidence about the pervasive impact of harmful sexual exploitation of vulnerable children by individuals with power – in families, communities, churches, schools, sports and entertainment.

A family and group treatment programme was established at Great Ormond Street Children's Hospital in 1981,[20] providing diagnosis and treatment for children, male and female victims, young people, protective mothers and abusive young people and parents. A rehabilitation approach based on family systemic principles was initiated, including, where possible, individuals in prison, who could take responsibility directly for abusive behaviour, albeit with stringent safeguards. A BBC *Horizon* documentary 'Prisoners of

Incest' in 1984 demonstrated the approach but was controversial from feminist perspectives that raised concerns about an inappropriate accommodation to perpetrators, who were at risk of continuing abusive behaviour.

Public Recognition of Maltreatment

The reality of child maltreatment was brought home by the tragic case in 1974 of Maria Colwell, a child subjected to extensive physical abuse.[21] This was the first in a series of thirty public inquiries into serious child maltreatment, with the most recent being Victoria Climbié in 2000 and 'Baby P' in 2009. There was extensive media coverage, detailed accounts about what had gone wrong and questioning of the current state of policy and practice. Social work professionals who had been made responsible for child protection were named, vilified and harshly criticised for accommodating to parents, failing to recognise and not using their statutory powers to protect children.

The secrecy and threat associated with sexual abuse make diagnosis through interviews and physical examination complex and challenging. In 1986, the paediatricians Hobbs and Wynne described a series of sex rings in a northern city and the criteria for diagnosis of boys and girls who had sustained anal abuse.[22] The Cleveland affair in the summer of 1987 focused on the work of two paediatricians and a social worker.[23] More than 100 children had been removed from their families over a short period, based in part on physical findings associated with possible sexual abuse. The findings were fiercely criticised as dubious in the media and parliament. The widely reported inquiry that followed highlighted the risk of professional intervention on questionable grounds and criticised the 'over-enthusiastic' use of medical science. The inquiry supported the rights of parents, in practice, undermining the attempts of practitioners to find ways to amplify the voice of the child who had been silenced. Our facilitative approach to interviews using anatomically correct dolls was also challenged.

Social Context: The Children Act

Implicit in the narrative of failure, incompetence and 'over-zealous' approaches to protect children were a criticism of social welfare approaches. The 1980s were characterised generally by an increasing disillusionment with the ability of the social democratic state to manage the economy and overcome a range of social problems. There was a rise in violence and a decline in social discipline. An alternative, individualised concept of relationships and market forces was advanced, aimed at shrinking the state. The family was seen as a predominantly private domain, excluding the state unless violence was being perpetrated.

This thinking underpinned the establishment of the Children Act 1989.[24] The Act provided a legal framework which emphasised the importance of providing support for families and established criteria for a child being at risk of 'significant harm' to justify removal from a parent's care. Mental health professionals played a key role in helping the courts understand the risks, the prospects for rehabilitation, the provision of treatment services and the possibility of the need for alternative care or, ultimately, adoption.

In parallel, the United Nation's Convention on the Rights of the Child (1989) was established to ensure that services were provided to enable children to participate in society, to have a voice and to be protected from violence and exploitation.

Consolidation of Mental Health Services for Children, Adolescents and Young People: 1990s to 2010

Social Policy Context

This period was marked by the last phase of Thatcherism, which extended market rationalities and focused on the individual rather than governing through society.[25] New Labour from 1997 to 2009 espoused the 'third way', combining individualism and egalitarianism and thus reconciling apparently conflicting cultural projects: personal self-realisation and rights to autonomy; and membership and community. Initiatives focused on reversing social exclusion, stressing the need for early intervention and prevention, including the Sure Start and Children's Fund programmes. Despite significant investment, there was no full-scale attempt to reduce social inequality, although more than a million children were lifted out of poverty. The final year of this period, following the financial crash, saw the re-election of a Conservative–Liberal Democrat coalition government destined to pursue a programme of austerity, a reduction in public services, shrinking of the state and a further drive towards the privatisation of public services.

Development of Services

By the 1990s, child and adolescent mental health had a higher profile in both the public and the professional worlds. More academic chairs and departments of child and adolescent psychiatry were established, and training and accreditation programmes were developed. Research developed across the fields, including in genetics, molecular biology and neurobiology (see also Chapter 16).[26]

A four-tiered framework of CAMHS (Children and Adolescent Mental Health Services) as a health service was established in 1995, replacing child guidance clinics:

Tier 1 Advice and treatment provided by practitioners working in a variety of settings in the community, in general practice, in schools and in agencies working with maltreated children – e.g. the NSPCC (National Society for the Prevention of Cruelty to Children).

Tier 2 Generic multidisciplinary teams – providing core community services for children, adolescents and young people.

Tier 3 Specialist multidisciplinary services.

Tier 4 Highly specialised services providing outpatient and inpatient care for young people presenting with early psychotic illness, eating disorders or displaying sexually harmful behaviour.

A highly specialised service that attracted much attention and controversy was the establishment of the Tavistock Gender Identity Development Service in 1989.[27] Following rigorous assessments and therapeutic help, a young person's wish to transition and develop their gender identity could be facilitated through medical and psychological intervention. During the controversy, it was asserted on the one hand that, lacking maturity, the deeply held wishes of young people should not be supported until they reached adulthood; on the other hand that there should be respect for the emerging individuality and autonomy of the young person.

The NHS organisation NICE (the National Institute for Clinical Excellence, later renamed as the National Institute for Health and Care Excellence) was established in

1999 and recommended the most effective approaches to help children and young people with mental health problems. The IAPT (Improving Access to Psychological Treatment) programme provided access to these effective therapies and was introduced to adult services in 2008 and children's services in 2011.[28] MindEd training was introduced to complement IAPT and to provide online training in emotional and behavioural 'first aid' and essential therapeutic skills.

One of the treatments recommended by NICE was the extensively researched CBT, with the risk that other modalities would be dismissed. Later research demonstrated that well-structured family/systemic or psychodynamic approaches were equally effective. In addition, much research focused on single disorders. The reality is that comorbid disorders are the rule rather than the exception. An alternative has been the development of *integrative approaches*, bringing different modalities together.[29] The *common treatment element approach* identified and categorised common features of treatments which can be integrated to meet complex needs,[30] an approach we adopted to reduce the harmful effects of all forms of maltreatment.[31]

Young Offenders Services

Young Offenders Services were established in 1998, with special school, youth courts, residential care and young offender institutions. However, the age of criminal responsibility remained at ten years. The world's press had heard a blow-by-blow account of the killing of James Bulger by two vulnerable eleven-year-olds in 1993 in an adult court. Popular judgement was that the children were 'evil' and 'devious' and deserved to be in prison for life. Growing knowledge was ignored about the way the young person's brain matures and responds to earlier trauma, undermining their capacity for judgement and control of impulsivity.

Our follow-up study of sexually abused boys demonstrated that sexually harmful adolescent or adult behaviour was more likely if they had also witnessed violence and suffered rejection.[32] Attempts to change the age of criminal responsibility have been firmly resisted. The aggressive behaviour of adolescents and young people has continued to be a societal and media preoccupation – with gangs, knife crimes, bullying and 'children who kill'.

Developments in Child Protection: Trauma-Informed Care

In 1988, in describing adverse childhood experiences (ACEs), Felitti and colleagues extended the concept of maltreatment to include household dysfunction and instability resulting from domestic violence; parental substance abuse; mental illness; imprisonment; and separation.[33] They found that the more types of ACEs that individuals reported in their childhood (e.g. emotional, physical or sexual abuse; physical or emotional neglect; mother treated violently; household substance abuse or mental illness; incarcerated household member; and parental separation or divorce), the greater their risks of health-harming behaviours (e.g. smoking or sexual risk-taking) and both infectious and non-communicable diseases (NCDs), including substance abuse, mental health problems and violent behaviour.

The *Framework for the Assessment of Children in Need and Their Families*, in 2000, broadened the approach and provided a model for practitioners across children's social care to describe the child's needs in the context of parenting, individual and community factors. We were commissioned to develop and provide training in evidence-based approaches to assessment, analysis and intervention.[34] *Trauma-informed care in the community* was introduced in 2005, integrating policies, procedures and practices as well as identifying potential paths for recovery.

The Internet: Beneficial and Harmful Influences

The World Wide Web, launched in 1989–90, gained massive popularity in the mid-1990s and was a near-instant communication aid and way of registering knowledge and information.[35] The development of online therapeutic work and training has grown. Young people embraced the Internet, using it for social networking, communicating, expanding their interests, enriching their lives, entertainment, gaming, connecting and learning. Important issues, including gender identification as male, female or transsexual, could be debated. The Internet gives a voice to children and young people and may provide informal support and advice about managing specific problems, for example self-harm and anorexia.

The harmful impact of the Internet has also dominated social discourse, including exposure to age-inappropriate material online, pornography, violence or hate speech. Child pornography is circulated on the Web, and children may be groomed into creating and circulating images of sexual activities. Perpetrators have falsified their identities and groomed young people as a way of meeting and exploiting them sexually. Self-harm, suicide or anorectic behaviour can be encouraged online. Children and young people can abuse each other by sexting (sending sexual images, thus risking blackmail), cyber-bullying, harassment, disclosure of personal information or threats of social exclusion may trigger self-harm and suicidal responses.

The issue of the safety and control of the Internet is a constant and continuing theme. Childline, established in 1986, currently receives multiple calls about abuse over the Internet. Offenders can be helped anonymously to break the addictive cycle through 'Stop it Now'.[36] Children, young people and parents can be helped to understand the beneficial and harmful risks associated with internet use.

Conclusion

In their masterly review of the history of child and adolescent mental health 1960–2010 Rutter and Stevenson concluded: 'there has been an amazing revolution in child and adolescent psychiatry … As a consequence, the body of knowledge, and the range of therapeutic interventions have increased in a way that would have seemed scarcely conceivable 50 years ago.'[37] This review has confirmed these conclusions, focusing on the interface between society and mental health; promoting developments in therapeutic approaches and services to the community; and identifying and managing the pervasive and lifetime harmful impact of child maltreatment and adversity.

Key Summary Points

- From the 1960s to the 1980s, in parallel to societal changes from welfarism to the counterculture, the legacy of the child guidance movement and psychodynamic approaches gave way to more active, transparent and fast-moving therapies. Family/systemic therapy involved the whole family and trained practitioners from all disciplines. Cognitive behavioural therapy (CBT) was developed as a new, effective psychological treatment.

- Different longitudinal and epidemiological research approaches developed, providing a variety of ways of measuring the presence and impact of mental health problems. Conditions such as anorexia nervosa of childhood, self-harming and neurodevelopmental disorders – autism and ADHD – have been identified. These developments established a significant profile of child and adolescent mental health in professional practice and public awareness.
- Despite attempts to 'shrink the state' in the 1980s, a continuing theme has been the recognition of the hidden yet pervasive traumatic impact of maltreatment many children suffer. The concept has been enlarged through the recognition of adverse childhood experiences (ACEs), adding exposure to family dysfunction and instability. There is a lifespan impact of adversity on mental and physical health and a need for a trauma-informed care approach.
- Fostered by an investment in social inclusion in the 1990s to the 2000s, multidisciplinary Children and Adolescent Mental Health Services (CAMHS) were established, providing general to highly specialised treatment. Academic units promoted training and research in genetics and neurobiology. The National Institute for Clinical Excellence, later renamed the National Institute for Health and Care Excellence, gathered the growing research information on intervention and recommended best practice.
- The introduction of the Internet in the 1990s has been both beneficial and harmful. The voice of the child as a person can be amplified, including the right to determine their gender. However, the Internet may also provide a route for some people to gratify inappropriate sexual interests in children and young people and to hurt them physically and emotionally. Safety and protection require constant vigilance.

Notes

1. M. Rutter and J. Stevenson, Developments in child and adolescent psychiatry over the last 50 years. In M. Rutter, D. Bishop and D. Pine et al., eds, *Rutter's Child and Adolescent Psychiatry* (5th ed.), 1–17. Oxford: Blackwell Science, 2008.

2. T. Judt, *Postwar: A History of Europe Since 1945*. London: Heinemann, 2005.

3. W. Ll. Parry-Jones, The history of child and adolescent psychiatry: Its present-day relevance. *Journal of Child Psychology and Psychiatry* (1998) 30: 3–11.

4. E. Rous and A. Clark, Child psychoanalytic psychotherapy in the UK National Health Service: An historical analysis. *History of Psychiatry* (2009) 20: 442–56, https://doi.org/10.1177/0957154X08338338.

5. D. W. Winnicott, *Therapeutic Consultations in Child Psychiatry*, London: Hogarth Press, 1971.

6. P. Stratton and J. Lask, The development of systemic family therapy for changing times in the United Kingdom. *Contemporary Family Therapy* (2013) 35: 257–74, https://doi.org/10.1007/s10591-013-9252-8.

7. L. Courtney, M. A. Benjamin and M. Connor et al., History of cognitive-behavioural therapy (CBT) in youth, *Child and Adolescent Psychiatric Clinics of North America* (2011) 20: 179–89, https://doi.org/10.1016/j.chc.2011.01.011.

8. J. Bowlby, *Maternal Care and Mental Health*. Geneva: World Health Organization, 1951.

9. Rutter and Stevenson, Developments in child and adolescent psychiatry over the last 50 years.

10. Ibid.

11. M. Rutter, J. Tizard and K. Whitmore, *Education, Health and Behaviour*. London: Longmans, 1970.

12. Rutter and Stevenson, Developments in child and adolescent psychiatry over the last 50 years.

13. Ibid.

14. Ibid.

15. C. H. Kempe, F. N. Silverman and B. F. Steele et al., The battered-child syndrome. *JAMA* (1962) 181: 17–24.

16. J. Gray, A. Bentovim and P. Milla, The treatment of children and their families where induced illness has been identified. In J. Howarth and B. Lawson, eds, *Trust Betrayed Munchausen Syndrome-by-Proxy, Inter-Agency Child Protection and Partnership with Families*. London: National Children's Bureau, 1995.

17. N. Parton, Social work, child protection and politics: Some critical and constructive reflections. *British Journal of Social Work* (2014) 44: 2042–56, https://doi.org/10.1093/bjsw/bcu091.

18. D. Finkelhor, H. Turner, S. Hamby and R. Ormrod, *Polyvictimization: Children's Exposure to Multiple Types of Violence, Crime, and Abuse*. Office of Juvenile Justice and Delinquency Prevention (OJJDP) bulletin, October 2011, www.ojp.gov/pdffiles1/ojjdp/235504.pdf.

19. A. Bentovim, A. Elton, J. Hildebrand, M. Bentovim and E. Vizard, *Child Sexual Abuse within the Family: Assessment and Treatment*. Bristol: Wright and Butterworth, 1988.

20. Ibid.

21. Parton, Social work, child protection and politics.

22. C. J. Hobbs and J. M. Wynne, Buggery in childhood: A common syndrome of child abuse. *Lancet* (1986) 2: 792–6, https://doi.org/10.1016/S0140-6736(86)90310-7.

23. Parton, Social work, child protection and politics.

24. Ibid.

25. Ibid.

26. Rutter and Stevenson, Developments in child and adolescent psychiatry over the last 50 years.

27. D. Di Ceglie and D. Freedman, eds, *A Stranger in My Own Body: Atypical Gender Identity and Mental Health*. London: Karnac Books, 1998.

28. S. Hamilton, A. Hicks, R. Sayers et al., A User Focused Evaluation of IAPT Services in London. Report for Commissioning Support for London, March 2011.

29. A. Bentovim and W. Kinston, Focal family therapy: Joining systems theory with psychodynamic understanding. In A. S. Gurman and D. P. Kniskern, eds, *Handbook of Family Therapy*, Vol. 2. New York: Brunner Mazel, 1991.

30. B. F. Chorpita and E. L. Daleiden, Mapping evidence-based treatments for children and adolescents: Application of the distillation and matching model to 615 treatments from 322 randomized trials. *Journal of Consulting and Clinical Psychology* (2009) 77: 566–79.

31. A. Bentovim and I. Elliott, Targeting abusive parenting and the associated impairment of children. *Journal of Clinical Child and Adolescent Psychology* (2014) 43: 270–85.

32. D. Skuse, A. Bentovim, J. Hodges et al., Risk factors for development of sexually abusive behaviour in sexually victimised adolescent boys. *British Medical Journal* (1998) 317: 175–9.

33. V. J. Felitti, R. F. Anda and D. Nordenberg, Relationship of childhood abuse and household dysfunction to many of the leading causes of death in adults: The adverse childhood experiences (ACE) study. *American Journal of Preventative Medicine* (1998) 14: 245–58.

34. A. Bentovim, A. Cox, L. Bingley Miller and S. Pizzey, *Safeguarding Children Living with Trauma and Family Violence: Evidence-Based Approaches to Assessment and Planning Intervention*. London: Jessica Kingsley, 2009.

35. P. Greenfield and Z. Yan, Children, adolescents and the Internet: A new field of inquiry in developmental psychology. *Development Psychology* (2006) 42: 391–4, https://doi.org/10.1037/0012-1649.42.3.391.

36. A. Brown, N. Jago, J. Kerr et al., *Call to Keep Children Safe from Sexual Abuse: A Study of the Use and Effects of Stop it Now! UK and Ireland Helpline*. London: NatCen Social Research: 2014.

37. Rutter and Stevenson, Developments in child and adolescent psychiatry over the last 50 years.

Changing Generations II: The Challenges of Ageism in Mental Health Policy

Claire Hilton

Introduction

In 1960, mentally disturbed people over about sixty years of age were widely assumed to have irreversible senility. Little attention was paid to Martin Roth's research which showed conclusively that mentally unwell older people were not all senile but suffered from a range of disorders. In the nomenclature of the time, those were affective psychosis, late paraphrenia, acute confusion and arteriosclerotic and senile dementia.[1] Only two hospitals in the UK routinely offered older people thorough psychiatric assessment and treatment. One was a ward at the Bethlem Royal Hospital led by Felix Post, primarily for people suffering from 'functional' illnesses, mainly depression, schizophrenia and other psychoses. The other was a comprehensive old age psychiatry service, including day hospital, outpatient and domiciliary services, plus assessment, infirmary and long-stay wards, which Sam (Ronald) Robinson established at Crichton Royal Hospital, Dumfries.

This chapter aims to explain how Roth's, Post's and Robinson's ideas gradually influenced clinical practice and service provision across the UK, shifting from typical custodial inactivity and neglect of patients assumed to be irreversibly senile to the creation of proactive 'psychiatry of old age' (POA) services. The chapter comprises two sections: 1960–1989 and 1989–2010. The first focuses on the development of the specialty until it was formally recognised by the Department of Health in 1989. It was the subject of my PhD thesis.[2] Regarding the second section, I started as a senior house officer in POA in 1989. For this section, I have also drawn extensively on the Royal College of Psychiatrists' (RCPsych) Old Age Faculty commemorative newsletter '21 years of old age psychiatry' published in 2011.[3] Although the essence of much National Health Service (NHS) policy is UK-wide, specific details and implementation plans may relate to one or more of the constituent countries. Given the brevity of this chapter, I have focused mainly on developments in England.

1960–1989

Liberal ideas about personal autonomy, choice and independence emerged internationally in the 1960s. New legislation in the UK on suicide, race relations, homosexuality and abortion reflected this. Changing agendas permitted younger people to make choices, even if risky, but older people were perceived as inevitably vulnerable and, despite their experience of life, their wishes were frequently ignored. According to Pat Thane, retirement was a mid-twentieth-century change which 'increasingly defined old people as a distinct social group defined by marginalisation and dependency'.[4] Alongside negative public perceptions, retirement was associated with a marked fall in personal income and reliance on the state pension.[5] With poverty came disadvantageous health inequalities.[6]

In the early 1960s, more than a third of psychiatric hospital beds were occupied by people aged over sixty-five. The social scientist Peter Townsend identified many older people in long-stay accommodation who 'possess capacities and skills which are held in check or even stultified. Staff sometimes do not recognise their patients' abilities, though more commonly they do not have time to cater for them.'[7] The sheer size of wards with up to seventy beds made providing satisfactory standards of nursing care almost impossible. These wards compared unfavourably with hotbeds of activity on those for younger people which used state-of-the-art medications, psychosocial, rehabilitative and therapeutic community approaches, and planned for discharge. After the Mental Health Act 1959 (MHA), with steps taken to begin to close the psychiatric hospitals and develop alternative services in the community and in district general hospitals (DGHs), younger people were discharged leaving older people behind.

For older people, clinically and scientifically, things edged on, albeit slowly. In 1961, Russell Barton and Tony Whitehead at Severalls Hospital, Essex, established a service based on Robinson's at Crichton Royal. In 1962, Nick Corsellis demonstrated that senile dementia had the same pathology as Alzheimer's disease: senility was therefore not just a worn-out ageing brain but a disease process requiring further research, aiming for prevention and cure. The same year, Post published an optimistic follow-up study of 100 older patients treated for depression.[8] In 1965, his textbook of old age psychiatry,[9] the first of its kind, was published, and the World Psychiatric Association (WPA) hosted an international symposium in London, *Psychiatric Disorders in the Aged*.[10] These developments provide insights into clinical, epidemiological and neuroscience achievements at the time and indicate mounting interest in older people's mental well-being. Neuropathology was discussed in terms of air encephalograms, post-mortems and electron microscopy. There were no validated brief cognitive assessment tools, and antidepressants consisted of tricyclics, monoamine oxidase inhibitors and electroconvulsive therapy. The WPA event included remarkable and charismatic leaders such as Post, Roth and Robinson, Tom Lambo (a Nigerian psychiatrist) and V. A. Kral of 'mild cognitive impairment' fame (who had survived incarceration in Theresienstadt Nazi concentration camp). Among the delegates were junior doctors Tom Arie, Klaus Bergmann, Garry Blessed and Raymond Levy, all inspired by the people they met and by the academic content.

Reports of scandalously low standards of care on long-stay wards in geriatric and psychiatric institutions reached the headlines in 1967 when Barbara Robb published *Sans Everything: A Case to Answer* (see also Chapter 7).[11] Arie, dual trained in social medicine and psychiatry, and shocked by the *Sans Everything* revelations, applied for a consultant psychiatrist post to work with older people at Goodmayes Hospital, Essex ('an unposh place ... Most people thought I had taken leave of my senses!').[12] Arie's team had a low hierarchical structure and high morale, able staff were eager to join it and patients began to get better.[13] Arie wrote in 1971: 'I have never before been in a professional setting where intellectual and emotional satisfaction go more closely hand in hand.'[14]

Arie and a few other newly appointed POA consultants, including Bergmann, Blessed, Whitehead and Brice Pitt – a 'happy band of pilgrims' as Pitt called them – began to meet as a 'coffee house' group. The group was in the right place at the right time: in the wake of *Sans Everything*, the government was taking more interest in the mental well-being of older people. Through Arie's social medicine links, including being personally acquainted with the chief medical officer, the group 'heavily influenced' a Department of Health and Social Security (DHSS) blueprint, *Services for Mental Illness Related to Old Age* (1972).[15] For the growing number of old age psychiatrists, this declaration of intentions became a bargaining tool to use with the DHSS or local NHS authorities when they failed to respond to identified needs.

Since, in most hospitals, younger people were discharged and older people were not, by 1973 almost 50 per cent of psychiatric hospital patients were over sixty-five,[16] far in excess of the 14 per cent in the general population. Almost two decades after Roth's research, undiagnosed but potentially treatable conditions contributed to this, particularly depression. This was also a personal tragedy, as Whitehead explained in the *Guardian*:

> Old people may spend their last years in dreadful misery because severe depression has been wrongly diagnosed as senile decay . . . If you are anxious and depressed, and more and more people start treating you as if you were a difficult child, and you are finally incarcerated in a ward full of other elderly people who are being treated in the same way, it is likely that in time you will give up and take on the role of not just a child, but a baby.[17]

Two events in 1973 were central to the development of POA services: the coffee house group became the RCPsych Group for the Psychiatry of Old Age (GPOA; which in 1978 became the Section for the Psychiatry of Old Age (SPOA); later the Faculty) and the international economy took a turn for the worse with the oil crisis, the stock market crash and curbs on public sector expenditure. Promises of new services for an undervalued sector of the community were particularly vulnerable to political and economic fluctuations. Reduced public spending generated competition for resources rather than collaboration. For older mentally ill people, this was further complicated by ambiguities about who should take responsibility for their care – geriatricians, general psychiatrists or old age psychiatrists. Responsibility for the care of patients with long-standing severe mental illness who had grown old in hospital was a bone of contention between old age and general psychiatrists who were 'dead keen to get us to take their old schizophrenics', recollected Pitt many years later. Both general psychiatrists and geriatricians were happy when old age psychiatrists took mentally disturbed older patients off their hands. Categories of 'dementia horizontalis' and 'dementia verticalis' (i.e. more mobile, restless and often disturbing to other patients, requiring much POA nursing expertise) were one way of determining who should manage which patients, but the British Geriatrics Society and RCPsych jointly created more robust guidelines for collaborative working.[18]

Despite liaising closely with the DHSS, POA was not officially recognised as a NHS specialty. As a result, relevant age-based mental health data were not collected because 'sub-specialty' statistics were 'ignored . . . coded under the appropriate main specialty'.[19] This resulted in excluding POA from plans, such as for training psychiatrists and appointing staff. In 1978, for example, the DHSS recommended five consultants in 'adult' psychiatry and one in child psychiatry for a district of 200,000 people, with no mention of POA.[20] Building projects for DGH psychiatric units also overlooked older people's needs and innovative architectural designs to promote their independence.[21] Sometimes, the DHSS admitted to only including older people when it feared that not doing so would leave them 'wide open to severe criticism'.[22] A different sort of data predicament arose when statistics derived from death certificates were used as a proxy for morbidity and health needs and underpinned NHS resource distribution; 'dementia' was generally subsumed under 'old age' making it invisible.

The government's discussion paper *A Happier Old Age* (1978) acknowledged that services were 'often less than satisfactory, making effective treatment or care difficult' and that older people should be more involved in decision-making related to their health and social care.[23] The Royal Commission on the NHS (1979) recommended additional resources for older people, but these were couched negatively in terms of 'the immense burden these demands would impose', a reiterated defeatist sentiment likely to discourage provision. In 1979, the new Conservative government was committed to controlling inflation, reviving the economy and holding back on public spending;[24] and two years later, the DHSS's *Care in the Community* was subtitled *A Consultative Document on Moving Resources for Care*, its real objective. The emphasis was on the role of the community, self-help and families to 'look after their own'. This was unrealistic. The challenges for carers of people with dementia were well known,[25] central to the origins of the Alzheimer's (Disease) Society (founded 1979) and reflected in the title of the book *The 36-Hour Day*.[26]

Establishing POA services was entwined with policy, politics, public opinion and stereotypes (Figure 22.1), and its leaders had to fight for every penny. Economic analyses of NHS provision tended to blame the difficulties on more older people living longer,

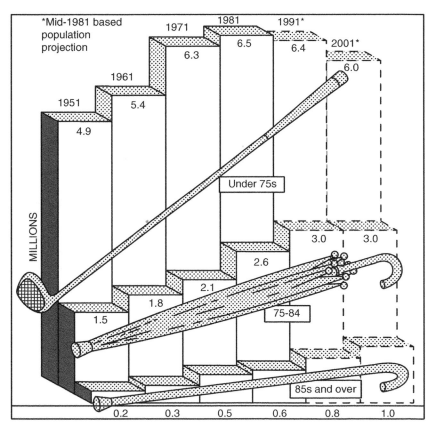

Figure 22.1 Official ageist stereotyping: 'numbers of the elderly by broad age groups', 1951–2001. Source: Office of Population Census and Surveys, *Census Guide 1: Britain's Elderly Population: 1981 Census.* London: HMSO, 1984, 1. (Crown copyright, reproduced under Open Government Licence v3.0.)

ignoring other factors, such as rising costs of staff salaries, drugs, health technology and the cost of high dependency and palliative care at *any* age. They ignored increasing longevity which allowed older people to be active for more years, often contributing to the economy despite not being formally employed. The government, however, attributed rising costs of health care to remediable inefficiency within the NHS,[27] which required administrative reorganisation.[28] Sir Roy Griffiths, managing director of Sainsbury's supermarkets, led a NHS management inquiry and introduced solutions from the commercial sector, particularly 'general management' with professional managers responsible for planning, implementation and control of performance (see also Chapter 12).[29] This was particularly abhorrent to POA which had evolved almost entirely through clinical leadership. The restructuring, like NHS reforms before and since, offered rhetoric about providing for older people rather than the means to do so.

Amid the gloom, the ever enthusiastic and determined POA leadership found beacons of light. In neuroscience, the acetylcholine hypothesis of Alzheimer's disease emerged and the Alzheimer's Society helped push dementia higher in public awareness and onto national policy and research agendas. Clinical POA became more multidisciplinary, adding strength to services and to previously medically led arguments on the need for them.[30] The British Psychological Society established their old age special interest group in 1980. Geriatricians established the first memory clinic in 1983 at University College Hospital, London.[31] Old age psychiatry was putting down academic roots, with four professors by 1986: Arie in Nottingham and Levy, Pitt and Elaine Murphy in London. Murphy became editor of the first dedicated POA academic journal, the *International Journal of Geriatric Psychiatry*, from 1986. Some hospitals established joint geriatric-psychiatric units, based on the model Arie devised and used in his professorial unit. However, the Royal College of Physicians (RCP) recommended that geriatric medicine should integrate more closely with general medicine, partly because of recruitment difficulties, and this took precedence over a holistic approach to older people's health care.[32] In 1987, older people's mental disorders were still not routinely included in nurse training, neither were they discussed in the Royal College of General Practitioners' *Preventive Care of the Elderly*. Older people were also excluded from much medical research, hazardous in the context of them being likely beneficiaries of that research.[33]

Each step forward had to be fought for. With the DHSS reluctant to create old age services, and with responsibility delegated to professional managers, undervalued specialties were easy to neglect. Inadequate data, ambiguities over responsibility for health care in old age, the DHSS and the main body of psychiatrists prioritising younger people before older, as well as the tendency for the NHS to prioritise physical over mental illness, ensured, intentionally or otherwise, that psychogeriatric services lagged behind. Nevertheless, the specialty grew, from a handful of old age psychiatrists in 1970, to 120 in 1980 and 280 in 1989. Old age psychiatrist Professor John Wattis, by his spurious use of statistics, commented humorously: 'You could draw a graph which showed that the number of old age psychiatrists was increasing exponentially and by the year 2000 there would be no doctors who were not old age psychiatrists!'[34] Inspiring teachers and a charismatic leadership – such as Arie, Wattis, David Jolley and Nori Graham – demonstrated POA's truly holistic approach to health and social care and the rewarding nature of the work and drew keen recruits into it. The SPOA wanted their specialty to be recognised by the DHSS to ensure dedicated data collection, training schemes and allocation of resources but the DHSS argued against it. One reason was their fear of recruitment difficulties for an 'unpopular' specialty but that was incompatible with evidence of more POA consultants leading more services.

There was little movement within the RCPsych to support official recognition of POA. However, the RCP was disgruntled about older, mentally unwell people on medical wards. Sir Raymond Hoffenberg, its president, established a working party about POA services. The outcome: a recommendation by the RCP and RCPsych for specialty recognition to facilitate service developments, education, training and research. The DHSS could hardly ignore the joint recommendation.

1989–2010

In 1990, the NHS and Community Care Act enshrined the NHS purchaser/provider split and the role of social services in assessing need while delegating care to the expanding private sector (see also Chapter 10). Instead of unifying old age services, it fragmented them, especially tricky for older patients who required coordinated multidisciplinary, cross-agency care. Despite ongoing challenges, old age psychiatry services multiplied across the country but many organisational goals and individuals' needs were still unmet. Greater provision was required.[35] By 1995, more than 400 POA consultants in the UK worked mainly in comprehensive catchment area and domiciliary-based services, a tried, tested and successful model of care.

The model of service provision began to change after the first acetylcholinesterase inhibitor for Alzheimer's disease, donepezil, was licensed in 1997. It was expensive, around £1,000 per patient per year. Dementia was prevalent, the population ageing, the potential demand excessive and the NHS required it to be rationed. In 2001, the National Institute for Clinical Excellence (now the National Institute for Health and Care Excellence (NICE)) ensured this happened by recommending that donepezil be 'initiated' by a specialist. This was widely interpreted to mean making the diagnosis and prescribing the medication in secondary care. Memory clinics multiplied. From being mostly research-based in a few university centres, they became local diagnostic and treatment services countrywide. More technology and 'real medicine' may have helped to reduce stigma and encourage public discussion. However, memory clinics also had drawbacks. These included transferring people with uncomplicated dementia into secondary care rather than developing skills in primary care as for other common disorders such as depression, diabetes and hypertension. They also diminished time available for expert staff to provide the mainstay of psychosocial interventions required by patients with the most complex and distressing dementias. More resources from a finite pot going into dementia services also detracted from providing services for older people with functional mental illnesses. This was worrying when dementia affected 5 per cent of people over sixty-five at any one time, while depression alone among the functional disorders affected more than 20 per cent.[36]

The pattern of officialdom allowing older people's mental health service provision to lag behind that for younger adults persisted. The *National Service Framework for Mental Health* (1999) was for 'working-age' adults. Substantial extra funding accompanied it. The *National Service Framework for Older People* arrived eighteen months later. It was comprehensive, including functional disorders and dementia, but without the money attached to facilitate implementation. Observing improvements made in services for younger patients caused much frustration among old age psychiatrists.

The POA leadership had to advocate persistently for older people to receive appropriate levels and ranges of care equitable with those provided for younger adults. In 2005, the RCPsych Faculty of Old Age Psychiatry pointed out that 'liaison psychiatry' (psychiatric services for physically unwell patients in general hospitals) for working-age adults had ninety-three dedicated consultant posts in the British Isles but, for older people, consultant liaison input was additional to their general catchment area responsibilities.[37] In 2006, a joint RCPsych and RCP report stated: 'Ageist neglect of older people with mental illness must stop.'[38] It did not stop and more inequity of provision followed, such as the Improving Access to Psychological Therapies (IAPT) programme (2008). IAPT was based on the premise that improved treatment of anxiety and depression for working-age adults would reduce their unemployment rates and thus pay for itself, or even generate notional surplus. IAPT excluded people over the age of sixty-five, even though they could benefit from the treatments offered. There was no acknowledgement that alleviating their mental symptoms could enable them to contribute more to society, such as in voluntary roles, and enhance independence, thus reducing the need for statutory support services, all of which could benefit the economy.

Other changes affected care for mentally unwell older people. The Mental Capacity Act (MCA) 2005 came into force in 2007. It provided a statutory framework to empower and protect vulnerable people who were unable to make their own decisions. Although idealistic and important for older people, implementing it, particularly the Deprivation of Liberty Safeguards, brought new layers of bureaucracy at great financial expense, removing resources from direct care.

The financial crisis of 2008 preceded another much-needed and well-intentioned initiative, the National Dementia Strategy,[39] and probably hampered its outcome. The Strategy aimed to help people 'live well with dementia', by encouraging early diagnosis; improving education and research; and attending to the needs of people with dementia and their carers in the community, care homes and general hospitals. It had money attached: £150 million over two years to support implementation. This was very welcome. However, in the context of direct costs of health and social care for dementia of around £8.2 billion annually, it was a drop in the ocean. Early problems with the Strategy included a baffling range of organisations – statutory, private, not-for-profit, health and social care – and a flurry of vaguely titled new job roles such as 'advisors', 'navigators' and 'co-ordinators', hardly straightforward for people with dementia and their carers to negotiate. The POA activists Professors Susan Benbow and Paul Kingston observed this and commented:

> sexy new solutions implemented by managers can have the opposite effect to that intended. We need to stop our headlong rush into implementation and look at the evidence for these new roles, to consider what added value they bring, and how they can be governanced and supported. Only then will we do justice to the people and families living with a dementia.[40]

In the wake of the Strategy, NHS England appointed Professor Alistair Burns as National Clinical Director for Dementia. Potentially beneficial, this added to the worries of many in the field of POA: should dementia be syphoned off as a separate entity, and what about the rest of old age psychiatry? Depression and psychosis in old age, key concerns for POA, were barely talked about outside specialist circles. The Strategy's protagonists had hoped that the issue of dementia would spearhead developments to benefit older people's mental health, well-being and dignity more broadly. The sentiments were admirable but the outcomes complex, multifaceted and mainly after 2010, so outside the scope of this chapter.

The Equality Act 2010 proved to be a hindrance as well as a help for POA: it could not abolish deep-rooted societal ageist attitudes. These contributed to (mis)interpreting the Act in ways which affected service provision, such as by depriving older people with non-dementia mental illnesses of specialist facilities and treatment and placing them instead in 'all-age' or 'ageless' services. This failed to take into account their needs which differed from those of younger people, including frailty; multiple comorbidities; risks from drug side effects and polypharmacy; different presentations of the same disorders; and different psychosocial, cultural and financial contexts.

Conclusion

Major drivers of change included dictates of fashion, supposed economy and non-validated theoretical perspectives, often imposed from a top-down template. Policies and implementation patterns derived from managerial rather than POA clinical leadership demonstrated ageist perspectives. National directives advocating uniformity of service provision could be good, ensuring access to an agreed range of services at acceptable standards and avoiding a postcode lottery. However, uniformity ignored the need for variation to fulfil local needs and undermined innovative service delivery responses. It also destroyed morale, particularly when it led to the dismantling of trusted service components which fostered expertise and humane practice, such as joint geriatric-psychiatric units, services for ethnic minority populations and long-stay NHS units for people with the most difficult to manage mental disorders. Some dismantled services required painful reconstruction when policy changed.

By 2010, there was unease about the future of the specialty. Baroness Elaine Murphy commented that some social care services, essential in POA, were in 'meltdown',[41] and Professor Robin Jacoby wrote an article on POA called 'Of pioneers and progress, but prognosis guarded'.[42] Ageism, despite the Equality Act, plus fiercer NHS business models of health care and seeking to maintain a corporate image, contributed to the difficulties. Despite the challenges, the rewards of making the lives of older people and their families more hopeful, dignified and fulfilling, by combining individual care and aiming to improve service delivery and linked to new frontiers of neuroscience research, exemplified the interactions between *Mind, State and Society* and continued to attract dedicated clinicians.

In 2018, a RCPsych report was entitled, *Suffering in Silence: Age Inequality in Older People's Mental Health Care.*[43] In 2020, NHS England's website stated ambiguously that older people's mental health 'is embedded as a "silver thread" across all of the "adult" mental health Long Term Plan ambitions.'[44] Both *Suffering in Silence* and the 'silver thread' blow an icy wind of ongoing ageism and under-resourcing, failing to allow older people to have the most humane treatment and failing to learn from history.

Key Summary Points
- Liberal ideas about personal autonomy, choice and independence emerged internationally in the 1960s. Changing agendas permitted younger people to make choices, even if risky, but older people were perceived as inevitably vulnerable and, despite their experience of life, their wishes were frequently ignored.
- For older people, clinically and scientifically, things edged on, albeit slowly.

- Promises of new services for an undervalued sector of the community were particularly vulnerable to political and economic fluctuations.
- The POA leadership had to advocate persistently for older people to receive appropriate levels and ranges of care equitable with those provided for younger adults.
- Ongoing and ageist themes over the fifty years have included prioritising services for younger patients; the double whammy of stigma of mental illness plus old age; and policy decisions based on short-term economic calculations rather than likely health and well-being outcomes.

Notes

1. M. Roth, The natural history of mental disorders in old age. *Journal of Mental Science* (1955) 101: 281–301.

2. C. Hilton, The development of psychogeriatric services in England c.1940 to 1989. Unpublished PhD thesis, King's College London, 2014. https://kclpure.kcl.ac.uk/portal/files/39505448/2014_Hilton_Clair e_1050674_ethesis.pdf.

3. C. Hilton and D. Jolley, eds, Special issue: 21 years of Old Age Psychiatry, *Old Age Psychiatrist* (2011) 53, https://catalogues.rcpsych.ac.uk/FILES/Spring%202011,%20Number%2053.pdf.

4. P. Thane, *Old Age in English History: Past Experiences, Present Issues*. Oxford: Oxford University Press, 2000.

5. P. Townsend, *The Family Life of Old People*. Harmondsworth: Penguin Books, 1963; British Medical Association (BMA), *All Our Tomorrows: Growing Old in Britain*. London: BMA, 1986.

6. E.g. DHSS, Inequalities in Health: Report of a Research Working Group (Black Report) [1980]. In P. Townsend and N. Davidson, eds, *Inequalities in Health: The Black Report*, 31–213. Harmondsworth: Penguin Books, 1992; Organisation for Economic Co-operation and Development (OECD), Pensions at a glance, OECD.Stat, https://stats.oecd.org/index.aspx?queryid=69414.

7. P. Townsend, A national survey of old people in psychiatric and non psychiatric hospitals, residential homes, and nursing homes. In H. Freeman, ed., *Psychiatric Hospital Care: A Symposium*, 223–32. London: Baillière, Tindall and Cassell, 1965.

8. F. Post, *The Significance of Affective Symptoms in Old Age: A Follow Up Study of 100 Patients*. London: Oxford University Press, 1962.

9. F. Post, *The Clinical Psychiatry of Late Life*. London: Pergamon Press, 1965.

10. World Psychiatric Association, *Psychiatric Disorders in the Aged*. Manchester: Geigy, 1965.

11. B. Robb, *Sans Everything: A Case to Answer*. London: Nelson, 1967.

12. E. Murphy, A conversation with Tom Arie. *International Journal of Geriatric Psychiatry* (1996) 11: 671–9.

13. T. Arie, The first year of the Goodmayes psychiatric service for old people. *Lancet* (1970) 2: 1179–82.

14. T. Arie, Morale and the planning of psychogeriatric services. *British Medical Journal* (1971) 3: 166–70.

15. DHSS, *Services for Mental Illness Related to Old Age*. London: HMSO, 1972.

16. DHSS, *Psychiatric Hospitals and Units in England: In-Patient Statistics from the Mental Health Enquiry for the Year 1973*. London: HMSO, 1976.

17. T. Whitehead cited in Anon, Aged 'could be spared misery'. *The Guardian*, 7 October 1974: 6.

18. Anon, Guidelines for collaboration between geriatric physicians and psychiatrists in the care of the elderly. *Psychiatric Bulletin* (1979) 3: 168–9.

19. DHSS memo, K. Robinson to R. Jenkins, 28 November 1988 (MH 154/935, The National Archives, TNA).

20. DHSS, *Medical Manpower: The Next 20 Years*. London: HMSO, 1978.

21. M. Kemp, Accommodation for elderly patients with severe dementia. Typescript with GPOA minutes, 28 March 1974 (RCPsych Archives).

22. Worcester Development Project, meeting 12 July 1973 (MH 154/953, TNA).

23. DHSS, *A Happier Old Age: A Discussion Document on Elderly People in our Society*. London: HMSO, 1978.

24. DHSS, *Growing Older*. Cmnd 8173. London: HMSO, 1981.

25. J. Grad and P. Sainsbury, An evaluation of the effects of caring for the aged at home. In *WPA, Psychiatric Disorders in the Aged*, 225–36. Manchester: Geigy, 1965.

26. N. Mace and P. Rabins, *The 36-Hour Day: Caring at Home for Confused Elderly People*. London: Hodder & Stoughton and Age Concern, 1985.

27. DHSS, *Care in the Community: A Consultative Document on Moving Resources for Care in England*. London: DHSS, 1981.

28. DHSS, *Care in Action*. London: HMSO, 1981.

29. R. Griffiths, *National Health Service Management Inquiry Report*. London, HMSO, 1983.

30. Hospital Advisory Service (HAS), *The Rising Tide: Developing Services for Mental Illness in Old Age*. Surrey: HAS, 1982.

31. T. Van der Cammen, J. Simpson, R. Fraser, A. Preker and A. N. Exton-Smith, The memory clinic. *British Journal of Psychiatry* (1987) 150: 359–64.

32. Anon, How to rescue geriatrics. *Lancet* (1977) 1: 1091–5.

33. Medical Research Council, *The Health of the UK's Elderly People*. London: MRC, 1994.

34. C. Hilton, ed., *The Development of Old Age Psychiatry in Britain 1960–1989* (Guthrie Trust Witness Seminar 2008). Glasgow: University of Glasgow, 2009, www.gla.ac.uk/media/media_196526_en.pdf.

35. A. Bebbington and H. Charnley, Community care for the elderly: Rhetoric and reality. *British Journal of Social Work* (1990) 20: 409–32.

36. NHS Digital, *Health Survey for England – 2005: Health of Older People*, https://files.digital.nhs.uk/publicationimport/pub01xxx/pub01184/heal-surv-heal-old-peo-eng-2005-rep-v4.pdf.

37. Faculty of Old Age Psychiatry, *Who Cares Wins: Improving the Outcome for Older People Admitted to the General Hospital*. London: RCPsych, 2005.

38. Faculty of Old Age Psychiatry, *Raising the Standard: Specialist Services for Older People with Mental Illness*. London: RCPsych, 2006.

39. Department of Health, *Living Well with Dementia: A National Dementia Strategy*. 2009, www.dh.gov.uk/en/Publicationsandstatistics/Publications/PublicationsPolicyAndGuidance/DH_094058.

40. S. Benbow and P. Kingston, Developing the dementia workforce: Numerus turbatio – 'Total confusion'. *Dementia* (2010) 9: 307–10.

41. E. Murphy, A word from the House of Lords. In C. Hilton and D. Jolley, eds, Special issue: 21 years of Old Age Psychiatry. *Old Age Psychiatrist* (2011) 53: 47–8, https://catalogues.rcpsych.ac.uk/FILES/Spring%202011,%20Number%2053.pdf.

42. R. Jacoby, Of pioneers and progress, but prognosis guarded. In C. Hilton and D. Jolley, eds, Special issue: 21 years of Old Age Psychiatry. *Old Age Psychiatrist* (2011) 53: 32–3, https://catalogues.rcpsych.ac.uk/FILES/Spring%202011,%20Number%2053.pdf.

43. Faculty of Old Age Psychiatry, *Suffering in Silence: Age Inequality in Older People's Mental Health Care*. Report No. CR211. London: RCPsych, 2018.

44. NHS England, *Older People's Mental Health*, www.england.nhs.uk/mental-health/adults/older-people/#:~:text=Older%20people's%20mental%20health%20(OPMH,and%20liaison%20mental%20health%20care.

23 Changing Services I: Clinical Psychiatric Perspectives on Community and Primary Care Psychiatry and Mental Health Services

Trevor Turner

The transition from asylum life to the everyday world is a stage of peculiar difficulty with the recovered patient. The home and family life to which he returns may be unsuitable or unsympathetic; employment may be hard to obtain, and friends may be unable or unwilling to help.

Royal Commission of 1924–6[1]

Introduction

The social and organisational development of community psychiatry in the UK has been covered in other chapters in this book (see also Chapters 10, 30 and 31). The best overall description of the meaning of 'community psychiatry', however, was provided by Douglas Bennett and Hugh Freeman in their magisterial 1991 textbook in which they outlined its principles, its origins and its progress.[2] Key features of the latter were, of course, the 1959 Mental Health Act; the process of 'normalisation' in the asylums; the discovery of chlorpromazine and other effective psychotropic medications; and the social underpinnings of whatever was meant by the term 'community'. The rising critique from the anti-psychiatry movement, and the notion that psychiatric illnesses were understandable reactions to social stress (rather than formal illnesses that could be medicalised), became a dominant theme (see also Chapter 20). Yet different localities proceeded at a different pace in terms of developing actual community care resources, there being no formalised process. Stumbling out of the fog of change came the Community Mental Health Teams (CMHTs) and, more specifically, in 1991, the Care Programme Approach (CPA),[3] developed by the government's managerialist Department of Health. Likewise, evaluating the effectiveness of community care teams has been extremely difficult and often very localised. Numerous thoughtful papers on the process of community care have been published (e.g. 'Deinstitutionalisation: From hospital closure to service development' by Graham Thornicroft and Paul Bebbington)[4] and there have been endless policy papers published (e.g. *Better Services for the Mentally Ill* in 1975)[5] as well as the *National Service Framework for Adult Mental Health* (NSF) in 1999,[6] these rarely involving or consulting frontline practitioners (see also Chapter 12).

As a result, the term 'community care' has come to be mocked in, for example, TV comedies and public attitudes and has been associated with public homelessness (see Chapter

26) and inquiries into homicides (see Chapters 27, 28 and 29) as well as being considered as indicating the neglect of psychiatric services. In a 2001 paper, Julian Leff asked, 'Why is care in the community perceived as a failure?'[7] Having developed the model TAPS project for the closing down of Friern Barnet Hospital in North London,[8] he admitted that 'a comprehensive community psychiatric service, catering to all the needs of the catchment area population, exists nowhere in the British Isles and will never be achieved'. He noted at the time that few people were aware that 'of the 130 psychiatric hospitals functioning in England and Wales in 1975, only 14 remain open, with fewer than 200 patients in each'.

From the point of view of a practising consultant psychiatrist working in the system, this chapter will therefore be an impressionistic understanding of how community care has developed and not developed and the extent to which it can be seen as a success or failure. The former is reflected in patients' greater personal freedoms in choosing their daily lifestyles and the latter in the doubling of the prison population over the last forty years as well as the concomitant institution of numerous medium-secure forensic health units. This process has been labelled 'reinstitutionalisation'.[9] There has also been a rise in the use of the Mental Health Act and the pernicious development of 'risk assessment' as the driving factor in working with patients (see Chapter 27). This is despite the fact that there is no evidence that risk assessment protocols show any effectiveness in terms of predicting who will or will not go on to become a 'mentally disordered offender' (see also Chapter 29). One could even consider that the primary role of the asylums, to deal with the neglect and corruption of the private madhouses, has now been reversed, in that private provision for the seriously mentally ill has become dominant.

Moving into the Community

There is no clear definition of 'community psychiatry' apart from the belief that it is not hospital-based. The original term for it was 'extramural', and the initial programme involved the gradual sizing down of the asylums (often many thousand strong) into smaller units with the development of general hospital psychiatric units. Thus, in 1974, if you developed a serious mental illness in Hackney in East London you were put in an ambulance and taken to one of the larger Surrey hospitals/'bins' outside to the southwest of the capital or possibly to Friern Barnet in North London. By 1975, the link between Hackney and the large asylums had been broken, with the setting up of specific, local psychiatric wards in Hackney Hospital. This hospital was an old workhouse infirmary and looked as grim as anything could, but it was local.

A feature of this development was also the need to establish clear catchment area limitations for any psychiatric hospital unit, a local responsibility arrangement harking back to the old parish responsibilities of the nineteenth century. This was because the theorisation of community psychiatry seems to have forgotten that a key feature of psychiatric treatment, particularly in the inner city, was the use of the Mental Health Act for patients lacking insight into their condition and their needs – the application of the Act requiring the engagement of local social services. Thus, variably unwilling asylum physicians had to move into general hospitals (often to the dismay of fellow consultants) and try to look after CMHTs, which in themselves were undefined and variably developed. The practicalities of doing this were never carefully outlined and, although the asylum bed numbers declined gradually, the detention rates soared and the shortage of psychiatric beds (illustrated by often being 120 per cent occupied!) became a dominant concern, particularly from the 1980s onwards.

In Manchester, for example, in the late 1990s, it was reported that there were more than twenty patients detained under the Mental Health Act but awaiting admission.[10] NHS resources often could not fund proper bed availability, this depending on the extent to which psychiatric professionals (especially consultants) were able to bully managers into making appropriate provision; and although CMHTs were primarily focused on looking after those with psychotic conditions ('the new long-stay'), there grew a rising demand for the treatment of common mental health problems, which some dismissed as the concerns of 'the worried well'. These patients were asking for help with depression and anxiety in the context of heavily advertised new antidepressant medications such as Prozac and the better recognition of the meaning of depression.

In essence, therefore, the process to deinstitutionalise and move towards community care was stumbled upon by accident, rather like the British Empire. A number of charismatic psychiatrists had led the way, for example Maxwell Jones at Belmont (his book *Social Psychiatry* was published in 1952; see also Chapter 20).[11] Yet the practical problems of setting up a CMHT depended substantially on the goodwill between NHS and local social services. Trying to get community psychiatric nurses (CPNs), consultant psychiatrists, psychologists, occupational therapists, social workers, senior and junior, and the 'lowly' support workers to live and work together required immense time and effort and there were often fractures in the teams, who differed in terms of background culture, training and pay grades. Latterly, the primacy of primary care in terms of funding local resources has generated a particular demand from GPs to have CPNs and psychologists working for their primary care resource, thus further depriving specialist mental health services of staff who might otherwise have been available.

Another key feature of community care has been the regularity of shocking newspaper exposés – for example, the 1980s articles by Marjorie Wallace in *The Times* and the relentless publication of homicide inquiries (e.g. the report on Christopher Clunis produced by Ritchie in 1987).[12] In this regard, whenever a lurid headline or TV news report announced yet another murder by a psychotic patient in the community, every thinking psychiatrist's first reaction was to find out where the event had taken place (hoping it wasn't in their catchment area). Fear of being called to appear before an Untoward Incident Inquiry, therefore, became part and parcel of being a consultant psychiatrist, certainly in the inner city, and the ultimate insult was when the process of inquiries was in itself privatised.

Homicide Inquiries

Homicide inquiries became the hallmark of psychiatric care in the 1980s and 1990s, gradually fading out only as pressure on the newspapers not to publish them too often started to work. This was achieved in terms of anti-stigma campaigns. The most offensive of these inquiries was the Luke Warm Luke case,[13] running to some £75,000 in costs (thanks to the chair, Baroness Scotland) and several volumes of standardised prose, largely rewriting the CPA and adding nothing new to our understanding of the management of serious mental illness. The incident was due to the girlfriend of a psychotic patient refusing CMHT advice that she not visit him at home and her ending up murdered by the patient. As noted, however, the most influential report was the inquiry into the care of Christopher Clunis,[14] which outlined all the problems of providing care in the community in a fractured framework of varying local mental health provision (see also Chapters 28 and 30).

Christopher Clunis was first detained in hospital in Jamaica (see Tables 23.1 and 23.2) and diagnosed with paranoid schizophrenia. Subsequently, however, he was detained in a number of different hospitals, mainly in London, with diagnoses changing constantly. Like many

Table 23.1 The Clunis inquiry: diagnoses, 1986–92

1986	paranoid schizophrenia
29.6.87	schizophrenia with negative symptoms
2.7.87	schizophrenia or drug-induced psychosis
24.7.87	depression
1.1.88	drug-induced psychosis, or manipulation for a bed
29.3.88	psychotic or schizoaffective illness
3.5.88	schizophrenia, drug-induced psychosis or organic illness
7.6.89	paranoid schizophrenia
23.7.91	schizophrenia
5.5.92	paranoid psychosis
14.8.92	paranoid schizophrenia
26.8.92	(diabetes)
10.9.92	normal mental state, abnormal personality

Table 23.2 The Clunis inquiry: lengths of stays, 1986–92

1986	Bellevue Hospital, Jamaica	Not known
1987	Chase Farm Hospital	25 days, 4 days
1988	Chase Farm Hospital	3 days, 4 days
	King's College Hospital	7 days
	Dulwich North Hospital	9 days
	Brixton prison	21 days
	Dulwich North Hospital	169 days
1989	St Charles Hospital	110 days
1991	St Thomas's Hospital	21 days
1992	Belmarsh Prison	24 days
	Kneesworth House Hospital	80 days
	Guy's hospital	34 days

difficult patients, he ended up with being 'diagnosed' as having a 'personality disorder'. Records showed his constantly assaultive behaviours were noted but tended to improve with appropriate medication. Like many insightless patients with paranoid schizophrenia, however, he would not continue medication on discharge from hospital, and one night in North Finsbury station (in North London) he stabbed Jonathan Zito in the eye, killing him. This assault very much reflected Clunis's own psychotic experience of feeling that people were somehow interfering with him by looking at him, and he had assaulted a number of other people in the eyes beforehand.

The Clunis case can be seen as a template for the problems in community care. None of the members of the teams standing in the rain outside his front door trying to assess him in North London on more than one occasion had ever seen him before, thus he was able to walk out of the house without being recognised. The disjunctions of care between South and North London were noted, as was the tendency of mental health staff to downplay assaultive behaviours and their significance. The subsequent criticisms directed at the team ultimately landed with assessing him were unfair (they had minimal information and none of them had ever assessed him before), but the outline of the problems of community care was well adjudged. An important corollary was the development of a voluntary organisation called the Zito Trust (led by Jayne Zito, wife of the murdered man) which developed a full review of homicide inquiries, some 120 reports having been published by 2002, summarising and outlining them to a helpful degree.[15] Like many other such voluntary organisations, for example Marjorie Wallace's development of SANE, the general view of the concerned public was that asylums should not have been closed so quickly and that there should be more hospital beds. As noted, bed shortages have been, perversely, the dominant theme in the community care debate.

The impact of homicide inquiries on the morale of CMHTs was substantial. Staff felt stigmatised by their work and reports regularly considered failures in communication and the inappropriate use of CPA documentation as problematic. The use of complex forms to be filled in at every assessment became a negative, however, with some CPA documents taking up nine to ten pages and requiring regular reiteration when each clinical review was carried out. This was despite there being no evidence at all that filling in such a form correctly predicted the outcome for individual patients. Homicide inquiries were infused with the problems of hindsight and the counterfactual thinking generated thereby.

Along with the development of CPA and risk assessment, there was an attempt by the government in 1999 (Patients in the Community Act)[16] to introduce supervision registers. These required doctors to fill in a form to determine the risk of every patient in their care, a bit like filling in the 'proscription' levels as noted in ancient Rome or being asked to identify potential Jews in your locality in Germany in the 1930s. Such central government impositions on practice were driven by a managerialism that has become intrinsic to NHS organisations, with little input from frontline clinicians, whether nurses, doctors, psychologists or social workers. The notion of community care as 'outdoor relief' or the transferring of care away to untrained staff on part-time contracts became increasingly part of our understanding of 'care in the community', CMHTs generally having to work out their own ways of managing patients. Heroically, supervision registers were mainly ignored.

Later Developments

In 1999, the Blair Labour government introduced the National Service Framework (NSF),[17] this demanding that Trusts set up specific teams for the assessment of crisis intervention (for acute and severe mental health problems), early intervention (for patients with first-episode psychosis) and assertive outreach (for those patients whose mental ill health was thought to cause serious concern but who were not engaging with mental health services follow-up). From the organisational point of view, the need to develop a series of teams that could be specific and could not be diluted by other NHS demands (as many mental health initiatives have been) enabled the NSF and funding for it to be forced through the NHS system (see also Chapters 10 and 11). This was a clever piece of government initiative but it imposed significant limitations in terms of how mental health teams operated. In particular, the dividing up of the CMHTs into these sub-teams generated arguments as to who looked after whom and created unrealistic expectations in those given, for example, early intervention services. After being moved on from their early intervention service (with its high inputs and regular support), they were in fact referred on to the badly resourced CMHTs.

While the government's introduction of these specialist teams was welcomed in terms of funding and resources, the role of the standard CMHT remained deracinated and uncertain. Furthermore, the crisis intervention teams took on the burden not only of seeing people in crisis (however defined) but also of being the 'gatekeepers' to admission to hospital. This led to arguments with consultant psychiatrists, who had known patients for many years, who were advised they had to resort to a nurse and social worker (relatively untrained compared to them) in a crisis care team to allow admission. The earlier difficulties of putting together multidisciplinary CMHTs were recreated and psychiatrists were deskilled, as their clinical activities became limited to certain interventions such as crisis management or early intervention. The ability to look after a patient right across their lifestyle and their lifetime, whether as an inpatient or outpatient, reviewed in the community, became limited. This fragmentation of services went against the standard findings of all homicide inquiry reports, namely that there should be connected services right across the spectrum.

Debates about the value of specialist teams went on in community care forums, with considerable division as to whether they were effective or not. A number of psychiatrists enjoyed the limitations of, for example, just doing assertive outreach, despite losing their skills in terms of managing patients with depression, anxiety and other non-schizophrenic disorders. Many assertive outreach teams became essentially rehabilitation teams, and a number have been gradually phased out in this context.

Overall, therefore, while the NSF engendered increased funding for psychiatry, the break-up of CMHTs generated limitations in the kind of work that could be provided. For example, new trainees found themselves either just in a crisis team or in an assertive outreach team or in an early intervention team and not seeing the overall picture in terms of management of patients with a range of conditions, in the community and in hospital wards. Thus, they missed out on being part of what has been called the 'general psychiatry' attitude. This imposition of excessive specialisation has been amplified by the hiving off of forensic psychiatric care into locked units (indoor psychiatry) and the push for many practitioners now to just conduct 'primary care psychiatry'.

Primary Care Psychiatry

Regarding primary care psychiatry, this again has developed in a patchwork way, depending on the willingness of GPs to have psychiatrists in their surgeries. As a keen young psychiatrist in the 1980s, my offer to see patients at GP surgeries was met with varying degrees of perplexity and receptivity. A number of thoughtful practices were very welcoming but other smaller practices found it difficult to accept having another doctor sitting in their offices (and often there was no room to do so). While GPs have been known to be at the front line of psychiatric services for many years,[18] their main engagement has been with patients with non-psychotic conditions and meeting the requirements of advice as to therapy as well as the best antidepressants and anxiolytics to prescribe. There could also have been a fruitful exchange of information between GPs and psychiatrists, in terms of the complex social and physical conditions that patients present with and the appropriate use of medications or other treatments. However, it is not untypical to review a patient's GP notes (a rich source of information) and find that they have been prescribed three or four different antidepressant selective serotonin reuptake inhibitors (SSRIs) over the years, with limited benefit and with no review of the patient's compliance or underlying mental state. Many patients asked about old prescriptions will often say they did not take the pills for very long, if at all.

Fortunately, the improvements generated by the IAPT (Improving Access to Psychological Therapies) programme have helped very much with the provision of cognitive behavioural therapy (CBT) for common mental conditions (see also Chapters 10 and 33). Resources, however, have varied from area to area. This has been one of the genuine positives of community care. The fact that many GPs, having undergone a psychiatric attachment in their rotation, are now trained in identifying and managing mental health problems has also enhanced the ability to develop appropriate psychiatric services in conjunction with GPs. This is in contrast with the failure of the Royal College of Physicians and the Royal College of Surgeons to embrace psychiatric education as any part of their training programmes.

Conclusion

The development of community care in the UK has been haphazard, deriving from theory rather than practical consideration. The human resource problems of putting together CMHTs in different areas have been little understood by central government, and the development of such teams has largely been based on the goodwill of local professionals to ensure communication and provide office space and support. The regular negative views of community psychiatry in the public perception have further limited the development of services. The impositions of paperwork and additional documentation based on risk management have led to many CMHT members spending half their day at their desks doing paperwork. This over-engagement in paperwork is well known throughout the NHS, and one only has to review a typical patient's GP notes to realise that most of what is written there is reduplicated and not clinically necessary. For example, blood test findings are mentioned under various different categories. The notion that 'every form filled out means a kindness foregone' can be seen as a key difficulty of community-based care.

As ever, psychiatry has been substantially undermined by the persistence of stigma (see also Chapter 27) and the intrusions of a powerful, socially generated belief that mental distress can be distinguished from mental illness. The battle to get mental illness back on the agenda has been prolonged, but a number of Trusts continue to downplay the need for a formal diagnosis and it is now possible to have an assessment for your mental health needs carried out by an individual who has no training as a psychiatrist but who may well be called a 'high intensity practitioner'. While the diminution of the consultant psychiatrist's role from their predominance in the old asylums has its benefits, in terms of introducing other expertise into the management of those with mental health problems, the need for expertise in psychiatric diagnosis, the management of psychopharmacology and leadership of a team with many diverse backgrounds is central to what a psychiatrist has to do whether in hospital or in the community care sphere.

The rise of risk management has been a dreadful negative, in terms of looking at the role of a consultant psychiatrist and in terms of the importance of carrying out an appropriate mental state assessment and diagnostic review. The prevalence of criminalised drug usage (e.g. cannabis and cocaine in particular) has further complicated matters. Given the vulnerability of mentally ill patients using drugs to improve their mood or lower their anxiety, this drugs 'prohibition' policy has major negative effects in terms of criminalising the mentally ill (see also Chapters 28 and 29). The extension of low-secure and medium-secure mental health units (often privatised) reflects the reinstitutionalisation of mental health care generated by a risk avoidance strategy and a more punitive attitude towards those with mental illness. The extraordinary rise in the number of prisoners in the UK (as noted in the Introduction to this chapter) is a key reflection of Penfold's theory that there is an inverse relationship between prison and asylum care.[19] Visiting HMP Pentonville in the late 1990s, I was advised by one of the senior prison officers that 'this is the largest medium secure unit in the country'. This imprisonment of the mentally ill is against the background that the number of homicides committed by mentally disordered offenders has not increased since the 1950s,[20] by contrast to the numbers of homicides committed by 'normal' citizens, which has increased markedly.

Key Summary Points

* The process of de-asylumisation into a community care–based mental health system has been a messy business, a social crusade rather than a clinically thought-out process.
* Concomitants like modern psychopharmacology and the effects of the Royal College of Psychiatrists' anti-stigma campaigns have helped but care has varied substantially in quality across the country.
* Community care has relied on the qualities of individual psychiatrists and CMHT members, as well as local GP and/or social services support, and generally has not been helped by the numerous government White Papers.
* The reversion to medium-secure mental health units and reinstitutionalisation has been a core feature, publicly unrecognised.
* Mental health services have coped to varying degrees despite their core asylum resource being stolen from them, and the key need now is for the elimination of the primacy of risk assessment and the maintenance of the generality of general adult psychiatry.

Notes

1.   The Royal Commission of 1924–1926 (the Macmillan Commission) quoted in K. Jones, *Asylums and After: A Revised History of the Mental Health Services from the Early 18th Century to the 1990s*. London: Athlone Press, 1993, p. 133.

2.   D. H. Bennett and H. L. Freeman, eds, *Community Psychiatry: The Principles*. London: Churchill Livingstone, 1991.

3.   Department of Health Circular, HC(90)23/LASSL(90)11, London, 1990.

4. G. Thornicroft and P. Bebbington, Deinstitutionalisation: From hospital closure to service development. *British Journal of Psychiatry* (1989) 155: 739–53.

5. Department of Health and Social Security (DHSS), *Better Services for the Mentally Ill*, Cmnd 6233. London: HMSO 1975.

6. Department of Health, *National Service Framework, Mental Health*, London: HMSO 1999.

7. J. Leff, Why is care in the community perceived as a failure? *British Journal of Psychiatry* (2001) 179: 381–3.

8. Team for the Assessment of Psychiatric Services (TAPS), *Preliminary Report on Baseline Data from Friern and Claybury Hospitals*. North East Thames Regional Health Authority, 1988.

9. S. Priebe, A. Badesconyi, A. Fioritti et al., Reinstitutionalisation in mental health care: Comparison of data on service provision from six European countries. *British Medical Journal* (2005) 330: 123–6.

10. Personal communication.

11. M. Jones, *Social Psychiatry: A Study of Therapeutic Communities*. London: Tavistock Publications, 1952.

12. M. Wallace, A caring community? The plight of Britain's mentally ill. *Sunday Times Magazine*, 3 May 1986: 25–38; J. Ritchie, D. Dick and R. Lingham, *The Report of the Inquiry into the Care and Treatment of Christopher Clunis*. London: HMSO 1994.

13. P. J. Scotland, H. Kelly and M. Devaux, *The Report of the Luke Warm Luke Mental Health Inquiry*. Lambeth, Southwark and Lewisham Health Authority, 1998.

14. Ritchie, Dick and Lingham, *The Report of the Inquiry into the Care and Treatment of Christopher Clunis*.

15. D. Sheppard, *Learning the Lessons: Mental Health Inquiry Reports Published in England and Wales between 1969 and 1996 and Their Recommendations for Improving Practice*. ZitoTrust: 1996.

16. Mental Health (Patients in the Community) Act 1995.

17. Department of Health, *National Service Framework, Mental Health*.

18. M. Shepherd and D. L. Davies, *Studies in Psychiatry*. London: Oxford University Press, 1968.

19. L. S. Penrose, Mental disorder and crime: Outline of a comparative study of European statistics. *British Journal of Medical Psychology* (1939) 18: 1–15.

20. P. Taylor and J. Gunn, Homicide by people with mental illness: Myth and reality. *British Journal of Psychiatry* (1999) 174: 9–14.

Changing Services II: From Colony to Community – People with Developmental Intellectual Disability

Peter Carpenter

Introduction

The fifty years since 1960 cover one of the major periods of change in services for people with intellectual disability as the service model based on colonies, with isolation and 'protection', was dismantled and a new model of care in the community enforced. This required a massive change in public attitudes, policy, funding, professional roles and training and in medical and social infrastructure. These various facets have not operated in synchrony, so it has been a prolonged journey through some turbulent waters which has not yet reached the tranquil lake. This chapter briefly discusses some of these issues but concentrates on the policies of England and Wales. The terminology has changed over time from mental deficiency to mental handicap, learning difficulties, learning disabilities and the current intellectual disabilities or disorders of intellectual development. The terminology at the time discussed is used in this chapter, even though the terms used then are seen today as objectionable. The reason for using the terms used at the time is that they referred to varying concepts and subgroups.

Where Did We Start From?

From 1913 to 1959, the model of care was dominated by the 1913 Mental Deficiency Act, derived from the 1908 Royal Commission on the Care and Control of the Feeble Minded.[1] It concentrated on the need to identify 'mentally defective' persons who were not adequately supervised in the community and maintain them in 'colonies' operated by local authorities. The purposes of the colonies were later stated in their nurses' manual to be:

1. A training school for mentally defective children or adults for whom suitable training outside is not available.
2. A shelter for those who are homeless, neglected or otherwise in need of a home and protection.
3. A hospital for those who are of low grade or physically helpless or epileptic and who require nursing care which cannot be provided in their own homes.
4. A place of control for those who are mischievous, destructive or harmful or who are a danger to themselves or to others if left in the community.[2]

With the formation of the NHS, the colonies were removed from the local authorities and transferred to the NHS in 1948 as hospitals. This immediately reinforced the assumption that 'mental deficiency' was a mental health condition and not a social concept. In addition, having the entire health budget for the country in one pot made governments reluctant to face the increasing cost of need while also facilitating the diversion of longer-term care monies to bail out the more prominent and bankrupt acute hospitals.

The 1957 Royal Commission on Mental Health Law recommended community care and a change in the law. The resulting 1959 Mental Health Act changed the legal concept of social defectiveness contained in 'mental defective' to that of 'mental subnormality', excluding many who were previously included. It also changed the assumption of compulsory admission to that of voluntary admission. The change of law changed the clinical concept. At the start of the 1960s, many of the more able patients became voluntary patients who immediately left hospital and lost contact with their services as they created their own lives in the community.

In 1960, most people with 'mental subnormality' lived in the community but almost all state-provided care for them came via special schools or 'subnormality' long-stay hospitals. These 'hospitals' commonly held 200–400 residents each, but there were 5 reaching more than 2,000. In these, men, women and children were still segregated as in the old Victorian workhouses. Most wards housed 50–60 patients with 2 staff to care for them. Staff would be sacked for mistreatment but keeping order relied on institutional intimidation. Everything had to happen in groups – patients queued for baths or shaving (razor blades changed only after a set number of people had been shaved); there was no personal clothing; and work was mundane. Abuse was widespread. Families were not allowed to visit the wards but were assured their loved ones were well cared for.

1960–1980: The Need to Act and First Steps

By 1960, the pressure to change was international and reforms started that still dominate the system. John F. Kennedy's family experiences enabled key legislation in the United States such as the 1963 Maternal and Child Health and Mental Retardation Planning Amendments.

The principles of 'normalisation' were being developed in Scandinavia with Bengt Nirje of the Swedish Association for Retarded Children at the forefront. In 1971, the United Nations' Declaration on the Rights of Mentally Retarded Persons stated such people should have the same rights as others *as far as feasibly possible*, should have economic security and should live in the community with their families.

In the UK, the 1960s saw campaigns for better services for people in the community taking hold. Local authorities started to create large institutional day centres (often called training centres) as well as respite hostels. Activities were structured like a continuation of school, but many centres emulated the new industrial therapy ideas of mental health with the more able attendees spending much of their week on simple assembly lines. The hospitals had lost a lot of the people who operated their farms, cleaned their wards and cared for the less able but were refilled from the long waiting lists of families desperate for care. The inpatient population became more demanding at a time when there were still usually only two staff per sixty residents. They were also universally overcrowded, often holding 20 per cent more patients than designed for. Scandals started to proliferate.

On 20 August 1967, the *News of the World* published allegations of abuse at Ely Hospital in Wales. Farleigh Hospital near Bristol was visited by the police in December 1968. Each triggered a formal inquiry that fed the newspapers sensational news of abuse. These scandals continued through the 1970s with inquiries at Coldharbour by Sherbourne in 1973; South Ockenden in Essex in 1974; Brockhall in Lancashire in 1975; St Ebba's in Epson in 1976; Mary Dendy in Lancashire in 1977; and the Normansfield in 1978. In addition, the media published various investigations inspired by the scandals. On 29 May 1972, the prime-time television programme *24 Hours* showed a devastating 20-minute programme on the state of Stoke Park Hospital, showing staff struggling against all odds. The senior staff described parts of the hospital as a slum, comments that echoed around the country. The message was clear and reinforced over ten years: relatives were no longer to trust the old institutions or the reassurances that their loved ones were well cared for. Things had to change.

In England, four new policies emerged:

- The Local Authority Social Services Act of 1970 brought together many of the social care services under the responsibility of local authorities to enable more coordinated care.
- The Education Act of 1971, which in accordance with the UN declaration explicitly included all children as the responsibility of the local authorities' education boards and no longer excluded 'subnormal' children who were in hospital training centres.
- The 1974 reorganisation of the NHS into district health authorities ended the local management separation of the mental handicap hospitals from the acute general hospitals. Local budgets were dominated by the needs of the acute hospitals, but this enabled closer co-ordination with general hospitals and with the coterminous local authorities.
- These structural changes underpinned implementation of the 1971 White Paper *Better Services for the Mentally Handicapped* which set out the new direction for all services. It included the principles of non-segregation, access to 'stimulation, social training and education and purposeful occupation' and wanted residences to be as homely as possible.

The White Paper recommended a large increase in the residential care provided in the community and training centres, alongside halving the hospital beds. It promulgated new 24-bed hospitals scattered around the community with new local authority homes of a similar size. No new hospital should exceed 100 beds and no old large site should be added to (except with temporary buildings to relieve current overcrowding).

At the time, this was a radical plan to move to a lifestyle closer to the ideology of normalisation, but it was still based on using rather large low-staffed units only half the size of the usual long-stay hospital villas. In addition, the White Paper looked only at 'mental handicap' services and did not consider whether the generic services were able to provide a non-discriminatory service.

In 1975, the government created the National Development Team for the Mentally Handicapped to advise their social service planners. Several pamphlets were published, including one describing the creation of Community Mental Handicap Teams and several local services were visited when requested to advise on local service developments. It was recognised that any move from long-stay hospital to local authority residential care would involve the development of care expertise in local authority settings. There were attempts to move nursing staff, along with the smaller health service hostels/hospitals, to local author-ities, but this was resisted by the unions, despite the 1979 Jay Report declaring an end to mental handicap nursing.[3]

The changes of the 1970s reflect the impact of scandals in hospital care which produced pressure for local authorities to develop services in the community and to close hospital wards or at least improve them with temporary buildings. However, they occurred in a decade of financial crisis, so resources were limited. Despite this, by 1980 new financial structures for community care were developing alongside day services and some Community Mental Handicap Teams (using hospital staff). In addition, there were some hospital improvements and some reductions in hospital numbers, particularly removing children from long-stay hospitals.

1980–2000: In Search of a New Model As the Old Hospitals Close

In 1980, the Department of Health and Social Security (DHSS) published a review of progress since the 1971 White Paper.[4] It concluded that it had overestimated the need for hospital places and estimated that 3 out of 1,000 of the general population needed special mental handicap services. It noted the problems of finance and the need to explore alternative models of transitioning. The next decade saw investment for new academic departments researching models of care. As a result, the policymakers had more evidence about specific models attracting public campaigns.

The pressure from campaigning groups trying to shape policy increased. The Campaign for the Mental Handicapped (CMH) had responded to the 1971 White Paper by publishing *Even Better Services for the Mentally Handicapped*. In 1981, it published *The Principle of Normalisation: A Foundation for Effective Services* by John O'Brien and Alan Tyne. O'Brien published his five principles in 1991 and they dominated service design in Britain for the next decade, being cited in almost all local policy and planning documents. The King's Fund also published a series of influential booklets and project papers, including *An Ordinary Life* in 1980 and *People First* in 1984. In 1984, the self- advocacy group People First was founded as the voice of people with 'learning difficulties' – and it was increasingly referred to by government when developing policy. Their campaign, summed up in the 1990s by *Nothing About Us Without Us*, became accepted by most policy organisations. In response to their campaign, the government abandoned the term mental handicap for the new term *learning disability* (LD). The general message from these campaigns was clear: the old colony 'mental defectives' were now *people with learning disabilities* (PWLDs) who were to be treated as equal members of the community and therefore would want to live in ordinary houses and integrated within the community, with useful employment. However, there were alternative voices: The National Society for Mentally Handicapped People in Residential Care (Rescare) was established in 1984 as the national voice of many League of Friends for the old hospitals. They expressed fears about their loved ones moving into the harsh community and advocated turning the hospital sites into residential campuses.

Alongside this, there was a new Education Act of 1981, inspired by the 1978 Warnock Report, with needs assessment to secure the resources to enable a child with learning difficulties to be educated in mainstream schools with additional support or in special schools. This was an advance in integration, which was set back later when school attainment tests reduced the popularity of low-performing pupils. Higher education colleges were also financially encouraged to admit students with severe learning difficulties, though cuts in the next millennium reduced this incentive as well.

The 1980s saw the active planning for closure of most of the large old long-stay hospitals. After ten years of planning, the first large hospital to close was Darenth Park in 1988.[5] Financial pressures and bureaucratic problems delayed other closures or forced some closures to include decanting patients to more local hospitals or large homes.[6] Nevertheless, by 2000 most of the large hospitals had closed or were near to closure.

In the 1980s, central government awarded a standard sum to people moving into community care homes to fund their care and community services. This was independent of need and encouraged many new small care settings, owned by ex-hospital staff, to take the more able out of hospitals. The escalating costs of the funding system changed with the 1990 NHS and Community Care Act, making it the responsibility of local authorities to assess the care and support needs of people and to fund according to need after means testing. The Act also brought in the purchaser/provider split (see also Chapter 10), ending the provision of care by local authorities and enabling a plethora of care providers to develop.

In 1992, the media reported one of the first major care scandals in a community care home. It was revealed that residents of the Long Care group in Buckinghamshire had been systematically physically, emotionally and sexually abused by some staff.[7] The main outcome was to remove inspection from local authorities to a new national social care inspectorate – which, after many reorganisations, has become part of the current Care Quality Commission.

2000–2010: Gaining Rights and Tackling Mainstream Services

In this decade, the persistent attitudes of the public and mainstream services came under the spotlight and the rights of PWLDs were consolidated. The White Paper *Valuing People* was published in 2001 (Scotland had published *The Same As You* a year earlier). Both emphasised the need for equality and inclusion in the mainstream community, including in all health services, education, work and accommodation. Person-centred care planning was mandated and advocacy promulgated. *Valuing People* highlighted the fact that most health care for PWLDs had always come from mainstream health services. Now GPs were financially encouraged to identify their patients with LD and to carry out annual health checks. Liaison LD nurses were recommended to facilitate access of PWLDs to mainstream health services. In 2004, the *Green Light Toolkit* encouraged mainstream mental health services to audit how they served PWLDs, as many had continued to see this as the only responsibility of specialist services.

In 2006–7, Mencap publicised how LD patients were neglected by mainstream services and criticised staff attitudes there. The publication of *Their Death by Indifference* forced the government to commission a systematic review of deaths of PWLDs, which confirmed the high rate of potentially avoidable premature deaths. There was also a growth in the number of care scandals in the community. Several NHS Trusts had seconded their staff to community homes rather than transferring their employment and now a series of reports showed the dangers of this producing poor surveillance and allowing institutional abuse.[8]

The 2000s witnessed the growth of supported living as the model for meeting the residential needs of PWLDs. In some cases, this meant care homes legally changed into being blocks of rented bedsits. People with high support needs were often placed in individual placements with dedicated 24-hour staffing. The pressure on local authority budgets escalated dramatically. Day care also followed the trend for more individual services with day care centres being replaced by individually supported activities, though financial constraints often limited the hours and range of activities provided.

There were other legal changes. The Mental Capacity Act of 2005 (changed from the Mental Incapacity Act after pressure from People First) set out a clear legal basis for deciding care when a person does not have the capacity to decide. The Convention on the Rights of Persons with Disabilities was adopted by the United Nations in 2006 and came into force in 2008. This promulgated the rights of PWLDs to equality of opportunities in education, employment and family life. Its oversight committee advocated supported decision-making rather than substituted decision-making as occurs in the UK. The end of the decade saw the Autism Act 2009 – the only specific disability Act in England. The Equalities Act 2010 highlighted the need to make reasonable adjustments to enable equality of opportunity.

By the end of 2010, all the old long-stay hospital beds had closed, though some of the old sites had forensic beds or new 'assessment and treatment' units. There was a rapid increase in private hospital beds concentrated on a few sites for those PWLDs with mental health and/or behavioural problems and challenging needs. As an example, in the Bristol area the 3,400 hospital beds of 1960 had reduced to 12 NHS beds and 24 private hospital beds. In 2011, those private beds in Winterbourne View were closed following widely publicised reports of abuse. This triggered the national Transforming Care project to close most of the remaining private and NHS specialist beds for PWLDs. By 2015, there were no specialist hospital beds in the Bristol area.

Staff Changes with Community Care

The roles of staff working with people with 'mental deficiency' were defined by the operational needs of the colonies. With their closure, professionals working there were forced to redefine their role to work in the community. This was most marked for psychiatry and nursing.

Psychiatry

The colonies were supervised by the same national board that supervised the psychiatric asylums. This board required a psychiatrist to be in charge of a colony/hospital as in psychiatric asylums. However, the colonies dealt with training and supervision and did not deal with comorbid psychiatric disorders. If you needed psychiatric treatment, you went to the asylum.

When the new Royal College of Psychiatrists was created in the 1970s it considered abandoning 'mental handicap' as a psychiatric specialty, as the hospitals were closing. It was decided to transform the specialism into the mental health aspects of 'mental handicap'. Publications on the special features of mental illness in 'mental handicap' started to appear during the 1970s,[9] and over the following years the psychiatry of mental handicap became a flourishing specialty within psychiatry, with its own training schemes, and a subspecialty within child psychiatry was created during the new millennium.[10] However, the specialty has remained defined by its treatment of people with intellectual disability rather than its more general skills in neurodevelopmental psychiatry.

Nursing

Mental deficiency nursing first became a specialty in 1919 when the Medico-Psychological Association (MPA) developed a training course and qualification. A nursing manual was published in 1931,[11] known as the Green Book to distinguish from the Red Book of psychiatric nurses. The book was mainly concerned with causes of mental deficiency, basic concepts of training inpatients and ward management. Mental illnesses such as depression and dementia were not mentioned in the book and epilepsy took up less than a page.

Nurses were seen as ward managers and carers.[12] The consequence was the 1979 Jay Report into the future of mental handicap nursing, which recommended the specialism change with community care to one based on a certificate in social services. As the hospitals closed, this change seemed inevitable as care homes did not advertise for registered nurses and few could maintain their nursing registration when working in care homes.

However, the Community Mental Handicap Teams still needed nurses, albeit ones who were more versatile. The early teams comprised only a nurse, a social worker and a part-time psychiatrist. Other clinicians and professionals were added later as patients moved into the community. In addition, nurses with expertise in mental illness and learning disabilities were required for the new specialist mental health services and liaison services for physical medicine.

As a result, the profession was transformed. The training courses changed and many existing nurses underwent further training in mental health, epilepsy, dementia care or behaviour modification. Like psychiatry, the nursing specialism changed to be closer to that of other nurses, with additional expertise defined by the health needs of the population they treated.

Care in the Community

The fifty years covered in this chapter saw the development of a wide range of community services and supports by different organisations. Local authorities now assess and fund care needs and provide safeguarding services rather than direct care. However, few PWLDs are in employment, despite this having been a target for fifty years.

As the LD hospitals closed, the skills of generic health services provided in the community became an issue. GPs are now expected to be able to assess PWLDs. Salaried dentists have increased in number to cater for PWLDs as they present special issues and take longer to treat. Some general hospitals now have liaison nurses to support staff working with PWLDs requiring assessment and treatment.

The early Community Mental Handicap Teams have tended to divide into two: one service providing support to GPs and the work of social workers, usually based within community primary care services; and the other dealing with 'challenging behaviour' and/or mental health aspects of care, often based within mainstream mental health services.

Conclusion

Just as the name of their condition kept changing (we now have *disorders of intellectual development* in the eleventh edition of the *International Classification of Diseases*, or ICD-11), services for PWLDs were also radically transformed between 1960 and 2010. The service started as one based on the eugenic model of confining and training nuisance 'mental defectives' in institutions built large to reduce costs with little provision for those who lived in the community. Over fifty years, the model became one of total inclusion as equals in the community with equal opportunities in employment, accommodation and family life. Policymakers had to negotiate a massive change of policy, service provision and associated funding mechanisms to do this. The frequent scandals of care probably helped provide impetus and funding.

During this time, there was a massive development in ideological models, including self-advocacy and safeguarding, as well as research into the causes of LD and how to empower PWLDs. Now the issue is how people experience the dream in reality. The law requires equality of treatment and lack of discrimination, but it is not clear if this will eliminate negative attitudes held by others.

For the author, there have been cycles of care: I was first the psychiatrist for a 200-bed hospital but with no empty beds and with little support for community emergencies. Eventually, I had a large supportive community team and an admission unit. Then, the community team came under four different employers who relocated their staff and the inpatient service closed. Continuity of care was lost and admissions could be 100 miles away. Now PWLDs have individualised direct support but the services around them are more fragmented, as is the case for anyone living in the community.

Key Summary Points

• In 1960, services were based on 'hospitals' which had been mental deficiency 'colonies'.
• The 1970s saw the start of the recognition of a right to live in the community as equals.
• It took thirty years to close the old hospitals and develop an entirely community-based service. This needed changes to policy, funding agencies and the benefits system.
• This also involved changing the skills of previous staff and changing skills and attitudes in mainstream services.
• We now have a rights-based system, which is more fragmented and more challenging for PWLDs to negotiate.

Notes

1.   *Report of the Royal Commission on the Care and Control of the Feeble Minded*, 8 vols, Cd. 4215–4202. London: HMSO, 1908.

2.   *Manual for Mental Deficiency Nurses*. London: Bailliere, Tindall and Cox, 1931, p. 2.

3.   Jay Committee, *Report of the Committee of Enquiry into Mental Handicap Nursing and Care*, Cm. 7468. London: HMSO, 1979.

4.   Department of Health, *Mental Handicap: Progress, Problems and Priorities*. London: Department of Health, 1980.

5.   L. Wing, *Hospital Closure and the Resettlement of Residents: The Case of Darenth Park Mental Handicap Hospital*. Avebury, 1989.

6.   For a description of the local closure process, see N. Bouras, *Reflections on the Challenges of Psychiatry in UK and Beyond*. PavilionPublishing and Media, 2017.

7.   J. Pring, *Longcare Survivors: The Biography of a Care Scandal*. DisabilityNews Service, 2011.

8.   See, e.g., *Joint Investigation into the Provision of Services for People with Learning Disabilities at Cornwall Partnership NHS Trust*. London: Commission for Healthcare Audit and Inspection, 2006; and *Investigation into the Service for People with Learning Disabilities Provided by Sutton and Merton Primary Care Trust*. London: Commission for Healthcare Audit and Inspection, 2007.

9.   The first was F. E. James and R. P. Snaith, eds, *Psychiatric Illness and Mental Handicap*. London: Gaskell, 1979.

10. N. Bouras and G. Holt, eds, *Mental Health Services for Adults with Intellectual Disability: Strategies and Solutions* (Maudsley Monograph). London: Routledge, 2010.

11. *Manual for Mental Deficiency Nurses*.

12. Another good example is C. H. Hallas, *Nursing the Mentally Subnormal* (2nd ed.). Bristol: John Wright, 1962, which does cover mental illness over 8 of its 200 pages, as many as is devoted to 'discipline and special privileges'.

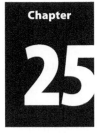

Chapter 25

Drugs, Drug Harms and Drug Laws in the UK: Lessons from History

Ilana Crome and David Nutt

Introduction

In the UK, the number of deaths due to substances far exceeds other preventable deaths such as melanoma, suicide, road traffic accidents and AIDS, which total around 10,000 per annum. The death rate due to drugs in the UK is now the highest in Europe: opiate and cocaine deaths are at an all-time high (Figure 25.1). Alcohol is responsible for approximately 25,000 deaths every year and is now the leading cause of death in men under fifty years of age. Tobacco still leads to 80,000 deaths every year. See Box 25.1 for definition of terms used in this chapter.

The health, social and criminal justice systems currently in place are not able to provide the flexible response in which the public can have confidence and to which they can adhere. Moreover, vindictive policies which criminalise people with substance dependence are therefore also unlikely to yield positive outcomes as addicts are suffering from a clinical disorder which requires treatment and support rather than indiscriminate sanctions.[1] Addictions exact a high price in preventable illness, disability and deaths and are a marker of deprivation and inequality.[2]

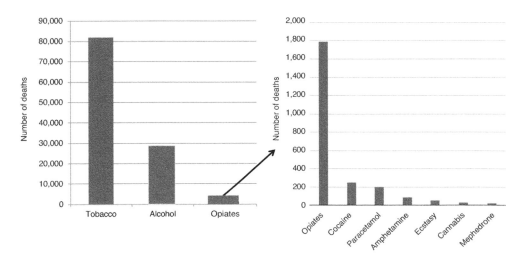

Figure 25.1 Deaths in the UK from different drugs
Source: 'Deaths related to drug poisoning in England and Wales: 2018 registrations', ONS data 2018.

Box 25.1 Terminology

The terms addiction and dependence will be used interchangeably, as will the terms 'drug' or 'substance'.

The terms 'drug' and 'substance' cover those psychoactive substances that are legal or licit and commercially available (tobacco and alcohol) as well as those that are illegal or illicit.

These terms will also be used to describe 'street' use of drugs which includes:

- drugs bought over the Internet;
- prescribed medication (e.g. benzodiazepines, opiate, opioid and gabapentinoid drugs) used in a manner not indicated or intended by a medical practitioner; and
- use of over-the-counter preparations such as codeine-based products (e.g. cough medicines, decongestants).

Illicit drugs include:

- cannabinoids (tetrahydrocannabinol or THC and cannabidiol) and synthetic cannabinoids ('spice');
- central nervous system depressants such as opiates and opioids (e.g. morphine, codeine, heroin; and buprenorphine, oxycodone, methadone, fentanyls);
- stimulants (e.g. cocaine, crack cocaine, amphetamines and 3,4-methylenedioxymethamphetamine, known as MDMA or ecstasy, khat);
- hallucinogens: lysergic acid diethylamide (LSD) and psilocybin (magic mushrooms); and
- novel psychoactive substances (NPS).

Social Epidemiology, Medical Treatment and Drug Laws: 1960–1990

Current policy ambition is to reduce use rather than the harms caused by substances, and tobacco consumption has decreased but alcohol consumption has doubled over the last fifty to sixty years. Deaths from liver disease have demonstrated a steep rise between 1970 and 2006, 80 per cent of which are alcohol related and 20 per cent due to viral hepatitis (see Figure 25.2). Alcohol consumption increased as it became more affordable and sales from corner shops and supermarkets for off-premises consumption became legal. The pattern of drug use, too, has changed markedly over the last 100 years. Between 1920 and 1960, drug use was very low and mostly by people with other conditions. The Dangerous Drugs Act prohibited the sale of drugs without a medical prescription.[3] Medical prescription to addicts was allowed as a last resort. This came to be known as the 'British System'.

From the 1960s, there was a new development: young drug users associated with the music scene appeared. Apart from the obvious link with entertainment, drugs such as cannabis, amphetamine or 'uppers' (in the form of an over-the-counter Benzedrine inhaler) and LSD came to symbolise their new 'alternative' identity with the hippy youth protest movement, its political values and new ways of dressing and behaving. This aroused suspicion and even anger in both the public and politicians. The Advisory Committee on Drug Dependence established the independent expert Wootton Committee review of cannabis and concluded that, despite the fact that the dangers of cannabis use had been exaggerated, it should stay illegal but in a lower class of the Misuse of Drugs Act 1971, that is, cannabis-related offending

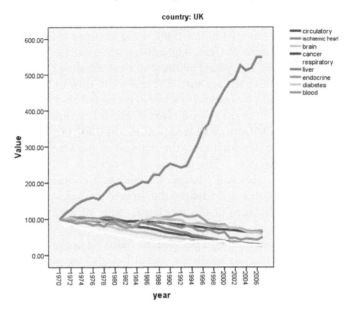

Deaths under age 65 from major diseases compared with 1970

country: UK

Figure 25.2 Standardised mortality rates from different diseases in the UK
Note the remarkable rise in deaths from liver disease as compared with other medical conditions: 80 per cent of these are due to excessive alcohol use and 20 per cent to viral hepatitis
Sources: British Beer and Pub Association (BBPA) Statistical Handbook 2008; Institute of Alcohol Studies Factsheet 'Trends in the affordability of alcohol in the UK'. Reproduced by permission of Professor Nick Sheron.

should be regarded as less serious than that related to opiates and cocaine and penalties be reduced.[4] This advice was ignored and some forms of cannabis stayed in Class A and the rest in Class B.

During this time, the Home Office spotted that notifications of cases of heroin addiction had increased from 50 in 1958 to 1,299 in 1967 and that 80 per cent of users were under the age of 29. They were mainly young men who injected intravenously and were perceived as some threat to society. As this new cohort differed markedly from the few older middle-class people who were treated under the 'British System', the second Brain Committee in 1964 concluded that heroin use was a 'socially infectious condition'.[5] Its recommendations included new specialist addiction treatment units (Drug Dependence Units, or DDUs) under psychiatric leadership; compulsory notification of new cases; licences for doctors to prescribe heroin or cocaine at these centres; and, importantly, abstinence rather than maintenance with heroin or a substitute medication. Withdrawal treatment became the treatment of choice, and when this failed, addicts sought alternative treatment or drugs. This strategy appeared to curb the drug problem to an extent but not entirely.

Cannabis remained popular and convictions increased. During the 1970s, injection of barbiturate drugs became the most common form of death from overdose, but this subsided when Southwest Asian heroin began to make an appearance on the black market and benzodiazepines replaced barbiturates as they were considered a safer and non-addictive sedative medication at the time. Furthermore, as prescribed injectable amphetamine and illicitly produced amphetamine powder, which was either snorted or injected, became available, it became the most widely used drug after cannabis. Services remained focused on heroin users but, because of the HIV/AIDS epidemic, all injecting drug users became an increasing cause for concern.

A new heroin epidemic emerged in the 1980s when cheaper black market heroin was imported from the Golden Crescent (Iran, Afghanistan and Pakistan). This cohort differed in that now it was adolescents and young adults who were inhaling ('chasing') heroin, and although this route of use protected against HIV, many did turn to injecting and suffered serious complications. Use of cocaine and crack also increased and intravenous use of the benzodiazepine temazepam emerged as a problem. While it is estimated that in 1994 there were about 67,000 people in treatment for drug misuse, by 2007 there were 195,000.[6]

Following on from these developments, the revision of the Dangerous Drugs Act led to the Misuse of Drugs Act 1971.[7] The Misuse of Drugs Act 1971 (MDAct 1971) has two separate dimensions, classes and schedules. Schedule 1 contains all drugs that have no medicinal value. Schedules 2–5 define the degree of safekeeping that different medicines require; this is because of the medicinal value of many 'misused' or recreational drugs.

Classes define the penalties for illegal possession. Three classes of drugs emerged: those continuing to enjoy recognition as medically useful but also associated with abuse (e.g. opioids, amphetamine); those that lost recognition as medicines and continued to be associated with abuse (e.g. cocaine, LSD, MDMA, magic mushrooms); and those that had never enjoyed recognition as medicines and continued to be associated with abuse (e.g. crack cocaine and ketamine analogues). Within each class, penalties intending to serve as deterrents differ in severity, depending on whether they are for possession for personal use, dealing, supply or importation. These penalties are meant to indicate the relative harms of the different drugs and act as a deterrent to use/supply. Severity of penalties is related to the potential of each drug for individual harm rather than cumulative social harm, which arguably would be more rational. They reflect the predominant UK policy of prohibition of recreational drug use that has been in place for nearly a century. As the costs of this undertaking in terms of social and personal damage are not inconsequential, there is a case for considering the proportionality of the penalty to the harms that may accrue both socially and individually.

Emergence of Public Health and Harm Reduction Approaches

There were a range of responses to the heroin epidemic of the 1980s, including the national campaign 'Heroin Screws You Up' aiming to prevent its initiation, and expansion of facilities for medical treatment. New multidisciplinary services offered residential rehabilitation. The objective was to persuade addicts to abstain. However, the epidemic of HIV/AIDS transformed this strategy. Accordingly, a flexible harm reduction policy was recommended by the Advisory Council on the Misuse of Drugs (ACMD). Implemented under the Thatcher government, it further expanded services and instituted needle exchange and methadone prescription. It was credited with the less than expected increase of HIV infections in drug users; in fact, the UK had the lowest in Europe. Despite these measures, during the 1990s heroin use continued to increase, especially among adolescents and young people, and ecstasy (MDMA) use started to materialise as part of the rave dance scene. This development caused significant disquiet and stirred up much debate within criminal justice, political and health settings.

Over the previous decades, illicit drug use itself was being increasingly conceptualised by younger people as 'normal' behaviour, while smoking was considered a more 'deviant' practice and perceived as a 'drug'. It was argued that, had tobacco been discovered at the same time, it would not have been a legal substance. Restrictions on smoking and drinking and relaxation of the drug laws began to be examined. Continuing recreational use of licit substances, such as prescription drugs, added increasing complexity.

A model of public health, derived from that applied to tobacco, began to influence thinking on drugs and alcohol. Epidemiology became the research tool which underpinned the investigation of alcohol and drug use at the population level and represented a steer away from a strictly 'medical' model.

Thus, alcohol policies, though led by psychiatrists, also embraced a more varied group of disciplines and organisations such as the voluntary sector, the law and the police. This was because alcohol was conceptualised as a problem of the many, not just the few severely affected by the 'disease' of alcoholism. A landmark study by Edwards and colleagues in 1977 compared the impact of structured, individual advice, with the full treatment paraphernalia in use at the time. Advice, by and large, did as well as the already prevalent more complex treatment at twelve-month follow-up.[8] Encouraging the general population to reduce both smoking and alcohol consumption by 'brief interventions', mainly in primary care, was promoted.

Following the election of the Conservatives in 1979, this became problematic for politicians who were wary of imposing restrictions on advertising, increasing taxation and introducing licensing. During this time drug treatment had moved from primary care–based treatment to that which was led by psychiatric specialists. This was underscored by the need to notify the Home Office (rather than the Department of Health) of new cases, much like infectious disease control, as drug use was considered a 'socially infectious disease'. Ideas around risk and the health of the population formed part of the thinking. Lifestyle, self-help and control as well as abstention were now entwined with the public health agenda. So, the impact of substance use on the whole population, as well as the individual who needed treatment, mattered.

This overall strategy of harm reduction was instituted after Labour came to power in 1997. It was implemented through an expansion of treatment programmes in 2000 which did reduce the rising death toll from opioids (see Figure 25.3). As penalties for drug offences were also rising, Drug Treatment and Testing Orders were introduced to engage users in treatment which meant that drug treatment became inextricably linked to criminal justice. In 2004, an Alcohol Harm Reduction Strategy was introduced to combat the massive rise in alcohol harms (e.g. Figure 25.2) and it was also based on the model of drug harm reduction.

In parallel, as the drug scene unfolded, since 1960 there had also been significant progress in the understanding of addiction and, to some degree, the associated harms to the individual and to society. The UK played an important role in the growth of this advancement. One key development in the 1970s was that novel terminology replaced the term 'addiction': the concept of 'dependence' was born and it could be applied to all substances. Dependence was defined by a set of criteria to diagnose or categorise the condition, be it because of drug, alcohol or tobacco use. Momentum around this conceptual breakthrough gathered so that, in due course, dependence came to be regarded as a chronic relapsing brain disorder.[9]

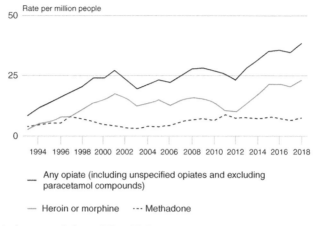

Age-standardised mortality rates for deaths by all opiates, heroin or morphine, and methadone, England and Wales, registered 1993 to 2018

__ Any opiate (including unspecified opiates and excluding paracetamol compounds)

— Heroin or morphine   ⋯ Methadone

Figure 25.3 Deaths from opioids from 1993 to 2018
Source: 'Deaths related to drug poisoning in England and Wales: 2018 registrations', ONS data 2018.

Towards an Understanding of Mechanisms and Harms: The Contribution of Neuroscience

Historically, addiction disorders have been portrayed – or understood – as a moral failing, a bad habit. Substance misusers may be treated in the acute phase of their illness in medical settings but, if left untreated, as they often are, they are then prone to poor medication adherence, poor control of common disorders such as hypertension and diabetes, increased risk of cancers and decreased effectiveness of treatments for pain. Substance misusers have not been considered worthy of first-class care compared to people with other preventable or treatable long-term conditions.

The remarkable contributions of neuroscience over half a century, 1960–2010, have demonstrated the biological basis of substance misuse, which can become a chronic medical condition, much like diabetes and hypertension. Recent research has demonstrated that a drug that induces dependence initially produces changes in reward neurotransmitters and neural circuitry which are (perhaps permanently) affected after repeated use. Eventually, the user loses control due to the development of negative physiological and emotional states and habit entrenchment. This neuroscience-based analysis in no way precludes an appreciation of the social, cultural and political factors that influence initiation and continuation of substance use.

Over this time, effective and innovative pharmacological treatments have forged ahead and continue to do so. There is a diversity of medications based on detailed knowledge about how they block the action of drugs such as opiates, stimulants, benzodiazepines and cannabis. Methadone has been and continues to be prescribed to those with heroin dependence and nicotine replacement to tobacco smokers. Newer medications such as buprenorphine and naltrexone for opiate dependence and acamprosate for alcohol dependence now form part of the pharmacological treatment options available. Psychological treatments, too, have found favour with service providers, and a combination of psycho-social interventions and medications are often recommended.[10]

It has become much clearer that the lack of response to treatment, rather than being due to poor character, lack of willpower or self-control, has very likely been rooted in an inadequate understanding of the nature of the problem. Refusing to recognise that the provision of resources to effectively treat, research and educate professionals and the public about addiction diminishes legitimate optimism derived from this substantial body of research.

As important are fair and appropriate drug policies, that is, public laws and regulations which can be expected to reduce harms to society while minimising unintended consequences. This stance recognises that psychological, social and political processes may lead to exacerbate and even thwart access and responsiveness to appropriate treatment. It also acknowledges that the biological and psychosocial drivers of addiction are unlikely to disappear even if abstinence is achieved. Understanding of brain mechanisms can be translated within the individual and wider social context.

Drug Laws in the UK: Lessons Learnt?

The justification for the illegality of many drugs is that they are harmful and hence criminal sanctions are necessary to reduce the harms to society and to individuals because they will act as a deterrent to their use.

For the last sixty years, the UK drugs policy has been controlled under two Acts of Parliament. Medicines are controlled under the Medicines Act and recreational drugs under the Misuse of Drugs Act 1971. In practice, many drugs – for example opioids, ketamine, benzodiazepines and stimulants – are controlled under both Acts which makes the position unnecessarily complicated as they come under the control of two different ministries of state.

Up until the early 1970s, rather than the policy debate around the drug laws centring on harms, it was focused on the morality of drug taking. In an attempt to redress this to some extent, the Misuse of Drugs Act in 1971 was introduced. This included understanding of the perceived harms caused by drugs, but they were not as well understood then as now. The ACMD was established to 'keep the drug situation under review and to advise ministers on the measures to be taken for preventing the misuse of drugs or for dealing with problems connected with their misuse'. One of its key objectives is to decide on the relative harms of drugs and so locate them within the classes A, B and C.

Since 1971, there has been some movement of drugs between classes. Ketamine and GHB have come under the control of the Act. Methamphetamine has moved from Class B to Class A. Magic mushrooms have been made Class A and benzylpiperazine Class C. Cannabis has moved from Class A/B to C and then back to Class B. Until 2009, all governments had followed the advice of ACMD, but then, for the first time, their recommendations about cannabis and ecstasy were not heeded.

The public, policymakers and scientists need to act in unison to produce an evidence-informed, balanced and workable response as substance use and misuse remain a feature of everyday life in the UK today. Arguably the most important example of the divergence between science and policy is in the classification of what constitutes a 'legal' or 'illegal' drug. Alcohol, which is, of course, legal and widely available, produces considerable harm. Tobacco, too, is highly addictive and harmful but legal. Cannabis, on the other hand, remains illegal in many countries following the ban in 1961 by the UN convention but does relatively little harm.[11] As another example, some 'drugs of abuse' have medicinal value – for example, opioids, benzodiazepines, amphetamines and constituents of cannabis – so the regulations make allowance for these. However, other drugs such as psychedelics (e.g. psilocybin) and MDMA with lesser harms and arguably with therapeutic potential for alcohol dependence, obsessive-compulsive disorder and PTSD (post-traumatic stress disorder) are not currently available legally.[12]

This issue has been examined in a multi-criteria decision analysis incorporating sixteen parameters of health and social harms of different drugs as illustrated in Box 25.2.[13] The results demonstrate a striking lack of correlation between harms and the degree of prohibition (see Figure 25.4). This has been internationally replicated in Australia and Europe.

One key element underpinning the value of systematic harm assessment of different drugs is that the availability of less harmful drugs leads to lower levels of harms to users. One of the most remarkable natural experiments that support this was the rise and subsequent fall of mephedrone in the UK (see Figure 25.5). This synthetic cathinone was legal in 2008 when it became popular in the UK. Within a few months, it had commandeered a significant part of the recreational stimulant market. This led to huge media hysteria with exaggerated claims of harms that, in effect, forced the Labour government to ban it just before the 2010 general election. Several years later, it became clear that mephedrone use had very significantly reduced deaths from cocaine and amphetamines. It appears that a significant proportion of the users of these drugs had switched to mephedrone, probably because it was legal, easily available and comparatively safe. Once mephedrone was made illegal, they switched back to their original stimulant and deaths from cocaine and amphetamine have reached all-time highs.

Box 25.2 Harms Related to Drug Use

Harms to users:
   Drug-specific mortality
   Drug-related mortality
   Drug-specific harm
   Drug-related harm
   Drug-specific impairment of mental functioning
   Drug-related impairment of mental functioning
   Loss of tangibles
   Loss of relationships
Harms to others:
   Injury
   Crime
   Economic cost
   Impact on family life
   International damage
   Environmental damage
   Decline in reputation of the community

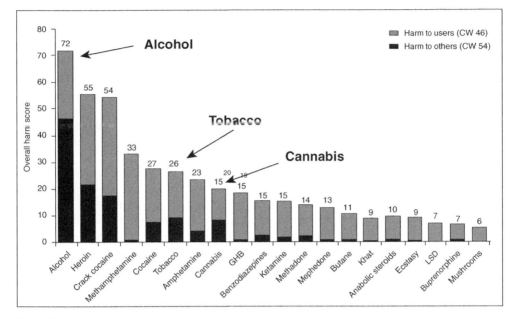

Figure 25.4 Drugs ranked according to harm

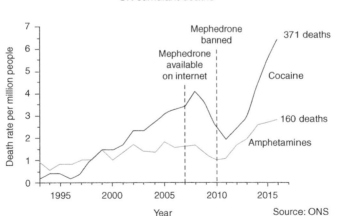

Figure 25.5 Death rates from cocaine and amphetamines before during and after the mephedrone episode
Source: Nutt from 'Deaths related to drug poisoning in England and Wales: 2018 registrations', ONS data 2018.

At this point, it is worth noting that the use of tobacco and alcohol products falls under separate age of purchase controls and taxation and are regulated food or commodities.

As the historical overview outlines, the profile of users changes as do the type and pattern of use of substances changes over time. Substance users can be very variable in terms of social status and health conditions. They have multiple needs, including being stigmatised, socially deprived and having traumatic life histories, mental health problems and living on the margins of society: the homeless, migrants, refugees and asylum seekers.

Substances are now commonly consumed in combination, and some combinations are more dangerous than others. New drugs emerge and, sometimes, if a particular drug becomes difficult to obtain because of either a change in the law or reduced supply, a more potent drug is developed. Several examples of this are cannabis and heroin which have been supplemented by synthetic cannabinoids or fentanyl. Very often users are not aware of what precisely is contained in the drugs they are using and so are not aware of the risk to which they are exposing themselves. Laws and policies need to take account not only of the type of drug and extent of use but also of these changing profiles of both drug and user.

Future Directions: 2010 and Beyond

In 2007, Sir David King, former UK chief scientific adviser, predicted improved treatments for addiction and other mental health disorders and the development of newer recreational drugs, some of which may lead to fewer harms and lower risks of addiction than the substances in use today.[14]

In 2009, one of us, David Nutt was dismissed as Chair of the Advisory Council for the Misuse of Drugs after pointing out that current government policy and the Misuse of Drugs Act 1971 were not evidence-based. Specifically, he commented that among the most harmful drugs in the UK were legal ones – that is, alcohol and tobacco – and the current government approach to focus on 'illegal' drugs was a missed opportunity to reduce overall drug harms. His removal was justified on the grounds that, as the chief government advisor, he should not be opposing government policy which failed to acknowledge that these were drugs.

Since then, with the advent of 'austerity', the UK has witnessed the decimation of treatment services for drugs, alcohol and smoking cessation, with numbers of consultant addiction psychiatrists and trainees dramatically reduced.[15] This is a false economy: the stark increase in deaths is a chilling reminder of the gravity of the state of play.

There have been new issues and new substances as well as new groups of substance misusers. While much of the debate has centred on younger people, including children and adolescents, attention has recently turned to older people who are misusing cannabis and heroin as well as over-the-counter and medically prescribed medications.[16] For example, there is now an appreciation that addiction is a lifetime problem for some and accumulating evidence that older people are vulnerable to the impact of legal and illegal use.[17] In addition, we see the emergence of an ever-growing number of designer 'novel' psychoactive substances, available through the Internet; the popularity of e-cigarettes (vaping) for many substances apart from nicotine; and the changes in the legal status of cannabis so that it can be prescribed as a medicine. There is exciting potential for the development of new pharmaceutical agents for the treatment of substance misuse.

What half a century has shown us is that, overall, deaths from substance use have risen. There are a broad range of factors that contribute to this sad situation. The last years can be characterised as having seen prohibitionist developments in UK drug laws, while those evidence-based policies that could reduce the use of alcohol, especially minimum unit pricing, have not been introduced universally. Scotland and, recently, Wales have introduced these changes and preliminary data from Scotland suggest a decrease in alcohol use and its harms. However, in England, encouraged by the drinks industry, the government has resisted any change. There have been some significant steps forward in that smoking advertising has been banned and there are restrictions on smoking in public places, bars and restaurants, but the alcohol industry has managed to avert similar controls. These strategies have failed to achieve their goal and sometimes have even led to the development and use of more harmful substances. Particularly disturbing perhaps is that the Schedule 1 controls make it very difficult to use certain drugs for medical research.[18]

As is the case in many countries now, policy regarding substances is best placed within health care departments rather than the Home Office. For example, in the Netherlands, testing and regulated access to some substances has largely eliminated deaths from new recreational drugs; and in Portugal, the provision of appropriate comprehensive treatment interventions and facilities has significantly reduced opioid deaths. Further examples include prescription of medicinal cannabis as an alternative to opioid analgesics and the development of safer injecting/drug consumption rooms for those who have tried other methods.

Conclusion

The last sixty years has been an extraordinarily dynamic period in terms of both the rapid march of scientific progress and the changing landscape of drug use, drug harms and drug policy. It is fitting to end with prescient excerpts from an interview by Griffith Edwards, the quintessential figure in addiction psychiatry in the UK between 1960 and 2010 and editor-in-chief of the journal *Addiction* between 1979 and 2004:

> Addiction science at its most productive knows no substance boundaries. There is great benefit in comparing across substances the mechanisms of dependence, distributions of consumption, treatment processes, policy and control responses.

He valued:

> Daring to provoke debate, but with respect for everyone's opinion.

He summarised key components as follows:

> Our agenda themes (include) to encourage debate on the ethical dimension (in journal publishing), the relationship between science and policy, to promote internationalism (and) enhancing the quality of science.[19]

Key Summary Points

- Substance use and misuse remain a feature of everyday life in the UK today. They are a cause of death and disability and a marker of deprivation and inequality. The health, social and criminal justice systems currently in place are not able to provide the flexible response in which the public can have confidence and to which they can adhere.
- While much of the debate has centred on younger people, including children and adolescents, attention has recently turned to older people who are misusing cannabis and heroin as well as over-the-counter and medically prescribed medications.
- The remarkable contributions of neuroscience over half a century, 1960–2010, have demonstrated the biological basis of substance misuse, which can become a chronic medical condition, much like diabetes and hypertension.

- There is exciting potential for the development of new pharmaceutical agents for the treatment of substance misuse.
- An aspiration we have is towards a new public understanding of addiction through education so that people can make informed choices based on realistic policies.

Notes

1. Royal College of Psychiatrists, *Drugs Dilemmas and Choices*. London: Gaskell, 2000.

2. A. Case and A. Deaton, Rising morbidity and mortality in midlife among white non-Hispanic Americans in the 21st century. *Proceedings of the National Academy of Sciences of the United States of America* (2015) 112: 15078–83.

3. The Dangerous Drugs Act 1964, www.parliament.uk/about/living-heritage/transformingsociety/private-lives/relationships/collections1/parliament-and-the-1960s/dangerous-drugs-act-1964/.

4. The Wootton Committee review, https://cashewnut.me.uk/Home/Wootton-Report.php.

5. The 1964 Brain Committee, www.dldocs.stir.ac.uk/documents/2nd-brain-report.pdf.

6. S. MacGregor, Policy responses to the drug problem. In S. MacGregor, ed., *Responding to Drug Misuse*, 1–19. London: Routledge, 2010.

7. Misuse of Drugs Act 1971, www.legislation.gov.uk/ukpga/1971/38/contents.

8. G. Edwards, J. Orford S. Egert et al., Alcoholism: A controlled trial of 'treatment' and 'advice'. *Journal of Studies on Alcohol* (1977) 38: 1004–31.

9. A. I. Leshner, Addiction is a brain disease, and it matters. *Science* (1997) 278, 45–7, https://doi.org/10.1126/science.278.5335.45.

10. D. Nutt, *Drugs without the Hot Air* (2nd ed.). Cambridge: UIT Cambridge, 2020.

11. R. Weissenborn and D. J. Nutt, Popular intoxicants: What lessons can be learned from the last 40 years of alcohol and cannabis regulation? *Journal of Psychopharmacology* (2012) 26: 213–20.

12. D. Nutt and A. T. McLellan, Can neuroscience improve addiction treatment and policies? *Public Health Review* (2013) 35, https://doi.org/10.1007/BF03391704.

13. D. J. Nutt, L. A. King and L. D. Phillips, Drug harms in the UK: A multicriteria decision analysis. *Lancet* (2010) 376: 1558–65.

14. D. King, Introduction. In D. J. Nutt, T. W. Robbins, G. V. Stimson, M. Ince and A. Jackson, eds, *Drugs and the Future: Brain Science, Addiction and Society*, xi. London: Elsevier, 2007.

15. C. Drummond, Cuts to addiction services are a false economy. *British Medical Journal* (2017) 357: j2704, https://doi.org/10.1136/bmj.j2704.

16. I. B. Crome and R. Williams, *Substance Misuse and Young People: Critical Issues*. London: Routledge, 2020.

17. Royal College of Psychiatrists, *Invisible Addicts*. Report No. 211. London: Royal College of Psychiatrists, 2018; S. MacGregor, Proposals for policy development. In I. B. Crome, L.-T. Wu, R. Rao and P. Crome, eds, *Substance Use and Older People*, 353–63. Chichester: Wiley Blackwell, 2015; Crome, Wu, Rao and Crome, eds, *Substance Use and Older People*.

18. D. J. Nutt L. A. King and D. E. Nichols, Effects of Schedule I drug laws on neuroscience research and treatment innovation. *Nature Reviews Neuroscience* (2013) 14: 577–85, https://doi.org/10.1038/nrn3530.

19. E. Griffith, Conversation with Griffith Edwards. *Addiction* (2005) 100: 9–18, https://doi.org/10.1111/j.1360-0443.2005.00954.x.

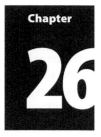

Chapter

26

Homelessness and Mental Health

Philip Timms

Introduction

Today, in the UK, homelessness is a hot topic. In 1960, it was not. One memory of my first few weeks in London in 1971 was of large numbers of men sleeping on the streets 'under the arches' in Charing Cross. Very few people at the time really seemed to view this as a problem. The prevailing view was that most homeless people were alcoholics who had chosen to live like that. There was, therefore, nothing you could do for them, so it was pointless to try. Unbeknown to me, there were thousands more homeless men (and some women) living in the deteriorating remnants of the workhouse system and nineteenth-century dosshouses for the poor. Insofar as homelessness and mental illness were thought of at all, they were seen as different phenomena, with little or no connection between them. Back then, mental health professionals were preoccupied with new developments in pharmacological and group interventions – and, of course, the issue of mental hospital beds, which had been closing since 1955.

Background

There is a historically documented association between homelessness and mental illness.[1] In England and Wales, throughout the nineteenth century some 20–25 per cent of all known pauper lunatics had been accommodated in workhouses rather than asylums.[2] However, in 1960 the stereotype of the single homeless man (for most homeless people at that time, then as now, were men) was that of the alcoholic. Most were not sleeping out on the street but were accommodated in one of the many large hostels for homeless men (and a few women) that punctuated the urban landscape.

Little research had been done in this area by psychiatrists or anyone else. Americans had suggested in 1939 that mental illness was more common in what they called 'the disorganised community'.[3] Two roughly equivalent descriptive classifications of the homeless were constructed, describing three categories of itinerant workers, itinerant non-workers and non-itinerant non-workers. An American sociologist called these respectively hobos, tramps and bums;[4] and, thirty years later, a French psychiatrist described such groups as 'errants, vagabonds and clochards'.[5] These arbitrary and stigmatising classifications served neither to clarify issues nor to provoke further thought or research. The few academic papers concerning the mental health of homeless people were focused on alcohol problems.

Hostels for the homeless were situated in the middle of working-class areas of housing. Local people had learnt to tolerate rather than love them. They might be 'reception centres' (see below), Salvation Army hostels or Rowton hotels, established in Victorian times for the working poor. There was usually no formal connection between these institutions and local health services, apart from the occasional appointment of a visiting GP at some of the larger hostels, such as the Camberwell Reception Centre. Their residents were often as hidden in these institutions as they would have been in any of the large mental hospitals.

The first sign of interest was a UK paper in 1956, which looked at psychiatric admissions to a south London observation ward.[6] Of these admissions, 8 per cent were of 'no fixed abode', a synonym for homelessness which continues to be used (and misused) to this day. This was a much higher proportion than would have been expected from the numbers of homeless men in the local area. A third were diagnosed as suffering from schizophrenia, mostly with delusional ideas; and those with this diagnosis tended to be living in the most impoverished circumstances, such as night shelters, rather than common lodging houses. The author suggested that

> When he falls ill, the down and out should, ideally, be treated in a separate institution ... where his environment was as near his normal habitat as possible. He would then be more likely to stay ... it would be an advantage if he could be committed to the institution for a definite period, and as so many appear in court, this should be possible.

This was the first clear acknowledgement of excess morbidity for psychosis in the homeless and the first call for a specialist service – but one that remained unheard for thirty years.

The 1948 National Assistance Act, passed by Attlee's Labour government, had formally abolished the Poor Law system that had existed for four centuries, where the only recourse for the indigent had been the workhouse. The Act established a safety net for those who could not work and could not pay national insurance contributions (such as the physically handicapped, unmarried mothers – and the homeless).

As part of this effort, it also established the National Assistance Board (NAB) so that 'persons without a settled way of living may be influenced to lead a more settled way of life'. In other words, it aimed to reduce or abolish homelessness. The Casual Wards of the old workhouses were rebranded as 'reception centres' to provide temporary accommodation The high levels of employment at the time and the provisions of the new welfare state meant that demand for such beds plummeted and the NAB closed 136 of the 270 centres it had taken over. By 1970, there were just seventeen left. However, echoes of the workhouse remained. There was still a 'work task' that had to be completed before an individual could leave after an overnight stay, and conditions were still miserable. A study of reception centres as late as 1968 revealed that residents had suffered from severe malnutrition.[7] Conditions in other large hostels were often no better.

The Act did theoretically have the power to keep people off the streets, but problems remained. In 1966, a pair of Birmingham psychiatrists reported that 23 per cent of men admitted to their urban acute psychiatric ward were of no fixed abode and that this proportion seemed to be rising quickly.[8] Of these homeless patients, 74 per cent had had previous hospital admissions. The authors were driven to comment that 'Their plight is evidence that the initial enthusiasm evoked by the new act (1959 Mental Health Act) for the discharge of psychotics into the community was premature and has resulted in the overwhelming of community services'. However, they acknowledged that this was not the whole story. They noted the housing shortage created by the closure of 'lodgings available for persons of no fixed abode'.

In 1968, Griffith Edwards and his team interviewed the entire population of the Camberwell Reception Centre – one of the largest homeless hostels in the country.[9] He found that 25 per cent of the residents had been previously admitted to a mental hospital – and this was equal to the proportion of those with alcohol problems. This was, perhaps, the first epidemiological evidence to challenge the idea that alcoholism was the cardinal mental health problem of the homeless man.

Although we are focusing on homeless men, it is worth mentioning the furore that was stirred up in 1966 by a BBC television play called *Cathy Come Home*. It portrayed a young working couple who, due to accidents and the rigidity of legislation and provision, move from a settled, self-sufficient domesticity to street homelessness and separation from each other and from their children. This created a media storm and encouraged support for Shelter, a housing charity that had been formed just before the programme was broadcast. It also prompted the foundation of the housing charity Crisis and was named in 2005 as the UK's most influential TV programme of all time.[10]

Yet, for all the concern this programme aroused, the only practical difference it really made was that homeless fathers could now stay with their wives and children in hostels. It did not really touch the single homeless person. One specific problem was the limited access to medical care in these institutions. This meant that mental health needs would not usually be identified unless the person were to behave in a violent or disruptive way. The subsequent response would usually have been ejection from the hostel rather than a referral for a medical assessment.

At the end of the decade, a survey of a Salvation Army hostel in 1969 noted that it had been 'conducted in an area with good psychiatric after-care services and an active local authority Mental Health Department. There is one psycho-geriatric hostel and one hostel for the subnormal, but no hostel for discharged psychiatric patients.'[11] The Salvation Army was serving as an unacknowledged, de facto aftercare service for many patients discharged from psychiatric wards (see Figure 26.1). They concluded: 'In our survey, 34 per cent of the residents had been in mental hospitals and 20 per cent were schizophrenic. It is surely not right to unload onto a voluntary organization, whose function is not to act as a therapeutic agency, patients who still need community care?' Willing but untrained housing workers were shouldering the burden of supporting those who should have been supported by mental health services.

1970s

Occasional enthusiasts continued to take an interest. A doorstep survey of two Salvation Army hostels for men found that 15 per cent of the residents had a diagnosis of schizophrenia and 50 per cent had a personality disorder.[12] On this occasion, both hospital and community care were criticised: 'The small number of schizophrenics who were receiving treatment suggests both a failure of community care and inappropriately early discharge.'

David Tidmarsh and Suzanne Wood restated the idea that there might be 'a need for services for the destitute men and women at present residing in common lodging houses and reception centres'.[13] They showed that, on a given night, around 150 men, mostly with schizophrenia and without contact with services, were sleeping in the Camberwell Reception Centre. Ironically, this 'invisible asylum' was just over a mile from the Maudsley Hospital, a major centre of British psychiatry.

Robin Priest's 1976 Edinburgh survey took a more sophisticated approach. He compared a general survey of the homeless population with those who were admitted to psychiatric hospital.[14] He noted the unusually high prevalence of schizophrenia in the homeless population (32 per cent) but also that the prevalence of schizophrenia

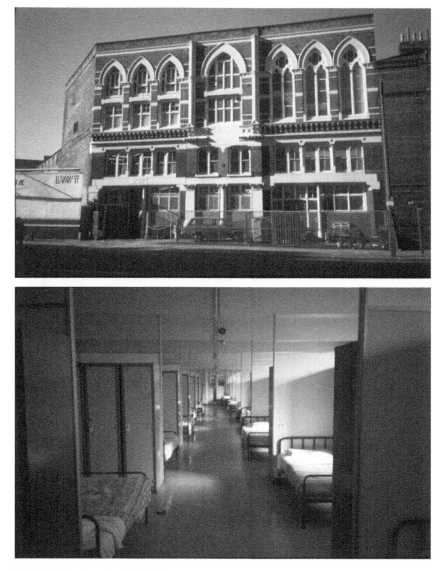

Figure 26.1 Salvation Army hostel, 1985

was greater in the general homeless population than in the subgroup that had presented to psychiatric services for treatment. Homeless men outside hospital were more likely to suffer from schizophrenia than those in hospital. So those with schizophrenia appeared to be less likely than their peers with other diagnoses to find their way to hospital treatment.

In 1977, parliament passed the Housing (Homeless persons) Act.[15] For the first time, this placed a statutory duty on local authority housing departments to permanently house some categories of homeless people, if that person had been found to be:

- In priority need (including vulnerability).
- Unintentionally homeless – that they had not made themselves homeless.
- Connected to the area – 'local connection'.

It sought to provide for:

- Those in 'priority need' for rehousing, regarded as 'fully homeless' and deserving of support. These were households with, or about to include, a dependent child.
- 'Vulnerable' lone people, or households without children, who could not reasonably be expected to fend for themselves, such as frail older people or those made homeless by an emergency – such as a fire or flood. Such households could be rehoused in local, funded social housing.

Under these criteria, people who were homeless, but did not appear particularly vulnerable (and did not have dependent children) were viewed as being able to support themselves. They came to be known as 'single homeless people' or as 'non-statutory homeless people', as they fell outside the main provisions of the new legislation and so were only entitled to advice and assistance from the local housing department. Homeless mentally ill people should have fitted well into the 'vulnerable' category, but three issues complicated matters, each of which I saw operating during my years of clinical practice:

- It was often hard to establish vulnerability in someone with a mental health problem, especially if they were not in contact with a psychiatric service.
- If, as a consequence of their mental illness, someone had behaved badly, not paid their rent or had neglected the care of their accommodation, it was easy for them to be viewed as having made themselves 'intentionally homeless'. They would then find themselves outside the provisions of the Act.
- Even if a person had been sleeping on the street in an area for many years, it could be argued that, as they did not have an address, then they did not have a local connection – and so, again, they fell outside the scope of the Act.

Moreover, the Act was only a general statute. A Code of Guidance was provided, but this left considerable room for interpretation. If you could not make your case, you were excluded from the provisions of the Act. This was particularly problematical with the criterion of not having made yourself intentionally homeless, containing as it did an echo of the notion of the 'undeserving poor'. The effectiveness of such provision was further challenged, in 1995, when it was ruled that local authorities could discharge their obligation by providing merely temporary accommodation.[16]

1980s

The Thatcher government of the 1980s created the right for tenants in England and Wales to buy their council flat. This was couched in terms of extending to everyone the right to have your own home, even those on low incomes. Although it was seen by many as a cynical attempt to buy working-class votes for the Tory party, it proved popular with those at whom it was aimed.[17] However, it also kick-started a drastic reduction in the social housing available to those who could not afford commercial rents, either because they were not employed or because they could not earn enough, even in full-time jobs. Thereafter, homelessness increased. Households accepted for assistance under the terms of the 1977 Act doubled from 53,110 households in 1978 to 112,730 in 1987 – and this rose to a peak of 144,780 in 1991.

At the same time, a silent and unpublicised process had begun – the closure of the large old hostels for homeless men and women. Much was written both for and against the closure of mental hospitals from the 1960s to the 1980s, and it was a matter of public knowledge and open debate. However, over the years from 1980 to 1995, the traditional large hostels for the homeless were also closed, with little public discussion or debate. This affected not only the Department of Health and Social Security (DHSS) reception centres/ resettlement units but also Salvation Army hostels, Rowton houses and night shelters. The closures took place for a variety of reasons, similar in many ways to those leading to the closures of mental hospitals.

In London, in 1981, there were 9,751 bed spaces in the wider network of direct-access hostels, 6,000 of these in large, traditional hostels for the homeless. The London Boroughs Association (LBA) described them as 'at once a resource and a problem':[18] a resource because of the shelter provided; a problem because of the often-appalling physical conditions and catastrophically inadequate staffing. This was illustrated by a crisis in 1983, when local authorities directed the owners to improve conditions in three Rowton houses – and the company promptly threatened to evict all the residents.[19] The local authorities subsequently bought the three hostels, intending to close them within five years.

Nationally, the DHSS had wanted to close resettlement units for some time.[20] It took the view that centrally funded institutions were inappropriate in an age of local social services and housing departments. Such large institutions were also seen as unsuitable places for influencing people 'to lead a more settled way of life', to use the original words of the NAB. So the decision was taken to close all the resettlement units and to replace them with locally run projects, with a system of grants to encourage voluntary sector organisations and local authorities to take on this task.[21] The closures started with the Camberwell Reception Centre, the largest of the old NAB reception centres, in September 1985.

The LBA report had recommended the opening of 600 beds each year to replace the old hostels but acknowledged the financial and planning difficulties that such schemes faced. Belated enforcement of fire regulations led some hostels to reduce in size and others to close. By 1985, the numbers of direct-access bed spaces had declined to 4,885 and, by 1990, to around 2,000.[22] The 900 beds of the Camberwell Reception Centre, all direct-access, were replaced by only 62 direct-access bed spaces, the rest being in specialist, referral-only, units. Across the board, 75 per cent of direct-access hostel spaces were lost during the 1980s. There was much good practice in the resettlement schemes for the existing residents of these hostels; but the loss of direct access beds without much in the way of equivalent provision did make it harder for a street homeless person, without resources, to get accommodation for the night.

There was, however, some official and academic interest now developing. *Helping Destitute Men* was a book written by a psychiatrist and a nurse and published in 1980. It commented on the presence of mental disorders in St Mungo's hostels but did not remark on them further, focusing instead on the sensible notion of rehabilitation for homeless hostel residents rather than simple containment.

Single and Homeless was a major report, commissioned by the Department of the Environment in 1982.[23] It covered a wide range of data and listed mental illness as a single category with no further details. It reported levels of mental illness which, if they included depression and anxiety, would have been unremarkable in a primary care sample. However, the methodology used meant that it would probably have missed much of the psychosis present in hostels. Their profiles of 'types of homeless people' included a drinker but no one with a mental illness. So an opportunity was missed for increasing awareness of the connection between homelessness and mental illness. However, across the Atlantic, there was a burgeoning literature developing which drew a strong connection between their process of deinstitutionalisation and excess rates of mental illness among their homeless populations.[24]

In the middle of this decade, and while this process of closure was going on, another Salvation Army hostel was found to have a third of both its residents and new arrivals with a diagnosis of schizophrenia;[25] however, some change was coming. In 1987, an outreach team to the large hostels in Lewisham and North Southwark in south London was established. The Psychiatric Team for Single Homeless People (PTSHP) consisted of two nurses, one psychologist, an occupational therapist and a trainee psychiatrist (me).[26] It provided a service to several of the large hostels that would soon be closing, but the question was asked, would this extra effort – or outreach as it has come to be known – be worth it? To answer this question, referrals were randomised into a treatment group – to whom the team would provide a clinical service – and an advice group – whom the team would assess and then advise the hostel nurse as to appropriate referrals to make. At the end of both three months and the year, the numbers remaining in the treatment group were significantly higher – as one would have hoped.

1990s

By 1990, Jeremy Corbyn – at that time a rebellious backbencher – was challenging Mrs Thatcher in parliament over the increasing levels of London street homelessness.[27] Although many felt that this was a consequence of the psychiatric deinstitutionalisation, the evidence suggested that it had more to do with the hostel closures of the 1980s.[28] The homeless mentally ill were clearly vulnerable both to deficits in health care and to inadequacies in other systems, such as housing. Whatever the cause, the Conservative government then decided to fund the Central London Homeless Mentally Ill initiative.[29] This consisted of several multidisciplinary mental health outreach teams in five locations across central and east London. Their scope was widened beyond hostels and incorporated the ideas of assertive outreach – but the work was directed at those who were not in touch with services at all.[30] Nurses, social workers and psychiatrists found themselves working in homeless day centres, squats, parks and even on the streets. This proved successful and three of the original teams are still functioning.

One of these, the START team, in south London, established a close working relationship with Thames Reach, a local homelessness charity (see Figure 26.2). Independently of the NHS, they had set up three housing projects in the same area, specifically for people with severe mental health problems who were sleeping out. The stage was set for a rich collaboration between the two agencies. A person with schizophrenia who was sleeping out could now be offered a small flat to move into without going through the usual accommodation 'ladder' – an almost 'housing first' set-up.[31]

A Labour government came to power in 1997 with a rather different set of ideas about social problems. Essentially, they drew on the notion of 'social exclusion', derived from French social science ideas about the nature of poverty.[32] This term might be assumed to be part of a set of left-wing or even socialist views of poverty. However, this version was, perhaps, a more a liberal-democratic idea. It viewed the marketplace as the weighted

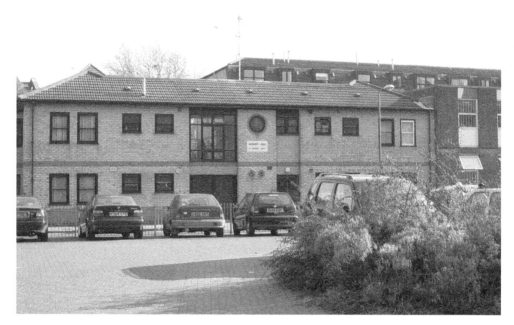

Figure 26.2 Thames Reach housing project, Bermondsey, 1994

centre of society – and proposed, at least in part, to 'improve' the marginalised so that they can now play a full (or fuller) part in society. So, although society may be reshaped to include the individual, there was also an emphasis on reshaping the individual to conform to society. Homelessness was defined as an element of social exclusion and major policies were put in place to counteract it,[33] including the formation of a Rough Sleepers Unit in 1999, with a target of reducing the number of rough sleepers by two-thirds by 2002. The target was met in 2001 and there were no increases in the number of people sleeping rough in England until 2010; but, of course, in the years since 2010 there has been marked deterioration.

2000s

There were few further important political or legislative changes during the first decade of the twenty-first century. Yet, professionally, those providing mental health services to homeless people began to look beyond psychosis and substance abuse. Psychologists came to the table and Nick McGuire in Southampton pioneered the use of cognitive behavioural therapy (CBT) in high-risk homeless populations.[34] John Conolly set up an outreach psychotherapy and 'pre-psychotherapy' service in Westminster;[35] and the notion of the psychologically informed environment began to be explored. Given the reluctance of many homeless and socially excluded people to engage with mental health services, it made more sense to provide psychological services in hostels and housing projects.[36] Other major cities such as Sheffield, Birmingham and Liverpool also set up mental health outreach teams for their homeless populations.

Conclusion

Attitudes and practices did change significantly between 1960 and 2010. Both homelessness and mental illness became increasingly matters of concern – and the high levels of mental disorder among homeless people were recognised.

At the beginning of this period, there was probably less visible street homelessness but this was because homeless people and people with mental illnesses were both, to a large extent, hidden. From the mid-1980s, increased recognition of the problem produced a range of high-quality and effective projects. Although these were mainly focused on psychosis, in the latter part of this period the psychological needs of those homeless people without psychosis were at last recognised and addressed, often using the explanatory idea of complex trauma.

Those of us working in the field have, I think, developed novel, flexible and user-centred services. What we have not been able to do is to change the economic and social forces that force people with mental disorders onto the street; and, perhaps, we have not changed the practice of psychiatry to the degree we would have wished. Patients are still discharged from psychiatric wards to the street and there is evidence that the majority of referrals to specialist mental health teams have previously been in touch with psychiatric services.[37] There is still much work to be done, especially as we have seen the subsequent years of austerity undo many of the achievements accomplished during the period described.

Key Summary Points

- Homelessness and mental health problems have been historically associated, but before the 1980s this connection was not generally recognised.
- For many people with mental health problems, the large hostels for the homeless formed a parallel system of institutionalisation to that of mental hospitals. Unlike mental hospitals, they were generally situated within working-class areas of housing.
- Attitudes and practices changed significantly between 1960 and 2010. Both homelessness and mental illness became increasingly matters of concern – and the high levels of mental disorder among homeless people were recognised.
- In 1990, homelessness and mental illness became a political issue because of the increasing numbers of people visibly sleeping out in London. Although it was linked to psychiatric deinstitutionalisation, the evidence suggested that it had more to do with the closures of the large hostels in the 1980s.
- From the mid-1980s, increased recognition of the problem produced a range of high-quality and effective projects which provided better access to mental health care for homeless people. These were initially focused on psychosis. In the latter part of this period, the psychological needs of those homeless people without psychosis were at last recognised and addressed, and the explanatory framework of complex trauma was introduced.
- The 'driver' factors that create homelessness have remained substantially unaddressed.

Notes

1. P. Timms, Homelessness and mental illness: A brief history. In D. Bughra, ed., *Homelessness and Mental Health*, 1996.

2. E. D. Myers, Workhouse or asylum: The nineteenth century battle for the care of the pauper insane. *Psychiatric Bulletin* (1998) 22: 575–7.

3. R. E. Faris and H. W. Dunham, *Mental Disorders in Urban Areas: An Ecological Study of Schizophrenia and Other Psychoses*. Chicago: University of Chicago Press, 1959.

4. N. Anderson, *The Hobo: The Sociology of the Homeless Man*. London: University of Chicago Press, 1923.

5. A. Vexliard, *Le clochard: Étude de psycholgie sociale*. Paris: Desclee de Brouwer, 1953.

6. J. S. Whiteley, Down and out in London: Mental illness in the lower social groups. *Lancet* (1955) 2: 608–10.

7. R. J. V. Ollendorff and A. Morgan, *Survey of Residents in Camberwell Reception Centre*. Unpublished report to the National Assistance Board, London, 1968.

8. C. Berry and A. Orwin, No fixed abode: A survey of mental hospital admissions. *British Journal of Psychiatry* (1966) 112: 1019–25.

9. Edwards et al., as above.

10. J. Deans, BBC evokes spirit of Cathy come home. *The Guardian*, 17 October 2005, www.theguardian.com /media/2005/oct/17/broadcasting.bbc3

11. B. Crossley and C. Denmark, Community care: A study of the psychiatric morbidity of a Salvation Army hostel. *British Journal of Sociology* (1969) 20: 443–9.

12. I. Lodge Patch, Homeless men in London: I. Demographic findings in a lodging house sample. *British Journal of Psychiatry* (1971) 118: 313–17.

13. D. Tidmarsh, Services for the destitute: Camberwell reception centre. In J. Wing and A. M. Hailey, eds, *Evaluating a Community Psychiatric Service. The Camberwell Register, 1964–1971*, 73–76. Oxford: Oxford University Press, 1972.

14. R. O. Priest, The homeless person and the psychiatric services: An Edinburgh survey. *British Journal of Psychiatry* (1976) 128: 128–36.

15. Housing (Homeless Persons) Act 1977, www.legislation.gov.uk/ukpga/1977/48/section/21/enacted.

16. House of Lords opinions of the Lords of Appeal for judgement in the case Regina v London Borough of Brent (Respondents), ex parte Awua (A.P.) 6 July 1995, www.casemine.com/judgement/uk/ 5a8ff85f60d03e7f57ebee75#1.

17. D. Foster, Right to buy: A history of Margaret Thatcher's controversial policy. *The Guardian*, 7 December 2015, www.theguardian.com/housing-network/2015/dec/07/housing-right-to-buy-margaret-thatcher-data.

18. GLC and LBA (Greater London Council and London Boroughs Association), *Hostels for Single Homeless in London*. Report. London: LBA, 1981. Report of a Joint Working Party on provision in London for people without a settled way of living.

19. GLC (Greater London Council), Four Victorian Hostels. London Borough of Havering: GLC, 1986.

20. J. Hewettson, Homeless people as an at-risk group. *Proceedings of the Royal Society of Medicine* (1975) 68: 9–13.

21. The Resettlement Units Executive Agency, *Annual Report and Financial Statement 1990/91*. London: HMSO, 1991.

22. M. Harrison, R. Chandler and G. Green, *Hostels in London: A Statistical Overview*. London: Resource Information Service, 1992.

23. M. Drake, M. O'Brien and T. Biebuyck, *Single and Homeless*. London: HMSO, 1982.

24. R. Lamb, Deinstitutionalisation and the mentally ill. *Hospital and Community Psychiatry* (1984) 35: 899–907.

25. P. Timms and A. Fry, Homelessness and mental illness. *Health Trends* (1988) 21: 70–1.

26. H. Brent Smith and R. Dean, *Plugging the Gaps: Providing a Service for Homeless Mentally Ill People*. London: Lewisham and North Southwark Health Authority, 1990.

27. A. Lusher, On this day: 1990 Jeremy Corbyn takes on Margaret Thatcher over 'disgrace' of UK homelessness. *The Guardian*, 8 May 2018.

28. T. Craig and P. Timms, Out of the wards and onto the streets? Deinstitutionalization and homelessness in Britain. *Journal of Mental Health* (1992) 1: 265–75.

29. T. Craig, E. Bayliss, O. Klein et al., *The Homeless Mentally Ill Initiative: Evaluation of 4 Clinical Teams*. London: Department of Health, 1995.

30. Assertive Outreach, *Sainsbury Centre for Mental Health*, London: Sainsbury Centre for Mental Health, 1971.

31. Croft-White. *Two Years On: An Evaluation of Lambeth High Street*. London: Thamesreach, 1997.

32. G. Room, *Beyond the Threshold: The Measurement and Analysis of Social Exclusion*. London: Policy Press, 1995.

33. Cabinet Office, *Rough Sleeping: Report by the Social Exclusion Unit*. London: Stationery Office Books, 1998.

34. N. Mcguire, Cognitive behavioural therapy and homelessness: A case series pilot study. *Behavioural and Cognitive Psychotherapy* (2006) 34: 107–11.

35. J. Conolly, Pre-treatment therapy approach for single homeless people. In P. Cockersell, ed., *Social Exclusion, Compound Trauma and Recovery: Applying Psychology, Psychotherapy and PIE to Homelessness and Complex Needs*, London: Jessica Kingsley Publishers, 2018.

36. R. Johnson and R. Haigh, Social psychiatry and social policy for the 21st century: New concepts for new needs – the 'enabling Environments' initiative. *Mental Health and Social Inclusion* (2011) 15: 17–23.

37. P. Timms and T. Craig, Letter re. Deinstitutionalisaiton, prison and homelessness. *British Journal of Psychiatry* (2016) 209: 349–50.

Chapter 27

From Fear and Pity to Parity: Politics and Public Mental Health

Peter Byrne

Introduction

Stigma, fear and pity are deeply intertwined with the history of psychiatry and mental health. This chapter reviews their continued impact during the years 1960–2010 and reasons and efforts to move beyond them towards respect, engaged relationships and social inclusion. It draws on the journey, individual and societal, of a social psychiatrist that began well before I started my first trainee psychiatrist job in Dublin in 1992, a seminal year for UK psychiatry as described in the section '1992: Jonathan Zito, Christopher Clunis and NHS Mental Health Services'. This journey includes thirteen years' experience as Associate Registrar at the Royal College of Psychiatrists.

I had learned at an early age that people with 'mental problems' were *different*. Back in the 1970s, my grandfather returned one day, upset, from a job as a draughtsman-builder at the local psychiatric asylum in midlands Ireland. He had grown up nearby in the rural poverty of 1920s Ireland, burying four of his six siblings to tuberculosis before they reached the age of eighteen, but even he was shocked by the living conditions he saw then in what locals called the 'looney bin'. His job was a short-term 'fixer-upper' for the wards, perhaps someone had written a bad report or an official was coming to visit. He said he had been told to do the bare minimum lest questions be asked about expenses, and he wanted to do more: 'these people have nothing.' I still have the photo of the outside of the building. We were not allowed in.

A year of two later, at my Dublin secondary school, a classmate reappeared following his first psychiatric admission for bipolar disorder. It should have been a low-key return. Instead, our chemistry teacher started to call him 'mentler'. Jim also used the term *looney bin* when he talked about it. I said nothing. The abuse continued from that teacher and fellow pupils and Jim did not finish school.

It was the 1970s and Ireland had public service TV ads urging its citizens to stop driving while intoxicated: 'if you give car keys to a drunk man, you might as well hand a loaded shotgun to a lunatic.' I heard language like this, and much worse, within my new profession for the seven years I trained in psychiatry. My last trainee job there was in North County Dublin, another old asylum. There were several long corridors with fresh-ish paint until the turns where the long-stay wards began – with bare, crumbling walls. Did they run out of paint, I asked? No, that is for when health ministers visit: they do not need to go beyond these points. My twenty-one years' experience as a full-time NHS consultant has been different but also similar. In north-east London, a senior manager declined a cup of tea on a visit to our day hospital because we offered her the same cup 'the patients' drink from.

What the Public Thinks It Knows about Mental Disorders

My interest developed into why having a mental illness was so less deserving of recognition/status/empathy than a physical one. I often asked people, well or unwell, what they thought about specific mental disorders, and talked to many psychiatrists and other health professionals, before I started to read the scientific literature. I met many Irish then UK-based colleagues who shared the same interest in public engagement with what we do and how our patients' lives are impacted by stigma and discrimination. One of my east London colleagues, Mark Salter, taught me that 'psychiatrists are the only branch of medicine that need to read the newspapers and go to the cinema'. There was much to review [1] I read 'factual' media pages (print and broadcast, online content) and was guided by fictional representations.[2] Rabkin reflected on responses to the three key messages of an innovative 1960s Canadian educational programme to promote understanding of mental disorders, namely that:

- the range of normal behaviours is wider than often believed
- deviant behaviour is not random but has a cause and can be modified
- normal and abnormal behaviour fall on a continuum and are not qualitatively distinct.[3]

She concluded that 'the third proposition was so unpalatable that the community eventually rejected the entire (six month) educational program(me)'.[4]

Taking Corrigan's definition that stigma is a prejudice based on stereotypes leading to discrimination,[5] one avenue of study is to explore the stated opinions of the general public towards people with mental disorders. To find out what public attitudes are, work has often used agreement with stereotypical statements as a measure of prejudice. Broader research examines other aspects of public negative attitudes, but here I focus on two: violence perceptions and pity.[6] Their consequence (discrimination) causes considerable distress to individuals. Even minor avoidance or subtle rejection of people with mental disorders is significant.

Reconceptualisations of psychosis allow for the possibility that stigma-mediated events play a role in relapses of psychosis through the ways these events are evaluated.[7] Appraisal of events is influenced by reasoning and attributional biases; dysfunctional schemata of self and the world; and isolated or adverse environments.[8] We can hypothesise similar end results in people with the common mental disorders: anxiety and depression (albeit through different mechanisms such as lowering self-esteem or increasing anticipatory anxiety).[9]

Courting Public Opinion

The Royal College of Psychiatrists (RCPsych) in the late 1990s funded an anti-stigma campaign led by the late Arthur Crisp, professor of psychiatry at St George's Hospital Medical School. It looked at available research and completed a pre-campaign UK-wide opinion survey.[10] *Changing Minds* (aka *Every Family in the Land*) was run from RCPsych from 1998 to 2003; other campaigns followed, the most enduring ones being *See Me* in Scotland and *Time to Change* across England and Wales. These latter two campaigns, or more accurately social movements, continue and do things differently and better: they are user-led (experts by experience) with training and support for people with mental health problems to do media work; they start within communities, not 'top-down', using social plus traditional media when necessary; and they achieve key alliances (celebrities, sporting

Table 27.1

20th Century	21st Century
Mental illness	Mental health
Psychiatric patient, patients	Service user, experts by experience
Family, husband/wife/partner	Carers
Schizophrenic	Person/people with schizophrenia
Psycho, lunatic, nut job, etc.[11]	Known to services, care in community

organisations, barbers, taxi drivers, artists). What is required is that, as a society, we now talk about mental disorders, *mostly* with a new progressive language (see Table 27.1).

Others have placed tackling practical discrimination at the centre of their campaigns, most notably Graham Thornicroft and his international collaborators.[12] After all, people learn how to conceal racist and other negative attitudes and what they might tell researchers can be at variance with what they believe and how they act. Some have argued that softer language is no practical gain – and some activities, for example challenging distasteful media items, are both stereotype suppression (implying an unwanted rebound) and a distraction from a rights-based approach to reducing stigma.[13] All great points but, three decades ago, we faced an even greater distraction.

1992: Jonathan Zito, Christopher Clunis and NHS Mental Health Services

Everything changed in 1992. On 17 December, Jonathan Zito (age twenty-seven) was changing trains at Finsbury Park Station (London) when a complete stranger, Christopher Clunis (age twenty-nine), approached him to fatally injure him without any provocation. In the subsequent Clunis Report,[14] multiple service failures were identified, principally that no service took responsibility to follow up Clunis to maximise his treatment engagement (see also Chapter 23).

I started my first consultant psychiatrist job in Kent, England, in 1999 and the only item left by my immediate predecessor on my office desk was that report.[15] The UK government fed on this. When mental health services were allocated extra resources from 1999 onwards (as were hospital accident and emergency departments (A&E), cardiology and cancer), it was to protect public safety and much less to treat mental disorders. The Zito Trust became one of several public bodies to call for more coercion in mental health services, and when it wound down its last chief executive said it had become a 'victim of its own success'.[16]

I acknowledge the sudden nature of the violent act that stole Jonathan Zito's life as well as the years of grief of his widow, family and friends. The aftershocks of the homicide, inquiries, government statements and media coverage combined, however, to turn community psychiatry into 'scare in the community'. Widespread assumptions about the violent unpredictability of all aspects of psychosis generalised to other mental disorders, and these stereotypes hardened public attitudes.[17]

Jonathan Zito's homicide spoke to the public's worst fears that severe mental illness (SMI) was hidden in 'normal people' (think Norman Bates in *Psycho*, 1960); that psychiatrists were 'too soft' to insist on confinement or coercion; and that our treatments don't work anyway. At the time, Brian Cooper called this the Iron Triangle of public anxiety and distrust of people with mental illness; an alienated tabloid press; and government policies focused on populist measures.[18] There was no public appetite for evidence of the declining rates of homicides by people with psychosis over forty years,[19] and so when the murders (sic) of Lin and Megan Russell occurred in 1998, committed by a stranger who had *no* psychosis, 'something had to be done'.[20] It remains hard to fathom the depth of government feeling during these years, such that politicians instructed the civil service (not clinicians) to invent a diagnosis and then legislated to treat it. The Dangerous Severe Personality Disorder (DSPD) diagnosis was conjured up and imposed on psychiatry and mental health. A couple of 'treatment' centres sprang up but, not long after, like the credibility of this 'diagnosis', vanished into a sad chapter of UK psychiatry (see also Chapter 28).[21]

A review of fifteen years of population-based public attitudes research identified differences between disorders, with worse attitudes towards addictions and schizophrenia than towards depression and anxiety. The key difference was perceived to be not 'deviant' behaviour but risk of violence.[22] The first challenge of public education/engagement was to facilitate empathy by shifting the focus away from violence. Every time there was a high-profile story, we at RCPsych have 'put out' a small group of media-trained clinicians to counter with arguments about actual incidence of these homicides,[23] with clear messaging on what is needed (well-resourced general adult psychiatry and community mental health services). Even 9/11 brought psychosis back into the bear pit of public opinion, when then home secretary Jack Straw called bin Laden 'psychotic' in an interview, adding that he 'was picking [his] words with care here because whenever you use the language of mental illness, you get letters from people'.[24] The same Jack Straw drove the DSPD agenda.

'Behaving Strangely'

This vague, informal two-word descriptor remains the referral headline from my A&E colleagues. Even within mental health services, clinical work is bedevilled by colleagues failing to differentiate, as evidence and professionalism demand, between functional psychoses (e.g. schizophrenia or bipolar disorder), acute confusional states caused by metabolic and similar abnormalities (delirium) and recreational substance-induced severe but transient mental disturbances; and sometimes also autism.

Successive government policies to outsource NHS addiction services to charities have undermined training in this area and compounded difficulties in both identification and treatment of related clinical problems. One of the clear empirical research messages about violence is that it is true that with stranger assaults the aggressor is far more likely to be intoxicated than be suffering from a functional psychosis. This actuarial statement is never an argument against people with addictions or addictions services. It is an argument in favour of evidence-based anti-alcohol policies such as minimum alcohol pricing.[25] At the time of writing (2021), only England has neglected to pursue this enlightened public health policy in the UK. In fact, resourced addiction treatment services that engage people, including treatment of comorbid mental disorders, are part of the solution to reduce societal violence due to alcohol and drugs).[26]

The core argument to reduce homicides by people with functional psychosis remains: work for less stigma and discrimination and people will be more likely to present to mental health services, engage well and take agreed medications. More stigma (hysterical media headlines, government legislative zeal) and they will more likely present to police than psychiatrists; take medication only under coercion; and use cannabis/other substances that increase the risk of violence. People will then present to services not 'because they are suffering but because they are insufferable'.

Existential Crisis within Psychiatry

As a clinician who works full-time as a general hospital psychiatrist, seeing patients referred from A&E and medical and surgical wards, my greatest frustrations relate to having responsibility without power. Often, I return patients home to unspeakable poverty with few or no supportive relationships in their lives. I document but cannot 'fix' their medium-term risks of suicide, coming to physical harm or, much less frequently, a future impulsive moment of violence to others. I am at once responsible but lack the power to make the right changes happen.

As the century began, NHS services in which I worked received 'new money' to assist us to set up five new early intervention in psychosis and general hospital liaison services but frustrations increased as that money dried up or was wasted on needless layers of management (see also Chapter 12). Professor Sir David Goldberg in his lecture on 'NHS psychiatry 1980–2006', referring to mental health services and the overemphasis on fear of psychiatric patients, concluded:

> This deterioration occurred despite (Treasurer) Gordon Brown's new money: £172 million a year between 2001 and 2005. Overall, the King's Fund estimate that 17 per cent of the new money was spent on local service developments, 32 per cent on pay and price infrastructure, and 46 per cent on the NHS Plan and modernisation funds. Furthermore, the National Survey of Investment 2004/2005 revealed a focus on forensic services at the expense of basic provision. Spending on secure and high dependency, access and crisis services and home support rose by 81 per cent, 79 per cent and 75 per cent respectively. The NHS invested far less on new buildings (17.0 per cent increase), CMHT (13.0 per cent), continuing care (11.0 per cent) and clinical services (10.0 per cent). In other words, the new money has been spent on the wrong things. Funds for forensic patients have been given marked preference over improving basic services.[27]

Hitting the Target but Missing the Point

More than half a century ago, Phillips speculated about the relationship of knowledge to stigma: 'the increased ability of the layman to identify certain behaviours as mental illness does not necessarily imply changes in the way he will act toward persons suffering from mental disease.'[28] Clinical experience has taught me that the A&E doctor who correctly identified psychosis among the behaving strangely cohort was never more empathic towards this group. Aimed at the public, from the biomedical corner, public talk of 'brain disorders . . . biochemical imbalances' was followed by a decade or so of raising awareness about mental health and well-being (whatever that is). It is hard to prove this hypothesis, but the more universally mental health has been discussed, and despite sound general advice (exercise more, value your friendships), the greater the distancing and neglect of people with SMI. A review of the literature has shown that the 'illness like any other' approach to the stigma of schizophrenia increases perceptions of violence and the public's desire for more social distance.[29]

'Beware Pity: It's About Parity'

More recently, and with fewer 'scares in the community' stories gaining media traction, we see new images, literally the stock photo images in print and online of what journalists/ subeditors think mental disorders look like – principally, 'headclutchers'.[30] These are individuals with their heads bowed, hiding their distress and their secrets in both hands, with fingers splayed. With a sense of mystery as to what led them to here and a loss of personhood, they evoke pity and discourage interaction with others. Anti-stigma campaigners have mounted a spirited response, and a BBC News account called for 'more sympathy (sic) for those affected'.[31] Even complementary newspaper articles that covered the former UK prime minister David Cameron's declared 'mental health revolution' in 2016 gave us another headclutcher.[32] This time, as usual, the money did not follow the rhetoric: anti-stigma talk was cheap.

My experiences of this decade in briefing journalists, lobbying in Westminster, and working with *some* trustees of UK mental health charities were similar. What I encountered was not rights-based, social justice mindsets but pity-led motivations. Perhaps as a short-term strategy asking for funding because 'these people have nothing' seems the only way to achieve what is needed. The public mood had changed (perhaps Jack Straw's 'letters from people' has evolved to censure in the social media) and 'these people' are now thought to deserve our sympathy and a better deal. However, listening to the warm words of journalists, politicians and charity grandees, there comes to mind Prince Lampedusa's response to Garibaldi's revolutionary campaign to unify Italy in the novel *The Leopard*: 'things must change so that they can stay the same.'

There is no need to read the stigma literature to know that high public perceptions of danger generate avoidance and more distance from people with psychosis. Equally, we would not like to be in a relationship or get a new job merely because someone felt sorry for us. Stigma-based discrimination is about social relationships, but those where there is a power differential (between stigmatiser and stigmatised): pity from powerful others is internalised and makes people more hopeless over time, just as it lowers self-esteem and has the potential to provoke depression.[33]

The employment example makes a wider point. Less than 15 per cent of people with SMI are in paid employment, lower even than low European comparisons. These scandalous rates are not about ability or potential; they reflect an abundance of employer sympathy ('this job might be too much for them') and a lack of empathy (to enquire of 'them' what adjustments might be needed, if any, to support them in this employment). We asked our early intervention patients with a recovered psychosis what they wanted. They said jobs, relationships and housing. Within the two multidisciplinary early intervention psychosis teams where I have worked with nurses, support workers and vocational rehabilitation specialists, I have seen many young people with psychosis achieve employment, often their first job. We assumed only that they would recover. On reflection, the very fact that we supported them to stay out of hospital, or the 'looney bin', helped employers see their potential not their deficits.

Pity Can Seriously Damage Your Health

Recent collaborations with ASH (Action on Smoking and Health) as part of the mental health smoking partnership have revealed another aspect of pity over parity. *The Stolen Years* report identified cigarette smoking as the main preventable cause of the seventeen-year average reduction in life expectancy among people with SMI. Seventeen years of life lost *and* the final years of life are blighted with cardiovascular disorders, stroke, respiratory illnesses and smoking-related cancers: the stolen years.[34] As mental health Trusts went smoke-free (banning smoking on their premises), some psychiatrists called for 'exceptions'. They cited human rights, but no one has a right to smoke in a hospital building. Next came the arguments that psychiatric patients were different from general hospital patients and that:

- 'I couldn't expect my patient to quit smoking during a crisis';
- 'If we grab their cigarettes, they will become violent'; and
- 'It's all they have . . . let them smoke'.

For me, this is three decades in one exchange: violence, pity and low expectations. In case I sound too severe, we do not ask people to give up (highly addictive) nicotine but are insisting that they do not smoke cigarettes in our hospitals. This is also about the rights of other patients and staff to healthy smoke-free environments. We provide nicotine replacement and multiple resources, including electronic cigarettes, as well as access to quit programmes that include varenicline. The evidence is clear: people with SMI want to quit just as much as any smoker and achieve high quit rates with the right options; and violence on psychiatric wards has reduced since the smoking ban.[35]

Conclusion

I was too young to interrogate my grandfather's response to the inhumane conditions cited in the Introduction to this chapter; was it pity or might it have been what Patrick Corrigan calls 'righteous anger'? Fifteen years after school made life hell for Jim, I met him when I was resident on call to the psychiatric unit where he had been sectioned (against his wishes). It was a quiet night for both of us and I made some tea. I did not tell him how sorry I felt for his life course, but I got the chance to apologise for my silence when others harassed him. He laughed it off and then told me some tales 'from the other end of the hypodermic needle'. The worst of his experiences were outside health services, and he set me on a path of learning about poverty and inequality.[36]

Effective community mental health services require an understanding of the communities we serve. This goes beyond cultural and subcultural beliefs. The community's main concerns (their safety, young people who self-harm, seeing 'homeless people' who look mentally unwell) will change over time. When governments and others exploit these attitudes, we (psychiatrists and other mental health professionals) need to call this out. The public wants to know and engage with psychosocial explanations of distress and mental disorders, even self-harm and suicide. Social psychiatry, now public mental health, encompasses an understanding of the factors (poverty and inequality, adverse childhood experiences, structural inequalities, discrimination and daily stress, etc.) that cause and perpetuate mental disorders. We must use this evidence to pursue prevention, ensure treatment plans are properly resourced and address underlying social causes of mental disorders.

Key Summary Points

- Historical fears of violence by people with mental disorders increased in the final years of the last century. Science demonstrated falling UK homicide rates by people with psychosis, but inaccurate perceptions drove UK government policy instead.

- As the public perception of violence subsides, we see increasing societal narratives of pity for people who lose their mental health; these will mostly serve to extend their exclusion and deepen inequalities. Pity makes people ill.
- Actions to highlight and reduce stigma and discrimination have softened some attitudes, but mental health awareness is no substitute for actual engagement with people who have mental disorders and sustainable funding for those that need state support (housing, income) or health services.
- Clinicians and partners in mental health reform have a duty to engage with local communities (and sometimes beyond) to achieve sufficient degrees of public engagement to prevent mental disorders by reducing the causes, principally poverty and inequality. These actions are just as important as providing fully integrated community mental health services.
- Parity of esteem is never having to say you are sorry (for someone) but to collaborate/advocate for their rights.

Notes

1. Personal communication (verbal) with Dr Mark Salter. See also P. W. Corrigan and B. Gelb, Three programs that use mass approaches to challenge the stigma of mental illness. Psychiatric Services (2006) 57: 393–8; P. W. Corrigan, A. C. Watson and F. E. Miller, Blame, shame, and contamination: The impact of mental illness and drug dependence stigma of family members. *Journal of Family Psychology* (2006) 20: 239–46; P. Byrne, Stigma of mental illness and ways of diminishing it. *Advances in Psychiatric Treatment* (2000) 6: 65–72; P. Byrne, Psychiatry and the media. *Advances in Psychiatric Treatment* (2003) 9: 135–43; G. Thornicroft, E. Brohan, D. Rose et al., Global pattern of experienced and anticipated discrimination against people with schizophrenia: A cross sectional survey. *Lancet* (2009) 373: 408–15.

2. Byrne, Psychiatry and the media.

3. J. Rabkin, Opinions about mental illness: A review of the literature. *Psychological Bulletin* (1972) 77: 153–71; E. Cummings and J. Cummings, *Closed Ranks: An Experiment in Mental Health.* Cambridge, MA: Harvard University Press, 1957.

4. Ibid.

5. Corrigan and Gelb, Three programs that use mass approaches to challenge the stigma of mental illness; Corrigan, Watson and Miller, Blame, shame, and contamination.

6. Corrigan and Gelb, Three programs that use mass approaches to challenge the stigma of mental illness; Corrigan, Watson and Miller, Blame, shame, and contamination; Thornicroft, Brohan, Rose et al., Global pattern of experienced and anticipated discrimination; M. Aichberger and N. Sartorius (2006); see the annotated bibliography of selected publications and other materials related to stigma and discrimination in *Publications (Books and Journals) of Members of the World Psychiatric Association's Section on Stigma and Mental Disorders (2006 to 2010)* as part of the World Psychiatric Association Global Programme to reduce the stigma and discrimination because of schizophrenia, www.queensu.ca /sites/default/files/assets/pages/principal/docs/WPAPublications2006to2010.pdf; M. C. Angermeyer and S. Dietrich, Public beliefs about and attitudes to people with mental illness: A review of population studies. *Acta Psychiatrica Scandinavica* (2006) 113: 163–79; A. H. Crisp, M. Gelder, S. Rix et al., Stigmatisation of people with mental illnesses. *British Journal of Psychiatry*, (2000) 177: 4–7; A. H. Crisp, M. Gelder, E. Goddard et al., Stigmatisation of people with mental illnesses: A follow-up study within the Changing Minds campaign of the Royal College of Psychiatrists. *World Psychiatry* (2005) 4: 106–13; L. Magliano, C. De Rosa, A. Fiorillo et al., National Mental Health Project Working Group: Perception of patients' unpredictability and beliefs on the causes and consequences of schizophrenia. A community survey. *Social Psychiatry and Psychiatric Epidemiology* (2004) 39: 410–16.

7. P. A. Garety, E. A. Kuipers, D. Fowler, D. Freeman and P. Bebbington, A cognitive model of the positive symptoms of psychosis. *Psychological Medicine* (2001) 31: 189–95.

8. Ibid.

9. A. W. Fominaya, P. W. Corrigan and N. Rusch, The effects of pity on self- and other-perceptions of mental illness. *Psychiatry Research* (2016) 241: 159–64.

10. Crisp, Gelder, Rix et al., Stigmatisation of people with mental illnesses.

11. D. Rose, G. Thornicroft, V. Pinfold and A. Kassam, 250 labels used to stigmatise people with mental illness. *BMC Health Services Research* (2007) 7: 97.

12. Thornicroft, Brohan, Rose et al., Global pattern of experienced and anticipated discrimination.

13. P. W. Corrigan, Lessons learned from unintended consequences about erasing the stigma of mental illness. *World Psychiatry* (2016) 15: 67–73.

14. J. H. Ritchie, D. Dick and R. Lingham, *The Report of the Inquiry into the Care and Treatment of Christopher Clunis*. London: HMSO,1994.

15. Ibid.

16. O. Bowcott, Jayne Zito: Why it's time to end the campaign. *The Guardian*, 17 May 2009.

17. Angermeyer and Dietrich, Public beliefs about and attitudes to people with mental illness; Crisp, Gelder, Rix et al., Stigmatisation of people with mental illnesses; Crisp, Gelder, Goddard et al., Stigmatisation of people with mental illnesses: A follow-up study; Magliano, De Rosa, Fiorillo et al., National Mental Health Project Working Group.

18. B. Cooper, Public health psychiatry in today's Europe: Scope and limitations. *Social Psychiatry and Psychiatric Epidemiology* (2001) 36: 169–76.

19. P. J. Taylor and D. Gunn, Homicides by people with mental illness: Myth and reality. *British Journal of Psychiatry* (1999) 174: 9–14.

20. Home Affairs Committee, *Managing Dangerous People with Severe Personality Disorder*, https://publications.parliament.uk/pa/cm199900/cmselect/cmhaff/42/4203.htm.

21. A. Feeney, Dangerous severe personality disorder. *Advances in Psychiatric Treatment* (2003) 3: 349–58.

22. Angermeyer and Dietrich, Public beliefs about and attitudes to people with mental illness.

23. Taylor and Gunn, Homicides by people with mental illness.

24. See Byrne, Psychiatry and the media. The fact that a serving Home Secretary did not know what psychosis is was also written up by Nicholas Watt in *The Guardian*: Watt, Bin Laden is psychotic, *The Guardian*, 6 November 2001, www.theguardian.com/politics/2001/nov/06/september11.uksecurity.

25. T. Babor, *Alcohol: No Ordinary Commodity: Research and Public Policy*. Oxford: Oxford University Press, 2010.

26. K. Bhui, P. Byrne, D. Goslar and J. Sinclair, Addiction care in crisis: Evidence should drive progressive policy and practice. *British Journal of Psychiatry* (2019) 215: 702–3, https://doi.org/10.1192/bjp.2019.158.

27. Goldberg lecture. Author's private collection. Goldberg makes similar comments and is cited in J. Turner, R. Hayward, K. Angel et al., The history of mental health services in modern England: Practitioner memories and the direction of future research. *Medical History* (2015) 59: 599–624, https://doi.org/10.1017/mdh.2015.48.

28. D. L. Phillips, Public identification and acceptance of the mentally ill. *American Journal of Public Health* (1966) 56: 755–63.

29. J. Read, N. Haslam, L. Sayce and E. Davies, Prejudice and schizophrenia: A review of the 'mental illness is an illness like any other' approach. *Acta Psychiatrica Scandinavica* (2006) 114: 303–18.

30. The quote in this section's subtitle is from Corrigan, Lessons learned. For examples of 'headclutcher' stock images, see the search results on Google Images for 'mental health stock photos': www.google.com/search?

source=univ&tbm=isch&q=mental+health+stock+photo&sa=X&ved=2ahUKEwju6p_q_KLrAhXlQUEAH
c6RAaYQsAR6BAgKEAE&biw=1513&bih=758.

31.   K. Hawkins, Mental health and the death of the 'headclutcher' picture. *BBC News*, 13 April 2005, www
.bbc.co.uk/news/blogs-ouch-32084441.

32.   T. Ross, David Cameron makes personal commitment to helping mental health sufferers. *The Telegraph*,
13 February 2016, www.telegraph.co.uk/news/politics/david-cameron/12156058/David-Cameron-makes-
personal-commitment-to-helping-mental-health-sufferers.html.

33.   Fominaya, Corrigan and Rusch, The effects of pity on self- and other-perceptions of mental illness.

34.   ASH (Action on Smoking and Health), *The Stolen Years: The Mental Health and Smoking Action Report*,
2016, https://ash.org.uk/information and-resources/reports-submissions/reports/the-stolen-years/.

35.   Ibid.

36.   P. Byrne and A. James, Placing poverty-inequality at the centre of psychiatry. *BJPsych Bulletin* (2020) 44:
187–90.

28

The Origins of the Dangerous and Severe Personality Disorder Programme in England

Peter Tyrer

It is lack of appreciation and understanding of this factor (psychopathic personality) which has often led to a great deal of prolonged, useless, faulty and even dangerous treatment.

David Henderson, 1951[1]

Introduction

The Dangerous and Severe Personality Disorder (usually abbreviated to DSPD) richly funded 'treatment' programme was introduced in the late 1990s by the then Labour government. It attempted to combine psychiatric diagnosis and treatment for severe personality disorder, but its main aim was public protection. Unsuccessful attempts were made to enshrine the 'treatment' programme in law. They met widespread resistance on human rights grounds by psychiatrists and other mental health professionals as well as service user–led organisations and all failed.

The exact origin of the concept of the DSPD programme remains an enigma. I will try to piece together the strands, focusing mainly on political actors, while appreciating that some will be left hanging in the air. What I hope to elucidate is that initiatives taken by government without the profession approving are rarely likely to succeed.

In this account, I am appreciative of all the contributions made by those listed in the Acknowledgements section of this chapter and also of the very detailed and scholarly account in Max Rutherford's *Blurring the Boundaries*, published by the Sainsbury Centre in 2010. This is one of a few documents published about the programme that can be regarded as completely unbiased. Most of the other published papers, including many from government sources, are tendentious and misleading. Although I would like to exclude our own published papers on the subject,[2] I feel even they, despite attempts to be neutral, have a tendency to overstate in their attempt to correct errors on the other side.

Early History

The story appears to start on 9 July 1996. Lin Russell, a mother aged forty-five, was walking home with her two daughters, Josie, aged nine, and Megan, aged six, and their dog down a quiet country lane near Canterbury in Kent after a school swimming competition.

Out of the blue, they were attacked. A man tied them up, blindfolded them and then beat them all indiscriminately. They all died apart from Josie, who after a rocky rehabilitation, has, gratifyingly, almost completely recovered.

The case was difficult to resolve, but in July 1997, Michael Stone, a heroin addict at that time on probation, was arrested and charged with murder. There is still great doubt that he was the murderer and Levi Bellfield, the man convicted of the murder of Milly Dowler in March 2002, has also been accused of the crimes.

The shocking case of Lin Russell and her family is said to be the stimulus behind the DSPD programme. Why was it that a man who was recognised to be unwell, with diagnosed antisocial or psychopathic disorder, was allowed to be at liberty and yet remain a big risk to the public. Psychiatrists regarded these people as untreatable, but were they right and what could be done to prevent it?

In all my enquiries, there has been one consistent feature in the timeline. It was the attack on the Russell family, followed by the widespread public reaction, that initiated the implementation of the DSPD programme.

Political Action between 1997 and 1999

In Chapter 9, I report on an interview with the former Conservative secretary for health and social services, Ken Clarke, who, while not involved in the Department of Health or the Home Office at this time, still knew a great deal about what was going on at the heart of government. He maintains that it was the Labour government who initiated the DSPD programme and that the earlier Conservative (John Major) government of 1992–7 had no part in this.

Yet it could be argued that this is not entirely true. Throughout the 1990s, in the context of psychiatric deinstitutionalisation, there had been concern in the UK about the number of homicides carried out by people with severe mental health problems. The frequency of such homicides was alleged to be increasing but analysis of official data showed the opposite; homicides had been reducing at the rate of 3 per cent per annum over many years.[3] It is not the purpose of this chapter to examine why the misleading impression was created but a considerable amount of responsibility can be placed on the publishers of tabloid news-papers who reported almost every homicide on three separate occasions: the time of the offence, the time of detention and a full and garish report of the trial. Because of the gap between each of these reports, the average reader would think that homicides were three times more frequent than they actually were.

Yet there had long been concern over the provision of services for mentally disordered offenders, and even Taylor and Gunn conceded: 'There appears to be some case for specially focused improvement of services for people with a personality disorder and/or substance misuse.'[4]

The Conservative government of 1992–7, in the last throes of its chequered existence, felt it had to do something to address the widely perceived notion that highly dangerous people were milling around the countryside looking for victims. They were in the same position as Mrs Ramsbottom, who, in the Stanley Holloway sketch,[5] following the unex-pected departure of her son Albert into the stomach of a lion, protested: 'Someone's got to be summoned! So that was decided upon.' This is not meant to be flippant. If there were going to be high-profile cases, the government needed to be able to point to action being taken.

The first summons came in the form of the Crime (Sentences) Act of 1997, introduced by the Conservative government but enacted by the Labour one. This introduced a new power for the courts, allowing them to attach a 'Hospital Direction' to a prison sentence. A new section was added to the 1983 Mental Health Act (45A) that allowed a prisoner to be moved to hospital from prison provided

(a) The patient is suffering from psychopathic disorder,

(b) The mental disorder (i.e. psychopathy) is of a nature or degree which makes it appropriate for the offender to be detained in a hospital, and

(c) Such treatment is likely to alleviate or prevent deterioration of the offender's condition.

The new Labour government passed this Act in 1997, but it is important to note there has always been a provision for prisoners to be transferred to hospital (currently sections 47–48). Section 45a was a hybrid order that authorised the court to send a sentenced prisoner directly to hospital and then on to prison if they became medically fit before the end of their sentence. The implication of a transfer to hospital was that treatment could be provided for the individual if the doctors agreed. This became 'the treatability clause dispute'. Put simply, the government's view was 'if a mental disorder exists and is treatable, why should this decision be left to psychiatric whim?'

Why the Treatability Clause Led Everyone Astray

When the Mental Health Act was passed in 1959 'severe personality disorder' was in nobody's mind but 'psychopathic personality' was prominent, mainly because of the influence of the Scottish psychiatrist and sometime president of the Royal College of Physicians (Edinburgh), David Henderson, who had done so much to bring it to public attention in his book *Psychopathic States*, published in 1939.[6] As it had such a powerful effect after twenty years, it influenced the wording of the Act, defining psychopathic personality as 'a persistent disorder or disability of mind (whether or not including sub-normality of intelligence) which results in abnormally aggressive or seriously irresponsible conduct on the part of the patient, and requires or is susceptible to medical treatment'. (It is important to note that this only referred to one of the three types of psychopathic personality that Henderson described: predominately aggressive; predominantly inadequate or passive; and predominantly creative.)

The problem was that this definition was, in the wording of its last clause, unworkable. It left unanswered a host of questions:

- Do all psychopathic personalities require medical treatment?
- Is psychopathic personality per se treatable?
- Do psychopathic personalities that are susceptible to treatment automatically require it (the ambiguous 'or' in the last clause suggests this is optional)?
- What does the Act suggest for those with psychopathic personality who are not susceptible to medical treatment?

It is this last question that led to much animosity. The argument came down to the level of psychiatric responsibility required for people with this disorder when not susceptible to treatment.

In 1998, Jack Straw, then Home Secretary, said on the BBC:

Twenty years ago psychiatrists were adopting what I would say what was a common sense approach to serious and dangerous persistent offenders. These days they have gone for a much narrower interpretation of the law. Quite extraordinarily for the medical profession, they have said they will only take on those patients they may regard as treatable. If that philosophy applied anywhere else in medicine there will be no progress whatsoever. It's time, frankly, that the psychiatric profession seriously examine their own practices and trying to organise them in a way that they have so far failed to do.[7]

Robert Kendell, then president of the Royal College of Psychiatrists, and well known for his plain speaking, responded robustly, if not entirely wisely under the circumstances:

'We are not very pleased with him, but even more important we are appalled by his ignorance. The Home Secretary cannot expect psychiatrists to do his dirty work for him.[8]

Yet Robert Kendell had an important point to make. Are all diagnosed patients required to be treatable and under care? One does not say to a palliative care physician looking after incurable patients, 'you are a physician, you have to treat these patients, you cannot just allow them to die, jump to it'. This broad generalisation also assumed that the responsibility for dealing with dangerous offenders lay mainly, if not entirely, with the medical profession.

The Joint Policy of the Department of Health and the Home Office

The focus on psychiatrists' practice only was soon realised to be a mistake and a joint approach was then suggested:

It is not just a problem for The Home Office but a problem for the Department of Health, for the prison service, for mental health services, and somehow or other we have to find a solution to that problem. The truth is we can only do that together.[9]

It was far from clear, however, who would lead on this. Someone had to take the initiative. It was Jack Straw at the Home Office, who recalls:

During my first eighteen months as Home Secretary I had seen a number of cases where obviously dangerous individuals were having to be released back into the community, notwithstanding the patent risk they posed, and the near certainty that they would commit further serious violence, because they had reached the end of their prison sentences, and could not be detained under the Mental Health Acts because their condition was not diagnosed as 'treatable'.[10]

Jack Straw also denied that the policy came from advisors as Ken Clarke has suggested (see Chapter 9):

I think you have to give the responsibility to the Labour government. The trouble is with policies like this is that you now have this semi-presidential system where everyone listens to advisers and so when public opinion gets sufficiently animated new policies are introduced without ever having been thought through.

Straw firmly contradicted this:

Ken is wrong in suggesting that this policy came from advisers, or from 'President' Blair. It came from me. I would have told Tony what I was doing, (probably in writing) but I don't recall any second-guessing from No 10. I was rather resistant to that, and in any event there was no need, as I was getting on to develop the policy.

He also underplays the influence of the health ministers in the generation of the programme:

At this stage I cannot say for certain whether I talked to Frank Dobson, but it is highly probable, as with Alan Milburn who took over from Frank in early 1999. I might too have discussed the matter with the Shadow Home Secretary. There was no reason why not.

In this area, support from the Conservative opposition was likely to have been forthcoming.

Straw also makes it clear that public protection was most prominent in his mind in introducing the DSPD programme and it was the Michael Stone case that initiated it:

> I thought (and still think) that it was irrational that whether someone really dangerous could be detained in hospital depended not on any objective analysis of the risk they posed to the public, but on the state of psychiatric understanding and diagnosis for the time being.

My recollection is that I initiated the review within government, probably prompted by concerns expressed in the Commons and in the press. I am pretty certain that the most prominent case was indeed the Michael Stone one.

Why Have a DSPD Programme When You Just Need to Change the Law?

The DSPD programme was bound to be coercive, although it is fair to add that, at its very beginning at HMP Whitemoor, the first prisoners volunteered for the programme. The normal process at this point is to change the law. I had a hint of this developing in March 1997. Ann Coffey, MP, then the Labour opposition spokesperson on health, was recommended to accompany me on my community visits in central London in March 1997. She said she wanted to see 'psychiatry in the raw'. This turned out to be rather more accurate than was envisaged. One of the patients we were visiting in Paddington was highly suspicious, banned the community nurse from seeing her and only allowed me and Ann to come into her basement flat, where the patient proceeded to take off all her clothes and run round the kitchen table saying she was a werewolf.

Afterwards Coffey and I discussed a new Mental Health Act being introduced if Labour came to power. She expressed concern about people with personality disorders not being covered by existing legislation and asked what the profession would think about this. I said I thought it would be unwise, as we already had too much coercion, and the conversation rested there. It was, however, clear as early as 1997 that there was a move towards legislation for this group. It was never enacted. Attempts were made to enshrine the DSPD programme in law but all failed. Why?

This is even odder to explain as, only a little further north in Scotland, perhaps still following the advice of their fellow Scot, David Henderson, they solved the legal matter expeditiously. As there was already a Crime and Punishment Hospital Act passed in 1997 (see above), psychiatrists could exercise discretion in regard to a 'hospital direction' (i.e. the transfer of personality disordered offenders to hospital from prison); and this was extended further by the devolved Scottish government by simply passing legislation to allow the detention of dangerous prisoners.

Conflict between Psychiatrists and Government

The government in England was in one way trying to be encouraging to the psychiatric profession by introducing the option of treatment programmes that could allow new approaches and ideas to be tested. Yet, by introducing the programme without proper consultation – in the end it was simply bulldozed – it was received very badly. Dr Dilys Jones, at the time medical director at the Special Hospitals Services Authority and clinical strategy director to the High Security Psychiatric Services Commissioning Board, was the main proselytiser of the advantages of the programme for both public protection and therapeutic gain, but she was in a very small minority.

The minister who bore the main brunt of the criticism was Paul Boateng, who was appointed parliamentary under secretary of state at the Department of Health in 1997 and subsequently minister of state at the Home Office and a privy councillor in 1999. He therefore had a foot in both the Home Office and the Department of Health camps and was well placed to defend the new programme. Yet, although he could be quite charming, he had a short temper and did not take kindly to being challenged by psychiatrists.

In my discussions with John Gunn, Emeritus Professor of Psychiatry, Institute of Psychiatry, Psychology and Neuroscience at King's College London, about these events, he fed back to me the essentials of a forensic faculty meeting in Cardiff where Boateng made it clear that the programme would be going ahead and if 'you won't play ball, we'll get the psychologists to do it'. A similar response was forthcoming at a subsequent debate at the Maudsley Hospital, as by that time the prospects of retreat had disappeared. The DSPD programme would go ahead and if these 'pesky psychiatrists' would not see its advantages they could peek in from outside and later take part if they behaved more reasonably.

Straw finally announced the introduction of the DSPD programme in January 1999:

> As to the future, my honourable friend the Secretary of State for Health has made it clear that alongside prison for those who are subject to serious personality disorder and to commit offences, and hospital for those who are categorisable under the Mental Health Act, we need a third approach, under which those who are suffering from severe personality disorders and pose a grave risk to the public can be kept in securer conditions as long as they continue to pose that risk.

The programme started at HMP Whitemoor and Broadmoor Hospital in 2001 and subsequently extended to HMP Frankland in County Durham. It was intended to include Rampton Hospital but this was abandoned. The initial cost was £128 million with operational costs amounting to £40 million per annum, and by 2010 it had cost £480 million. Jack Straw and Paul Boateng had their way and the treatment programme was developed and carried out almost entirely by psychologists using esoteric interventions that had no evidence base and whose outcome was not, and never will be, properly evaluated. The prison system still has a block when it comes to evaluation by randomised trials, even though we acknowledge they are difficult to carry out in secure settings. We carried out one but randomisation at times was deliberately overruled by prison staff because of 'operational requirements'.[11]

Cost-Effectiveness

One of the key aims of the DSPD programme at its outset was to make the intervention 'cost-effective'. This was a completely empty aim. The criminal justice system, at least at that time and almost certainly still at present, had no plans to carry out any form of economic evaluation worthy of the term, and the history of previous initiatives included only primitive measures of costs.[12] (This should not be tolerated now, and any future experiments of this nature will have to include a proper economic component, preferably carried out completely independently. Criminal justice is far too expensive to ignore its economics.)

Did the DSPD Programme Identify the Really Dangerous?

The government policy of identifying and detaining the 'really dangerous offenders' was given a further blow by a systematic review published by Alec Buchanan and Morven Leese in the *Lancet* in 2001,[13] which concluded that 'six people would have to be detained to prevent one violent act'. So, to prevent such acts, five out of six people would be inappropriately detained. This was a serious matter for human rights.

What Went Wrong?

In the late 1990s, there were no good links between the Royal College of Psychiatrists and the governments of the day and this impaired understanding and inhibited cooperation. Nevertheless, there was a vigorous response by the College coordinated by Mike Shooter (then president) and Tony Zigmond (vice president lead on mental health law) linked to the Mental Health Alliance formed to examine implications of a new Mental Health Act. Louis Appleby, the first national director for mental health ('mental health tsar'), appointed in 2000, was also involved; but although some in government may have listened, none were moved to intervene.

Vanessa Cameron, former chief executive of the College adds:

I do think the DSPD programme harmed the College's relationship with governments. With a few exceptions the College was rather amateur in its dealings with ministers. Things got better when during Sheila Hollins' presidency a Policy Unit, which included parliamentary monitoring, was created and professional staff employed.[14]

It is also fair to add that the later presidents of the College, Sheila Hollins and Dinesh Bhugra, were more mellifluous than Robert Kendell.

I personally think if there had been a minister of mental health at the time of the DSPD initiative matters might have turned out very differently. I think it very unlikely that such a programme could be introduced again without agreement with the key professionals who should have been intimately involved from the start. When one reflects on battles between governments and the doctors, there are virtually none in which the government has ultimately won. Ken Clarke managed to introduce the internal market to the NHS (see also Chapter 9) and did not give in to the British Medical Association (BMA) over pay, but he suffered greatly in his political standing in the process and probably scuppered his chances of becoming prime minister. The doctors then recovered their earning potential in 2004. In the DSPD programme debate, the doctors won in the end in that the programme was abandoned in favour of a much more modest offender pathway based in prisons. There is still room for compromise here, and how we combine public protection with psychiatric care effectively and humanely remains on the agenda. Until then, the statement by David Henderson at the beginning of this chapter remains just as true today as it was seventy years ago.

Conclusion

It would be wrong to say that the DSPD programme was a complete failure. It was a ridiculously premature experiment but it certainly improved engagement with prisoners, led to a serious review of the therapeutic environments of long-term offenders, which is described comprehensibly and well by Akerman and colleagues,[15] and focused attention on a very neglected group, if not always for the best reasons. It also helped to stress the importance of severity in the study of personality disorder, to the degree that a single dimension of severity constitutes the new classification of personality disorder.[16]

Through dint of careful planning and subtle manoeuvring, in which Alison Hooper (an unsung heroine from the civil service) played a very important part behind the scenes, funding was made available for the development of personality disorder services across England, and these now cover most of the country.[17] These developments still only provide a skeletal service in most areas, and many clamour for more, but I doubt whether they would have existed at all but for the DSPD programme. Perhaps if the acronym is regarded in the future as the Development of Services for Personality Disorder it will have achieved its best legacy.

Key Summary Points

- Throughout the 1990s, there had been concern in the UK about the number of homicides carried out by people with severe mental health problems. The frequency of homicides was alleged to be increasing but analysis of official data showed the opposite; homicides had been reducing at the rate of 3 per cent per annum over many years.
- The Dangerous and Severe Personality Disorder (DSPD) legislation and richly funded 'treatment' programme were introduced in the late 1990s by the then Labour government and aimed at the use of contrived psychiatric 'diagnosis' and 'treatment' to enhance public protection. The exact origin of the concept of DSPD programme remains an enigma but Jack Straw, secretary of state for the Home Office, and his Department played the leading role.
- The programme started at HMP Whitemoor and Broadmoor Hospital in 2001 and subsequently extended to HMP Frankland in County Durham. The initial cost was £128 million with operational costs amounting to £40 million per annum, and by 2010 it had cost £480 million in total.
- The legislation and 'treatment' programme were vigorously opposed by the Mental Health Alliance. The government policy of identifying and detaining the 'really dangerous offenders' was given a blow by a systematic review that concluded that, to prevent one significant violent act, five out of six people would have to be inappropriately detained.

Acknowledgements

The preparation of this chapter was a more complex assignment than first envisaged. I am particularly grateful to the politicians Jack Straw, Ken Clarke and Ann Coffey for their time and input and to Alastair Campbell for assisting in contacts. Max Rutherford's publication *Blurring the Boundaries* is a very balanced account of the history and context of the DSPD development and I have quoted extensively from this work. John Gunn, Tony Zigmond and Vanessa Cameron contributed valuable additions and corrections to the original draft, and the editors of his book have done so also, with aplomb. I am also thankful to my many colleagues who were involved in our own evaluation of the DSPD programme and gave me additional insights, particularly Deborah Rutter, Conor Duggan, Rick Howard, Barbara Barrett, Eddie Kane and Helen Tyrer. I have also had additional comments from colleagues in the prison service, who wish to remain anonymous, who inform me that the DSPD therapeutic programme is still active; the programme has not gone away.

Notes

1. D. K. Henderson, Psychopathic states. *British Journal of Delinquency* (1951) 2: 84–7.

2. P. Tyrer, S. Cooper, D. Rutter et al., The assessment of dangerous and severe personality disorder: Lessons from a randomised controlled trial linked to qualitative analysis. *Forensic Psychology and Psychiatry* (2009) 20: 132–46; P. Tyrer, C. Duggan, S. Cooper et al., The successes and failures of the DSPD experiment: The assessment and management of severe personality disorder. *Medicine, Science and the Law* (2010) 50: 95–9; P. Tyrer, R. Mulder, Y.-R. Kim and M. J. Crawford, The development of the ICD-11 classification of personality disorders: An amalgam of science, pragmatism and politics. *Annual Review of Clinical Psychology* (2019) 15: 481–502.

3. P. J. Taylor and J. Gunn, Homicides by people with mental illness: Myth and reality. *British Journal of Psychiatry* (1999) 174: 9–14.

4. Ibid.

5. M. Edgar, *The Lion and Albert* (Stanley Holloway Monologues). London: Francis, Day & Hunter, 1934.

6. D. K. Henderson, *Psychopathic States*. New York: WW Norton, 1939.

7. Jack Straw quoted in M. Rutherford, *Blurring the Boundaries*. London: Sainsbury Centre for Mental Health: 2010.

8. BBC News, Psychiatrists accuse Straw of ignorance. *BBC News*, 26 October 1998.

9. Alan Milburn, House of Commons Select Committee on Health, 2000, quoted in Rutherford, *Blurring the Boundaries*.

10. Jack Straw is quoted here and in what follows from personal communication between him and the author.

11. Tyrer, Cooper, Rutter et al., The assessment of dangerous and severe personality disorder.

12. B. Barrett, S. Byford, H. Seivewright, S. Cooper, C. Duggan and P. Tyrer, The assessment of dangerous and severe personality disorder: Service use, cost and consequences. *Forensic Psychology and Psychiatry* (2009) 20: 120–31.

13. A. Buchanan and M. Leese, Detention of people with dangerous severe personality disorders: A systematic review. *Lancet* (2001) 358: 1955–9.

14. Personal communication.

15. G. Akerman, A. Needs and C. Bainbridge, eds, *Transforming Environments and Rehabilitation: A Guide for Practitioners in Forensic Settings and Criminal Justice*. Abingdon: Routledge, 2018.

16. Tyrer, Mulder, Kim and Crawford, The development of the ICD-11 classification of personality disorders.

17. O. Dale, F. Sethi, C. Stanton et al., Personality disorder services in England: Findings from a national survey. *BJPsych Bulletin* (2017) 41: 147–53.

Chapter
29

Psychiatry and Mentally Disordered Offenders in England

John Gunn and Pamela Taylor

Introduction

In 1960, offenders with mental disorder were still sometimes treated by general psychiatrists but, more often, they were sent to prison, occasionally to special (high-security) hospitals where, in the 1960s, nursing staff dressed as prison officers. Consultant psychiatrists there were generally as isolated from mainstream psychiatry as their patients, neither specially trained nor recognised as trainers of future specialists. All that has changed.

In 1946, Aubrey Lewis became the first full-time professor of psychiatry at the Maudsley and took the Institute of Psychiatry into the University of London. He appointed first Norwood East, who gave lectures at the Maudsley before the war, and then Trevor Gibbens, returning from five years as a prisoner of war, as senior lecturers in 'forensic psychiatry'. Why 'forensic'? It is not what East wrote about – he was just treating criminals,[1] but the term has stuck. The East and Hubert report had advocated the development of a specialist psychiatric prison in England (Grendon),[2] although when it was finally opened in 1962 it did not, as he suggested, specialise in treating prisoners with psychosis but became a therapeutic community;[3] but he had long recognised the need to treat 'non-sane, non-insane' prisoners. They abound in every prison system in the world.

In 1960, the Department of Health recognised only two consultants in Britain as forensic psychiatrists: Trevor Gibbens, who became the first UK professor of forensic psychiatry, and Peter Scott, who was allowed to 'borrow' two general psychiatry beds at the Maudsley Hospital before acquiring a joint appointment between the Maudsley and Brixton prison, but this gave little scope for effecting prisoner transfers to hospital. Their clinical work was the assessment of juveniles who were before the courts.

The abolition of the death penalty in Britain allowed the proper development of assessment and treatment of offenders. The last executions were in 1964 and the death penalty was abolished even for treason in 1998. Until abolition, it was hard for psychiatrists to remain completely objective in reports for the courts, feeling, almost inevitably, involved in the grisly process of trying to save the lives of condemned individuals. Professor Denis Hill, an expert on epilepsy, assessed Derek Bentley, a young man with epilepsy and intellectual disability, who was hanged in 1953; though involved with a homicide, he did not actually kill anyone. This experience left Professor Hill determined to improve society's understanding of relationships between mental disorder and crime and to develop forensic psychiatry when he succeeded Sir Aubrey Lewis at the Institute of Psychiatry.

Professional Developments

In 1978, Trevor Gibbens's chair was established and, in 1988, an independent Department of Forensic Psychiatry was created at the Maudsley. Between 1990 and 2002, seven forensic psychiatry chairs were created around England, almost invariably funded by the NHS; but British universities were becoming business-oriented and their core funding was decreasingly available for developing academic subjects, like forensic psychiatry, which did not attract large grants. The Department of Health set up a Special Hospitals Research Unit in 1970, initially funding a special hospitals' case register but then, under the Special Hospitals Service Authority (SHSA), more wide-ranging projects and a new chair. As special hospital management was devolved, so the research monies passed into the National Programme on Forensic Mental Health. This both built knowledge and developed young academics across relevant disciplines, but success was rewarded with the removal of the protected streaming in 2007.[4] Since then, British academic posts generally have come under increasing threat,[5] thus hampering future research developments in psychiatry and, as a smaller specialty, forensic psychiatry is likely to suffer disproportionately.

The vision of specialist *clinical* development, however, began back in 1963, when the then two recognised forensic psychiatrists and thirteen others met, under the chairmanship of Dr Patrick McGrath, then medical superintendent of Broadmoor Hospital. They resolved to form a forensic subcommittee of the Royal Medico-Psychological Association. After the inauguration of the Royal College of Psychiatrists in 1971 this became a College section, holding its first two-day academic meeting in Birmingham, attended by tens of people. In 1997, it became a College faculty, now with an annual conference attendance of more than 400 people. Training continues, evolving alongside service development, with the three-year higher training curriculum under review at the time of writing.

Liberalising Legal and Institutional Systems

The Mental Health Act 1959, implemented in 1960, placed emphasis on voluntary psychiatric treatment. In 1961, the minister of health, Enoch Powell, launched the 'care in the community' policy – with one of his famous melodramatic speeches advocating the closure of hospitals and a drop in bed numbers of around 75,000 within 15 years.[6]

The care in the community ideal was that most psychiatric work would be done in the outpatient clinic or at home by visiting nurses, with rare need for short-term admissions to small general hospital units. This is probably the best approach if well-resourced and stable families can work with highly skilled staff, quickly available at any moment of crisis. It was hardly a novel idea. Towards the end of the eighteenth century, this is precisely how Mary Lamb was managed after killing her mother while psychotic.[7] Few families of people with severe mental disorders, however, have the emotional or social resources to do this and good community clinical care is expensive. Governments have never provided adequate resources nor apparently have understood the extent, complexity and durability of need. Worse, as care gaps opened in England, the then three special hospitals – Broadmoor, Rampton and Moss Side – were increasingly asked to take more patients, ironically because of the liberalising effect of the Mental Health Act 1959.[8] By the early 1970s, these hospitals were grossly overcrowded – with patients sleeping in corridors. A fourth was built – Park Lane (later combined with Moss Side, becoming Ashworth).

To some extent, such problems had been foreseen. In the same year as Enoch Powell's speech, the Emery Report recommended that regional hospital boards should include secure units in the range of local hospital provision – nothing happened.[9] In 1974, the Glancy Report recommended the building of a secure hospital unit in each NHS region of England and Wales, with approximately 20 secure beds per million population (about 1,000) – not implemented.[10]

Matters came to a head when Graham Young, admitted to Broadmoor hospital at the age of fourteen after poisoning several family members and perhaps suffering from autism, was released after nine years there.[11] His intense preoccupation with heavy-metal poisons continued, he found employment in a photographic works, with access to thallium, and he poisoned several colleagues. At his second trial, he was found fully responsible for his actions and imprisoned. The home secretary, Reginald Maudling, established two inquiries on the same day – an inquiry into discharge arrangements from special hospitals, to be chaired by Sir Carl Aarvold,[12] and a more wide-ranging inquiry into service provision, to be chaired by Lord Butler, a previous home secretary.

The Growth of Mental Health Services for Offenders

The Butler Report included recommendations for caring for and treating offenders with mental disorder.[13] The committee, which included Denis Hill, from the Institute of Psychiatry, other psychiatrists, a lawyer and a criminologist, found the overcrowding in the high-secure hospitals so serious that they issued an interim report in 1974, recommending a medium-security hospital unit for every health region, just as Emery and Glancy had done, but with twice the Glancy number of beds. Unlike its predecessors, the Butler Report was not ignored. The secretary of state for health and social services, Barbara Castle, accepted the urgent need and allocated funds for 1,000 medium-security beds. By 1978, some interim units had opened and, by the early 1980s, there was steady growth, although some regions resisted on the advice of their general psychiatrists, even diverting the money to general medical and surgical services. One real problem was training clinicians of all disciplines, especially psychiatrists, quickly enough to staff the units. By 1990, almost all regions had provided purpose-designed units.

The Butler Report is perhaps principally remembered for launching these developments, but it ranged much more widely. Around thirty years before Corston and Bradley,[14] it was advocating diversion from the criminal justice system for appropriate cases and calling for explicit care and treatment pathways. Frameworks for coercion and treatment contracts in the community were considered in depth; they expressed the need for research into the effectiveness of 'psychiatric probation orders', which applies also to their current counterparts – community sentences with treatment requirements. Indeed, Butler emphasised 'the need to plan evaluative studies as soon as any new regime or form of treatment has been decided on'. The report also said that '*the terms "psychopath" and "psychopathic disorder" are unsatisfactory*'. These have been removed from disorder classification systems and UK legislation, but they are still used casually and pejoratively. One recommendation belatedly taken up in the Criminal Justice Act 2003 was an indeterminate sentence for public protection (IPP). This proved to be a serious mistake and was repealed in 2012. A Channel 4 documentary, *Crime and Punishment*, captures the awful legacy of this experiment.[15]

A key recommendation that has borne fruit was on co-operation between professions. Forensic psychiatry embraced that most systematically under the Multi-Agency Public Protection Arrangements (MAPPA), introduced in the Criminal Justice and Court Services Act 2000 and strengthened under the Criminal Justice Act 2003. The Forensic Psychiatry Faculty of the Royal College provided guidance for clinicians.[16]

A further wide-ranging review,[17] chaired by Dr John Reed, included separate, supplementary reports on academic development, community treatment, finance, hospital provision, learning disability and autism, special service groups (e.g. women, under-eighteen-year-olds), prisons, research, people with special needs, staffing and training and services for people from black and ethnic minority groups. The enunciated principles still hold good:

> patients should be cared for [according] to the needs of individuals, as far as possible in the community, rather than institutional settings, under . . . no greater security than is justified by the degree of danger they present to themselves or others, in such a way as to maximise . . . chances of . . . an independent life, as near as possible to their own homes or families if they have them.

Also:

> there should be strong proactive equal opportunity policies relating to race and culture in all agencies involved. . . . ethnic minority communities should be involved in the planning, development and monitoring of services for mentally disordered offenders.

Elements of the review relating to people with mental illness and inpatient provision were generally followed through well. The Special Hospitals Service Authority assumed management of the high-security hospitals from direct Department of Health control between 1989 and 1996, before handover to local Health Trusts; the special hospital population was substantially reduced. The vision of better treatment of offenders with personality disorder was deferred to a new working group but that of reducing numbers of people with mental disorder in prison was not achieved. One recommendation has resonated forward:

> services dealing with mentally disordered offenders [should] take account of the needs of victims.

Perhaps inevitably, funding for the development of the new services created resentment among some other psychiatrists. Perhaps uniquely in the history of medicine, one pair called for forensic psychiatry to be *abolished*:

> forensic services, as they currently stand, primarily exist to fulfil political demands for a visible and coercive response to risk. . . . Meanwhile the poorly adherent, treatment resistant patients . . . come in and out of general acute wards, frequently abusing and hitting staff on their way . . . The reluctance of adult general psychiatry to accept low secure cases into this environment is often perceived as obstructive by forensic specialists. . . . General psychiatrists, in return, see forensic units as awash with resources and spoilt by the luxury of selectivity based on the specious definition of caseness.[18]

In fact, this outburst reflected old-fashioned attitudes towards mentally disordered offenders, implying that they should be treated in prisons,[19] and the problem that general psychiatry is under-resourced.

Prisons

While truly innovative work has occurred in prisons since 1960, the situation for the average prisoner has worsened. Grendon prison was opened as a therapeutic community in 1962, its first governor a senior prison doctor – William Gray. Essential criteria were that men had to volunteer and be violence-free or leave. Grendon was evaluated by the Institute of

Psychiatry;[20] prisoners were assessed before, during and after treatment. On all the main measures – psychiatric state, symptoms, personality and attitudes to authority figures and to self – large changes were found between the first and final assessments. At baseline, two-thirds of the men had clinically significant psychiatric disorder but just one-third at final assessment; cases of moderate/marked severity dropped from 37 per cent of the total to 18 per cent. Although criminal attitudes also changed substantially, a ten-year follow-up of reoffending was equivocal, but, of course, relevant continuation work had rarely been available to the men.[21] Subsequent studies confirmed positive effects.[22] That Grendon continues and a second therapeutic community was opened at Dovegate prison in 2001 also indicate success.

Other prison developments were less positive. In 1960, 25,000 people were in UK prisons. By 1972, there were 40,000 in England and Wales, when an Institute of Psychiatry study of their mental health needs found that about one-third were 'psychiatric cases'.[23] A second epidemiological study in 1990 suggested that about 45 per cent of the prison population needed psychiatric treatment, about 1,000 of them as hospital inpatients.[24] Later, an Office for National Statistics survey suggested that these figures were underestimates, reporting 7 per cent with psychosis, more than 60 per cent with 'personality disorder', 63 per cent with alcohol use problems and 66 per cent with other drug problems.[25]

By 2020, the prison population in England and Wales was about 83,000 but 40 per cent cuts to prison staff in 2013 in publicly run prisons in England and Wales undid some undoubted previous service improvements.[26] Following these cuts, prisoner suicide, self-harm and violence rates rose to the highest levels since recording began in 1978, with 57,968 incidents of self-harm in 2018/19 alone.[27] Her Majesty's Chief Inspector of Prisons (HMCIP), in his annual report of 2016–17, observed:

> By February this year we had reached the conclusion that there was not a single establish-ment that we inspected in England and Wales in which it was safe to hold children and young people.[28]

Qualitative evaluation of adult prisoner experience suggests that it is similar to the 'institu-tionalism' of the dying asylums.[29]

What was going well before this false cost-saving exercise? Prison officers had generally moved towards more truly safeguarding and respectful practices, perhaps a halo effect from the Grendon initiative. Indeed, HMCIP found this still true even when the environment was otherwise failing, citing 74 per cent of prisoners asserting they were being treated respectfully.[30] Medical services in prisons had changed radically. When the NHS was established in 1948, the prison medical service had remained separate and answerable to the Home Office. Standards of care were poor,[31] probably due to its isolation from the mainstream NHS.[32] In 2002, it was announced that budgets for health care in public sector prisons would be transferred to the Department of Health, with full commissioning responsibility to be devolved to primary care trusts in stages; this process was completed in 2006. In 2007, HMCIP concerns had shifted:

> When mental health in-reach teams rode to the rescue of embattled prison staff they found a scale of need which they had neither foreseen nor planned for.
>
> Four out of five mental health in-reach teams felt that they were unable to respond adequately to the range of need.

... [in prison] need will always remain greater than the capacity, unless mental health and community services outside prison are improved and people appropriately directed to them: before, instead of and after custody.[33]

The importance of a long-term, comprehensive approach was underscored in guidance published as the *Offender Mental Health Care Pathway*.[34] The Royal College of Psychiatrists set up a Quality Network for Prison Mental Health Services in 2015,[35] which many prisons have joined, and set up an 'enabling environments' award.

From 'Dangerousness' to 'Risk'

Until 1960, dangerousness was a popular concept in psychiatry. It was the preferred term for the Butler Committee in 1975, and the *British Journal of Psychiatry* carried Peter Scott's guidance for psychiatrists on 'assessing dangerousness in criminals'.[36] In the 1970s, criminologists were very interested in dangerousness, and the Howard League sponsored a report on it,[37] exposing flaws in attempts until then to measure dangerousness as an individual characteristic. The concept of 'risk' became more popular. Psychologists laboured to provide tools to help clinicians, but systematic reviews have pooled data to find their predictive value limited,[38] the popular psychopathy checklist (PCL-R) producing the lowest of all as a geographer,[39] working on the prevention of road accidents, observed:

Human behaviour will always be unpredictable; it will always be responsive to other human behaviour, including yours.[40]

Nevertheless, the psychologists' tools do give prompts, structure and transparency in coming to decisions. Providing that a risk assessment is used 'as an aid to clinical decision making and not a substitute for it',[41] in conjunction with appropriate risk management and regular re-evaluation, these tools are helpful, although we must remain mindful of advice from a US forensic psychiatrist:

A society sincerely concerned about reducing violence will seek broad measures that address both known risks for violence among persons both with and without mental health problems.[42]

Miscarriages of Justice

Forensic psychiatry and psychology in England became particularly concerned with false confessions after a 1972 incident in England when an eighteen-year-old with intellectual disability and two young teenagers were wrongly convicted of homicide or arson, largely on confession evidence.[43] A subsequent case series of sixty estimated that less than half of suspects have a normal mental state at the time of police interview.[44] A Royal Commission on Criminal Procedure followed, leading to the Police and Criminal Evidence Act 1984 (PACE).[45] This provided rules for police interviews, with a requirement for the presence of a 'responsible adult' in the event of mental illness or disability. Further serious miscarriages of justice followed, however, with a common thread of police under pressure to solve a notorious crime providing flawed evidence. The release of six men wrongly convicted of the Birmingham IRA pub bombings led to the 1993 Royal Commission on Criminal Justice.[46] James MacKeith and Gisli Gudjonsson provided clinical and research evidence for added safeguards.[47] A new Criminal Cases Review Commission was established.[48]

Psychological damage to victims of miscarriage of justice adds to the social turmoil and is particularly difficult to treat in the face of constant re-traumatisation as inquiries follow.[49] In personal experience of one case alone (PJT), hearings on compensation, inquiries into the miscarriage, criminal cases against lay witnesses and police and further inquiry into why the latter failed lasted nearly thirty years.

Victim-Centred Work

Recognition of the importance of work with victims of harmful behaviours has grown in terms of respect for their wishes and needs and also from the perspective of preventing further harms.

Countless studies have now linked adverse childhood experiences (ACEs) with later violence and/or mental disorder, but Cathy Spatz Widom pioneered prospective study relating to verified abuse.[50] The mystery is that about half of such children do not become violent – why? Caspi and Moffitt identified a moderating effect of MAOA-LPR polymorphism;[51] in the prospective Dunedin birth cohort study, 85 per cent of boys with a genotype conferring low MAOA levels who had suffered severe maltreatment became antisocial. In England, Walsh and colleagues showed the perhaps comparable vulnerability of people with severe mental illness to being violently attacked,[52] not unique to the UK.[53]

In 1985 Shapland and colleagues highlighted the travesty of treating victims of crime merely as witnesses.[54] Victim support services had been set up in the UK, probably the first in Bristol in 1971, but only tiny numbers of victims benefited.[55] The Home Office published a Victim's Charter in 1990, which established the centrality of victims' rights, and probation services developed expertise in victim support.[56] Eventually, the Domestic Violence, Crime and Victims Act 2004 put those rights into law and extended them to victims of offenders with mental disorder. Such victims have the right to know about tribunal hearing dates and to submit written or in-person evidence. For victims of offender-patients on Mental Health Act restriction orders, the system is adequate; but independent victim support is not guaranteed for unrestricted cases.

Over and above a duty of care to victims, we must learn from their experiences. The Crime Survey for England and Wales (formerly the British Crime Survey, now devolved) is a household survey giving a more accurate picture of criminal activity than criminal conviction statistics.[57] In psychiatry, we have learned from individual inquiries after homicide. These followed Jayne Zito's drive to have something of value emerge from her husband's killing in 1992 by a man with inadequately treated schizophrenia(see also Chapters 23 and 27).[58] The Zito Trust closed in 2009, considering its specific goals met; Hundred Families has taken up some of its roles,[59] including being a repository for individual inquiries after homicide. Early collective evidence from these confirmed that, even with hindsight advantage, perhaps only 25 per cent of the homicides could have been predicted, but two-thirds might have been prevented with adequate treatment.[60] This fits with a growing understanding that when psychosis confers added risk of violence it is when it is untreated.[61] Adequate, timely treatment is evidenced on economic grounds too.[62]

International Exchange

Services for mentally disordered offenders are, in some respects, more culture- and country-bound than other medical specialties. Law and practice and court structures differ even between constituent UK countries. A powerful instrument supporting positive change in the UK, however, has been the European Convention on Human Rights.[63] This has underpinned many legislative changes since 1970, including the right in mental health law to appeal against detention even after restrictions on discharge have been imposed by a criminal court.

Many countries have had to reappraise after some service lapses. In England, this has related mainly to high-security hospitals – Rampton and Ashworth both had inquiries after allegations of cruelty to patients and Ashworth again after finding children visiting a personality disorder unit.[64] The latter simply excoriated anyone even marginally involved, from the secretary of state on down. Another report on security at all three English *hospitals*, led by a former director of the prison service, resulted in controversial and high expenditure on extra walls or fences at two of the hospitals.[65]

As other countries faced problems, British experience was occasionally called in, for example when New Zealand had to respond to over-restrictive and impoverished practices in its then high-security hospital.[66] Service development followed on the Butler medium-security model – with relevant cultural modifications, from which we, in turn, now learn. In other areas, forensic psychiatrists themselves have identified service gaps and innovated. Paul Mullen left the UK for Australasia where, in addition to secure inpatient services, he set up specific problem-behaviour clinics for people who provoke avoidance behaviours in many clinicians – including vexatious litigants, the fixated, the morbidly jealous and stalkers.[67] This model has recently been brought back to the UK and developed further, for example in a National Stalking Clinic and new gaps met as required and spread further internationally.[68]

International academic collaborations have been fostered through the International Association of Forensic Mental Health Services from 2000,[69] showcasing interdisciplinary research worldwide, while in Europe the Ghent Group, established in 2004, provides support to psychiatrists assessing and treating mentally disordered offenders through an annual meeting discussing services, educational visits and a training programme.[70]

Conclusion

The period 1960–2010 has generally been one of growth for services for offenders with mental disorder. There have been errors and we are sensitive to ever present risks from both external threats and internal failings that could damage safety, trust and progress.

We have established the first charity dedicated to research in the field – Crime in Mind –.[71] The charity finds it difficult to attract funding for the same reasons that forensic psychiatry does not attract funding in universities but it has managed to start a small programme of seminars relating to research issues and even to develop small-scale research projects.

Key Summary Points

• By the 1960s, some psychiatrists had begun to specialise in work with mentally disordered offenders but the term 'forensic psychiatry' was not used anywhere except at the Maudsley Hospital. In the UK, such work has demonstrated a highly developed capacity for inter-agency working.

• In 1978, the first UK professorial chair was established and in 1988 an independent Department of Forensic Psychiatry was created at the Maudsley Hospital. Between 1990 and 2002, seven forensic psychiatry chairs were created around England, almost invariably funded by the NHS; but British universities were becoming business-oriented and their core funding was decreasingly available for developing academic subjects, like forensic psychiatry, which did not attract large grants.

- The Butler Report, in 1975,[72] included recommendations for caring for and treating offenders with mental disorder. A further wide-ranging review, chaired by Dr John Reed in 1992,[73] included separate, supplementary reports on academic development, community treatment, finance, hospital provision, learning disability and autism, special service groups (e.g. women, under-eighteen-year-olds), prisons, research, people with special needs, staffing and training and services for people from black and ethnic minority groups. One problem was training clinicians of all disciplines, especially psychiatrists, quickly enough to staff the units.

- In 1960, 25,000 people were in UK prisons. By 1972, there were 40,000 in England and Wales, when a study found that about one-third were 'psychiatric cases'. By 2020, the prison population in England and Wales was about 83,000 but 40 per cent cuts to prison staff in 2013 undid some undoubted service improvements. Following these cuts, prisoner suicide, self-harm and violence rates rose to the highest levels since recording began in 1978. Qualitative evaluation of adult prisoner experience in 2020 suggests that it is similar to the 'institutionalism' of the dying asylums.

- Psychological damage to victims of miscarriage of justice adds to the social turmoil and is particularly difficult to treat in the face of constant re-traumatisation as inquiries follow. Forensic psychiatry and psychology in England became concerned with false confessions. In general, recognition of the importance of work with victims of harmful behaviours has grown in terms of respect for their wishes and needs and also from the perspective of preventing further harms.

Notes

1. W. N. East, *Society and the Criminal.* London: HMSO, 1949.

2. W. N. East and W. H. Hubert, *Report on the Psychological Treatment of Crime.* London: HMSO, 1939.

3. J. Gunn, G. Robertson, S. Dell and C. Way, *Psychiatric Aspects of Imprisonment.* London: Academic Press, 1978.

4. K. Soothill, K. Harney, A. Maggs and C. Chilvers, The NHS forensic mental health R&D programme: Developing new talent or maintaining a stage army? *Personality and Mental Health* (2008) 2: 183–91, https://doi.org/10.1002/pmh.44.

5. Medical Schools Council, *Survey of Medical Clinical Academic Staffing Levels*, 2018, www.medschools.ac.uk/our-work/publications?Category=2265&page=1.

6. J. E. Powell, *Enoch Powell's Water Tower Speech*, 1961, www.studymore.org.uk.

7. K. Watson, *The Devil Kissed Her: The Story of Mary Lamb.* London: Bloomsbury, 2004.

8. P. Bowden, Review of Report on the work of the Prison Department, Home Office 1976 and Statistical Tables Cmnd. & Cmnd 6884, HMSO. *Bulletin of the Royal College of Psychiatrists*, 13–15 November 1977; T. Black, Broadmoor Hospital: A unique facility. *The Psychologist* (2013) 26: 908–10.

9. Ministry of Health, *Special Hospitals: Report of a Working Party* [Emery Report]. London: HMSO, 1961.

10. Department of Health and Social Security (DHSS), *Revised Report of the Working Party on Security in NHS psychiatric hospitals* [Glancy Report]. London: HMSO: 1974.

11. P. Bowden, Graham Young (1947–90); the St. Albans poisoner: His life and times. *Criminal Behaviour and Mental Health* (1996) Supplement: 17–24

12. C. Aarvold, D. Hill and G. Newton, *Report on the Review of Procedures for the Discharge and Supervision of Psychiatric Patients Subject to Special Restrictions*, Cmnd 5191. London: HMSO, 1973.

13. Home Office and DHSS, *Report of the Committee on Mentally Abnormal Offenders* [Butler Report], Cmnd. 6244. Final report. London: HMSO, 1975.

14. J. Corston, *A Report by Baroness Jean Corston of a Review of Women with Particular Vulnerabilities in the Criminal Justice System*. London: Home Office, 2007, www.newsocialartschool.org/pdf/Corston-pt-1.pdf; K. Bradley, *The Bradley Report: Lord Bradley's Review of People with Mental Health Problems or Learning Disabilities in the Criminal Justice System*. London: Department of Health, 2009, https://webarchive .nationalarchives.gov.uk/20130105193845/www.dh.gov.uk/prod_consum_dh/groups/dh_digitalassets/docu ments/digitalasset/dh_098698.pdf.

15. L. Martin, Crime and Punishment: What time it's on Channel 4 tonight and what to expect from the documentary series. *iNews*, 23 September 2019, https://inews.co.uk/culture/television/crime-and-punishment-when-its-on-c4-tonight-what-to-expect-from-the-doc-series-339167.

16. R. Taylor and J. Yakeley, *Working with MAPPA: Guidance for Psychiatrists in England and Wales*. Faculty Report No. FR/FP/01 2013, www.rcpsych.ac.uk/docs/default-source/members/faculties/forensic-psychiatry /forensic-fp-01–final2013.pdf?sfvrsn=a3c2ba8b_2.

17. Department of Health and Home Office, *Review of Health and Social Services for Mentally Disorder Offenders and Others Requiring Similar Services* [Reed Report], Cm2008. . London: HMSO, 1992.

18. T. Turner and M. Salter, Forensic psychiatry and general psychiatry: Re-examining the relationship. *Psychiatric Bulletin* (2008) 32: 2–6, https://doi.org/10.1192/pb.bp.106.009332.

19. Bowden, Review of Report on the work of the Prison Department; R. K. W. Reeves, Regional medium security units: Solution or disaster? *Bulletin of the Royal College of Psychiatrists*, Feb, 33–35, 1978.

20. Gunn, Robertson, Dell and Way, *Psychiatric Aspects of Imprisonment*.

21. G. Robertson and J. Gunn, A ten year follow-up of men discharged from Grendon prison. *British Journal of Psychiatry* (1987) 151: 63–38. https://doi.org/10.1192/bjp.151.5.674.

22. E. Genders and E. Player, *Grendon: A Study of a Therapeutic Prison*. Oxford: Oxford University Press, 1995.

23. Gunn, Robertson, Dell and Way, *Psychiatric Aspects of Imprisonment*.

24. J. Gunn, A. Maden and M. Swinton, *Mentally Disordered Prisoners*. London: Home Office, 1991.

25. N. Singleton, H. Meltzer, R. Gatward, J. Coid and D. Deassy, *Psychiatric Morbidity among Prisoners in England and Wales*. London: HMSO, 1998.

26. Ministry of Justice, *National Offender Management Service Workforce Statistics*, 2017, www.gov.uk/govern ment/collections/national-offender-management-service-workforce-statistics.

27. S. McAllister, *Prisons and Probation Ombudsman Annual Report 2018–19*. Open Government Licence CP175. 2019 https://s3-eu-west-2.amazonaws.com/ppo-prod-storage-1g9rkhjhkjmgw/uploads/2019/10/PP O_Annual-Report-2018–19_WEB-final-1.pdf.

28. HM Chief Inspector of Prisons, *Annual Report: 2016–17*. London: HM Inspectorate of Prisons, 2017. https:// assets.publishing.service.gov.uk/government/uploads/system/uploads/attachment_data/file/629719/hmip-annual-report-2016–17.pdf.

29. S. O'Connor, Z. Bezeczky, Y. Moriarty, N. Kalebic and P. J. Taylor, Adjustment to short-term imprisonment under low prison staffing. *BJPsych Bulletin* (2020) 44: 139–44, https://doi.org/10.1192/bjb.2020.2.

30. HM Chief Inspector of Prisons, *Annual Report: 2016–17*.

31. P. Scraton and P. Gordon, *Causes for Concern: British Criminal Justice on Trial*. Harmondsworth: Penguin, 1984; R. Ralli, Health care in prisons. In E. Player and M. Jenkins, eds, *Prisons after Woolf: Reform through Riot*. London: Routledge, 1994; HM Chief Inspector of Prisons, *Patient or Prisoner? A New Strategy for Health Care in Prisons*. London: Home Office, 1996. www.justiceinspectorates.gov.uk/hmiprisons/wp-content/upl oads/sites/4/2014/08/patient_or_prisoner_rps.pdf; J. Reed and M. Lyne, Inpatient care of mentally ill people

in prison: Results of a year's programme of semi structured inspections. *British Medical Journal* (2000) 320: 1031–4, https://doi.org/10.1136/bmj.320.7241.1031.

32.   R. Smith, Prisoners: An end to second class health care? Eventually the NHS must take over. *British Medical Journal* (1999) 318: 954, https://doi.org/10.1136/bmj.318.7189.954.

33.   HM Chief Inspector of Prisons, *The Mental Health of Prisoners: A Thematic Review of the Care and Support of Prisoners with Mental Health Needs*, 2007. www.justiceinspectorates.gov.uk/hmiprisons/wp-content/uploads/sites/4/2014/07/Mental-Health.pdf.

34.   Department of Health and National Institute for Mental Health in England. *Offender Mental Health Care Pathway*. London: Department of Health, 2005, https://bulger.co.uk/prison/mentalhealthpath.pdf.

35.   National Offender Management Service & NHS England, *The Offender Personality Disorder Pathway Strategy*, 2015, www.england.nhs.uk/commissioning/wp-content/uploads/sites/12/2016/02/opd-strategy-nov-15.pdf.

36.   P. D. Scott, Assessing dangerousness in criminals. *British Journal of Psychiatry* (1977) 131: 127–42, https://doi.org/10.1192/bjp.131.2.127.

37.   J. E. Floud and W. Young, *Dangerousness and Criminal Justice*. Cambridge: Cambridge University Press, 1981.

38.   A. Buchanan and M. Leese, Detention of people with dangerous severe personality disorders: A systematic review. *Lancet* (2001) 358: 1955–9, https://doi.org/10.1016/S0140-6736(01)06962-8; J. P. Singh, S. Fazel, R. Gueorguieva and A. Buchanan, Rates of violence in patients classified as high risk by structured risk assessment instruments. *British Journal of Psychiatry* (2014) 104: 180–7, https://doi.org/10.1192/bjp.bp.113.131938.

39.   J. P. Singh, M. Grann and S. Fazel, A comparative study of violence risk assessment tools: A systematic review and metaregression analysis of 68 studies involving 25,980 participants. *Clinical Psychology Review* (2011) 31: 499–513, https://doi.org/10.1016/j.cpr.2010.11.009.

40.   J. Adams, *Risk*. London: University College London, 1995.

41.   Department of Health, *Best Practice in Managing Risk. Principles and Evidence for Best Practice in the Assessment and Management of Risk to Self and Others in Mental Health Services*. London: Department of Health, 2007, http://webarchive.nationalarchives.gov.uk/+/www.dh.gov.uk/prod_consum_dh/groups/dh_digitalassets/@dh/@en/documents/digitalasset/dh_076512.pdf.

42.   D. Mossman, The imperfection of protection through detection and intervention: Lessons from three decades of research on the psychiatric assessment of violence risk. *Journal of Legal Medicine* (2009) 30: 109–40, https://doi.org/10.1080/01947640802694635.

43.   H. A. P. Fisher, *Report of an Inquiry by the Hon. Sir Henry Fisher into the Circumstances Leading to the Trial of Three Persons on Charges Arising out of the Death of Maxwell Confait and the Dire at 27 Doggett Road, London SE5*. London: HMSO, 1977.

44.   B. Irving and L. Hilgendorf, *Police Interrogation Research Study No 1. The Psychological Approach*. Royal Commission on Criminal Procedure. London: HMSO, 1980.

45.   Royal Commission on Criminal Procedure, *Report*, Cmnd 8092. London: HMSO, 1991.

46.   Royal Commission on Criminal Justice, [Runciman Report], Cm2263. London: HMSO, 1993, https://assets.publishing.service.gov.uk/government/uploads/system/uploads/attachment_data/file/271971/2263.pdf.

47.   G. H. Gudjonsson and J. MacKeith, Retracted confessions: Legal, psychological and psychiatric aspects. *Medicine Science and the Law* (1988) 28: 187–94, https://doi.org/10.1177/002580248802800302; G. H. Gudjonsson, *Suggestibility Scales*. London: Psychology Press, 2007.

48.   Wikipedia, Criminal Cases Review Commission.

49.   A. Grounds, Psychological consequences of wrongful conviction and imprisonment. *Canadian Journal of Criminology and Criminal Justice* (2004) 46: 165–82, https://doi.org/10.3138/cjccj.46.2.165.

50.   C. S. Widom, The cycle of violence. *Science* (1989) 244: 160–6, https://doi.org/10.1126/science.2704995; C. S. Widom and M. G. Maxwell, An update on the 'Cycle of Violence'. *National Institute of Justice Research in Brief*, February 2001: 1–8, www.ncjrs.gov/pdffiles1/nij/184894.pdf.

51. A. Caspi, J. McClay, T. E. Moffitt et al., Role of genotype in the cycle of violence in maltreated children. *Science* (2002) 297: 851–4, https://doi.org/10.1126/science.1072290.

52. E. Walsh, P. Moran, C. Scott et al., Prevalence of violent victimization in severe mental illness. *British Journal of Psychiatry* (2003) 183: 233–8, https://doi.org/10.1192/bjp.183.3.233.

53. L. A. Teplin, G. M. McClelland, K. M. Abram and D. A. Weiner, Crime victimization in adults with severe mental illness: Comparison with the National Crime Victimization Survey. *Archives of General Psychiatry*, (2005) 62: 911–21, https://doi.org/10.1001/archpsyc.62.8.911.

54. J. Shapland, J. Willmore and P. Duff, *Victims in the Criminal Justice System*. Aldershot: Gower, 1985.

55. R. I. Mawby and M. L. Gill, *Crime Victims: Needs, Services and the Voluntary Sector*. London: Tavistock, 1987; M. Hough and P. Mayhew, *Taking Account of Crime: Key Findings from the Second British Crime Survey*. Home Office Research Study No. 85. London: HMSO, 1985.

56. M. O. Rawsthorne, The probation service and victims of crime. *Criminal Behaviour and Mental Health* (1998) 8: 178–83, https://doi.org/10.1002/cbm.244.

57. C. Mirrlees-Black, *Confidence in the Criminal Justice System: Findings from the 2000 British Crime Survey*. Home Office Research Findings No. 137. London: Home Office, 2001.

58. J. Ritchie, D. Dick and R. Lingham, *The Report of the Inquiry into the Care and Treatment of Christopher Clunis*. London: TSO, 1994.

59. See Hundred Families website: www.hundredfamilies.org.

60. E. Munro and J. Rumgay, Role of risk assessment in reducing homicides by people with mental illness. *British Journal of Psychiatry* (2000) 176: 116–20, https://doi.org/10.1192/bjp.176.2.116.

61. R. Keers, S. Ullrich, B. DeStavola and J. W. Coid, Association of violence with emergence of persecutory delusions in untreated schizophrenia. *American Journal of Psychiatry* (2014) 171: 332–9, https://doi.org/10.1176/appi.ajp.2013.13010134.

62. M. Senior, S. Fazel and A. Tsiachristas, The economic impact of violence perpetration in severe mental illness: A retrospective, prevalence-based analysis in England and Wales. *The Lancet Public Health* (2020) 5: e99–e106, https://doi.org/10.1016/S2468-2667(19)30245-2.

63. European Court of Human Rights, *European Convention on Human Rights*, Strasbourg: Council of Europe, 2013, www.echr.coe.int/Documents/Convention_ENG.pdf.

64. Department of Health and Social Security, Report of the Review of Rampton Hospital, Cmnd. 8073. 11. London: HMSO, 1980; L. Blom-Cooper, M. Brown, R. Dolan, E. Murphy and Department of Health, *Report of the Committee of Inquiry into Complaints about Ashworth Hospital*, Cm.2028-1. London: HMSO, 1992; P. Fallon, R. Bluglass, B. Edwards, G. Daniels and Department of Health, *Report of the Committee of Inquiry into the Personality Disorder Unit, Ashworth Special Hospital*, Cm.4194-ii. London: TSO, 1999.

65. T. Exworthy and J. Gunn, Taking another tilt at high secure hospitals: The Tilt Report and its consequences for secure psychiatric services. *British Journal of Psychiatry* (2003) 182: 469, https://doi.org/10.1192/bjp.182.6.469.

66. K. H. Mason, H. Bennett and E. Ryan, *Report of the Committee of Inquiry into Procedures Used in Certain Psychiatric Hospitals in Relation to Admission Discharge or Release on Leave of Certain Classes of Patients* [Mason Report]. Wellington: Department of Health, 1988.

67. L. J. Warren, R. MacKenzie, P. E. Mullen and J. R. P. Ogloff, The problem behavior model: The development of a stalkers' clinic and a threateners' clinic. *Behavioral Sciences and the Law* (2005) 23: 387–97, https://doi.org/10.1002/bsl.593.

68. D. V. James, T. Kerrigan, R. Forfar, F. Farnham and L. Preston, The Fixated Threat Assessment Centre: Preventing harm and facilitating care. *Journal of Forensic Psychiatry and Psychology* (2010) 21, 521–36, https://doi.org/10.1080/14789941003596981; D. V. James, F. R. Farnham and S. P. Wilson, The Fixated Threat Assessment Centre: Implementing a joint policing and psychiatric approach to risk assessment and management in public figure threat cases. In J. Reid Meloy and J. Hoffman, eds, *International Handbook of Threat Assessment*. New York: Oxford University Press, 2014; A. Underwood, R. Key, F. Farnham et al., *Managing*

Perpetrators of Child Sexual Exploitation and Indecent Images of Children (IIOC): Understanding Risk of Suicide. London: Barnet, Enfield and Haringey NHS Mental Health Trust and NHS England, 2017, https://doi.org/10.13140/RG.2.2.35312.51204; F. R. Farnham and K. G. Busch, Introduction to international perspectives on the protection of public officials. *Behavioral Sciences and the Law* (2016) 34: 597–601, https://doi.org/10.1002/bsl.2266.

69.   See the International Association of Forensic Mental Health Services (IAFMHS) website: www.iafmhs.org.

70.   See the Ghent Group wesbite: www.ghentgroup.eu; J. Gunn and N. Nedopil, European training in forensic psychiatry. *Criminal Behaviour and Mental Health* (2005) 15: 207–13; P. J. Taylor, N. Wolfenden and N. Nedopil, Forensic psychiatry training in Europe. *Die Psychiatrie* (2013) 10: 181–7.

71.   See the Crime in Mind website: www.crimeinmind.org; P. J. Taylor, C. Chilvers, M. Doyle, C. Gumpert, K. Harney and N. Nedopil, Meeting the challenge of research while treating mentally disordered offenders: The future of the clinical researcher. *International Journal of Forensic Mental Health* (2009) 8: 2–8, https://doi.org/10.1080/14999010903014564; C. Duggan, Looking from the outside: No substitute for rigorous evaluation. *Criminal Behaviour and Mental Health* (2019) 29: 189–95, https://doi.org/10.1002/cbm.2129.

72.   Home Office and DHSS, *Report of the Committee on Mentally Abnormal Offenders* [Butler Report].

73.   Department of Health and Home Office, *Review of Health and Social Services for Mentally Disorder Offenders and Others Requiring Similar Services* [Reed Report].

Chapter 30

Community Psychiatry: A Work in Progress

Tom K. J. Craig

Introduction

The closure and reprovision of the hospital asylums in the last century led the fundamental transformation of psychiatric services across Europe, North America and Australia. Italy undertook the most radical change, barring admissions to public mental hospitals and replacing inpatient beds with community residential care.[1] The second fastest decant was in parts of North America where more attention went to closure than reprovision, with consequences of soaring numbers of mentally ill people in prison and of homeless on the streets of several major cities.[2] The British experience fell somewhere between the two, following a more gradual trajectory, doing quite well with reproviding for the asylum population but in trouble from the outset with how to manage the steady accumulation of new cases with multiple and enduring disabilities stuck on acute wards when transfer to the asylum was no longer possible. This chapter recounts some of the journey, focusing on the experience in England and Wales from 1960 to 2010. The major landmarks of this journey are summarised in Box 30.1.

Box 30.1 Major Landmarks in the Evolution of Community Psychiatry, 1960–2010

- **Launch of asylum closure, 1960–5:** Minister of Health Enoch Powell launches plans to replace hospital asylums with 60 beds per 100,000 population located in new district general hospitals (DGHs), with most mental illness managed in the community.[3] Encouragement from psychiatrists.[4]

- **Reconfiguration and aspirations, 1966–75:** Generic social work and 'sectorisation' aim at integrated care focused on the same population. Aspirational White Paper *Better Services for the Mentally Ill* published but stalls in context of NHS reorganisation and political upheaval.[5]

- **Expansion of community care but cracks appear, 1976–86:** Increased collaborative mental health services in primary care;[6] first Community Mental Health Centre (CMHC) opens.[7] Concerns that these developments are at the expense of people with severe mental illness. Health and local authority staff in community and residential services reluctant/unable to manage challenging behaviour and 'new long-stay' patients accumulate.[8] First asylum closes in 1986.

- **Fear and loathing, 1987–96:** Asylum closures accelerate with mostly beneficial outcomes for the resettled patients,[9] but increasing criticism by the public, media and politicians of mental health services' failure to provide adequate supervision for new cases requiring long-term care.[10] Introduction of care programme approach aimed at providing better management of risk.[11] NHS

---

reorganisation establishes NHS Trusts that are no longer coterminous with local authorities.

- **Specialisation of community care, 1997–2010:** Fears continue. Mental health staff pulled back to secondary care; National Service Framework (NSF) reconfigures Community Mental Health Teams (CMHTs) to provide assertive outreach (AO), early intervention and crisis resolution home treatment teams,[12] resulting in considerable service disruption and fragmentation; Mental Health Act revised to include Community Treatment Orders (CTOs). Introduction of IAPT (Improving Access to Psychological Therapies) services increases provision of psychological therapy for common mental disorders.[13] World economic crisis in 2008 and the subsequent austerity programme fell heavily on social care.

Closing the Asylum

The impetus for closing the hospital asylum and providing treatment close to where people live came from a combination of optimism, disquiet and financial concerns: optimism among psychiatrists who found that the introduction of social and occupational therapies and the advent of chlorpromazine allowed them to unlock the hospital doors, do away with physical restraint and close long-stay beds, successfully discharging patients to outpatient clinics and day hospitals;[14] moral outrage at the conditions in some asylums fuelled by empirical findings that many behavioural problems among incarcerated patients were consequences of institutional life;[15] and, finally, the cost of maintaining the old asylums that became difficult to justify as the model of care was increasingly discredited.

In 1961, the minister of health, Enoch Powell, addressed the National Association of Mental Health at its annual conference, in which he included all these themes and called on psychiatrists and wider health and welfare bodies to provide the variety of community services for people whose needs were 'little short' of what only a hospital could provide (see also Chapter 1).[16] Anticipating his speech, a report estimated that bed requirements could fall by as much as 70,000 by 1975.[17] The old asylums would be replaced by a network of district general hospitals (DGHs), each serving a population of around 100,000 with up to 60 beds supported by group homes, day centres and mobile teams, models of which were already emerging around the country. At Warlingham Park, in Surrey, the first community nursing posts were established to support patients discharged from the asylum (see also Chapter 31).[18] In Manchester, Maurice Silverman described a district service that prioritised outpatient clinics, domiciliary visiting and day care, relying on just 100 inpatient beds for a population of 254,000. Four out of eight psychiatrists in Manchester, each serving a population of approximately 250,000, said they no longer needed the large mental hospital.[19] In 1968, a reorganisation of social services recommended bringing together all providers of personal social care into new social services departments in local authorities and principles of 'sectorisation' were introduced in which health and social care focused on the same local population.

Powell had estimated a closure and modernisation process lasting fifteen to twenty years but in fact it all took much longer. A great deal of the delay had to do with the worsening economic situation and industrial unrest through the 1970s and 1980s. Successive governments struggled to cope with strikes by coal miners, ambulance drivers, grave diggers and refuse collectors. Along the way, a reorganisation of the NHS (amusingly described as written in incomprehensible 'mandarin managerial English')[20] contributed to the loss of senior managerial posts and amplified disquiet among nursing and medical staff (see also Chapter 12).[21] Consultants complained that they were being made to do more work with less support; nurses marched in protest over low wages and against private health care; and senior medical staff took medical action, 'working to rule' for almost four months. Somewhat surprisingly, amidst this chaos, Barbara Castle, Labour minister of health, published a White Paper, *Better Services for the Mentally Ill*,[22] setting out a vision for future community mental health care. Economic circumstances meant little of this could be realised. Pioneering studies such as those in Manchester proved difficult to replicate, not least because of the paucity of residential and day care capable of managing challenging behaviours (see also Chapter 26). Local authorities struggled with competing priorities, including improving children's services, while some of the funding allocated to mental health ended up bailing out financial crises in general hospitals. Asylum discharges to that point had largely been of the more able patient, with surveys reporting that several hundred patients identified for discharge remained in hospital.[23] Furthermore, as the impetus to close the asylums gathered pace, the option to transfer patients from the acute ward to long-term asylum care was cut off. While it was possible to shorten the length of hospitalisation for acute illness and manage some patients in acute day hospitals,[24] no new treatment had prevented the accumulation of people with persistent illness that now comprised up to a third of people in the new DGH psychiatric facilities, stuck there for a year or longer.[25]

By 1980, asylum reprovision had become the government's top health priority and pressure was put on regions to close and sell off the old hospital sites as the only way to free up resources to fund new community facilities. The first asylum to close was Banstead Hospital in 1986 and thereafter the quickening pace soon became an end in itself. Most closures followed the same 'train and place' approach in which patients practised various aspects of managing life in the community followed by placement in small groups into ordinary houses, accompanied by staff from the asylum who provided supervision at least daily and in some instances up to twenty-four hours. The homes were intended 'for life' – then considered a very important reassurance and safeguard. This resettlement process was evaluated in a longitudinal study of the closure of Friern Barnet and Claybury hospitals in north London.[26] Although patients showed little change in symptoms or behaviour, most preferred being out of hospital and had significant gains in terms of social and domestic skills, social networks and living conditions. Fears that the move might be associated with higher mortality and homelessness were not realised, although 38 per cent had subsequent readmissions with a third of these having very lengthy hospitalisations. Even the small number of patients with challenging behaviours who were initially transferred to secure accommodation on the edge of the old hospital site did well, many moving on to community group homes.[27]

Despite these positive results, there were concerns that employing ex-institutional staff to support patients simply perpetuated institutional practices that could only be solved by bringing in a new workforce not contaminated by history, while the notion of providing a 'home for life' was soon abandoned. On the other hand, there were 'not in my backyard' protests and opposition to resettlement by people anxious about the impact on the values of their properties and of risks to their children. These fears were fuelled by the practice (on grounds of confidentiality but also an attempt to avoid confrontation) of not giving neighbours prior notice before patients were moved to their new homes. An experimental programme showed that openness and preparation of neighbours resulted in greater acceptance and integration but came too late to have much effect on policy.[28] Finally, with hospital closures, many of the occupational and sheltered employment schemes provided by the old asylums also ended and were not replaced, leaving many patients idle and lonely.[sup29]

By 1993, just over a quarter of the 130 large asylums in England had closed and beds for mental illness had fallen by two-thirds to 50,278.[30] Yet pressures on acute inpatient beds continued unabated. Occupancy levels were frequently well above 100 per cent and patients were admitted to private hospitals that had seen the business opportunity and stepped in to plug the gap.

Community Care Takes Off

As outpatient services developed, some psychiatrists started running clinics in primary care or provided a consultation-liaison service to general practitioners. Some mental health professionals, particularly community psychiatric nurses, were seconded or directly employed in primary care.[31] Brief psychological therapies for common mental disorders, including counselling and behavioural and cognitive therapies, were increasingly available across professional groups.[32] Extending support to primary care was popular with general practice and some models had good empirical support, including reductions in hospital admission.[33] The approach also chimed with views that lay behind asylum closure, notably that mental health care would best progress when delivered in non-institutional, non-stigmatising settings by staff not tainted by the institution.

Later controlled trials confirmed the benefit of these approaches in primary care and, in many respects, were the success story of community mental health. In practice, however, they were overtaken by a different model that was shaped by concerns about failures in the management of severe mental illness. Borrowing a model from the United States, the first Community Mental Health Centre was established in south London with a generous grant from the Gatsby Charitable Foundation. Opened in 1978, the Mental Health Advice Centre (MHAC) comprised a multidisciplinary team based in a deliberately non-descript community location. It provided referral and walk-in access for anyone with mental health problems living in the local catchment area.[34] The service model was soon replicated elsewhere, with similar centres doubling in number in England every two years and with eighty-one centres open by 1987.[35] Yet the approach was not without problems. The walk-in service was swamped by people seeking help for problems of daily life, arguably at the expense of severe mental disorders.[36] A survey of the fate of people with severe mental illness, including those in the catchment area of the MHAC, found half continuing to experience severe symptoms and behavioural problems with, paradoxically, the least well-functioning receiving the lowest level of support.[37]

Concerns from politicians, the press and the public about psychiatry's apparent inability to manage risk accelerated through the 1990s as people with severe mental illness became much more visible in the community. Managing severe mental illness in the asylum had been relatively easy. Patients were in one geographical location, moved between the ward and on-site or nearby supervised occupational facilities, and institutionalisation was reflected in compliance with treatment and the asylum regime. It proved much more difficult to keep track of vulnerable patients in the community. There was a conspicuous rise in the number of homeless mentally ill people, attributed by some to the asylum closure programme but actually reflecting the revolving door 'new long-stay' population, changes to housing benefit regulations introduced by the Thatcher government and a less widely acknowledged closure of several large direct-access hostels in which many people with chronic mental disorders had long-term shelter.[38] In 1992, Christopher Clunis, suffering from paranoid schizophrenia and with a long history of repeated admissions, interspersed with poor engagement with outpatient services, stabbed a stranger in the eye, killing him – just one of 39 homicides and 240 suicides by severely mentally ill people in the subsequent 3 years (see also Chapters 23 and 27). A report of a confidential inquiry into these tragedies concluded that many might have been prevented if patients had been adequately supervised. Communication failures, confusion about responsibilities and inadequate use of care plans were all cited as contributory factors.[39] The Department of Health issued guidance establishing the 'care programme approach for people with a mental illness' in which patients in the community had detailed health and social care plans overseen by a named member of a Community Mental Health Team (CMHT).[40]

To cope with the demand, CMHTs revised their offer for common mental disorders, limiting access to people already known to the teams or by formal referral from general practice and pulling back staff working in primary care. Some CMHTs split into two sub-teams, one focused on assessment and treatment of common mental disorders and the other taking on the care co-ordination role for severe mental illness. Studies confirmed that patients preferred the less stigmatising CMHT over more traditional outpatient clinics, co-ordination across health and social care was improved and there were reductions in hospitalisation, resulting in lower costs.[41] In time, the CMHT model expanded to provide specialist services such as in-reach to hostels for the homeless, with this early work leading ultimately to the DH-funded Homeless Mentally Ill Initiative, which established specialist multidisciplinary teams for homeless people, some of which survive to this day (see also Chapter 26).[42]

Yet, despite evidence for the benefit of CMHTs, they still seemed unable to do anything to prevent continuing tragedies among a few patients. The DH guidance on care co-ordination was strengthened in 1995 to give the supervising clinician the right to convey people to hospital if necessary. In the meantime, in the United States, one model of co-ordinated care became hugely influential. This 'Assertive Community Treatment' (ACT), provided 24-hour support, 7 days per week, ensuring that patients were maintained on medication and received appropriate support for daily living. Community members (family but also police and landlords) were given advice and direction on how to support the individual and, where necessary, an individual was helped to leave unhelpful relationships. A clinical trial comparing this approach to usual care proved ACT to be cost-effective, with patients in the experimental arm spending less time in hospital and with better overall clinical and social functioning.[43] Around the same time, in Australia, another controlled study diverting acute patients from hospital to 24-hour crisis and aftercare support by a community team also showed significant reductions in hospitalisation.[44] In England, a research team at the Maudsley Hospital attempted to replicate these findings. Patients at the point of an acute admission were randomised to either hospitalisation and routine care or to experimental home-based care with assertive community support. Outcomes over eighteen months were superior in the experimental service, considerably reducing hospital admissions and length of stay, but the positive results were overshadowed by a tragic homicide in the experimental arm and, perhaps for this reason, the study did not achieve the influence it deserved.[45] Instead, other studies focused on aspects of the ACT model (the size of team caseload or recruitment of patients outside of acute crisis) and failed to show comparable benefit.[46]

Alongside these studies, prompted by concerns about whether new community staff had the skills they required for the job, attention was given to training the multidisciplinary team. Most CMHTs included psychologists and other professionals with skills in the delivery of cognitive behavioural therapy (CBT) and other psychological therapies but few of these were developed for the care of severe mental illness. New interventions seemed to offer some hope. These included 'compliance therapy', based on motivational interviewing techniques that in studies had achieved improvements in insight and medication adherence; family interventions that reduced relapse, and CBT for psychosis. Drawing on these, a postgraduate training course, the Thorn nurse training initiative, was established in London and Manchester to equip community psychiatric nurses with specific skills in risk assessment, medication management, family intervention and how to support aspects of daily living.[47] The principles of the course were taken up in several centres around the UK but, despite some early success, services struggled to maintain these interventions once the supervision and support provided by the training courses were stopped (see also Chapter 19).

The Specialisation of Community Care

In 1998, Frank Dobson, the then health secretary, responded to continuing public concern about dangerous mentally ill people in the community by saying he would introduce new regulations to increase places in secure units and change the law to give mental health professionals new Community Treatment Orders (CTOs) to enforce treatment and 'sweep the mentally ill off the street'.[48] At the same time, and at odds with the idea that mental health teams were not being sufficiently proactive, it was increasingly apparent that there were discrepancies in both the incidence and the treatment response for psychotic disorders between black minority ethnic groups and the indigenous white British population. Not only was incidence considerably higher but people from these backgrounds were more likely to be compulsory hospitalised and to access services through the criminal justice system.[49] There were challenges of bias in the diagnostic judgement of psychiatrists and allegations that the high rates of incarceration and coercion reflected institutional or even frank racism (see also Chapter 35).[50]

In 1999, the DH produced a National Service Framework (NSF) that recommended training psychiatrists in cultural awareness and introduced new specialist teams to better manage risk while reducing reliance on hospitalisation (see also Chapters 10, 23 and 27).[51] These new teams included assertive outreach (AO) based on ACT principles, 24-hour crisis resolution and home treatment as an alternative to acute hospital admission and dedicated early intervention services (EIS) for first-episode psychosis. At the time of publication of the NSF, there was scant evidence from UK research for any of these services. The NSF arrived with some force behind it. National groups of experts and champions formed to steer implementation and, at a local level, services went through a protracted and disruptive period of reconfiguration. Not only was there the challenge of identifying staff for the new service but it was also blindingly obvious that some kind of generic CMHT provision would have to persist, perhaps comprising those clinicians who, for whatever reason, had not made the cut for a position in one of the new specialist services.

The new services introduced structural discontinuities in care that were most likely bad for patients. Those with a first episode of psychosis would receive care from the new specialist early intervention team to a maximum of three years before transfer to the CMHT; people who engaged poorly with the CMHT were to be taken over by a specialist AO team but transferred back to the generic CMHT once adherent with treatment; and those in crisis saw different clinicians from those usually involved in their care – all as though the personal relationship developed with a staff member was inconsequential. These services also fuelled an existing trend for psychiatrists to be dedicated to inpatient or community services, radically changing the traditional approach in which patients were under the care of a consultant psychiatrist across both hospital and community. With the greater resource going to managing severe mental illness, CMHTs increasingly offered only time-limited courses of treatment for people with non-psychotic disorders and tried to maintain links with primary care through 'link workers' but, in practice, also focused on the most disabled and troubling patients.

Earlier scepticism about the value of ACT in the UK was reinforced by a controlled trial that failed to show AO had any advantage in terms of hospitalisation over that achieved by CMHT care,[52] and a systematic review concluded that well-resourced CMHTs persistently matched AO outcomes in the UK.[53] Many of the patients that ended up in AO teams had problems with substance abuse in addition to mental ill health. It was hoped that integrating treatments for both disorders within an AO model would be more effective than treatment by separate services but neither this integrated approach nor a much more intensive intervention of combined psychological therapies made any substantial impact on outcomes.[54] In contrast, EIS did reduce rehospitalisation and improve clinical and social functioning.[55] Ultimately, AO services disappeared from many parts of the country while EIS expanded albeit with concern that resources were being diverted from long-term care. Establishing the Crisis Resolution teams took longer, often starting with the rather easier task of facilitating discharge rather than the intended but much more challenging task of diverting the acute admission itself. Eventually, however, the model did get going and amassed some evidence in the UK.[56]

By the end of our epoch, the general public were far more accepting of the idea that mental health problems were common, could be spoken about and could be effectively treated. New models for delivering psychosocial help for common mental disorders emerged, notably Improving Access to Psychological Therapies (IAPT),[57] and for severe mental illness, new models of occupational support (particularly for paid work; see also Chapter 33)[58] as well as more proactive housing support encouraged progress towards independence, albeit with no evidence by way of controlled clinical trials.[59]

Dobson's proposals for CTOs eventually found their way into law, though in a less draconian form than originally envisaged. Even before their introduction, international research suggested these approaches had little benefit in terms of reduced rates of rehospitalisation or treatment adherence,[60] a view supported by a later UK study.[61] The policy also did little to halt a continuing growth in incarceration in forensic and other long-stay secure accommodation.[62] Involuntary hospitalisation, originally expected to shrink, instead increased with more rather than less use of locked doors and seclusion.[63] Important efforts to counterbalance coercion by greater involvement of patients in their care, including, for example, early experiments with the use of joint crisis care plans to reduce compulsion, peer support and 'personal recovery',[64] emerged to be further developed in the subsequent decade. In 2008, an international financial crisis originating in the United States put paid to much further development, particularly in social care.

Conclusion

There is little doubt that community care increased the 'reach' of psychiatry to bring effective treatments to much larger numbers of people in the wider population, sometimes at the risk of accusations that it has encouraged inappropriate medicalisation of the woes of everyday life. If that is one concern, the opposite is the accusation that psychiatry still relies too much on hospital care. Closing the asylum did not guarantee the elimination of institutional care, which remained in the longer-stay rehabilitation units and group homes that replaced the asylum. If added to residential forensic care and mentally ill people in prison, it has been argued that there are now as many people in some form of incarceration as there were in the old hospitals. Changes are also seen in the use of acute inpatient care where the rates of involuntary admissions have steadily risen since the mid-1980s, possibly due to reductions in acute beds or to changes in tolerance of risk among community teams.[65]

As noted by some of the earliest commentators, there is very little appetite in health or social care providers to develop to-scale community residential alternatives to hospitals to the extent done in Italy. There have been a few implementations of crisis houses,[66] but, typically, these have been for special patient groups not considered at particularly high risk or requiring involuntary care, some of whom would not be hospitalised in any event. Challenging behaviour is still viewed as too risky to be managed in community units, not least because of fears of getting hold of a sufficiently rapid and robust response in an emergency, with the result that, to this day, the model has never caught on as a serious alternative to acute hospitalisation. Similarly, while there are some rehabilitation units that can provide secure care, there is a reluctance to expand provision, as they are viewed as perpetuating institutionalisation. If mental health services should proceed, like in Italy, to radically reduce hospital care, it would need to do this 'at scale' with the full backing of authority and increased tolerance of risk. Such a development is yet to emerge.

Key Summary Points

- The closure of the old hospital asylums in Britain was driven by psychiatric optimism; moral outrage at overcrowding and poor quality of care; and concerns about the cost of maintaining the old buildings. Initial results were promising, and patients discharged from the asylum experienced a better quality of life with few adverse outcomes. At the same time, mental health care became more multidisciplinary and reached out to people with less disabling conditions.
- Problems emerged when the asylums could no longer accept new referrals of people with enduring disability whose needs for care were publicly visible and who were stuck on acute wards. Community residential facilities were unwilling to accept people with challenging behaviours.
- The prevailing social model was one of a progressive movement towards independence that spoke against the provision of long-stay accommodation. This left ambulatory mental health teams to provide intensive support that nevertheless failed to prevent tragedies, including suicide and homicide.
- The media and politicians claimed community care had failed and demanded more powers to enforce treatment. By the end of the epoch, calls for such draconian measures had ameliorated somewhat but the core dilemma of balancing personal independence with the need for care remained unresolved.

Notes

1. M. Tansella, D. De Salvia and P. Williams, The Italian psychiatric reform: Some quantitative evidence. *Social Psychiatry* (1987) 22: 37–48.

2. A. Gralnick, Build a better state hospital: Deinstitutionalization has failed. *Hospital and Community Psychiatry* (1985) 36: 738–41.

3. J. E. Powell, *John Enoch Powell Speech Archive.* http://enochpowell.info/wp-content/uploads/Speeche s/1957–1961.pdf.

4. Goffman, *Asylums*; Powell, *John Enoch Powell Speech Archive.*

5. Department of Health and Social Security, *Better Services for the Mentally Ill*, Cmnd 6233. London: HMSO, 1975.

6. M. Balestrieri, P. Williams and G. Wilkinson, Specialist mental health treatment in general practice: A meta analysis. *Psychological Medicine* (1988) 18: 711–18; P. Tyrer, N. Selvewright and S. Wollerton, General practice psychiatric clinics: Impact on psychiatric services. *British Journal of Psychiatry* (1984) 145: 15–19; L. Gask, B. Sibbald and F. Creed, Evaluating models of working at the interface between mental health services and primary care. *British Journal of Psychiatry* (1997) 170: 6–1.

7. D. I. Brough, N. Bouras and J. P. Watson, The Mental Health Advice Centre in Lewisham. *Bulletin of the Royal College of Psychiatrists* (1983) 7: 82–4.

8. S. A. Mann and N. Cree, 'New' long-stay psychiatric patients: A national sample survey of fifteen mental hospitals in England and Wales 1972/3. *Psychological Medicine* (1976) 6: 603–16.

9. Team for the Assessment of Psychiatric Services, *Preliminary Report on Baseline Data from Friern and Claybury Hospitals.* North East Thames Regional Health Authority, 1988; N. Treiman, J. Leff and G. Glover, Outcome of long stay psychiatric patients resettled in the community: Prospective cohort study. *British Medical Journal* (1999) 319: 13–167; J. Leff and N. Treiman, Long-stay patients discharged from psychiatric hospitals: Social and clinical outcomes after five years in the community. TAPS Project 46. *British Journal of Psychiatry* (2000) 174: 217–23; N. Treiman and J. Leff, Long-term outcome of long-stay inpatients considered unsuitable to live in the community. TAPS Project 44. *British Journal of Psychiatry* (2002) 181: 428–32.

10. Department of Health and Social Security, *Better Services for the Mentally Ill*; Royal College of Psychiatrists, *Report of the Confidential Inquiry into Homicides and Suicides by Mentally Ill People.* London: Royal College of Psychiatrists, 1996; Department of Health, *Caring for People: The Care Programme Approach for People with a Mental Illness Referred to Specialist Mental Health Services.* Joint Health/Social Services Circular, C(90) 23/LASSL(90)11. London: Department of Health, 1990; T. Burns, A. Beadsmoore, A. V. Bhat, A. Oliver and C. Mathers, A controlled trial of home-based acute psychiatric services I: Treatment patterns and costs. *British Journal of Psychiatry* (1993) 163: 49–54; D. Malone, S. Marriott, G. Newton-Howes, S. Simmonds, P. Tyrer and Cochrane Schizophrenia Group, Community mental health teams (CMHTs) for people with severe mental illnesses and disordered personality (Review), *Cochrane Database of Systematic Reviews* (2007), https://doi.org/10.1002/14651858.CD000270.pub2; P. W. Timms and A. H. Fry, Homelessness and mental illness. *Health Trends* (1989) 21: 70–1; T. Craig, E. Bayliss, O. Klein, P. Manning and L. Reader, *The Homeless Mentally Ill Initiative: An Evaluation of Four Clinical Teams.* London: Department of Health, 1995.

11. Department of Health, *Caring for People.*

12. Department of Health, *National Service Framework: Mental Health.* London: HMSO,1999.

13. D. M. Clark, R. Layard, R. Smithies, D. Richards, R. Suckling and B. Wright, Improving access to psychological therapy: Initial evaluation of two UK demonstration sites. *Behaviour Research and Therapy* (2009) 47: 910–20.

14. J. Harper, Out-patient adult psychiatric clinics. *British Medical Journal* (1959) 1: 357–60.

15. R. Barton, *Institutional Neurosis.* Bristol: Wright, 1959; E. Goffman, *Asylums: Essays on the Social Situation of Mental Patients and Other Inmates.* Harmondsworth: Penguin Books, 1961.

16. Powell, *John Enoch Powell Speech Archive.*

17. G. C. Tooth and E. M. Brooke, Trends in the mental hospital population and their effect on future planning. *Lancet* (1961) 1: 710–13.

18. S. Moore, A psychiatric outpatient nursing service. *Mental Health (London)* (1961) 20: 51–4.

19. M. Silverman, A comprehensive department of psychological medicine: A 12 months review. *British Medical Journal* (1961) 2: 698–701; S. Smith, Psychiatry in general hospitals: Manchester's integrated scheme. *Lancet* (1961) 1: 1158–9.

20. A. Paton, Reorganisation: The first year *British Medical Journal* (1975) 2: 729–39.

21. National Health Service Reorganisation Act. London: HMSO, 1973.

22. Department of Health and Social Security, *Better Services for the Mentally Ill.*

23. E. Fottrell, R. Peermohamed and R. Kothari, Identification and definition of long-stay mental hospital population. *British Medical Journal* (1974) 4: 675–7.

24. S. R. Hirsch, S. Platt, A. Knights and A. Weyman, Shortening hospital stay for psychiatric care: Effect on patients and their families. *British Medical Journal* (1979) 1: 442; F. Creed, P. Mbaya, S. Lancashire, B. Tomenson, B. Williams and S. Holme, Cost effectiveness of day and inpatient psychiatric treatment. *British Medical Journal* (1997) 314: 1381–5.

25. Mann and Cree, 'New' long-stay psychiatric patients.

26. Team for the Assessment of Psychiatric Services, *Preliminary Report.*

27. Treiman, Leff and Glover, Outcome of long stay psychiatric patients resettled in the community; Leff and Treiman, Long-stay patients discharged from psychiatric hospitals; Treiman and Leff, Long-term outcome of long-stay inpatients considered unsuitable to live in the community.

28. G. Wolff, S. Pathare, T. Craig and J. Leff, Community knowledge of mental illness and reaction to mentally ill people. *British Journal of Psychiatry* (1996) 168: 191–8.

29. E. W. Harley, J. Boardman and T. Craig Friendship in people with schizophrenia: A survey. *Social Psychiatry and Psychiatric Epidemiology* (2012) 47: 1291–9; D. A. Curson, C. Pantelis, J. Ward and T. R. E. Barnes, Institutionalism and schizophrenia 30 years on: Clinical poverty and the social environment in three British Mental Hospitals in 1960 compared with a fourth in 1990. *British Journal of Psychiatry* (1992) 160: 230–41.

30. G. Thornicroft and G. Strathdee, How many psychiatric beds? *British Medical Journal* (1994) 309: 970–1.

31. K. Gournay and J. Brooking, Community psychiatric nurses in primary health care. *British Journal of Psychiatry* (1994) 165: 231–8.

32. L. Mynors-Wallis, I. Davies, A. Gray, F. Barbour and D. Gath, A randomised controlled trial and cost analysis of problem-solving treatment for emotional disorders given by community nurses in primary care. *British Journal of Psychiatry* (1997) 170: 113–19; Balestrieri, Williams and Wilkinson, Specialist mental health treatment in general practice.

33. Tyrer, Selvewright and Wollerton, General practice psychiatric clinics; Gask, Sibbald and Creed, Evaluating models.

34. Brough, Bouras and Watson, The Mental Health Advice Centre in Lewisham.

35. E. Sayce, T. K. J. Craig and A. P. Boardman, The development of Community Mental Health Centres in the U.K. *Social Psychiatry and Psychiatric Epidemiology* (1991) 26: 14–20.

36. Ibid.

37. D. Melzer, A. S. Hale, S. J. Malik, G. A. Hogman and S. Wood, Community care for patients with schizophrenia one year after hospital discharge. *British Medical Journal* (1991) 303: 1023–6.

38. T. K. J. Craig and P. W. Timms, Out of the wards and onto the streets? Deinstitutionalisation and homelessness in Britain. *Journal of Mental Health* (1992) 1: 265–75.

39. Royal College of Psychiatrists, *Report of the Confidential Inquiry into Homicides and Suicides.*

40. Department of Health, *Caring for People.*

41. Burns et al., A controlled trial of home-based acute psychiatric services I; Malone et al., Community mental health teams.

42. Timms and Fry, Homelessness and mental illness; Craig, Bayliss, Klein, Manning and Reader, *The Homeless Mentally Ill Initiative*.

43. L. I. Stein and M. A. Test, Alternative to mental hospital treatment: I. Conceptual model, treatment program and clinical evaluation. *Archives of General Psychiatry* (1980) 37: 392–7.

44. J. Hoult, I. Reynolds, M. Charbonneau-Powis, P. Weekes and J. Briggs, Psychiatric hospital versus community treatment: The results of a randomised trial. *Australian and New Zealand Journal of Psychiatry* (1983) 17: 160–7.

45. I. M. Marks, J. Connolly, M. Muijen, B. Audini, G. McNamee and R. E. Lawrence, Home-based versus hospital-based care for people with serious mental illness. *British Journal of Psychiatry* (1994) 165: 179–94.

46. T. Burns, F. Creed, T. Fahy et al., Intensive versus standard case management for severe psychotic illness: A randomised trial. *Lancet* (1999) 353: 2185–9; F. Holloway and J. Carson, Intensive case management for the severely mentally ill: Controlled trial. *British Journal of Psychiatry* (1998) 172: 19–22.

47. S. M. Devane, G. Haddock, S. Lancashire et al., The clinical skills of community psychiatric nurses working with patients who have severe and enduring mental health problems: An empirical analysis. *Journal of Advanced Nursing* (2001) 27: 253–60; S. Lancashire, J. Haddock, N. Tarrier, I. Baguley, C. Butterworth and C. Brooker, Effects of training in psychosocial intervention for community psychiatric nurses. *Psychiatric Services* (1997) 48: 39–4.

48. R. Sylvester, Dobson acts to sweep mentally ill off streets. *The Independent*, 23 October 2011, www.independent.co.uk/news/dobson-acts-to-sweep-mentally-ill-off-streets-1184934.html.

49. G. Harrison, C. Glazebrook, J. Brewin et al., Increased incidence of psychiatric disorders in migrants from the Caribbeans in the United Kingdom. *Psychological Medicine* (1997) 27: 799–806; G. G. Rwegellera, Differential use of psychiatric services by West Indians, West Africans and English in London. *British Journal of Psychiatry* (1980) 137: 428–32.

50. F. W. Hickling, K. McKenzie, R. Mullen and R. A. Murray, Jamaican psychiatrist evaluates diagnoses at a London psychiatric hospital. *British Journal of Psychiatry* (1999) 175: 283–5; S. P. Sashidharan, Institutional racism in British psychiatry. *Psychiatric Bulletin* (2001) 25: 244–7.

51. Department of Health, *National Service Framework*.

52. H. Killaspy, P. Bebbington, R. Blizard et al., The REACT study: Randomised evaluation of assertive community treatment in north London. *British Medical Journal* (2006) 332: 815–20.

53. T. Burns, J. Catty, M. Dash, C. Roberts, A. Lockwood and M. Marshall, Use of intensive case management to reduce time in hospital in people with severe mental illness: Systematic review and meta-regression. *British Medical Journal* (200) 7: 335–6.

54. S. Johnson, G. Thornicroft, S. Afuwape et al., Effects of training community staff in interventions for substance misuse in dual diagnosis patients with psychosis (COMO study). *British Journal of Psychiatry* (2007) 191: 451–2; C. Barrowclough, G. Haddock, T. Wykes et al., Integrated motivational interviewing and cognitive behaviour therapy for people with psychosis and comorbid substance misuse: Randomised controlled trial. *British Medical Journal* (2010) 341: 1–12.

55. T. Craig, P. Garety, P. Power et al., The Lambeth Early Onset (LEO) Team: Randomised controlled trial of the effectiveness of specialised care for early psychosis. *British Medical Journal* (2004) 329: 1067–70.

56. S. Johnson, F. Nolan, S. Pilling et al. Randomised controlled trial of acute mental health care by a crisis resolution team: The north Islington study. *British Medical Journal* (2005) 331: 599; G. Glover, G. Arts and K. S. Babu, Crisis resolution/home treatment teams and psychiatric admission rates in England. *British Journal of Psychiatry* (2006) 189: 441–5.

57. Clark et al., Improving access to psychological therapy.

58. T. Burns, J. Catty, T. Becker et al., The effectiveness of supported employment for people with severe mental illness: A randomised controlled trial. *Lancet* (1997); 370: 1146–52.

59. R. Chilvers, G. Macdonald and A. Hayes, Supported housing for people with severe mental disorders. *The Cochrane Database of Systematic Reviews*, 4: CD000453.

60. R. Churchill, G. Owen, S. Singh et al., *International Experience of Using Community Treatment Orders*. London: Department of Health, 2007.

61. T. Burns, J. Rugkasa and A. Molodynski et al., Community treatment orders for patients with psychosis (OCTET): A randomised controlled trial. *Lancet* (2013) 381: 1627–33.

62. S. Priebe, A. Badesconyi, A. Fioritti et al., Re-institutionalisation in mental health care: Comparison of data on service provision from six European countries. *British Medical Journal* (2005) 330: 123–6.

63. P. Keown, S. Weich, K. S. Bhui and J. Scott, Association between provision of mental illness beds and rate of involuntary admissions in the NHS in England 1988–2008: Ecological study. *British Medical Journal* (2011) 343: 196–204.

64. On compassion, see K. Sutherby, G. I. Szmukler, A. Halpern et al., A study of 'crisis cards' in a community psychiatric service. *Acta Psychiatrica Scandinavica* (1999) 100: 56–61; on peer support, see T. Craig, I. Doherty, R. Jamieson-Craig, A. Boocock and G. Attafua, The consumer-employee as a member of a Mental Health Assertive Outreach Team: I. Clinical and social outcomes. *Journal of Mental Health* (2004) 13: 59–69; on personal recovery, see M. Slade, *Personal Recovery and Mental Illness: A Guide for Mental Health Professionals*. Cambridge: Cambridge University Press, 2009.

65. Keown et al., Association between provision of mental illness beds and rate of involuntary admissions.

66. L. Howard, C. Flach, M. Leese et al., Effectiveness and cost-effectiveness of admissions to women's crisis houses compared with traditional psychiatric wards: Pilot patient-preference randomised controlled trial. *British Journal of Psychiatry* (2010) 197: s32–s40.

Chapter 31

UK Deinstitutionalisation: Neoliberal Values and Mental Health

Andrew Scull

Introduction

The year 2021 marks the sixtieth anniversary of Enoch Powell's Water Tower speech – a famous or infamous occasion depending upon one's assessment of deinstitutionalisation and the advent of community care. Powell, the minister of health in Harold Macmillan's Tory government, was a superb orator and a man not known to mince his words. In 1968, his 'Rivers of Blood' speech on immigration would cost him his position on the Opposition front bench and essentially end his political career (see also Chapters 1 and 2). In 1961, however, he was seen as a formidable figure in the Conservative Party and a possible future prime minister. Delivered at the annual conference of the National Association for Mental Health, the Water Tower speech announced a radical shift in mental health policy. Since the passage of the Asylums Act in 1845, which made construction of county lunatic asylums at taxpayer expense compulsory, Britain, like the rest of the Western world, had placed primary emphasis on institutionalisation as the preferred solution to the problems posed by serious mental illness. That era, Powell announced, was coming to a close.[1]

Neoliberal Dawn

The shift in policy was couched in the apocalyptic tones that Powell preferred. 'There they stand,' he intoned, 'isolated, majestic, imperious, brooded over by the gigantic water-tower and chimney combined, rising unmistakable and daunting out of the countryside – the asylums our forefathers built with such immense solidity to express the notions of their day. Do not for a moment underestimate their powers of resistance to our assault.' Yet assault them he would. The government's plans 'imply nothing less than the elimination of by far the greatest part of this country's mental hospitals'. It was, he acknowledged, 'a colossal undertaking'. Within fifteen years, however, half of the existing beds, 75,000, should be gone: 'if we are to have the courage of our ambitions, we ought to pitch the estimate lower still, as low as we dare, perhaps lower.' Mistakes might be made, but 'if we err, it is our duty to err on the side of ruthlessness. For the great majority of these establishments there is no, repeat no, appropriate future use.'

Powell granted that vast sums had been spent on these edifices, and in the past decade much treasure had been expended to make them 'less inadequate'. Those sunk costs were proffered as one argument against radical change. Other objections could be expected from the 'hundreds of men and women who have given years, even lifetimes, to the service of a mental hospital or group of hospitals … have laboured devotedly, through years of scarcity and neglect, to render conditions in them more tolerable'. Too bad. The mental hospitals were 'doomed'; and Powell volunteered to be 'the first to set the torch to the funeral pyre'. In the following year, the NHS *Hospital Plan* began the process of enacting these proposals.

Powell spoke like an Old Testament prophet, and a prophet he proved to be. Though the asylums did not begin to vanish from the scene until the 1980s under Margaret Thatcher, their population did shrink significantly throughout the 1960s and 1970s. On an average day in 1960, the population of England's mental hospitals was just over 140,000. By 1970, the census had fallen to 106,000 and, a decade later, to just over 79,000. Under administrations of all political stripes, Conservative, Labour and Coalition, the remorseless run down of institutional populations has continued apace. When David Cameron took power in 2010, the inpatient population had fallen to less than 23,000, and, while most mental hospitals remained open into the 1980s, notwithstanding the shrinking inpatient population, during the second half of Thatcher's term in office they were largely abandoned. Some, like the massive Friern Hospital in north London, were converted to upscale flats for the nouveau riche (the building's past coyly hidden as it became the Princess Park Manor); while others, like the old Devon County Asylum at Exeter, contaminated with asbestos and heavy metals, proved too costly to repurpose and were left to rot. 'For dust thou art, and into dust shalt return', as one of Powell's favourite books would have it.

As Powell's speech should make clear, deinstitutionalisation was no accident. It was a consciously chosen policy, pursued relentlessly over many decades, even as evidence materialised that the alternative to the hospital – 'community care' – was largely a figment of politicians' imaginations, a phrase that sought to obscure the fact that there was little in the way of community to which most mental patients could return and still less in the way of care. Community care is, as I have suggested elsewhere, a shell game in which there is no pea.[2] Those suffering from serious forms of mental illness have been cast into the wilderness – a wilderness that has little time for those with few resources of their own; for people who lack the capacity to function in a neoliberal environment whose architects regard them as little more than a drain on the public purse; and for 'unfortunate creatures' chronically dependent on the not-so-tender mercies of a shrinking welfare state, doubly stigmatised for their illness and because they show no signs of reform or recovery.

Psychiatrists have embraced the myth that the mass discharges of patients reflected advances in therapeutics, most especially the psychopharmacological revolution that began in 1954, with the marketing of Largactil (chlorpromazine). That, coincidentally, is the year in which the mental hospital census in England and Wales reached its zenith. The reality, however, is that the number of patients resident in many hospitals had begun to decline several years before antipsychotics arrived on the scene. Leading British psychiatrists such as Sir Aubrey Lewis and Michael Shepherd were rightly sceptical about the relationship between pharmacology and hospital discharges, and a host of later scholarship has confirmed their suspicions (see also Chapter 2).[3] Drugs may have soothed professional anxieties when psychiatrists were asked to discharge long-stay patients, and the effects of Thorazine (chlorpromazine) and its copycat drugs on florid symptomatology may have made a difference at the margin, notwithstanding the tendency of disturbed patients to be non-compliant about taking their medications. Most awkwardly, though, for the advocates of the notion of a technological fix as the source of deinstitutionalisation, they have no way of accounting for the pattern of accelerated discharge that manifested itself from the 1970s onwards, a period where no breakthroughs in psychopharmacology materialised.

The record demonstrates that it was policy choices, not drugs, that fundamentally underpinned deinstitutionalisation, whose impetus did not come from the ranks of psychiatry. Indeed, the shift from the hospital to the community occurred largely behind the backs of the profession and independent of its predilections and actions. Political preferences ruled and, by and large, the profession followed along.

Deinstitutionalisation was not a uniquely British phenomenon, of course. Strikingly similar patterns can be observed in the United States and, later, in most advanced industrial societies. The mental hospital, once touted as 'the most blessed manifestation of true civilization the world can present',[4] was now dismissed as a 'total Institution' on a par with such places as prisons and concentration camps, an anti-therapeutic engine of degradation that fomented chronicity rather than cured its inmates.[5] That focus on the defects of the institution and its malign effects on those it purported to treat accounted for much of the support the new policy drew from civil libertarians and those concerned with patients' rights (see also Chapters 3, 4, 13 and 20). Yet it substituted for careful assessment of what alternatives were being prepared, if any, for those discharged back into society at large.

Long before the principle that medical care would be provided free and as a right for all British citizens had been established, the special problems associated with serious mental illness had prompted the state to pay for the confinement and treatment of the overwhelming majority of mental patients. Such care, well into the twentieth century, had come at the price of being labelled a 'pauper lunatic', but the costs of housing and providing for the tens of thousands of patients who crowded the wards had long constituted a major draw on the public purse. Nor did that change much with the advent of the NHS in 1948. Mental hospitals continued to exist as a separate system, independent of the health service that dealt with physical ill health. The end of that separation was forecast in the 1962 *Hospital Plan* but only became a reality during the 1970s. No longer were the mental health services a separate administrative and financial system, and in the fight for resources, the generally low priority placed on mental illness has left the advocates for resources in a parlous position. Worse still, the incurable tendency of the political classes to reorganise and 'reform' the health services has repeatedly added to the chaos. Particularly pernicious in this regard was the 1990 National Health and Community Care Act, which passed responsibility for community care on to local authorities. Uneven and inadequate provision has been the inevitable result. No resources were allocated to the local authorities to provide for these new responsibilities, and the dislocations associated with establishment of NHS Trusts then compounded the problem (see also Chapters 10 and 30).

Neoliberal Supremacy

The 1970s saw the breakdown of the post-war consensus in British politics, which had seen both parties embrace a strong role for the government in the economy, an expanded welfare state and a major role for trade unions.[6] Though they would be exacerbated by the external shock of the sharp rise in oil prices in 1973, the structural problems that already plagued the economy were exacerbated even further by the increasingly fractious state of labour relations. Unions flexed their power. Massive strikes, both official and unofficial, appeared to render Britain almost ungovernable. The country's difficulties were made worse by the weakness and fecklessness of the politicians of both parties who ruled Britain during this decade.[7] The miners' strikes of 1972 and 1974, and the resultant blackouts and forced move to a three-day work week, brought the collapse of the Heath government, but Labour under Callaghan proved equally inept and incompetent in the face of industrial turmoil and political unrest. The 'Winter of Discontent' of 1978/9 saw more massive strikes, particularly by public sector trade unions, as Callaghan vainly sought to rein in rampant inflation. Bodies went unburied, rubbish uncollected and flying pickets restricted hospitals to taking emergency patients only. Public services appeared to be on the brink of collapse, as did the economy itself.

The sick man of Europe responded by electing a Conservative Party led by Margaret Thatcher in May 1979. Blessed with a thumping majority, her pro-market and neoliberal instincts, and visceral hostility to both unions and the public sector, would dominate British politics for decades. Within two years, she had ejected most of the one-nation Tories from her government and embarked on a radical reconstruction of the British economy and the British state. By the time Tony Blair brought 'New Labour' out of the political wilderness and back into power, following more than a decade and a half of Conservative rule, trade unions had been neutered as a political force, economic inequality had widened sharply and the parameters of political discourse and public policy had been altered, if not permanently, then certainly for the foreseeable future. Blair's 'Brave New Britain' in many ways continued to embrace key plans of Thatcherite orthodoxy, albeit while putting a softer, more emollient face on its policies.[8]

Someone who could announce with a straight face (and meaning it) that 'there is no such thing as society', and who proceeded to amplify her meaning by insisting that 'It is our duty to look after ourselves', was not inclined to show much support for those who depended upon public provision of services for their very survival. Scornfully, in the same interview Thatcher noted that 'we have gone through a period when too many children and people have been given to understand "I have a problem, it is the Government's job to cope with it!" ... they are casting their problems on society.'[9] It was a view for which she evinced no sympathy. At best, she saw a role for Victorian charity, *de haut en bas*: 'There is a living tapestry of men and women and people [sic] and the beauty of that tapestry and the quality of our lives will depend upon how much each of us is prepared to take responsibility for ourselves and each of us prepared to turn round and help by our own efforts those who are unfortunate.' Victims of misfortune who sought collective, public responses to the difficulties they confronted were out of luck. Hers was not an administration who viewed such supplicants with favour. Handouts were to be in short supply.

In Thatcher's view, British citizens had become far too dependent on the state, losing their sense of responsibility for their own lives. For her, the key to reviving Britain was to restore economic incentives and the discipline of the marketplace, rolling back the frontiers of the state and reducing expenditure on welfare, confining it to those in 'real need'. Social security payments steadily eroded in value, and sickness and unemployment benefits were cut. The upshot was a doubling of the relative poverty level by the time she resigned in 1990, when 28 per cent of British children were found to be living below the poverty line (3.3 million, up from 1.7 million when she took office) – statistics that grew even worse under her successor, John Major. Levels of inequality showed no signs of declining under New Labour and have worsened still further since.[10] Neoliberalism, in other words privatisation, the deification of individualism, the destruction of union power, economic liberalisation and increased ideological hostility to the collective provision of public goods became the hallmarks of her tenure in office and have perceptibly changed the terms of political debate ever since. Welfare 'reform', in Britain as in the United States, has become a term of art disguising repeated assaults on the social safety net and the demonisation of those dependent upon it.

Neoliberal NHS and Mental Health Services

The sole and singular exception to this sustained ideological attack on the welfare state in the UK has been the NHS. Thatcher ostentatiously chose private health care, but this is one area where her ideology encountered stiff resistance (see also Chapter 9). At least at the level of rhetoric, governments of all stripes since she was forced from office have genuflected to the NHS and promised to protect it, a reflection of its overwhelming popularity among the public at large. Under Labour, the rhetoric was matched for a time with an attempt to boost resources for the health services, though little of this new money found its way into the mental health sector. The promised 'parity of esteem' for physical and mental health remained a slogan without substance. The great bulk of the additional money provided to the NHS was directed at physical illness, though administrative obfuscation and the fragmentation of service provision have made quantifying where the money went extraordinarily difficult.[11] Moreover, though serious violence among those living with schizophrenia and psychosis is quite rare,[12] media-inspired moral panics surrounding this issue have exercised a lopsided influence over public policy and have meant that such increases in resources for mental health provision as did occur under Labour were disproportionately spent on mitigating these risks – a distortion of policy that found legislative recognition in the new category of 'Dangerously Severe Personality Disorder' (DSPD) in the 2007 Mental Health Act (see also Chapters 23, 27 and 28). Labour's decision to have the NHS Trusts mimic the marketplace, a standard feature of neoliberal policy, added additional layers of administration and increased the strain on the system, to no good effect.

Whatever slight progress towards improving the lot of the seriously mentally ill that had accompanied Labour's thirteen years in power has since been reversed. David Cameron had given notice prior to wining the general election and entering a coalition with the Liberal Democrats in 2010 that 'the age of irresponsibility was going to be giving way to the age of austerity'. With the enthusiastic support of his chancellor, George Osborne, he was as good as his word. The transfer of welfare to the private and voluntary sectors – a key part of the Thatcherite agenda – was soon under way. Over the ensuing decade, local authorities had their funding from Whitehall cut by 60 per cent. At the same time, caps were introduced on increases in council tax, placing local government under increasing fiscal strain. Under the 1990 legislation, local authorities bore primary responsibility for the community care of the mentally ill. What meagre provision they had previously made for their needs was increasingly threatened. Simultaneously, sharp cuts of the social care budget and the essential abandonment of any pretence to provide social housing worsened the situation further. Nor were these to be temporary measures to cope with the economic shock of the Great Recession. That provided the initial excuse for the cuts, but by 2013 (by which time public spending had already been cut by 14.3 billion pounds compared to 2009–10), Cameron announced that he had no intention of reversing the changes when and if the economy improved. The reduced commitment of the state was to be a permanent feature of Britain's future.

The NHS was supposedly to be protected from austerity; its funding 'ring-fenced'. Though this was true in nominal terms particularly as demands increased with the ageing of the population, the health service has suffered drastic cuts in real terms. Cash increases that averaged 1.4 per cent per year adjusted for inflation were entirely inadequate to meet demand. Forced to prioritise day-to-day expenditures, capital budgets were neglected, which led to rapid deterioration of both buildings and equipment. Over 32,000 overnight beds were lost in a decade. Waiting times for services of all sorts lengthened, despite promises to reduce them. And, as usual, in the face of this deteriorating fiscal environment, mental health care suffered disproportionately. The gap between needs and services available took another turn for the worse, and deeper cuts in social services added to the problems faced by those with serious mental illness.

The idea that we bear a collective moral responsibility to provide for the unfortunate – indeed, that one of the marks of a civilised society is its determination to provide as of right certain minimum standards of living for all its citizens – has been steadily eroding since Thatcher came to power. In its place, we have seen the resurgence of an ideology far more congenial and comforting to the privileged: the myth of the benevolent 'Invisible Hand' of the marketplace, and its corollary, an unabashed moral individualism. There is little place (and less sympathy) within such a worldview for those who are excluded from the race for material well-being by chronic disabilities and handicaps – whether physical or mental disease, or the more diffuse but cumulatively devastating penalties accruing to those belonging to racial minorities or living in dire poverty.

The punitive sentiments directed against those who must feed from the public trough extend only too easily to embrace those who suffer from the most severe forms of psychiatric misery. Those who seek to protect the long-term mental patient from the opprobrium visited upon the welfare recipient may do so by arguing that the patient is both dependent and sick. But I fear this approach has only a limited chance of success (see also Chapter 27). After all, despite two centuries of propaganda, the public still resists the straightforward equation of mental and physical illness. Moreover, the long-term mental patient in many instances will not get better, and often fails to collaborate with his or her therapist to seek recovery. Such blatant violations of the norms governing access to the sick role in our societies make it unlikely that people with severe and enduring mental ill-health will be extended the courtesies and exemptions accorded to the conventionally sick (see also Chapter 3).[13] Instead, even those incapacitated by psychiatric disability all too often find themselves the targets of those who would abolish social programmes because they consider any social dependency immoral.

Conclusion

Seen in this larger context, the neglect that has been the hallmark of the shift from the asylum to community care should come as no surprise. Among those with more noticeable continuing impairment, ex-patients placed with their families seem overall to have fared best. It would be a serious mistake, though, to suppose that even here deinstitutionalisation has proceeded smoothly and has proved unambiguously beneficial. Quite early in the process, John Wing expressed 'surprise' that, in view of the greatly increased likelihood of someone with schizophrenia living at home instead of in a hospital, so little research was being done on the problems experienced by their relatives.[14] His own work, and that of his associates demonstrated that 'the burden on relatives and the community was rarely negligible, and in some cases, it was intolerable' (see also Chapter 2).[15] A good deal of the distress and misery continues to remain hidden because of families' reticence about complaining, a natural tendency, but one which has helped to sustain a false optimism about the effects of the shifts to community treatment. As George Brown pointed out, 'relatives are not in a strong position to complain – they are not experts, they may be ashamed to talk about their problems and they have come to the conclusion that no help can be offered which will substantially reduce their difficulties'.[16] Such conclusions may have a strong factual basis, in view of the widespread inadequacies or even absence of after-care facilities, and the reluctance, often refusal, of the authorities to countenance rehospitalisation. Long delays in receiving appointments, the absence of any provision for respite care, and the lack of co-ordination among service providers compound the problems families face, and eventually many give up the struggle.

Many psychotic patients are thus left to shuffle between flop-houses, homelessness, and short periods in jail, when their illness and dependency cause them to commit what are usually minor offences. Misery and poverty remain their lot, till most of them succumb to an early death. Given the thrust of public policy for the past sixty years, it should come as no surprise to learn that those afflicted with serious mental illness have a life expectancy of between fifteen and twenty-five years less than the rest of us.[17] It is, nonetheless, a disgrace.

Key Summary Points

- The number of patients resident in many hospitals had begun to decline several years before antipsychotics arrived on the scene.
- The population of asylums did shrink significantly throughout the 1960s and 1970s, though mental hospitals did not begin to vanish from the scene until the 1980s under Margaret Thatcher.
- Deinstitutionalisation was no accident. It was a consciously chosen neoliberal policy, pursued relentlessly over many decades.
- Welfare 'reform,' in Britain as in the United States, has become a term of art disguising repeated assaults on the social safety net and the demonisation of those dependent upon it.
- 'Community care' in the era of neoliberal politics has turned out to be an Orwellian euphemism, masking a nightmare existence for all too many of those afflicted with serious psychoses and for their families.

Notes

1. E. Powell, Address to the Mental Health Association, 1961. The Papers of Enoch Powell, GBR/0014/Poll. Churchill Archives Centre, Cambridge, Poll 4/1/1, 9/3/1961.

2. A. Scull, *Decarceration: Community Treatment and the Deviant: A Radical View*. Englewood Cliffs, NJ: Prentice-Hall, 1977.

3. P. Lerman, *Deinstitutionalization and the Welfare State*. New Brunswick, NJ: Rutgers University Press, 1982; W. Gronfein, Psychotropic drugs and the origins of deinstitutionalization. *Social Problems* (1985) 32: 437–53; S. Rose, Deciphering deinstitutionalization: Complexities in policy and program analysis. *Milbank Memorial Fund Quarterly* (1979) 57: 429–60; A. Scull, The decarceration of the mentally ill: A critical view. *Politics and Society* (1976) 6: 173–212.

4. G. Paget, *The Harveian Oration*. Cambridge: Deighton, Bell, 1866, pp. 34–5.

5. E. Goffman, *Asylums: Essays on the Social Situation of Mental Patients and Other Inmates*. New York: Doubleday, 1961.

6. K. O. Morgan, Britain in the seventies – our unfinest hour? *French Journal of British Studies* (2017) 22, https://doi.org/10.4000/rfcb.1662.

7. D. Sandbrook, *Seasons in the Sun: The Battle for Britain*. London: Penguin Allen Lane, 2012.

8.   J. Gray, Blair's project in retrospect. *International Affairs* (2004) 80: 39–48.

9.   M. Thatcher, Interview with *Women's Own*, 23 September 1987.

10. A. Shephard, Income inequality under the Labour government. Briefing Note No. 33. London: Institute for Fiscal Studies, 2003; C. J. Belfield, J. Cribb, A. Hood and R. Joyce, *Living Standards, Poverty and Inequality in the UK, 2016*. London: Institute for Fiscal Studies, 2016.

11. G. Thompson, NHS expenditure in England. Research Briefing SN/SG/724, 7. London: House of Commons Library, 2009.

12. S. Fazell, G. Gulati, L. Linsell, J. R. Geddes and M. Grann, Schizophrenia and violence: Systematic review and meta-analysis. *PLoS Medicine* (2009) 6: e1000120. https://doi.org/10.1371/journal.pmed.1000120.

13. T. Parsons, *The Social System*. New York: Free Press, 1951.

14. J. K. Wing, Planning and evaluating services for chronically handicapped psychiatric patients in the United Kingdom. In L. I. Stein and M. A. Test, eds, *Alternatives to Mental Hospital Treatment*. New York: Plenum Press, 1978.

15. J. K. Wing and G. W. Brown, *Institutionalism and Schizophrenia*. Cambridge: Cambridge University Press, 1970.

16. G. W. Brown, M. Bone, B. Dalison and J. K. Wing, *Schizophrenia and Social Care*. London: Oxford University Press, 1966.

17. S. Brown, Excess mortality of schizophrenia: A meta-analysis. *British Journal of Psychiatry* (1997) 171: 502–8; S. Saha, D. Dent and J. McGrath, A systematic review of mortality in schizophrenia: Is the mortality gap worsening over time?. *Archives of General Psychiatry* (2007) 64: 1123–31; T. M. Laursen, Life expectancy among persons with schizophrenia or bipolar affective disorder. *Schizophrenia Research* (2011) 131: 101–4; J. F. Hayes, L. Matson, K. Waters, M. King and D. Osborn, Mortality gap for people with bipolar disorder and schizophrenia: UK-based cohort study 2000–2014. *British Journal of Psychiatry* (2017) 211: 175–81.

32

Dealing with the Melancholy Void: Responding to Parents Who Experience Pregnancy Loss and Perinatal Death

Hedy Cleaver and Wendy Rose

Introduction

I go about my domestic duties in mourning, sighing over the melancholy void that death has made ... There sits her empty cradle ... I shall never see her sleeping there again.[1]

This was one woman's reaction to the death of her baby in the first half of the nineteenth century. Her grief and despair are timeless. However, the understanding and compassion shown to miscarriage and perinatal death is now very different.

Although such loss does not respect age, previous fertility or wealth, women living in poverty are at most risk.[2] The impact on the mental health of parents depends on a number of variables, including prior mental health, relationship between partners, culture, gender identity, medical and social support and religion. This chapter explores how the support provided to those experiencing loss reflects many of the seismic societal changes taking place on a broader canvas from the 1960s onwards.

Contribution of Legislation in Marking Change

Legislation in the last fifty years has marked both advances in medical science and changing attitudes towards pregnancy, parenting and the loss of a baby. It continues to do so. Stillborn babies had no legal existence prior to 1927 in England and 1939 in Scotland. 'The stillborn were thus treated as if they had never existed, and registered as neither a birth nor a death.'[3] The Stillbirth (Definition) Act 1992 extended the definition of stillborn from lost after the twenty-eighth week of pregnancy to lost after the twenty-fourth week. Those born earlier are not registered and there is no legal requirement for burial or cremation. Attitudes, however, continue to change. 'In recent years, with greater understanding of the significance of the death of a baby at any stage of pregnancy, more babies born before 24 weeks have been formally buried or cremated.'[4]

Medical terminology and its wider use have evolved; abortion originally described pregnancy loss without clarifying whether it was spontaneous or induced. Change began with the Abortion Act 1967, allowing women greater legal access to abortion services and the Guidance on the Act was updated in 2014.[5] Women who experienced a spontaneous miscarriage were thus able to talk to their doctor without fear of being criminalised and those seeking terminations could be referred to expert and safe clinical services. It was not until the 1980s with the development of ultrasound, enabling the foetus to be seen, that doctors consciously began using the term miscarriage to refer to early pregnancy loss.[6]

Prevalence of Pregnancy and Perinatal Loss

The rate of conception in England and Wales has, over the past half century, shown considerable variation. In 1969 conception was estimated to be 832,700 for women of all ages, falling to 686,400 in 1977 and by 2010 had risen to 909,200. Since then there has been a steady decrease. Scares over the safety of the contraceptive pill between 1976 and 1996 may have contributed to increases in conceptions due to the use of less reliable contraceptive methods.[7]

Not all conceptions lead to a live birth. It is estimated that today one in four pregnancies in England and Wales ends in miscarriage.[8]

A foetus may be lost because of an ectopic pregnancy. The recorded incidence increased between 1966 and 1996, 'probably due to a sexually transmitted agent' and has remained stable since.[9] It currently accounts for around one in every ninety pregnancies in the UK.[10] Some women decide to terminate their pregnancy. The recorded abortion rate increased from 6 per 1,000 resident women in England and Wales in 1970 to 20.8 per 1,000 in 2010. Of these, 1 per cent were performed in 2010 because of a substantial risk of foetal abnormalities.[11] The rate of perinatal mortality in the UK has been declining, falling from 11.8 deaths per 1,000 total births in 1981 to 7.5 deaths in 2011.[12]

There is now greater interest in monitoring and understanding pregnancy and perinatal loss. MBRRACE-UK undertakes regular perinatal surveillance reports to identify trends in stillbirth, neonatal and perinatal mortality rates.[13] The reports have informed the NHS Long Term Plan covering maternity and neonatal services, aimed at reducing stillbirth, neonatal mortality and serious brain injury.[14]

Attitudes to Motherhood and Fertility

It might be expected that widely held views on the imperative of motherhood would have undergone major changes over the last fifty years, thanks to family planning, the development of medical fertility techniques and greater economic independence.

Post-war advertisers targeted women as mothers and homemakers, mirroring the prevalent view in society. Women were expected to bear children and, in the mid-twentieth century, 'doctors who believed that female infertility was a psychosomatic condition recommended adoption as a "cure"'.[15] Even now, the prioritising of motherhood continues. The results of a recent UK survey are surprising. 'Around four in five British women say being a mother is "more important" than having a career, while only 6% put having a career first'.[16]

Although women are expected to become mothers, there has been a major change in the public response to pregnancy. In the 1960s and 1970s, it was often seen as a rather embarrassing condition and any evidence was disguised. Today the stigma and shame are disappearing, pregnant women can remain in the workforce, they are featured and celebrated in the media and clothes are designed to emphasise the baby bump. Fertility is also no longer seen as the prerogative of young women: 'Fertility in the over-forty age group has trebled since the 1980s, and there are now more women giving birth in their forties than in their teens.'[17]

Views on single parenthood have gradually been overturned. In the 1960s and 1970s, secrecy and shame surrounded unmarried motherhood,[18] attitudes perhaps reinforced by John Bowlby's influential work on attachment, which stressed the two-parent family and the stay-at-home mother as the bedrock of social stability. Change started in the 1970s with the wider availability of oral contraception and continued in 1984 with the licensing of the 'morning-after pill'. This meant that to have a baby as a single woman became largely a matter of choice. Language has also changed; terms such as 'bastard', 'illegitimacy' and 'living in sin' are now rarely used except by the fiercely religious. Yet policy progress has been slow and remains dogged by political and media rhetoric of 'the feckless poor' and 'problem families'.[19]

Attitudes towards same-sex partnerships and members of the LGBT community have shifted radically; the number of people who think same-sex relationships are 'not wrong at all' has gone from 17 per cent in 1983 to 65 per cent in 2018.[20] The many changes in the law around same-sex relationships since 1967, when sex between two men over the age of twenty one in England was decriminalised, have kept pace with public opinion. Views on the LGBT community continue to shift, including their equal rights to parenthood (see also Chapter 34). A discussion on the impact of pregnancy and baby loss must take a broader perspective on parenthood than would have been assumed fifty years ago.

Fear and Hope in Pregnancy and Perinatal Loss

Pregnancy evokes a variety of emotions: for some, it will produce feelings of joy, excitement and hope for the future; for others, anxiety, dread and guilt; but for many the emotions will be mixed. Women's reactions will be predicated on whether pregnancy was wanted and planned and the underlying mental health of the parent – issues that will subsequently shape their reaction to losing the pregnancy or baby.

Until relatively recently, many women still feared childbirth, knowing a mother or baby who had died in the process. Today most women trust that technology will minimise risk and they will have a problem-free pregnancy and give birth to a perfect child. Once the pregnancy is established, many women start to plan their future with the yet unborn child and a bond is formed stimulated by foetal activity.

In the mid-twentieth century, the pervasiveness of eugenic beliefs and fear of an 'abnormal' child led to couples being advised to feel fortunate if they experienced a miscarriage because the foetus would have been malformed. Although parents' unhappiness was recognised, grief was not emphasised; what was stressed was the possibility of future success. 'Doctors and science writers exuded confidence in medicine's abilities to give all women babies . . . Follow directions and there is no reason you should not have a fine, full-term baby'.[21] To achieve medicine's promise of a healthy baby, a woman might have been required to submit to repeated examinations, long stays in bed, abstaining from all physical activities and ingesting pharmaceuticals.

The medical advancements of the 1960s strengthened the belief that women who miscarried would give birth to a healthy child if they followed their doctor's advice. Yet this is not always the case; 1–2 per cent of women have three miscarriages in a row, classified as recurrent miscarriage.[22] Half of these result from chromosomal anomalies where the embryos would not survive; others are due to a wide variety of issues such as anatomical defects, infections and haematological disorders.[23] Nonetheless, three-quarters of women who experience recurrent miscarriage go on to have a successful pregnancy, and there is no evidence that 'lifestyle adaptation' increases the likelihood of success.[24]

Impact of Loss on Women's Mental Health

In the mid-twentieth century, miscarriage was a private affair that was rarely spoken of. Attitudes are changing due to the campaigns of vocal groups such as the Miscarriage

Association and Mumsnet with its Miscarriage Care Campaign. Baby loss is now treated with greater sensitivity and parents are offered choices, including funerals and other types of ceremonies, for a foetus that would previously have been quickly removed for disposal.

Although miscarriage is now more openly discussed, it could be argued that only certain voices are heard. Miscarriage is expected to evoke grief and trauma. Yet for women who were distressed rather than delighted at becoming pregnant, a miscarriage may be seen as good news. Other would-be parents, particularly those who have experienced recurrent miscarriage, may suffer intense grief that will not be resolved for years. When a much-wanted pregnancy is lost, women tend to be at risk of depression, anxiety, post-traumatic stress disorder, guilt and self-blame.[25]

> I was shocked. I had no idea that a miscarriage could happen so quietly, without bleeding or pain. Instead of going home clutching pictures of our baby, we left the hospital with instructions on how to shed its dead body.[26]

Research for the Stillbirth and Neonatal Death Society (Sands) found women who had experienced intrauterine death or stillbirth shared similarly profound emotions. The parents expressed a sense of 'overwhelming loss of what might have been. This was felt not only in relation to the baby as a physical presence, but also the loss of joy, of celebration, of parenthood and, in some cases, of their sense of self'.[27] Redshaw and colleagues' study of the impact of neonatal death and stillbirth showed similar results, practically a third of women reported symptoms of anxiety and a quarter reported depression.[28] These findings were substantiated by a meta-analysis of the negative psychosocial impact of stillbirth.[29]

There is general agreement that terminating a pregnancy is associated with increased risks of mental health problems,[30] with some groups of women at greater risk of negative outcomes.[31] When the termination is for reasons of foetal abnormality, it can have a profound impact on both parents because of the existence of choice and the potential for self-blame.[32]

For same-sex partners, losing a pregnancy or baby may be amplified because of the complex processes involved in becoming pregnant and the emotional and material investment. They may also face heterosexism and prejudice from health professionals. 'Some health professionals seemed unable to understand my partner's distress at losing her child ... I don't think they understood what it meant for my partner, that she was a parent and she had lost her baby too.'[33] Lesbian partnerships experience loss in similar ways to heterosexual women, but the impact on mental health appears to last for longer.[34]

Perhaps most devastating is when a baby is lost due to failures in clinical practice, systems or culture. There have been several investigations into preventable perinatal deaths at maternity units over the past few years.[35]

Silent Partners in Grief

Masculinity has been characterised by emotional detachment, silence and rationality. Traditionally, men have been excluded from all aspects of pregnancy and childbirth. Popular media portrayed their role as the 'anxious father' allaying his fears in the company of friends (often in the pub) while waiting to toast the arrival of a healthy baby. Changes began in the 1970s with more women giving birth in hospital and the belief that they should be allowed to choose whether to have their partner with them. By 2010, would-be fathers were expected to accompany their partner for the ultrasound, take an active role in antenatal classes and be present at the birth. Public recognition of fathers' more active parental role was marked finally by the introduction of paternity leave of up to two weeks in 2003.

Recent research has focused on men's experiences of baby loss. Qualitative studies reinforced by meta-studies have identified key themes.[36] This body of work suggests men react in similar ways to women, experiencing guilt and blame, regret, fear and grief as well as shame, stigma and post-traumatic stress disorder.[37] 'I will never forget what I saw. I can't. It's burned into my mind forever'.[38]

Many men felt grief and a deep sense of loss not only for their baby but also for their lost dreams of fatherhood. Because the woman experienced the event biologically, men felt less entitled to feel or to communicate their emotions. Many assumed the traditional role of protector, putting aside their own emotions to support their grieving partner; others buried their grief by taking on practical tasks. They 'expected themselves, and were expected by others, to be unaffected by the loss: yet, they recounted feelings, uncertainties, and desire for support beyond anything they would have anticipated'.[39]

Parenting after Miscarriage or Baby Loss

Awareness that the experience of losing a pregnancy or baby can affect parents' relationships with existing or future children is being acknowledged. Losing a pregnancy is associated with an increased likelihood of women experiencing sadness, low mood and excessive worry during any subsequent pregnancy, emotions that subside once the baby is born.[40] However, the arrival of a healthy baby may cause conflicting emotions as parents struggle to bond with their new baby while still grieving for the baby lost. A widely held misconception is that pregnancy and baby loss are far more prevalent for first-time mothers. The evidence suggests otherwise; just under half of neonatal deaths and 41 per cent of stillbirths occur following a previous successful delivery.[41]

The Missing Sibling

Following a miscarriage or stillbirth, a proportion of women will experience mental health problems that affect their capacity to care about themselves and their existing children. Men may deal with their grief by an increased use of alcohol or drugs, a coping strategy that makes them less available to their children.[42] Children will be directly affected by the loss and their reactions may be complicated as jealousy may have vied with excited expectation.

> When a baby is stillborn, it is a tragic event not only for the parents but also for older siblings who are waiting for their little sister or brother.[43]

A Swedish study identified several themes that helped parents and children deal with such loss. These include making the stillborn baby and the loss a reality for the sibling: providing honest, age-appropriate information, creating memories, recognising and acknowledging the child's grief and being able to show how they feel themselves.[44] When parents are unable to provide the support and understanding children need, children will self-interpret the loss of their sibling and the risk of pathological reactions can be high.[45]

Research suggests that, by supporting parents through the grieving process and facilitating the sharing of the loss within families, the emotional well-being of children can be better protected.[46] The debate has now moved into the political arena in the UK. The impact on children was acknowledged and fundraising for counselling applauded in the government's debate on baby loss in 2017.[47]

Professional Practice in Response to Baby Loss

Fifty years ago, all evidence of miscarriages and stillborn babies was immediately removed from the labour ward and parents had no opportunity to see or hold their baby.

> When they rushed my baby out of the room, I assumed I'd given birth to a monster, something that was too awful to look at. That thought haunted me for many years. Now I realise that he probably looked perfect, just as if he was asleep.[48]

It was generally believed at the time, both within the medical professional and wider society, 'that parents could, and should, forget their babies, and that it was best to carry on as though nothing had happened. Expressions of grief were discouraged.'[49]

While stillborn babies have been registered since 1927, even as late as the 1960s and 1970s many parents were not provided with a death certificate and few knew what happened to their baby's body. The 1970s heralded a gradual change in attitudes and practices, changes led by the work of Sands and other similar organisations. As a result, since the mid-1980s parents of a stillborn baby are consulted about funeral arrangements.[50]

The remains from a miscarriage continue to be classified as 'medical waste' and the Human Tissue Act 2004 made no distinction between the disposal of pregnancy remains and that of other tissue from a living person. Attitudes are beginning to change. The Guidance provided by the Human Tissue Authority in 2015, although acknowledging that parental consent is not required for the disposal of pregnancy remains, stresses that hearing the wishes of the parents 'are of paramount importance and should be respected and acted upon'.[51]

The NHS review identified the different responses of parents who suffer pregnancy loss, 'some wanted to remember their baby whatever the gestation and should have the opportunity to do so'.[52] The review found that 'compassion and attitude of the staff have a lasting impact on the experience' but that high workloads and competing priorities could hamper this important work.[53] The review also identified the relevance of the environment:

> due to shortage of beds I was moved to the maternity department where I was put in a side room and forgotten about. All through the night I lay awake and crying to myself as the new born, very new born baby next door cried all through the night as if it was in my own room.[54]

Health professionals are more aware of the impact of losing a baby and parents are offered opportunities to see and hold the baby, to take photos and collect keepsakes. Research on the impact of making memories is nuanced. For example, Crawley and colleagues found no direct relationship between maternal mental health and memory making, but the sharing of memories with partners, families and friends, along with the time since the baby died and professional support, were factors associated with improved mental health.[55] Watson's autobiography provides an illustration of the difference support can make to grieving parents. Recorded on a thank-you card in a neonatal intensive care unit was the following message:

> To Maddie, the bereavement midwife. You helped us through the worst time of our life. We will treasure the memories you let us make during Annabelle's short time. Thank you is not enough. But there are no words.[56]

Developments in Perinatal Mental Health and Community Services

How individuals experience losing a pregnancy or baby is personal and it would be wrong to assume that one type of response would suit everyone.[57] The type of support available can depend on the stage of pregnancy. Busy health professionals who deal with early pregnancy loss on a regular basis may normalise the event and fail to recognise its possible profound psychological impact. Women are routinely discharged quickly from hospital and often return home in a state of shock: many mothers and fathers may leave with undetected and unresolved psychological symptoms.[58]

Our understanding of the process of grieving over the last fifty years has influenced the development of preventive and community mental health services. Some parents will not need or want professional or community support while for others it will be a lifeline. For a few women, a stillbirth will have long-lasting effects. A better understanding of the experience and access to psychosocial support may benefit some women and their families to deal with the impact.[59] Gaps in the provision of maternal mental health services have been identified,[60] as has the lack of accessible support services for men that acknowledge and validate their experience of grief.[61]

As in the nineteenth century with child welfare services, charitable organisations have played an instrumental part since the 1970s in changing the landscape through campaigning; working with health professionals; raising funds for research; promoting good practice; providing information and advice; and, above all, supporting grieving parents and their families. Their role underpins the advances made in the last fifty years, and they are often founded by bereaved parents, devastated by their own loss and the lack of understanding of its significance and impact on their lives. Each with their own distinctive missions, these organisations have shown drive and resilience and continue to be strongly active. Bliss, Sands, Miscarriage Association, Tommy's, Lily Mae Foundation and Mariposa Trust are among many organisations providing new models of bereavement care and support. They engage with the NHS to bring about much-needed specialist and expert resources to help parents in their contact with the NHS and at home in the community.

Parliamentary engagement in the issues and NHS England's action plan are more recent advances. The All Party Parliamentary Group on Baby Loss made a commitment to providing high-quality bereavement care through their initiative *Safer Maternity Care*.[62] The Parental Bereavement (Leave and Pay) Act 2018 provides for the first time in the UK's history a legal right for bereaved parents to have leave from work, bereavement pay and employment protection. NHS England is engaged in improving women's access to perinatal mental health support through the establishment of new services and targeted funding.[63]

Conclusion

Advances in medical science and major changes to the law have influenced and reflected wider society's changing attitudes to pregnancy and parenthood. Consequently, single parents draw less condemnation and same-sex partnerships are legal. Attitudes towards miscarriage and perinatal death have benefited from these changes. What was previously a very private affair is talked about more openly, revealing the profound and long-term impact such loss can have on the mental health of would-be parents and existing children. This has resulted in health professionals managing miscarriage and stillbirth with greater compassion, enabling parents to have the opportunity to hold their baby and create memories. Fifty years ago, parents were sent home from hospital to cope with their grief alone; charities and voluntary groups, working in conjunction with health professionals, now fill the gap and provide information and a range of support. Although much has been accomplished, there is certainly scope for further advances.

Key Summary Points

- Any discussion on the impact of pregnancy and baby loss must take a broader perspective on parenthood than would have been assumed fifty years ago.
- Loss of a baby can affect any woman, irrespective of age, previous fertility or wealth, although those living in poverty are most at risk.
- Grief and despair for women at the loss of a baby were historically seen as a private affair. The need for health services to offer sensitivity and choice in coping with loss is now better recognised.
- The consequences of loss are far-reaching for all family members, including existing children. Some may not cope, which can have a profound effect on their mental health and well-being, if not addressed.
- Community mental health and voluntary organisations offer greater compassion and support to grieving families but the need for easily accessible and responsive local services remains.

Notes

1. S. D. Hoffert, 'A very peculiar sorrow': Attitudes toward infant death in the urban Northeast, 1800–1860. *American Quarterly* (1987) 39: 601–16, 601.

2. H. Cleaver, W. Rose, E. Young and R. Veitch, Parenting while grieving: The impact of baby loss. *Journal of Public Mental Health* (2018) 17: 168–75.

3. G. Davis, Stillbirth registration and perceptions of infant death, 1900–60: The Scottish case in national context. *Economic History Review* (2009) 62: 629–54.

4. Sands, *Long Ago Bereaved*. London: Sands, 2014, p. 12.

5. Department of Health, *Guidance in Relation to Requirements of the Abortion Act 1967*. London: Department of Health, 2014, https://assets.publishing.service.gov.uk/government/uploads/system/uploads/attachment_data/file/313459/20140509_-_Abortion_Guidance_Document.pdf.

6. A. Moscrop, 'Miscarriage or abortion?' Understanding the medical language of pregnancy loss in Britain; a historical perspective. *Medical Humanities* (2013) 39: 98–104.

7. ONS (Office for National Statistics), *Conceptions in England and Wales: 2018*. ONS Statistical Bulletin, 2020, www.ons.gov.uk/peoplepopulationandcommunity/birthsdeathsandmarriages/conceptionandfertilityrates/bulletins/conceptionstatistics/2018.

8. Tommy's, Miscarriage statistics: 2020, Tommy's website, www.tommys.org/miscarriage-stats.

9. M. Rajkhowa, M. R. Glass, A. J. Rutherford et al., Trends in the incidence of ectopic pregnancy in England and Wales from 1966 to 1996. *BJOG* (2000) 107: 369–74, 369.

10. NHS, *Long Term Plan*, 2019. www.longtermplan.nhs.uk.

11. Department of Health and Social Care, *Abortion Statistics, England and Wales: 2010*. London: Department of Health, 2011.

12. ONS, *Child and Infant Mortality in England and Wales: 2011*. ONS Statistical Bulletin, 2013. www.ons.gov.uk.

13. MBRRACE-UK, *Perinatal Mortality Surveillance Report: UK Perinatal Deaths for Births from January to December 2017*. Leicester: The Infant Mortality and Morbidity Studies, Department of Health Sciences, University of Leicester, 2012, www.npeu.ox.ac.uk/downloads/files/mbrrace-uk/report/MBRRACE-UK%20Perinatal%20Mortality%20Surveillance%20Summary%20Report%20for%202017%20-%20FINAL.pdf.

14. NHS, *Long Term Plan*.

15. T. Loughran, Infertility through the ages – and how IVF changed the way we think about it. *The Conversation*, 2018. www.theconversation.com/.

16. W. Jordan, Most women put motherhood ahead of career. *YouGov*, www.yougov.co.uk.

17. C. Watson, *The Language of Kindness. A Nurse's Story*. London: Chatto & Windus, 2018, p. 76.

18. P. Thane, Unmarried motherhood in twentieth-century England. *Women's History Review* (2011) 20: 11–29, https://doi.org/10.1080/09612025.2011.536383.

19. W. Rose and C. McAuley, Poverty and its impact on parenting in the UK: Re-defining the critical nature of the relationship through examining lived experiences in times of austerity. *Children and Youth Services Review* (2019) 97: 134–41.

20. M. Albakri, S. Hill, N. Kelley and N. Rahim, Relationships and gender identity. In J. Curtice, E. Clery, J. Perry, M. Phillips and N. Rahim, eds, *British Social Attitudes: The 36th Report*, 114–41. London: The National Centre for Social Research, 2019.

21. L. J. Reagan, From hazard to blessing to tragedy: Representations of miscarriage in twentieth-century America. *Feminist Studies* (2003) 29: 357–78, www.jstor.org/stable/3178514.

22. K. Duckitt and A. Qureshi, Recurrent miscarriage. *British Medical Journal: Clinical Evidence* (2015) 10: 1409, www.ncbi.nlm.nih.gov/pmc/articles/PMC4610348/pdf/2015-1409.pdf.

23. Y. B. Jeve and W. Davies, Evidence-based management of recurrent miscarriage. *Journal of Human Reproductive Science* (2014) 7: 159–69, https://doi.org/10.4103/0974-1208.142475.

24. S. Kilshaw, How culture shapes perceptions of miscarriage. *Sapiens*, 2017. www.sapiens.org/body/miscarriage-united-kingdom-qatar/.

25. J. Farren, M. Jalmbrant, L. Ameye et al., Post-traumatic stress, anxiety and depression following miscarriage or ectopic pregnancy: A prospective cohort study, *BMJ Open* (2016) 6, https://doi.org/10.1136/bmjopen-2016-011864.

26. Kilshaw, How culture shapes perceptions of miscarriage, p. 2.

27. S. Downe, E. Schmidt, C. Kingdon and A. Heazell, Bereaved parents' experience of stillbirth in UK hospitals: A qualitative interview study. *BMJ Open* (2013), https://bmjopen.bmj.com/content/bmjopen/3/2/e002237.full.pdf.

28. M. Redshaw, R. Rowe and J. Henderson, *Listening to Parents after Stillbirth or the Death of Their Baby after Birth*. Oxford: Policy Research Unit in Maternal Health and Care, 2014, www.npeu.ox.ac.uk/research/listening-to-parents-stillbirth-neonatal-death-248.

29. C. Burden, S. Bradley, C. Storey et al., From grief, guilt pain and stigma to hope and pride: A systematic review and meta-analysis of mixed-method research of the psychosocial impact of stillbirth. *BMC Pregnancy and Childbirth* (2016) 16: 1–12, https://core.ac.uk/download/pdf/33131729.pdf.

30. D. Fergusson, J. Horwood and J. Boden, Abortion and mental health disorders: Evidence from a 30-year longitudinal study. *British Journal of Psychiatry* (2008) 193: 444–51, https://doi.org/10.1192/bjp.bp.108.056499.

31. D. Reardon, The abortion and mental health controversy: A comprehensive literature review of common ground agreements, disagreements, actionable recommendations and research opportunities. *SAGE Open Medicine* (2018) 6: 1–38, https://doi.org/10.1177/2050312118807624.

32. A. Kersting and B. Wagner, Complicated grief after perinatal loss. *Dialogues in Clinical Neuroscience* (2012) 14: 187–94.

33. E. Peel, Pregnancy loss in lesbian and bisexual women: An online survey of experiences. *Hum Reproduction* (2010) 25: 721–7, 726, https://doi.org/10.1093/humrep/dep441.

34. Ibid.

35. M. Buchanan and J. Melley, East Kent hospitals: Baby death parents, heartbreak over errors. *BBC News*, 23 January 2020.

36. J. O'Leary and C. Thorwick, Fathers' perspectives during pregnancy, postperinatal loss. *Journal of Obstetric, Gynecologic Neonatal Nursing* (2006) 35: 78–86, https://doi.org/10.1111/j.1552–6909.2006.00017.x; M. S. Chavez, V. Handley, R. Jones et al., Men's experiences of miscarriage: A passive phenomenological analysis of online data. *Journal of Loss and Trauma* (2019) 24: 664–77, https://doi.org/10.1080/23802359.2019.1611230; H. Williams, A. Topping, A. Coomarasamy et al., Men and miscarriage: A systematic review and thematic synthesis. *Qualitative Health Research* (2019) 30: 133–45, https://doi.org/10.1177/1049732319870270.

37. S. Murphy and J. Cacciatore, The psychological, social, and economic impact of stillbirth on families. *Seminars in Fetal and Neonatal Medicine* (2017) 22: 129–34, https://doi.org/10.1016/j.siny.2017.02.002.

38. Chavez, Handley, Jones et al., Men's experiences of miscarriage, 671.

39. Williams, Topping, Coomarasamy et al., Men and miscarriage, 136.

40. Ibid.

41. Redshaw, Rowe and Henderson, *Listening to Parents*.

42. Cleaver, Rose, Young and Veitch, Parenting while grieving.

43. P. Avelin, K. Erlandsson, I. Hildingsson et al., Make the stillborn baby and the loss real for the siblings: Parents' advice on how the siblings of a stillborn baby can be supported. *Journal of Perinatal Education* (2012) 21: 90–8, 90, www.ncbi.nlm.nih.gov/pmc/articles/PMC3400252.

44. Ibid.

45. J. H. Fanos, G. A. Little and W. H. Edwards, Candles in the snow: Ritual and memory for siblings of infants who died in the intensive care nursery. *Journal of Pediatrics* (2009) 154: 849–53, https://doi.org/10.1016/j.jpeds.2008.11.053.

46. C. Chojenta, S. Harris, N. Reilly et al., History of pregnancy loss increases the risk of mental health problems in subsequent pregnancies but not in the postpartum. *PLos ONE* (2014) 9: e95038, https://doi.org/10.1371/journal.pone.0095038; J. Warland, J. O'Leary, H. McCutcheon and V. Williamson, Parenting paradox: Parenting after infant loss. *Midwifery* (2011) 27: 163–9, https://doi.org/10.1016/j.midw.2010.02.004.

47. Baby Loss Awareness Week debated in the House of Commons on 10 October 2017. Hansard, HC, Vol. 629, Cols. 267–300, https://hansard.parliament.uk/commons/2017-10-10/debates/FF772C31-1540-436B-BF50-8E4DD352458A/BabyLossAwarenessWeek.

48. Sands, *Long Ago Bereaved*, p. 6.

49. Ibid.

50. Ibid.

51. Human Tissue Authority, *Guidance on the Disposal of Pregnancy Remains Following Pregnancy Loss or Termination*, March 2015, www.hta.gov.uk/sites/default/files/Guidance_on_the_disposal_of_pregnancy_remains.pdf, p. 2.

52. NHS, *A Review of Support Available for Loss in Early and Late Pregnancy*, February 2014, p. 7, www.england.nhs.uk/improvement-hub/wp-content/uploads/sites/44/2017/11/Available-Support-for-Pregnancy-Loss.pdf.

53. Ibid, p. 22.

54. Ibid.

55. R. Crawley, S. Lomax and S. Ayers, Recovering from stillbirth: The effects of making and sharing memories on maternal mental health. *Journal of Reproductive and Infant Psychology* (2013) 31: 195–207, https://doi.org/10.1080/02646838.2013.795216.

56. Watson, *The Language of Kindness*, p. 148.

57. F. A. Murphy, A. Lipp and D. L. Powles, Follow-up for improving psychological wellbeing for women after a miscarriage. *Cochrane Database of Systematic Reviews* (2012) 3, https://doi.org/10.1002/14651858 .CD008679.pub2.

58. E. Clossick, The impact of perinatal loss on parents and the family. *Journal of Family Health* (2016) 26: 11–15, 13.

59. J. Cacciatore, The unique experiences of women and their families after the death of a baby. *Social Work in Health Care* (2010) 49: 134–48, https://doi.org/10.1080/00981380903158078.

60. M. Bavetta and M. Walker, Maternal mental health: Everyone's business. *Journal of Health Visiting* (2015) 3, https://doi.org/10.12968/johv.2015.3.11.500.

61. K. L. Obst, C. Due, M. Oxlad et al., Men's grief following pregnancy loss and neonatal loss: A systematic review and emerging theoretical model. *BMC Pregnancy and Childbirth* (2020) 20, https://doi.org/10.1186 /s12884-019-2677-9.

62. Department of Health, *Safer Maternity Care: Progress and Next Steps*. Policy Paper, November 2017, www .gov.uk/government/publications/safer-maternity-care-progress-and-next-steps.

63. NHS England, *Next Steps on the NHS Five Year Forward View for Mental Health: One Year On*, Report, February 2017, www.england.nhs.uk/wp-content/uploads/2017/03/NEXT-STEPS-ON-THE-NHS-FIVE-YEAR-FORWARD-VIEW.pdf.

Work, Unemployment and Mental Health

Jed Boardman and Miles Rinaldi

Introduction

Work or, more broadly, activity has been of interest to medical practitioners over the centuries.

Activity or exercise, rest, relaxation and leisure have been seen as health promoting and a core part of medical practice, from the Graeco-Roman tradition, Ayurveda and Chinese medicine to modern times. The place of work as physical labour in medical regimes is a more recent development, emerging towards the end of the eighteenth century and playing a significant role in the daily lives of inmates of the large asylums.[1] For psychiatric practice and the study of mental health/ill health in the twentieth century, the focus has been on the role of work in rehabilitation and the health risks associated with unemployment and the conditions of employment. In this chapter, we focus on these two areas.

Work, Employment and Leisure

What we mean by work is not easy to define; it is a shifting and contradictory concept that has varied over history and with the development of more complex societies.[2] Our contemporary view of work has its origins in the development of capitalism and the creation of a free labour market. This has dominated our conception of work and differentiated it from leisure and the home. It has allowed for the distinction between the employed and the unemployed (and children and retired people) but has also raised questions about work that does not receive renumeration, particularly that of housework and the work of carers. In practical terms, we may see 'work' as an activity that involves the exercise of skills and judgement, taking place within set limits prescribed by others.[3] It is something you 'do' for other people, whereas in most leisure activities you can 'please yourself'. 'Employment' is seen as work you get paid for, thus clarifying that many activities (childcare, housework, looking after elderly or sick relatives, for example) involve 'work' but do not usually attract formal payments and so are not 'employment'.

The Benefits of Work

Work may be viewed as being a uniquely human quality, essential not only for our material subsistence, growing needs and the wealth of nations but also for our psychological needs and sociability. It is a normative concept defined by the customs of society, but it is fundamentally relational and assists in defining who we are and our relation to others. It plays a central part in personal identity, gives a structure and purpose to the day and provides opportunities for socialisation and friendship. The social networks established in the workplace often extend beyond it and are a core component of social capital.

The potential magnitude of these beneficial effects (and by implication their ill effects) is brought home to us when we consider that our working lives represent the single longest period of the human lifespan, amounting to some forty to fifty years. This is the greater part of our adult lives, a time when many are raising families with the consequent responsibilities of dependents and effects on subsequent generations.

Employment, Worklessness and Their Ill Effects

Changes to the working life of Britons brought about by the industrial revolution revealed dangers of work on physical health in the hazardous conditions of the factories and mines during the nineteenth and into the twentieth century. During the twentieth century, however, the effects of unemployment and working conditions on our mental health emerged.

Economic cycles and crises during the twentieth century brought with them periods of high unemployment. During the Great Depression in the late 1920s and 1930s we saw the social and psychological effects of mass and long-term unemployment. These were documented in the classic studies of Marie Jahoda and colleagues examining the effects of the closure of the 'Marienthal' factory on the population of the Austrian village of Gramatneusiedl in 1929 and the subsequent studies of mass unemployment in the United States.[4] The morale of people suffers during periods of prolonged unemployment, and those without employment experience emotional instability, depression, hopelessness and apathy. These psychological effects can, in a vicious cycle, reduce social engagement and the likelihood of future employment and may blur the distinction between those who are unemployed and those removed from the job market for health reasons.[5] They also contribute to other social and interpersonal problems, including family and domestic discord.

The rising rates of unemployment in the UK during the 1980s prompted a revival of studies on the health effects of worklessness. These provided further evidence of the link between unemployment and poor mental health.[6] Studies typically find higher rates of anxiety and depression, alcohol and substance use and alcohol-related deaths among the unemployed than among those in work, even after taking account of age and sex. Suicide rates, especially among the long-term unemployed, are greater than among those in work. This association between unemployment and poor mental health seems to be bidirectional – being made unemployed can be a direct cause of poor mental health but mental illness or poor mental health can result in loss of employment. Continuing poor mental health can be a barrier to regaining employment, but re-entry into employment can result in an improvement of mental health.

The recognition of a link between suicide rates and rapid social change and economic depression has been noted since the nineteenth century.[7] By now, we can be confident about the association between unemployment and suicidal behaviour and the tendency for suicide rates to increase during economic crises.[8] The longer the duration of unemployment, the greater the risk of suicide or suicide attempts.[9] There is evidence for a direct causal relationship between unemployment and suicide, although most of the effects are related to the presence of mental health conditions.[10] This relationship is complicated and, like many psychosocial phenomena, dependent on a range of socioeconomic factors, including the strength of social safety nets and the degree of social fragmentation.[11]

The mental health conditions associated with unemployment are predominantly those that have become known as 'common mental health' disorders (or the studies used a measure of mental well-being). That these disorders were 'common' has been revealed by many population and primary care studies carried out since 1945. The emerging relationship between poor mental health, suicide and joblessness exposes the role of broad social, economic and political factors in determining the nation's health.

While employment may be beneficial to health, what emerged in the late twentieth century was evidence that the exposure to a range of psychosocial hazards can also put workers at risk of poor mental health.[12] Jobs can be poorly paid or provide people with insufficient or overly long working hours. They may be temporary or insecure or place people at risk of job loss or redundancy. They may also provide exposure to conditions of low psychosocial quality that affect the mental health of workers. Several large population studies of workforces in Europe and Australia have contributed to this body of evidence and the two British Whitehall studies conducted on populations of UK civil servants showed that adverse psychosocial conditions were associated with less satisfaction and well-being, a greater prevalence of mental health conditions and predicted poor mental health over a five-year period.[13] Low psychosocial quality includes conditions of a 'high-strain' working environment where the high demands on workers are combined with conditions of low control, such as little autonomy and reduced decision-making or conditions in which the effort to perform the job is not met by commensurate rewards in terms of money, esteem, career opportunities or job security.

UK Health and Social Policy since 1945

The cross-national studies on unemployment (or recessions) on mental health and suicide have noted a modulating effect of the strength of national social security programmes: countries with the weakest welfare states showed a greater impact of unemployment on rates of suicide.[14]

The provision of services and income transfers by the state to meet the welfare needs of the UK population and the concomitant expenditure grew in the twentieth century. These provisions include personal social services; services for health, education and housing; and income transfers such as pensions and out-of-work payments. Following the Second World War, the UK established reforms to create a more comprehensive and universal welfare state with an increase in resources to extend benefits and coverage which were associated with a commitment to economic growth and full employment (see also Chapter 3). These were accompanied by improvements in provisions for people with disabilities, including those for people with mental health conditions and intellectual disabilities. These welfare state developments facilitated the rundown of the large asylums and the development of community-based facilities for people with severe and long-term mental health conditions and improved access to primary care for those with common mental health conditions (see also Chapters 23 and 30).[15]

The golden age of the UK's welfare state declined in the 1970s, and the 1980s saw a period of retrenchment and recalibration with an abandonment of full employment and cuts to welfare provision, despite continuing growth in public expenditure. This was set against a background of increasing income and wealth inequality. In the late 1990s and 2000s, the New Labour government's vision for welfare was for a system that enabled rather than provided. The challenge was to reduce worklessness and introduce new benefits and tax credits as well as work support schemes. The recession in 2008 and the election of the coalition government in 2010 brought in a period of austerity and the introduction of further welfare reforms in 2012. The squeeze on expenditure and the roll-out of the new benefits continue to this day.

Contemporary Changes to Conditions of Work and Employment

In high-income countries, the labour market has changed dramatically over the past seventy years. In Britain, many traditional, large national employers such as the coal mining and motor manufacturing industries that were at the heart of the economy are long gone, radically reduced in scale or have been sold to global corporations. These dominant industries have been largely replaced by financial, service and hospitality industries, with many manual labour tasks replaced by automation.

In more recent years, there has been a movement away from the standard employment model in which workers earn wages or salaries in a dependent employment relationship with their employers, jobs that usually offer a stable contract and employment as well as labour law and social security protection.[16] In high-income countries, including the UK, while the standard employment model is still dominant, there has been a move towards increasing labour market flexibility and a weakening of regulations and protective policies. Associated with this has been an increase in forms of 'precarious' employment which may include 'flexible employment,' 'temporary work', 'casual work', 'zero hours contracts' and 'gig economy work'. In the UK, before the 2007 recession, we began to see an increase in 'underemployment' (employed persons who have not attained their full employment level) and a rise in 'in-work poverty' (households with incomes below the poverty line) which, along with precarious employment, has since increased. Working in insecure employment has a detrimental effect on psychological well-being and somatic health,[17] as does living below the poverty line.[18]

The labour market and the conditions of work or lack of work reflect and reinforce health inequalities and can have knock-on effects for future generations. High-pay conditions are protective of health, but poor-quality conditions in the workplace are more likely to be experienced by people from disadvantaged socioeconomic groups.[19] Certain jobs are more likely to expose people to these poor working environments, including elementary jobs, sales and customer services, plant and machine operatives and caring, leisure and other service occupations.[20] People who are in danger of unemployment are those who are looking for (or have previously worked in) jobs which carry the greatest risk to their health. There are stark regional differences in poor-quality work in England with the north of the country faring worst.[21]

Employment in People with Mental Health Conditions

People with mental health conditions are more likely than others in the general population to be out of work. Across the Organisation for Economic Cooperation and Development (OECD) countries, the employment rate of people with a mental disorder is between 55 per cent and 70 per cent, 10–15 per cent lower than for people without a mental disorder.[22]

While many people with common mental health conditions are in work, about 300,000 people with a long-term mental health condition lose their jobs every year in the UK and do so more frequently than those with physical health conditions.[23] People with mental health conditions now represent the largest group receiving out-of-work sickness benefits. One reason for this labour market disadvantage is that many people experience their first episode of a mental health problem in their teens or early adulthood, with serious and often enduring consequences for their education and employment prospects. Stigma and discrimination also contribute to these reduced employment opportunities (see also Chapter 27). In addition, they have a lower re-entry rate into the labour market, particularly in economic downturns.

Employment rates in people with common mental health conditions, while lower than the general population, are much higher than those with psychoses.[24] In the UK, between 10 per cent and 20 per cent of people with schizophrenia are in some form of employment.[25] These rates may have fallen over the years, as before 1990 employment rates of 20–30 per cent were reported.

Developments in Vocational Rehabilitation for People with Mental Health Problems

The view that occupation was an integral part of treatment and the subsequent development of vocational rehabilitation were influenced by the rise of 'moral treatment' in the early 1800s. However, despite the growth of patients working within the confines of nineteenth-century asylums, this was less about moral therapy and rehabilitation but more a matter of filling the patient's day, reducing idleness and providing free labour for the hospital farm, kitchens and laundry, with a view to reducing costs and raising funds for the running of the institution.[26]

This changed during the early-to-mid twentieth century as work became seen as enabling, valuable to good physical and mental health and part of a patient's rehabilitation. We saw the development of industrial workshops and creative therapies as well as the profession of occupational therapy.[27] The reforms after 1945 facilitated the idea that hospital-based work might be a stepping stone to eventual resettlement and were supported by research findings.[28] In the industrial workshops, which attempted to provide realistic conditions of employment, patients were paid for their labour and their work exceeded the expectations of staff. However, as the asylums diminished, the hospital workshops relocated to the community, patients' earnings were capped and workshop numbers dwindled. It became obvious that few people from these settings went on to get paid 'open' employment in the labour market.

In the United States, during the late 1970s, a new conceptual model emerged for the development of community-based treatment programmes for patients with mental health problems who would typically have been inpatients in large psychiatric hospitals. This took a multidisciplinary team approach and delivered integrated community-based treatment, rehabilitation and support services to help people with severe and persistent mental health problems to avoid psychiatric hospitalisation as well as to live independently in natural community settings. This approach gave patients sustained and intensive assistance in finding a job or a sheltered workshop. When in the job, staff retained contact with patients and their supervisors or employers to help with on-the-job problem-solving. Those who received this new approach spent significantly less time unemployed, spent more time in sheltered employment and earned a significantly higher income in open employment than those receiving the control intervention.[29] These new models of community-based treatment programmes seemed radical at the time but have since evolved into one of the most influential service delivery approaches in community mental health. Regrettably, when these new models of community-based treatment programmes were implemented in the UK, the presence of supporting people with longer-term mental health problems into work did not translate into practice.

Changes in the Emphasis of Vocational Rehabilitation

During the 1980s, also in the United States, new forms of vocational rehabilitation were being developed. These models of vocational rehabilitation were based on a 'train and place' approach – people with longer-term mental health problems would typically go through a stepwise approach of skills training and development in a segregated and sheltered environment, with a view that these new skills would enable them to gain and retain jobs in the open labour market. A variety of different models were developed ranging from pre-vocational training programmes through to clubhouses which were developed alongside other models of community mental health rehabilitation for people with longer-term mental health problems. The choose–get–keep model of rehabilitation began the shift from viewing work solely as a form of therapy to one that viewed it as a personal goal of the patient.[30] This approach defined the process both from the mental health practitioner's point of reference and from that of the person served. The practitioner's role was to facilitate rehabilitation: choosing, getting and keeping were what the individual did to attain their goals.

In 1993, Becker and Drake published the first manual of the Individual Placement and Support (IPS) approach to vocational rehabilitation.[31] The IPS approach is a form of supported employment and differed from previous approaches to vocational rehabilitation. Moving away from 'train and place', it adopted a 'place and train' approach, in which the primary goal of the approach was to directly find a job and then provide continued support. Its approach was fundamentally 'person-centred'. In 1996, the first randomised controlled trial (RCT) of the IPS approach was published and showed that people with longer-term mental health problems could be directly supported to gain and retain open employment without the use of pre-vocational training.[32] By 2001, a Cochrane systematic review of vocational rehabilitation for people with severe mental illness found that supported employment was significantly more effective than pre-vocational training,[33] and there are now twenty-seven RCTs supporting the efficacy of IPS compared to standard vocational rehabilitation.[34]

The ten-year plan of the National Service Framework for Mental Health contained several targets in which work was important, including 'action needed for employment, education or training or another occupation' (Standard 5) and the requirement of health and social services to 'combat discrimination against individuals and groups with mental health problems and promote their social inclusion'. The associated development of early intervention teams in the early 2000s provided a focus for vocational rehabilitation to support young people with a first episode of psychosis in education, training and employment.[35]

In 2003–4, the UK government undertook a cross-government review into mental health and social exclusion. The term 'social exclusion' was initially used as a simile for poverty but grew to acquire a wider interpretation. It encompassed unemployment, poor-quality housing or homelessness, limited social networks and restricted participation in social, economic and political life. The *Mental Health and Social Exclusion* report examined the connections between mental health problems and social exclusion.[36] It noted that mental health problems often led to and reinforced social exclusion, stigma and discrimination, owing to low expectations of what people with mental health problems can achieve; lack of clear responsibility for promoting vocational and social outcomes; lack of ongoing support to enable them to work; and barriers to engaging in the community. This report provided a catalyst for the development of vocational rehabilitation services for people with longer-term mental health problems and for the promotion of the IPS approach.

Two important developments occurred during this time. First, the Convention on the Rights of Persons with Disabilities was adopted on 13 December 2006. Rather than viewing persons with disabilities as 'objects' of charity, medical treatment and social protection, it saw persons with disabilities as 'subjects' with rights, who can claim those rights and make decisions based on their free and informed consent as well as being active members of society. The Convention dealt with the right to work and employment, stating that priority should be given to participation in the open labour market and all efforts should be done, through reasonable accommodations, to achieve this. The other development was the emergence of the recovery approach within mental health services in England.[37] At its heart, the recovery approach is a set of values about a person's right to build a meaningful life for themselves, with or without the continuing presence of mental health symptoms. Recovery is based on ideas of self-determination and self-management. It emphasises the importance of 'hope' in sustaining motivation and supporting expectations of an individually fulfilled life. Many of the ideas underpinning the recovery philosophy were not new. The main impetus came from the consumer/survivor movement in the 1980s and 1990s. The emergence of the recovery approach brought a renewed focus on the personal goals that were important to those with longer-term mental health problems and a focus on functional outcomes for mental health services.

Yet, despite these developments, annual surveys conducted in England between 2004 and 2008 repeatedly showed that, of those who use mental health services and were unemployed, more than half would have liked help in gaining employment but mental health services had not offered such help.[38] By 2010, there was evidence that the IPS approach could be effectively implemented within mental health services in England.[39]

Conclusion

This brief look at work and mental health perhaps tells us more about developments in psychiatry and its relation to history and social and economic factors than is immediately obvious.

First, it reflects the change in what has come under the psychiatric gaze during the twentieth century. The predominant interest in the nineteenth century was in severe mental illness located in the asylums. In the twentieth century, particularly after 1950, this shifted to include those with more prevalent conditions, common mental health disorders. In the development of mental health services, this extended gaze has increased the tensions related to the planning of services, particularly when we consider the size of the financial cake and its apportioning.

Second, the predominant emphasis for those with severe and enduring conditions has been on vocational rehabilitation, viewing work as part of therapy. Historically, this has been based on a more optimistic view of outcomes for this groups of people, from moral therapy to post-war enthusiasm and the recovery movement. More recently, we have seen a shift from 'work' as therapy to 'work' as a human right. Recent developments in vocational rehabilitation, notably IPS, have a firm and well-established evidence base but remain poorly implemented.[40] For those with common mental health conditions, the realisation of their increasing costs to the welfare benefit bill led the New Labour government (and subsequent UK governments) to adopt a series of welfare reforms to move these groups back into work. The evidence for the efficacy of these approaches has been poor but they continue. The initial business case for IAPT (Independent Access to Psychological Treatment) assumed that the receipt of cognitive behavioural therapy (CBT) would result in people returning to work but few did (see also Chapter 11).

Third, we see how economic cycles or crises and changes in labour markets have significant effects on the mental health of populations and on rehabilitation services.[41] Improvement to vocational services for people with serious mental illness (SMI) may mean increased spending on community rehabilitation services; but improving the quality of the working environment and alleviating the effects of unemployment require improvements to occupational health services and a public health or preventative approach to reducing health inequalities to 'create fair employment and good work for all',[42] as well as wider employment and welfare benefit reforms. This means taking action to reverse the fundamental causes, prevent the harmful environmental influences and mitigate the negative impact on individuals.

Key Summary Points

- There is an association between unemployment, poor mental health and suicidal behaviour. There is a modulating effect of the strength of national social security programmes: countries with the weakest welfare states showed a greater impact of unemployment on rates of suicide.
- While employment may be beneficial to health, exposure to a range of psychosocial hazards can also put workers at risk of poor mental health.
- People with mental health conditions now represent the largest group receiving out-of-work sickness benefits. In the UK, rates of employment of people with schizophrenia may have fallen.
- Supported employment is significantly more effective than pre-vocational training. The initial business case for IAPT (Independent Access to Psychological Treatment) for common mental disorders assumed that the receipt of cognitive behavioural therapy (CBT) would result in people returning to work but few did.
- More recently, we have seen a shift from 'work' as therapy to 'work' as a human right. Annual surveys conducted in England between 2004 and 2008 repeatedly showed that, of those who use mental health services and were unemployed, more than half would have liked help in gaining employment but mental health services had not offered such help.

Notes

1.   W. Ernst, *Work, Psychiatry and Society, c. 1750–2015*. Manchester: Manchester University Press, 2016.

2.   K. Thomas, *The Oxford Book of Work*. Oxford: Oxford University Press, 1999.

3.   D. Bennett, The value of work in psychiatric rehabilitation. *Social Psychiatry* (1970) 5: 224–30.

4. M. Jahoda, P. F. Lazarfeld and H. Zeisel, *Marienthal: The Sociography of an Unemployed Community*, trans. J. Reginall and T. Elsasser. London: Tavistock, 1974; P. Eisenberg and P. F. Lazarfeld, The psychological effects of unemployment. *Psychological Bulletin* (1938) 35: 358–90.

5. A. Sen, Social exclusion: Concept, application, and scrutiny. Social Development Papers No. 1, Office of Environment and Social Development, Asian Development Bank. Manila, Philippines, 2000.

6. G. Murphy and J. Athanasou, The effect of unemployment on mental health. *Journal of Occupational and Organisational Psychology* (1999) 72: 83–99.

7. J.-P. Falret, *De l'hyponchondrie el du suicide*. Paris, 1822; E. Durkheim, *Suicide*. London; Routledge and Kegan Paul, 1952. (Originally published in 1897.)

8. S. Platt, Unemployment and suicidal behaviour: A review of the literature. *Social Science and Medicine* (1984) 19: 93–115; D. Gunnell, J. Donovan, M. Barnes et al., *The 2008 Global Financial Crisis: Effects on Mental Health and Suicide*. Policy Report No. 3. University of Bristol, 2015.

9. A. Milner, A. Page and A. D. LaMontagne, Long-term unemployment and suicide: A systematic review and meta-analysis. *PLoS ONE* (2013) 8: e51333, https://doi.org/10.1371/journal.pone.0051333.

10. T. A. Blakely, S. C. D. Collings and J. Atkinson, Unemployment and suicide. Evidence for a causal association? *Journal of Epidemiology and Community Health* (2003) 57: 594–600.

11. T. Norström and H. J. Grönqvist, The Great Recession, unemployment and suicide. *Journal of Epidemiology and Community Health* (2015) 69: 110–16.

12. S. B. Harvey, M. Modini, S. Joyce et al., Can work make you mentally ill? A systematic meta-review of work-related risk factors for common mental health problems. *Occupational and Environmental Medicine* (2017) 74: 301–10.

13. S. A. Stansfeld, F. North, I. White and M. G. Marmot, Work characteristics and psychiatric disorder in civil servants in London. *Journal of Epidemiology and Community Health* (1995) 49: 48–53; S. A. Stansfeld, R. Fuhrer, M. J. Shipley and M. Marmot, Work characteristics predict psychiatric disorder: Prospective results from the Whitehall II study. *Occupational and Environmental Medicine* (1999) 56: 302–7.

14. Norström and Grönqvist, The Great Recession.

15. N. Rose, Historical changes in mental health practice. In G. Thornicroft, G. Szmukler, K. T. Mueser and R. E. Drake, eds, *Textbook of Community Mental Health*. Oxford: Oxford University Press, 2011.

16. International Labour Office, *World Employment and Social Outlook 2015: The Changing Nature of Jobs*. Geneva: International Labour Office, 2015.

17. H. De Witte, J. Pienaar and N. De Cuyper, Review of 30 years of longitudinal studies on the association between job insecurity and health and well-being: Is there causal evidence? *Australian Psychologist* (2016) 51: 18–31.

18. Joseph Rowntree Foundation, *UK Poverty 2019/20*. York: Joseph Rowntree Foundation, 2020.

19. Marmot Review Team, *Fair Society, Healthy Lives: Strategic Review of Health Inequalities in England Post-2010*. London: Marmot Review Team, 2010.

20. NHS Health Scotland, Good work for all. Inequality Briefing No. 2. Edinburgh: NHS Health Scotland, 2016.

21. Public Health England, *Local Action on Health Inequalities: Promoting Good Quality Jobs to Reduce Health Inequalities*. London: Public Health England, 2015.

22. Organisation for Economic Cooperation and Development (OECD), *Mental Health and Work: United Kingdom*. Paris: OECD Publishing, 2014, www.oecd.org/els/emp/mentalhealthandwork-unitedkingdom.htm.

23. P. Farmer and D. Stevenson, *Thriving at Work: The Independent Review of Mental Health and Employers*. London, 2017.

24. S. McManus, P. Bebbington, R. Jenkins and T. Brugha, eds, *Mental Health and Wellbeing in England: Adult Psychiatric Morbidity Survey 2014*. Leeds: NHS Digital, 2016.

25. S. Marwaha and S. Johnson, Schizophrenia and employment. *Social Psychiatry and Psychiatric Epidemiology* (2004) 39: 337–49.

26. Ernst, *Work, Psychiatry and Society*.

27. Ibid.

28. J. K. Wing and G.W. Brown, *Institutionalism and Schizophrenia*. Cambridge: Cambridge University Press, 1970.

29. L. I. Stein and M. A. Test, Alternative to mental hospital treatment: I. Conceptual model, treatment programme and clinical evaluation. *Archives of General Psychiatry* (1980) 37: 392–7.

30. K. S. Danley and W. A. Anthony, The choose–get–keep model: Serving severely psychiatrically disabled people. *American Rehabilitation* (1987) 13: 27–9.

31. D. R. Becker and R. E. Drake, *A Working Life: The Individual Placement and Support (IPS) Program*. Concord, NH: Dartmouth Psychiatric Research Center, 1993.

32. R. E. Drake, G. J. McHugo, D. R. Becker, W. A. Anthony and R. E. Clark, The New Hampshire study of supported employment for people with severe mental illness. *Journal of Consulting Clinical Psychology* (1996) 64: 391–9.

33. R. Crowther, M. Marshall, G. R. Bond and P. Huxley, Vocational rehabilitation for people with severe mental illness. *Cochrane Database of Systematic Reviews* (2001) 2: CD003080, https://doi.org/10.1002/14651858 .CD003080.

34. B. Brinchmann, T. Widding-Havneraas, M. Modini et al., A metaregression of the impact of policy on the efficacy of individual placement and support. *Acta Psychiatrica Scandinavica* (2020) 141: 206–20.

35. E. Killackey, J. Smith, M. Rinaldi et al., Meaningful lives: Supporting young people with psychosis in education, training and employment: An international consensus statement. *Early Intervention in Psychiatry* (2010) 4: 323–6.

36. Social Exclusion Unit, *Mental Health and Social Exclusion*. London. Office of the Deputy Prime Minister, 2004.

37. G. Shepherd, J. Boardman and M. Slade, *Making Recovery a Reality*. London: Sainsbury Centre for Mental Health, 2008.

38. Healthcare Commission, *National NHS Patient Survey Programme: Survey of Users of Community Mental Health Services 2004–2008*. London: Healthcare Commission, 2008.

39. M. Rinaldi, T. Montibeller and R. Perkins, Increasing the employment rate for people with longer-term mental health problems. *The Psychiatrist* (2011) 35: 339–43.

40. J. Boardman and M. Rinaldi, Difficulties in implementing supported employment for people with severe mental health problems. *British Journal of Psychiatry* (2013) 203: 247–9.

41. R. Warner, *Recovery from Schizophrenia: Psychiatry and Political Economy* (3rd ed.). Brunner-Routledge, 2004.

42. Marmot Review Team, *Fair Society, Healthy Lives*.

Sexual Diversity and UK Psychiatry and Mental Health

Annie Bartlett

Introduction

While the stories of sexual diversity did not begin in 1960 there is no doubt that the fifty years that followed saw radical changes in thinking about sex, gender and sexual practice. To be alive now is to live in interesting times, ones in which new categories of meaning about sexuality and gender are proliferating. These provide individuals with innovative ways of explaining themselves to each other and to themselves. That idea of self-definition, rather than definition by experts, including psychiatrists, is a key shift; much of that movement happened between 1960 and 2010. This was a period in which UK psychiatry was part of the wider debate about gender and sexuality but also a period where its contribution to the evolution of thinking about sexual diversity and its capacity to provide appropriate services to sexual minorities came under considerable scrutiny.

The premise of the chapter is that what happened within UK psychiatry and mental health did not do so in a social vacuum. So it documents key changes, judged in terms of what does or does not and should not constitute a mental disorder as well as corresponding amendments to legal rights and restrictions, as they relate to different genders, sexual identities and practices. Yet that is only part of the story. Psychiatry between 1960 and 2010 has been practised largely within the NHS with a smaller number of mental health practitioners operating psychiatric or psychological services either privately or within voluntary sector groups. Practitioner views are important in shaping care and they have not been static. Equally, both research and practice over this period of time have led to a broader understanding of the mental health issues encountered by individuals from sexual minorities and to a prevailing view that many of these difficulties stem from the negative responses of the wider community (including family and school) rather than being intrinsic to the minority identity. Research has, perforce evolved, so that it has investigated the nature and frequency of mental health problems within what is now, but was not earlier, the LBGTQI community. This new focus could be characterised as a move from being the problem to having problems. This forms a local, UK-centred, backdrop to the patchwork quilt information on the experiences of those accessing services for mental health difficulties, be that voluntarily or involuntarily, be they statutory services or from voluntary sector or private providers.

This contribution is limited in scope but necessarily draws on work describing events in other countries but known to those of us living and working in the UK. Social historians in the UK have set the wider scene in which the changes described here occurred and it would be absurd not to acknowledge the relationships between psychiatry, liberalisation in public attitudes, campaigning, legislative change and the ongoing internal conflicts within major religions on their position in relation to sexual minorities. The presumption here is that these do relate to the overall impetus within psychiatry to keep abreast of changing thinking rather than to direct it.

Nor are these essentially social debates confined to single jurisdictions. The social situation of sexual minorities varies in the West and internationally. In July 2020, Poland re-elected a president opposed to gay rights. There are a number of countries in the world with records of state violence against gays, some with legislation that allows for the death penalty for consensual same-sex sexual expression between adults. The Royal College of Psychiatrists has members from all over the globe and this issue continues to challenge it even as the UK basks within a socially liberal atmosphere, albeit one that is only recently acquired. The delicacy of the position of the College is that it risks a neocolonialist position when speaking to an international audience, in which old tropes about the hegemony of Western-inspired categories of meaning can be dusted off. At the same time, as the rest of the world dances to its own tunes,[1] indigenous concepts of gender identity and sexual expression can be and are reworked for modern times by those for whom such identities are their life, often drawing on historical models of multiple genders.[2]

Writing about sexual diversity in earlier decades could incur the wrath of the censors.[3] This remains the case. The judgements of the next generation on today's thinkers may be unkind. The previously radical figure Germaine Greer and, more recently, the internationally renowned author J. K. Rowling have found out that, regardless of their intent, it is easy to invoke opprobrium.[4] This chapter will attempt to tread carefully, speaking about, not for, but it enters a hot debate, most obviously today in relation to transgender politics and health care.

Sexual Diversity: Concepts, Categories and Contemporary Currency

Underpinning this discussion is the tricky issue of categories. What constitutes sexual diversity has long been contested. Central to this chapter is the balance of power between those who have been heavily pathologised by prevailing psychiatric concepts and the institution of psychiatry and its practitioners. The real story of the last sixty years is the reclaiming of autonomy and the move to self-definition by those of us who do not find ourselves sitting comfortably in a heteronormative, gender binary culture. What has not changed is the penchant, indeed enthusiasm, for categories. Sexual diversity continues to provide many conceptual categories, functioning as coat hangers on which individuals can hang their own experience of themselves, or not.

In the 1960s, the main focus in the UK was homosexuality, to use the term of the day. The Wolfenden Committee had reported on homosexuality (and prostitution, strange bedfellows from the perspective of 2020) in 1957.[5] The history of the word 'homosexuality' is instructive. Weeks argues that it was only one of a number of terms emerging in the late nineteenth century as writing on sexual preference emerged from private diaries into a public spotlight.[6] Despite its centrality to Wolfenden, he suggests it was not owned by those who saw themselves as 'queer'. Lesbianism and Sapphism had an obvious connection to the island of Lesbos and the poetry of Sappho, invoking a notionally golden past of communities of women with same-sex desires. These terms were superseded in time in part by the word 'gay', a word adopted by both men and women but which has never entirely replaced the word 'lesbian'. Medical discourse on same-sex sexuality stuck firmly to homosexuality, often ignoring women.[7] The *British Journal of Psychiatry* currently contains 127 papers on homosexuality, 17 on lesbians and a rather confusing 35 thrown up by 'gay' in the search engine, many of the latter being nothing to do with sexuality.

The messy history of vocabulary, where words have currency in different and overlapping social arenas, says much about what happened as political activism, both male and female, took private struggles to a visible, political front line. Events such as the Stonewall riots in 1969 and the abseiling of women into a TV studio to protest against Section 28 of the Local Government Act 1988, derived and owed much to a motley crew of local and national groups campaigning and creating safer social spaces for what was increasingly, but not necessarily accurately, called a community.[8] Derogatory terms, or words that indicated some degree of self-loathing, such as 'dyke' or 'poof', became at least contested and in part reclaimed as the voice of the 'community' grew louder and more confident. While explicitly gay organisations, such as Gay Liberation Front (GLF), did much to support the daily life of often isolated gays and lesbians, this was more true for men than women who also found a home in the women's movement. There, concepts such as lesbian feminism and compulsory heterosexuality were debated alongside lesbian motherhood, men's use of pornography and other aspects of the patriarchy.[9]

The arrival of AIDS in the early 1980s both contributed to this public identification of an emerging gay community and vilified gay men. It can be understood, however, as a turning point, not only for AIDS but also for medicine as demands to be involved in treatment trials in a different way paved the way for greater patient involvement in care and research.[10] An era of sexual experimentation and hedonism turned to personal tragedy for many and this sobering experience also highlighted the absence of basic rights within gay relationships.

It is salutary to note that the voice of bisexual and transgender people was noticeably absent for much of this period. The pioneering academic work of Charlotte Wolff is one of few attempts to document the experiences of bisexuals at that time.[11] The subjectivity of trans individuals was publicly aired intermittently or privately rehearsed over decades.[12] It is only in the twenty-first century, partly assisted by campaigning organisations such as Stonewall and Mermaids,[13] that trans issues have come to the fore really. The cinderellas of sexual minority activism have perhaps had their territory invaded by the plethora of new subjectivities emerging which challenge conventional understandings of both gender and sexuality. Non-binary, gender queer, gender fluid and third gender contest the concept of binary gender and themselves may or may not sit under a transgender umbrella, all with a range of sexual expressions. This is happening now and will in time generate its own history when the extent to which a significant portion of the population will adopt and amend these understandings of themselves will be clearer.

Sexual Diversity: Counting Changing Concepts

Estimates of the presence of individuals from sexual minorities in the overall population have been problematic. Methodological concerns about individuals' willingness to disclose stigmatised identities to the state or to research are reasonable in the context of identities that in sixty years, less than the average lifetime of a UK citizen, have gone from being illegal or pathological or both to being at least intermittently celebrated.[14] The government could find no recent reliable estimate of LGBT numbers in the population in 2018.[15] ONS experimental statistics indicate 2.3 per cent of the population are LGB, with many more young people identifying as such.[16] As terminology changes and new categories achieve prominence, historical comparisons become harder. Older studies from the 1990s have generated range of figures, for example 5–12 per cent men and 3–5 per cent of women in the UK as gay,[17] 5 per cent of the UK population gay, lesbian or bisexual.[18] Data on transgender are not collected as part of the annual population surveys, but the consultation on the Gender Recognition Act reported an estimate of between 200,000 and 500,000 and it is anticipated that the 2021 census will include a question on gender identity.[19]

The advent of civil partnerships (2004), legislation allowing same-sex couples essentially the same rights as heterosexual marriage, resulted in 53,415 couples (roughly equal numbers of men and women) using the legislation by 2011, five times the original government estimate.[20] Only a small percentage (2.2 per cent for men and 4.6 per cent for women) of these partnerships are dissolved.

Family composition is varied in the UK. Official estimates suggest that in 2012 there were 18.2 million families of which 69,000 were same-sex cohabiting couples (of which 6,000 had dependent children) and 60,000 civil partnerships (of which 6,000 had dependent children). In 1996, prior to civil partnerships (and now gay marriage) there seemed to be far fewer, only 16,000 same-sex cohabiting couples (and 1,000 with dependent children).[21] Gay couples have been able to adopt since 2002 and account for a rising percentage of adoptions.[22]

Legislation in the UK: From Crime to Weddings

It is tempting to see the half-century of change, post-1960, in which this linguistic, conceptual and real-life journey has taken place, as moving inexorably in the direction of liberalisation, de-pathologisation and openness. In fact, it is more complex.[23] Many legal changes took decades to materialise and were fought for every step of the way. Equally, there was a hardening of attitudes towards homosexuality in the 1980s. In 1987, only 11 per cent of the population thought same-sex relationships were 'not at all wrong', a figure that had changed to 47 per cent in 2012 and 64 per cent in 2016,[24] which allowed for the introduction of Section 28 in the Local Government Act . This effectively censored sex education in schools, arguably making it harder to counteract homophobic bullying and jeopardising the local groups supporting LBGT individuals in local communities by restricting the activities of local authorities. The extent to which statute law has changed is striking and indisputable. The sheer volume of legislation in this area, as opposed to legislation about women or those from black and minority ethnic groups, is remarkable (see Chapters 15 and 35).

Key Legal Changes in the UK

The journey encapsulated in Box 34.1 is not yet complete. Sexual practices among gay men have been decriminalised; hate crimes against the LGBT community are recognised; the inequality in the age of consent has been rectified; and the state recognises personal commitment between people of the same gender and allows someone to define their gender as they think fit (although this requires medical action). All areas of life have been affected by legal change so that inroads have been made to what happens in schools, workplaces and elsewhere.

It is also noticeable that the tone and vocabulary of government documents are very different; these have conspicuously adopted the self-defining terms used within the LGBT and wider community and in their very use speak to the depth of change since the Wolfenden Report. However, the debate about trans rights, for example, continues.

Box 34.1
1957 Wolfenden Committee on Homosexuality and Prostitution
1967 Sexual Offences Act decriminalises consensual sexual acts between men over twenty-one years of age in private (England and Wales)
1988 Local Government Act Section 28
1994 Legal recognition of male rape
2000 European Court of Human Rights (ECHR) challenge to law on gross indecency
2001 Equal age of consent regardless of sexual orientation
2002 Equality in the Mental Health Act with regard to 'nearest relative' (case law)
2003 Homophobic assault is recognised as a hate crime
2003 Repeal of Section 28 of the Local Government Act
2003 Repeal of Victorian laws on gross indecency and buggery
2004 Gender Recognition Act
2005 Civil Partnership Act (for same-sex couples only)
2010 Equality Act (creating a range of 'protected characteristics', including sexual orientation)
2013 Same-sex marriage (England, Wales and Scotland 2014; 2019 in Northern Ireland)
2017 'Turing's Law' in the Policing and Crime Act 2017 posthumously pardons men who were convicted for having sex with men prior to 1967 where the offence is no longer a crime

Aspects of this are acrimonious and unresolved at the time of writing, although the government has committed to further separate consultation with non-binary and intersex people.[25]

Psychiatry and Diagnostic Indecision

Much of the thinking and many of the changes in the understanding and experience of sexual diversity since 1960 have occurred independent of psychiatry but the concepts within mental health and associated practices within mental health care have also been profoundly affected. Drescher has documented the evolution of diagnostic thinking within both the *International Classification of Diseases* (ICD) and the *Diagnostic and Statistical Manual of Mental Disorders* (DSM) over the second half of the twentieth century to the present day.[26] As a gay psychiatrist who has lived and worked through many of the changes, it is a relief no longer to be a diagnosis. The self-belief of a profession which viewed the application of terms such as 'sexual deviation' or 'pathological personality' to gay individuals as reasonable jars with modern sensibilities.[27] The individuals have not changed but the profession and the terminology certainly have.

In 1973, the American Psychiatric Association (APA) removed 'homosexuality' from DSM-II. This was done on a vote, a democratic approach rather than a scientific one, and based on a small constituency, few of whom were gay.[28] ICD dragged its feet in comparison. In 1965, 'lesbianism' and 'sodomy' were added to the ICD-8 collection of sexual deviations already featuring homosexuality. ICD-9, in 1975, hedged its bets and, while 'homosexuality' was still a diagnosis, it was less clear that it was construed as a mental disorder.[29] Not until 1992 did 'homosexuality' per se finally disappear, with ICD-10 featuring 'ego dystonic sexual orientation' instead. 'Gender identity disorder' appeared for the first time, having been in DSM since 1994.[30]

The tension between wanting to help someone with a problem and pathologising them is evident in the history of psychiatry and all things LGBT.[31] Access to health care can depend on having a diagnosis. While being a diagnosis resulted in gay men and women being sent to doctors (notably to psychiatrists) for help in what could and can be a hostile world, the sense of negative difference engendered by the diagnostic process is unavoidable. This is now being played out in the UK more markedly in relation to transgender individuals where the role of medicine in the current Gender Recognition Act is very clear and constrains a person's capacity for positive self-definition.

Mental Health Problems and Sexual Minorities

psychological and sociological research this century has almost always attempted to uncover sickness, psychological difficulty and unhappiness as intrinsic to homosexuality. Little heed is paid to the social context of the lives of gays and lesbians.[32]

It was not until 2003 that the first robust UK-based study was able to suggest that some mental health problems were more common in lesbian and gay individuals than in straight counterparts,[33] echoing research done in north America. Gay men and lesbians had higher levels of psychological distress, greater exposure to recreational drugs and higher rates of self-harm and were more likely to have consulted mental health professionals as a result. These findings have persisted over time and now include similar information on bisexual, non-binary and transpeople.[34]

The uncoupling of distress from identity and the identification of an external set of societal stressors – for instance, LGBT hate crimes and bullying at school – is an important paradigm shift and echoed what gay people had been saying themselves.[35] King and colleagues argued that both societal prejudice and restricted lifestyle opportunities contributed to their findings.[36] Hunt and Minsky had earlier argued persuasively that, for the LGBT community, simply considering sexual orientation was inadequate and the inter-sectionalities with age, disability, youth issues and membership of a BAME community also mattered.[37] The salience of this observation is evident in the later work that highlights the increased rates of mental health difficulties among LGBT young people, BAME individuals, disabled individuals and within lower-income households.[38] Only with this more nuanced grasp of health needs and their origins can health services meet needs appropriately.

Professional Practice with Sexual Minorities

Medicine has an overt obligation to try and meet the health needs of the whole population without prejudice and LGBT people use health care like everybody else, perhaps more so.[39] Unlike visible difference, LGBT status may not always be recognised by health care practitioners, regardless of their own sexual orientation or gender identity. There is substantial evidence that health services in general and mental health services in particular have historically failed to live up to the General Medical Council (GMC) standard. Patients perceived staff as holding negative views about their sexuality and connecting it with their mental health problems as well as responding negatively to self-disclosure by the patient. Bisexuals in particular reported negative experiences.[40] In this context, a reluctance to be 'out' to health care professionals, an avoidance of health care and a wish to see LBGT clinical staff are understandable.

Treatment issues have compounded this for LGB individuals and now in a related but also different way for transpeople. The history of the treatment of 'homosexuality' and its current manifestation as conversion or reparative therapy of LGBT people, endeavours which have involved mental health services but which are by no means confined to them, have caused pain and generated mistrust over much of the twentieth century.[41] Psychodynamic theory and practice were often directed to changing sexual orientation in men and women, using a model of compulsory heterosexuality.[42] With the same aim, behavioural theory and practice,[43] for instance aversion therapy using electric shocks, was principally directed at gay men, sometimes those who had fallen foul of the courts. Individuals sought treatment mainly because of negative social or family attitudes towards their sexuality. More recently, there was further evidence, from a survey of 2,000 psychiatrists, psychologists and psychotherapists, that 4 per cent of these professionals were still prepared to offer treatment directed at altering sexual orientation from gay to straight where clients requested this and 17 per cent had done so previously.[44] In 2018, 5 per cent of a large sample of LGBT individuals had at some earlier point in their lives been offered reparative therapy and 2 per cent had undergone it (half within faith groups but one in five from health care professionals).[45] A systematic review of psychological therapies in the UK and elsewhere found that early studies revealed that concern about LGBT identity precipitated contact with therapy but that was less true in recent studies.[46] LGBT affirmative therapy was becoming ordinary and therapy was positively experienced unless an attempt to change sexual orientation was attempted.

A proportion of transpeople will seek help from primary care and specialist services for a number of aspects of their gender identity, including hormone treatment and surgery. Much recent material on transpeople's experience of care falls outside the historical scope of this chapter but suggests that specialist services are hard to access, transpeople will often avoid general health care and they often do not feel understood by health care services.[47] Given the need for access to specialist services for a person's gender recognition, their long waiting times are unhelpful.

UK Psychiatry and Sexual Minority Issues

Sporadic work in the UK on attitudes in psychiatry to LGBT issues suggested that psychiatrists were influenced by disease models of sexual preference more than GPs.[48] Bhugra and King found the opposite in a survey undertaken just before the AIDS crisis.[49] Both these studies predate the removal of homosexuality form ICD-10. Current attitudes are uninvestigated. It is also far from clear how rigorous the approach is taken within either basic medical training or psychiatric training such that practitioners are culturally competent with LGBT patients. Without this information, it is debatable whether psychiatry knows enough about lifestyle, sexual practices and contemporary identity to provide an inclusive service for an LGBT patient; material from patients suggest that problems remain.

Against a background of political change, alterations to the diagnostic systems and anecdotal concern about homophobia against colleagues, support within the membership led the Royal College of Psychiatrists to endorse the formation of a Lesbian and Gay Special Interest Group (SIG) in 2001. In 2012, its remit expanded to include trans issues and it was renamed the Rainbow SIG. The original remit of this group was determined by the membership and was 'to promote discussion and research, provide expertise within the College and contribute to education'.[50] Its regular appearance at mainstream College meetings and periodic workshops gave it a profile that allowed isolated psychiatrists to identify its activities and created the possibility of a broader audience for its work. It has provided a forum to discuss patient-focused issues – the broader social context of LGBT life, for example parenting, discrimination and intersectionality – in a clinical context, for instance by working with older LGBT people, and also to provide support to colleagues. Its advisory role within the College led to two position statements: one essentially in tandem with other mental health organisations on the lack of evidence for conversion therapy and another, more recently, on trans issues.[51] This is in some contrast to the earlier work in the United States on diagnosis, perhaps because the College lacked a coherent LGBT voice until the formation of the SIG, long after many of the most difficult discussions on diagnostic entities had taken place. It may be that the NHS is better placed to transform organisations to provide inclusive environments for staff and patients. In 2020, only one mental health services Trust, Central and North West London (CNWL), is in the Stonewall Top 100 Employers list; no other NHS organisations are listed, suggesting that there is more to do; this is in line with recent evidence of experiences of care.

Conclusion

History, whether of psychiatry or not, does not have bookends. The focus of this contribution has necessarily been principally on the experiences of gays and lesbians in relation to psychiatry, as it was those issues that dominated the years from 1960 to 2010. Yet, as identities alter over time, there has been some space to acknowledge the mental health issues and experiences of those with a less well-rehearsed sense of self, for instance bisexual and trans-people, non-binary and intersex individuals whose voices have come to the fore only recently.

The historical period in question has been one of profound change, experienced as such by those of us affected by changing social attitudes, protection in the workplace and the street, public recognition of our relationships and stability for our children. Psychiatry, and UK psychiatry in particular, seems both central and peripheral: central because embedded in its previous way of thinking was a wholesale and widely shared sickness model of LGBT sexuality which has been overthrown; peripheral because it is hard to argue that psychiatry did anything more than follow where the emerging LGBT community and its influencers bravely led, backed up academically by a handful of social scientists, historians and psychologists.[52]

Questions remain about the proper role of psychiatry going forward. Some may argue that this is a dismal history and in future there is no place for psychiatrists in relation to LGBT matters; but, as mental health services are used by many of the LGBT community, UK psychiatry can play a role, if it chooses to do so. However, if this chapter tells us anything, it is that psychiatry should adopt an unaccustomed humility that sits uneasily with the intrinsic power and authority of the profession.

Key Summary Points

- The sickness model of LGBT people was dominant within UK psychiatry and its impact was still apparent years later, despite the removal of homosexuality from ICD-10 in 1992.
- Conversion and reparative therapies were important aspects of psychiatrists' and other mental health practitioners' approaches to LGBT people, despite the lack of a credible evidence base.

- More positive, gay-affirming therapeutic approaches have been developed and adopted by mental health practitioners, although many LGBT people report concerns about their experience of mental health care.
- Social changes (liberalisation in public attitudes and law) were brought about through complex social processes that owed nothing to UK psychiatry.
- The history of LGBT people in relation to psychiatry raises important questions about the legitimacy of psychiatric power and authority.

Notes

1. S. Nandy, The hijras of India: Cultural and individual dimensions of an institutionalised third gender role. In E. Blackwood, ed., *The Many Faces of Homosexuality: Anthropological Approaches to Homosexual Behaviour*, 35–54. London: Eurospan and Harrington, 1988; C. Callender and L. Kochems, Men and no-men: Male gender mixing statuses and homosexuality. In Blackwood, *The Many Faces of Homosexuality*, 165–78.

2. Hijras shake it! YouTube, 31 January 2014, www.youtube.com/watch?v=Vl2BOiBtRio; BBC News, Pre-colonial communities' history of gender fluidity. *BBC News*, 28 July 2020, www.bbc.co.uk/news/av/world-53573764/pre-colonial-communities-history-of-gender-fluidity.

3. D. Souhami, *The Trials of Radclyffe Hall*. London: Weidenfeld and Nicholson, 1998.

4. BBC News, Germaine Greer: Transgender women are not women. *BBC News*, 24 October 2015, www.bbc.co.uk/news/av/uk-34625512/germaine-greer-transgender-women-are-not-women; J. K. Rowling, J. K. Rowling writes about her reasons for speaking out on sex and gender issues. J. K. Rowling website, 10 June 2020, www.jkrowling.com/opinions/j-k-rowling-writes-about-her-reasons-for-speaking-out-on-sex-and-gender-issues/.

5. J. Wolfenden, *Report of the Committee on Homosexual Offences and Prostitution* [Wolfenden Report]. London: Home Office Scottish Home Department, 1957, www.parliament.uk/about/living-heritage/trans formingsociety/private-lives/relationships/collections1/sexual-offences-act-1967/wolfenden-report-/.

6. J. Weeks, *Coming Out: The Emergence of LGBT Identities in Britain from the Nineteenth Century to the Present* (3rd ed.). London: Quartet, 2016.

7. See, for example, C. Allen, *Homosexuality Its Nature Causes and Treatment*. London: Staples Press, 1958.

8. E. Grinberg, How the Stonewall riots inspired today's Pride celebrations. *CNN*, 28 June 2019, https://edition .cnn.com/2019/06/28/us/1969-stonewall-riots-history/index.html.

9. A. Rich, Compulsory heterosexuality and lesbian existence. In A. Rich, *Blood, Bread, and Poetry: Selected Prose, 1979–1985*, 1986; A. Stewart-Park and J. Cassidy, *We're Here: Conversations with Lesbian Women*. London: Quartet; J. Dixon, Separatism: A look back at anger. In B. Cant and S. Hemmings, eds, *Radical Records Thirty Years of Lesbian and Gay History*, 69–84. London: Routledge, 1988.

10. T. Bereczky, Patient advocacy and the HIV community, *BMJ Opinion* (blog), 9 January 2017, https://blogs .bmj.com/bmj/2017/01/09/tamas-bereczky-patient-advocacy-and-the-hiv-community/.

11. C. Wolff, *Bisexuality: A Study*. London: Quartet, 1977.

12. J. Morris, *Conundrum*, London: Faber & Faber, 1974; D. Souhami, *No Modernism without Lesbians*. London: Head of Zeus, 2020, pp. 111–212, Bryher.

13. See the Stonewall website: www.stonewall.org.uk; and the Mermaids website: https://mermaidsuk.org.uk.

14. E. Price, *LGBT Sexualities in Social Care Research*. London: School for Social Care Research, 2011, www .sscr.nihr.ac.uk/wp-content/uploads/SSCR-methods-review_MR002.pdf.

15. Government Equalities Office, *National LGBT Survey: Summary Report*. July 2018, https://assets .publishing.service.gov.uk/government/uploads/system/uploads/attachment_data/file/722314/GEO-LGBT-Survey-Report.pdf.

16. Office for National Standards (ONS), *Sexual Orientation, UK: 2018*. Statistical Bulletin, 2020, www .ons.gov.uk/peoplepopulationandcommunity/culturalidentity/sexuality/bulletins/sexualidentityuk/2018.

17. K. Wellings, J. Field, A. Johnson et al., *Sexual Behaviour in Britain*. London: Penguin,1994.

18. A. M., Johnson, C. H., Mercer, B. Erens et al., Sexual behaviour in Britain: Partnerships, practices and HIV risk behaviours. *Lancet* (2001) 358: 1835–42.

19. Government Equalities Office, *Reform of the Gender Recognition Act 2004 Consultation 2018*. London: HMSO, 2018, https://assets.publishing.service.gov.uk/government/uploads/system/uploads/attachment_ data/file/721725/GRA-Consultation-document.pdf.

20. ONS, *Civil Partnerships in the UK: 2012*. Statistical Bulletin, 2013, www.ons.gov.uk/peoplepopulationand community/birthsdeathsandmarriages/marriagecohabitationandcivilpartnerships/bulletins/civilpartnership sinenglandandwales/2012–07–31.

21. ONS, *Families and Households in the UK: 2012*. Statistical Bulletin, 2013, www.ons.gov.uk/peoplepopulatio nandcommunity/birthsdeathsandmarriages/families/bulletins/familiesandhouseholds/2012–11–01.

22. Adoption Plus, www.adoptionplus.co.uk/LGBT-Gay-Adoption-UK.

23. Horsfall 1988.

24. National Centre for Social Research, *Moral Issues: Sex, Gender Identity and Euthanasia*. In *British Social Attitudes*, Vol. 34, www.bsa.natcen.ac.uk/media/39147/bsa34_moral_issues_final.pdf.

25. Government Equalities Office, *Reform of the Gender Recognition Act 2004*; Government Equalities Office, *LGBT Action Plan: Improving the Lives of Lesbian, Gay, Bisexual and Transgender People*. London: HMSO, 2018, https://assets.publishing.service.gov.uk/government/uploads/system/uploads/attachment_data/file/72 1367/GEO-LGBT-Action-Plan.pdf; J. Doward, Polarised' debate on gender recognition is harming UK, says equalities chief. *The Guardian*, 8 August 2020, www.theguardian.com/society/2020/aug/08/polarised-debate- on-gender-recognition-is-harming-uk-says-equalities-chief.

26. J. Drescher, Queer diagnoses: Parallels and contrasts in the history of homosexuality, gender variance, and the *Diagnostic and Statistical Manual*. *Archives of Sexual Behavior* (2010) 39: 427–60, https://doi.org/10.1007 /s10508-009-9531-5; J. Drescher, Queer diagnoses revisited: The past and future of homosexuality and gender diagnoses in DSM and ICD, *International Review of Psychiatry*, 2015, 27: 386–95, https://doi.org/10.3109/0 9540261.2015.1053847.

27. World Health Organization (WHO), *International Classification of Diseases and Related Health Problems* (6th revision). Geneva: WHO,1948; WHO, *International Classification of Diseases and Related Health Problems* (7th revision). Geneva: WHO, 1955.

28. Drescher, Queer diagnoses.

29. WHO, *International Classification of Diseases and Related Health Problems* (8th revision). Geneva: WHO, 1965; WHO, *International Classification of Diseases and Related Health Problems* (9th revision). Geneva: WHO, 1975.

30. WHO, *International Classification of Diseases and Related Health Problems* (10th revision). Geneva: WHO, 1990.

31. M. King and A. Bartlett, British psychiatry and homosexuality. *British Journal of Psychiatry* (1999) 175: 106–13.

32. Ibid.

33. M. King, E. McKeown, J. Warner et al., Mental health and quality of life of gay men and lesbians in England and Wales: Controlled, cross-section study. *British Journal of Psychiatry* (2003) 183: 552–8.

34. M. Plöderl and P. Tremblay, Mental health of sexual minorities: A systematic review. International Review of Psychiatry (2015) 27: 367–85, https://doi.org/10.3109/09540261.2015.1083949; C. L. Bachmann and B. Gooch, *LGBT in Britain: Health Report*. London: Stonewall, 2018, www.stonewall.org.uk/system/files/lg bt_in_britain_health.pdf.

35. L. Trenchard and H. Warren, *Something to Tell You: The Experiences and Needs of Young Lesbians and Gay Men in London*. London: London Gay Teenage Group,1984.

36. King, McKeown, Warner et al., Mental health and quality of life of gay men and lesbians.

37. R. Hunt and A. Minsky, *Reducing Health Inequalities for Lesbian Gay and Bisexual People: Evidence of Health Care Needs*, London: Stonewall, 2006, www.ilga-europe.org/sites/default/files/reducing_health_inequalities_for_lesbian_gay_and_bisexual_people_evidence_of_health_care_needs.pdf.

38. Bachmann and Gooch, *LGBT in Britain.*

39. Good Medical Practice (GMC), *Good Medical Practice*. Guidance, March 2013, www.gmc-uk.org/-/media/documents/good-medical-practice–english-20200128_pdf-51527435.pdf?la=en&hash=DA1263358CCA88F298785FE2BD7610EB4EE9A530.

40. E. McFarlane, *Diagnosis: Homophobic. The Experiences of Lesbians, Gay Men and Bisexuals in Mental Health Services*. London: PACE, 1997; J. Golding, *Without Prejudice: Mind – Lesbian, Gay and Bisexual Mental Health Awareness Research*. London: Mind, 1997; M. King and E. McKeown, *Mental Health and Social Wellbeing of Gay Men, Lesbians and Bisexuals in England and Wales: A Summary of Findings*. London: Mind, 2003, www.mindout.org.uk/wp-content/uploads/2012/06/SummaryfindingsofLGBreport.pdf.

41. King and Bartlett, British psychiatry and homosexuality; G. Smith, M. King and A. Bartlett, An oral history of treatments for homosexuality in Britain since the 1950s: I. The views of patients. *British Medical Journal* (2004) 328: 427–9; M. King, A. Bartlett and G. Smith An oral history of treatments for homosexuality in Britain since the 1950s: II. The views of professionals. *British Medical Journal* (2004) 328: 429–32.

42. A. Storr, *Sexual Deviation*. Harmondsworth, Penguin, 1965; M. Glasser, Homosexuality in adolescence. *British Journal of Medical Psychology* (1977) 50: 217–25; I. Rosen, *Sexual Deviation*. Oxford: Oxford University Press, 1996; J. MacDougall, Homosexuality in women. In J. Chasseguet-Smirgel, ed., *Sexuality and New Psychoanalytic Views*, 171–212. Ann Arbor: Michigan University Press; A. Bartlett, M. King and P. Phillips, Straight talking: An investigation of the attitudes and practice of psychoanalysts and psychotherapists in relation to gays and lesbians. *British Journal of Psychiatry* (2001) 179: 545–9; P. Phillips, A. Bartlett and M. King, Psychotherapists' approach to gay and lesbian patients/clients: A qualitative study. *British Journal of Medical Psychology* (2001) 74: 73–84.

43. M. J. McCulloch and M. P. Feldman, Aversion therapy in management of 43 homosexuals. *British Medical Journal* (1967) 2: 594–7; J. Bancroft, Aversion therapy of homosexuality: A pilot study of 10 cases. *British Journal of Psychiatry* (1969) 115: 1417–31.

44. A. Bartlett, G. Smith and M. King, The response of mental health professionals to clients seeking help to change or redirect same sex sexual orientation. *BMC Psychiatry* (2009) 9: 11, https://doi.org/10.1186/1471-244X-9-11.

45. Wellings, Field, Johnson et al., *Sexual Behaviour in Britain.*

46. M. King, J. Semlyen, H. Killaspy et al., *A Systematic Review of Research on Counselling and Psychotherapy for Lesbian, Gay, Bisexual & Transgender People*. London: British Association for Counselling and Psychotherapy, 2007, www.bacp.co.uk/media/1965/bacp-research-relating-to-counselling-lgbt-systematic-review.pdf.

47. S. Bridger, M. Snedden, C. L. Bachmann and B. Gooch, *LGBT in Britain: Health Report*. London: Stonewall, 2018, www.stonewallscotland.org.uk/sites/default/files/lgbt_in_scotland_-_health_report.pdf.

48. P. A. Morris, Doctors' attitudes to homosexuality. *British Journal of Psychiatry* (1973) 122: 435–6.

49. D. Bhugra and M. B. King, Controlled comparison of attitudes of psychiatrists, general practitioners, homosexual doctors and homosexual men to male homosexuality. *Journal of the Royal Society of Medicine* (1989) 82: 603–5.

50. Royal College of Psychiatrists, *Annual Report to Council 2016*. LGB Special Interest Group, www.rcpsych.ac.uk/docs/default-source/members/sigs/rainbow/rainbow-sig-annual-report-2016.pdf?sfvrsn=726ec7e3_4.

51. Royal College of Psychiatrists, *Royal College of Psychiatrists' Statement on Sexual Orientation*. Position Statement No. PS02/14, April 2014, www.rcpsych.ac.uk/docs/default-source/improving-care/better-mh-policy/position-statements/ps02_2014.pdf?sfvrsn=b39bd77c_4; Royal College of Psychiatrists, Supporting Transgender and Gender-Diverse People. Position Statement No. PS02/18, March 2018,

www.rcpsych.ac.uk/docs/default-source/improving-care/better-mh-policy/position-statements/ps02_18 .pdf?sfvrsn=af4d4aad_4.

52. See, for example, E. M. Ettore, *Lesbians, Women and Society*. London: Routledge and Kegan Paul, 1980; C. Wolff, *Love between Women*. London: 1971; K. Plummer, *The Making of the Modern Homosexual*. New York: Barnes & Noble.1981; C. Kitzinger, *The Social Construction of Lesbianism*. London: SAGE, 1987.

Chapter 35

Race, State and Mind

Doreen Joseph and Kamaldeep Bhui

Introduction

This chapter examines the experience of black and minority ethnic communities and the way their mental health needs were understood, recognised, prioritised, discussed and tackled by service providers and commissioners in the UK in the period 1960–2010. The chapter begins with the section 'Doreen's Narrative and the Research Evidence', an experiential narrative account from Doreen Joseph, placed alongside research evidence. This attends to black, Asian and minority ethnic (BAME) children, young people and their families in and against the youth (criminal) justice system. The issues are situated within a broader context of racism derived from a legacy of slavery, colonialism and postcolonialism. BAME people have felt this impact on their education, employment, housing, social circumstances, citizenship and health. To understand how these experiences emerged in a historical, social and political context, we then consider responses from practitioners and policymakers to health inequalities.

Doreen's Narrative and the Research Evidence

Growing up as a teenager in west London in the UK during the 1970s, I noticed the problem of Black youth falling into the criminal justice system. I saw Black youths being slammed against cars while policemen searched them under the 'sus' laws. This was the 'search under the suspicion' of criminality. This concerned the Black community because of the distress and shame it brought to parents who were law-abiding citizens and its occurrence in a racist and political climate of oppression.

BAME youth in contact with the criminal justice system is one element of a broader context of culture and politics which determines who gets what resources to live in society and how much. Racism is one of the tools that is used to ensure that 'the rich get richer, and the little that the poor man has is taken away' in accord with the so-called Matthew effect of cumulative advantage,[1] named after the parable of the talents or minas in the biblical Gospel of Matthew. The inverse of this is cumulative disadvantage and trauma, which lead to cumulative harms, including for health.[2] Poverty and dispossession drive some Black youth into criminality to survive. However, historical, economic and political factors are major determinants for this outcome, more so than individual 'bad' choices or deviant behaviour. Wider issues of immigration, citizenship, (mis- or under)education, (un)employment, housing and detention/incarceration, fuelled by racism, are pertinent. Ultimately, more structural fairness and equity of opportunity and choice would reduce poverty and disadvantage as well as consequent pathways to criminality. Although I look at the experience of the UK, it also applies worldwide where the legacy of slavery and colonialism has continued through racist policies and legislation.

Marginalisation

Racism has a long history that defines relations between different races, where there is a white hegemony over black people, but it was not always so. Black Africans had the ascendancy from ancient times up until the fifteenth century when Western exploration of Africa took off. Black Africans were powerful and respected; the Egyptians influenced the Greeks and Romans of antiquity. During these black civilised ascendancies, the colour black was equated with good representations and white with evil spirits. 'Black meant "life", and white "death".'[3] The situation reversed when Europeans joined in the Arab slave trade of black people in Africa and began to construct representations of themselves as 'superior' to the 'rest' of the world, separating 'us' from 'them'.

Demonology

In the eighteenth century, the Roman Catholic Church identified the colour black with evil. Black was made an emotional partisan colour, alluding to danger, repulsion and other negative connotations.[4] Travel stories from the 'dark continent' informed conceptions of Europeans in the Enlightenment by contrast with 'others' from the Orient.[5] They equated their 'whiteness' with being beautiful, enlightened, cultured, knowledgeable, progressive and modern. The demonology of Black people emerged as a result. Black people were portrayed as lazy, servile, untrustworthy, 'mad, bad and dangerous'.[6] The transatlantic slave trade in the fifteenth to nineteenth centuries displaced Africans. Racist views were exacerbated by plantocracy in the British colonies in the Caribbean. The nineteenth-century pseudoscientific racist 'ranking of races' chose skin colour, rather than hairiness, to demarcate separation.[7]

Racism is embedded in many economic, political and power relations between the 'white' 'West and the rest' of the diverse ethnicities of the world.[8] Western powers colonised many parts of the world, and immigrants from the Caribbean in the 1950s to 1980s; the Kenyan and Ugandan Asians in the 1980s; Ghanaians and Nigerians; those fleeing wars in Sudan, Somalia, the dissolved Czechoslovakia in the 1990s and Afghanistan and Syria today all mean that the world has come to Britain and it has become multiracial, multicultural, multi-ethnic, multifaith: cosmopolitan. White Britons at certain historical moments have been intolerant and tensions have overspilled. Right-wing racism and discrimination are very visible even today but are dressed up as neoliberal policies and practices designed to obscure the ways in which inequalities are generated and power relations sustained.

Criminalised

Immigration policy has been the mechanism by which Britishness and foreignness were defined. Creating a hostile environment to deter immigration was a response to public protests of scarce resources, perceived threats to British culture and perceived relatively liberal immigration policies. This hostile response was started in 2007 by Labour's home secretary John Reid and continued by the Conservative home secretary Theresa May from 2010 to 2016. This hostile response included criminal justice system actions to criminalise, legally identify and remove those coming to the UK; importantly, many who were unable to produce proof of the right to remain were also denied citizenship. When the UK was seeking workers from Commonwealth countries, the variety of visa options under which people could come and work often denied them and their children the right to remain and to full citizenship, resulting decades later in disputes about citizenship rights.

The Windrush generation arrived in the 'Mother Country' as invited members of the Commonwealth but were met with culture shock – there were no gold streets but hostility – 'no Blacks, no dogs, no Irish'.[9] Blatant racism and oppressive discrimination meant life was a challenge; and employment was often only available in low-level, low-skilled positions in factories, in the newly formed NHS, in the transport system or in construction to rebuild the infrastructure of post–Second World War Britain.

They 'sent' for their children from the Caribbean, while some children were born in Britain. Those who had been educated in the British colonial West Indies education system (to a high standard) now found that they were subjected to racism in British schools. Although some attended grammar schools and achieved O levels and A levels, others found themselves relegated, unjustly, to so-called educationally subnormal (ESN) schools.[10] Efforts were made to correct 'The Miseducation of the Black Child' through supplementary Saturday schools.[11] Hazel V. Carby's chapter 'Schooling in Babylon' in the edited volume *The Empire Strikes Back* and Gus John's book *Taking a Stand* show how the Black community were 'taking a stand' to address this travesty.[12]

The trajectory, however, was already set. Many were demoralised and disaffected. Ignored or undereducated by teachers, left to their own devices – listening to 'ghetto blaster radios' at the back of the classroom – some would stray into more deviant behaviour. The Black community and Black teachers tried to ameliorate antagonistic race relations by introducing 'multiculturalism' in schools but that too suffered a backlash.[13]

These developments occurred against a backdrop of rebellion and revolution in the 1960s and 1990s, with colonies gaining independence, the civil rights movement, the rise of Black Consciousness, Black Power and the reformed self-image of 'Black Is Beautiful'. As young people, we began to learn about Black History from courageous white and black historians.[14] Simultaneously, many youth were turning to Rastafarianism,[15] alienated from Christianity, which they associated with oppression and slavery. Hopes were raised for recognition of Black Power and values when apartheid (1948–94) was overthrown in South Africa and Nelson Mandela was released after twenty-seven years' imprisonment (1990) to later become the president of South Africa (1994–9). However, some felt that Mandela might have been brainwashed because he was no longer militant but followed Christian values of forgiveness, paving the way for reconciliation.

Social control was being exerted by government policies, causing division between races and social classes. This process of racist segregation starts very early on in the education system.[16] Indeed, in 1979 Coard stated that black (and mixed-race) children (and poor, white working-class children) would be minimally educated to maintain the 'social hierarchy' and 'an abundant' supply 'of unskilled labour'.[17] A white 'career' offender claimed that, instead of places of reform, 'prisons were colleges for criminals', where young offenders are taught more criminality from seasoned inmates.[18]

Education according to state strategies was (and still is) 'more for social control of black youth' and of black people in general.[19] In recent decades (2000–19), black children have been placed in Pupil Referral Units (PRUs), decried by some because schools and local councils received up to four times as much funding for each pupil as they would in mainstream schools, yet there are few teaching resources and the children are left to their own devices. Is history repeating itself? Epidemic proportions of black children are being excluded from schools, especially in inner cities. Parents are desperate, as they have little disposable income and must work so they can't supervise or teach their children. More determined parents resort to homeschooling, which is a challenge because the schools and councils refuse to release the funds that are rightfully for each pupil, so parents are forced to pay for costly private tuition.

Returning to black–white race relations, with rising unemployment, unions striking and far-right factions taking root, racism resurfaced, culminating in clashes, riots, racial attacks and injustice from the 1960s to the latest riot in 2011. I remember the battles between white and BAME youths as extreme racists went 'Niggah hunting' or 'Paki bashing'. During that time, Asians allied themselves to Black people as having a common enemy and seeking racial equality and justice. The police, however, were often 'too' ready to arrest Black youth whom they suspected of vagrancy and, in later years, of possession of illegal substances or weapons. The 'sus' law, which began under the 'suspected persons' stop-and-search section of the Vagrancy Act 1824, was used increasingly on Black youth during the 1970s and 1980s and was acutely felt in the post-Powell (racist) climate. Modern-day stop-and-search disproportionately targets black people today. Some things just do not change but are dressed up and justified in contemporary discourse and rationales that are clearly discriminatory but politically pushed through. After the riots in 1981 the Criminal Attempts Act repealed the sus law; but this was reversed in 1984 by the Police and Criminal Evidence Act (PACE), in effect reinstating sus. In 2000, section 44 of the Terrorism Act legitimated the racially profiled sus; but, in 2010, it was ruled illegal under the human rights agenda, though it continues under section 60.

Because of riots, Black youth were portrayed in the media as 'savages, rapists and rampagers'.[20] Van Djik avers that sources were only quoted because they fit into the dominant discourse and confirm general attitudes about Black people.[21] Soon, many Black youths found themselves in youth offender centres or prisons.

Victimised

In addition to sus on the streets, police often raided 'house' parties, nightclubs, 'shebeens' and homes where they suspected cannabis (or 'weed', 'ganja') was being used. The emergent Rastafarian community were often targeted, even though their young people were more well behaved than deviant. The 'crimes' diversified as more 'Black on Black' violence became prominent, and knife and gun crimes have become more prevalent today, with increasing numbers of young people killed year on year – 132 in London in 2019, the bloodiest in a decade. Rather than examine the history and social conditions and legacies of violence and oppression, modern commentators still resort to cultural and racial pathology, proposing that black people need to take care of their addictions, mental illnesses and propensities to join gangs rather than that these are manifestations of clustered disadvantage and geopolitical drivers of multiple problems.[22]

Nevertheless, some of the killings were racial, as notably the thirteen Black teenagers who died in a fire at a house party in Newcross, south London, in 1981, which sparked protests.[23] As was the fatal stabbing of eleven-year-old Damilola Taylor in 2000 and of eighteen-year-old Stephen Lawrence in 1993. In the latter case, it took eighteen years for his mother to get justice and hold the police and judiciary up to scrutiny and obtain a new ruling. A change in legislation to partially revoke the rule of not being able to prosecute for the same offence twice (double jeopardy) eventually enabled two of the defendants to be convicted and imprisoned. In the MacPherson Report in 1999 of the inquiry on the Stephen

Lawrence case, there are 382 mentions of the word 'racist'. In his inquiry report, MacPherson said that 'institutional racism' had hampered the investigations. Since then, this term has then been applied as a lens through which to consider inequalities in other public services. More recently, 'unconscious racism or bias' has been proffered to explain (excuse) racial harassment cases.[24] It is regrettable that racism in health care remains a concern and some still dispute its relevance.[25]

Such processes are unacceptable to Black communities when members are attacked, maimed or killed by police – police who are supposed to protect citizens. In 1985, three Black women, Cynthia Jarrett, Cherry Groce and Joy Gardner, were maimed or shot by police during raids on their homes who were allegedly searching for suspected criminals. Riots broke out in Tottenham's Broadwater Farm Estate and in Brixton, south London.[26]

The world was shocked in August 2011, when riots erupted in London and other UK cities, as well as arson attacks in Croydon, south London, after minicab passenger Mark Duggan was shot dead, 'execution-style', by police marksman. The police said it was drug-related; but whether it was or not surely arrest and then a fair trial is the usual route, not 'shoot first and ask questions later'?[27]

Invisibilised

'Disappear or become invisible' seems to be the underlying desire of racists towards Black people. Queen Elizabeth I expressed this sentiment. Called the greatest English monarch, her wealth and success came from slavery and sea battles in the West Indies. Yet, in 1596 and 1601, she issued proclamations to expel 'those kind of people', namely 'blackamoors' and 'nears' from 'her realm'.[28] Her attempts at immigration control failed and this has been a contentious issue, since I contend that Black people are considered too 'visible' in British society. Gary Craig also argues that the lack of focus on race has led to the 'invisibilising' of race within current policy.[29]

This I realised in 1998 when a Brazilian told me that Brazil had paintings where Black people were painted without defining features. They would have faces but no eyes, nose or mouth – dehumanising or 'invisibilising' them. The Roman Catholic Church in the Middle Ages behaved 'schizophrenically' in their apparent 'memory loss of the very real and influential presence of Moors (Moslem Africans), who invaded, conquered and ruled the Iberian peninsula, especially Spain, for 700 years from AD 711. The church gleaned the superior knowledge and science from the Moors who had established or influenced universities in Europe and in Oxford, England, but hid this from the masses because they feared the loss of church power and influence. Shakespeare's play Othello also evidences Black influence.[30]

The Windrush generation were not the first Black people in Britain, but decades of race relations have not brought them or their descendants closer to a sense of being welcome or 'belonging' here. However, their British-born children and grandchildren expect to be treated the same as other British people, to have an equal share in the society's resources and equal life chances.

State initiatives to forcibly assimilate immigrants have had little success and are resisted. Naturalisation tests (2005) and citizenship tests (2007) were introduced, and immigrants were put under extreme duress and financial burden to 'prove' their 'worthiness' to be accepted as British citizens. These policies would require that BAME people 'forsake all that makes them out as culturally distinct, before real Britishness can be guaranteed'.[31]

Furthermore, fear aroused from 9/11 in the United States and 7/7 in London exacerbated hostilities along religious, cultural and racial lines.

Pathologised

Another concern for Black youth is that they are pathologised, with some sent to mental institutions. Diagnosed by psychiatrists (with 'unconscious biases' or susceptible to 'institutional racism') or 'misdiagnosed',[32] they are sectioned, (over)medicated or incarcerated, disproportionately, in forensic and medium-secure mental institutions for lengthy periods. There is no natural explanation grounded in genetics or race, as such notions are scientific nonsense. The histories, legacies and conditions of life are responsible and yet ignored. Even following the experience of mental illness, black people receive coercive care, more medication and biological treatments rather than psychotherapy or sufficient social intervention.

Notable cases of Black men who have died in custody include David 'Rocky' Bennett, Sean Rigg and many more. Rigg's family published a list of 3,180 people who had died in police custody, prison, mental hospitals or immigration detention camps in the UK between 1969 and 2011.[33] Bennett's sister's campaign inspired the Delivering Race Equality (DRE) initiative and the Race Equality Cultural Capability (RECC) training (2005–10) to raise race and cultural awareness and minimise racist practices.

Black children's homes are regarded as 'dysfunctional' and 'not good enough' by social services, who remove children and put them into foster care or up for adoption, usually to white parents. The stereotypical Black family is perceived to be matrifocal or matriarchal, denoting the 'absence' of fathers because of the preponderance of 'baby mothers'. However, this does not acknowledge the part slave owners played in separating families and siring illegitimate mixed-race children themselves, which have left single parenting as its legacy into modern times.[34] Traditional African families say that 'it takes a village to raise a child'. However, slavery destabilised this family structure; and other deliberate ways to degrade and disable Black people, and keep them ignorant of their history, their moral and scientific principles, through sexually charged and violent music, are orchestrated by controlling factions (hip-hop's Professor Griff, 2010).[35]

Identity, Aspirations and Resolve

Given all these factors, it is not surprising that Black youth may be confused on issues of belonging, identity, self-image, self-esteem and worth. With a barrage of negativity through media, society and community, they may have internalised this,[36] which may explain how 'self-hatred' and 'Black on Black' violence have taken hold. Whether they want protection, 'respect' from 'olders', or father figures, to be feared or want to make 'quick money', more Black youth have joined gangs.

They also identify with 'celebrity' music artists (hip-hop rappers, grime or drill) who talk about experiences they can relate to. Rastafarian 'Black conscious' reggae songs promoted Black pride and positive self-image. Black youth can reject the negative impositions on their identity and reach out for a universal humanity that fosters justice, equality and equity.[37]

Research Evidence and New Directions

The narratives of oppression are supported by much evidence on ethnic inequalities of incidence and experience of mental health systems in which some black minority groups and migrants experience more coercive care.[38] This includes more adverse pathways to care through criminal justice systems, police involvement and use of the Mental Health Act. Part of the challenge is a reductionist approach that sees mental illness as a product of individual failings or exposures to risk factors rather than a dynamic balance of resilience and risk factors over the life course and that in specific social contexts is too simplistic. That is, assets have a positive influence cumulatively and likewise risk factors a negative influence. Indeed generations of traumatic experiences (genocide, slavery, religious, ethnic or racial persecution) continue to have evident impacts on future generations. These are transmitted through narratives of identity and how these are often shaped by histories of persecution. A further problem is the web of causation, including social divisions and status; stratification by poverty, employment and housing; and safety and trust in neighbourhoods. These rarely feature as structural factors that offer potential explanations for why some groups continue to suffer greater adversity, thus leading to poor mental health (see also Chapters 3 and 5).

A historical perspective on life in Britain during the period 1960–2010 therefore becomes important. Historical documents can reveal prevailing attitudes to mental health care and mental illness and attitudes towards migrants and minorities not only in official policy and practice but also in popular culture. Boxes 35.1 and 35.2 present, respectively, British health policies during this time, and as a way of tapping popular culture, situation comedies during the same approximate period. The documents and shows listed in Boxes 35.1 and 35.2 could be examined, interrogated and explored for popular cultural stereotypes and for information on how ethnicity, race and cultural diversity were viewed. The situation comedies openly show racist language, ostensibly to call out bigots but reinforcing common attitudes towards minorities and not considering the power imbalances (e.g. Spike Milligan's Paki-Paddy from *Curry and Chips*). More recent decades have seen black actors and comedians reverse this situation by taking leading roles and directing and writing the material for comedies in an attempt to share both the ironies and the realities of their lives (e.g. *The Fosters*, *Desmond's*, *The Kumars at No. 42* and *Goodness Gracious Me*).

Certainly, in the 1960s, we have the incredible movement of deinstitutionalisation, which led to the closure of the asylums and the call for community care, greater social care and support in ordinary places, as well as a recognition of the importance of the environment and social space in both causation of mental illness and recovery. It is ironic that, at the end of the National Service Framework (NSF) in 1999, specialised services to support community care have been stripped back, resulting, ultimately, in crisis-only services with little space for rehabilitation and adequate place-based social care (see also Chapters 23 and 26). Health inequalities in general were identified by the Black Report and the review by Michael Marmot; and ethnic inequalities were profiled more recently by the Synergi Collaborative Centre.[39] These inequalities persist and have not seen a coordinated set of actions by successive governments.

There is no sustained and consistent action on systems change to impact care practices. At the same time, during the period of interest Powell's 'Rivers of Blood' speech stoked hostility towards migrants and minorities, and the ramifications are still felt today, with contentions around whether racism was and is a helpful term, specifically institutional racism. Furthermore, the legacy of the Windrush generation has not been overlooked, when, even recently, a hostile environment for immigrants under the May government appears to have been repeated and expressed past colonial attitudes. Historical moments

Box 35.1 Relevant Health Policies, 1959–2020[40]

1959   Mental Health Act

1975   *Better Services for the Mental Ill* White Paper

1976   Joint Care Planning, Health and Local Authorities

1981   *Care in Action: A Handbook of Policies and Priorities*

1982   Korner Report: collecting NHS data

1983   Mental Health Act

1986   Making a Reality of Community Care

1988   *Community Care: An agenda for Action.* Sir Roy Griffiths's report into the care of Sharon Campbell

1990   NHS & Community Care Act

1992   Mental Health as a Key Area in Health of the Nation/Joint Home Office and Department of Health review on care of mentally disordered offenders (MDO)

1993   Mental Illness: Key Area Handbook/Mental Health and Britain's Black Communities

1994   Richie Report on care of Christopher Clunis/Guidance on Supervision Registers, aftercare of MDO and care in the community/Mental Health Taskforce in London and regions; Black Mental Health: A dialogue for change; NHS letter mandating collection of ethnic group data for inpatients; establishment of NHS ethnic health unit

1995   Mental Health Patients in the Community Act/Mental Health: Information booklet on ethnic minorities service users and carers

1997   The New NHS Modern, Dependable

1999   National Service Framework

1999   Stephen Lawrence inquiry

2000   Race Relations Amendment Act

2002   Commission for Race Equality: guidance for organisations

1998–2003   Inside Outside: Improving Mental Health Services to Black and Minority Ethnic Communities in England

2007   Ethnicity and Health. Parliamentary Office of Science and Technology

2005–2010   Delivering Race Equality

2007   Government decides to not use the term 'institutional racism' or 'racism'

2010   Equality Act. Silence and Invisibility as DH and many government bodies removed the term 'institutional racism' from official vocabularies and policy

2018   Synergi Collaborative Centre established

2019   Independent review of the Mental Health Act

2019/20   Covid legislation and crisis

lead to products that show an underlying default of hostility towards perceived aliens, often the underclasses and the poorer and most vulnerable in society. The visibility of historical moments, monuments even to British identity, fluctuates and some consider these events as irrelevant to modern life in Britain, contrary to the lived experience of being black in Britain.

> **Box 35.2** Popular Television Reflecting Societal Attitudes to Race and Immigration: Using Comedy to Attack the Bigot
>
> 1965   *Till Death Us Do Part*
>
> 1968   *Carry On Up the Khyber* (same year as the 'Rivers of Blood' speech)
>
> 1969   *Curry and Chips* (with Spike Milligan's Paki-Paddy)
>
> 1972   *Love Thy Neighbour*
>
> 1974   *It Ain't Half Hot Mum*
>
> 1974   *Rising Damp*
>
> 1976   *The Fosters* (first comedy with black characters)
>
> 1977   *Mind Your Language*
>
> 1984   *The Cosby Show*
>
> 1989   *Desmond's*
>
> 1995   *Porkpie*
>
> 1998   *Goodness Gracious Me*
>
> 2001   *The Kumars at No 42*

Policy and Research Discourse

The language of policy and research lacks ambition or motivation, being grounded in modest recognition of inequalities in society, given the challenge these pose politically and the necessary additional spend required. Most research provides evidence for the majority which may then be applied to minorities, or those with clustered disadvantage. Ambivalence and divergent political, policy, research and clinical perspectives tend to favour the advantaged, the least unwell, the most well off who are already well placed and make best use of the interventions; thus these actions widen inequalities.[41]

Psychiatry and Culture

Psychiatric practice and research made incredible advances in the 1960s-1990s, but since then there seems to be little innovation in terms of pharmacological or social or psychological interventions (see Chapters 2, 17). Work continues to repurpose medication, develop better and more cost-effective psychological therapies, and consider the social drivers of poor mental health. The role of race and culture has a more chequered history with psychiatry and psychology being implicated in early research and practice as being racist, culture blind, and reinforcing stereotypes. Indeed, the very power structures of society are replicated in institutions, and psychiatrists are increasingly seen as public servants who act for the government and the socially constructed public good.

Wittkower established a newsletter in 1956 called Transcultural Research in Mental Health Problems creating a new field of Transcultural Psychiatry, from McGill University Canada, since when Cultural Psychiatry (as it is more commonly called these days) has been established in several countries as a distinct approach. In the UK, the Transcultural Special Interest Group of the Royal College of Psychiatrists is the nearest to a membership society that has stood the test of time; others have come and gone, including NGOs, and charity partners, ethnicity and health units. The World Psychiatric Association has a Transcultural Section and the World Association of Cultural Psychiatry was formed in 2008. Initially Transcultural Psychiatry, as it was originally termed, was dominated by anthropological research methods and, more recently, additional qualitative and quantitative approaches are applied for the same purpose, to better understand cultural influences in the expression and presentation of mental disorders, and across distinct cultural groups, ethnic groups, and races. The latter as a focus of concern is especially common in North American discourse but has had an uneasy existence in the UK, where notions of racism and race equality remain contentious, provoking ambivalence amongst government, policy makers, commissioning bodies and research leaders.

British psychiatry did not reflect on its own contributions to racist practices and poorer outcomes for some until Julian Leff, Roland Littlewood and Maurice Lipsedge debated and contested psychiatric cultures, followed by Suman Fernando, Dinesh Bhugra, Kwame McKenzie, as well as active members of the Transcultural Special Interest Group of RCPsych (Parimala Moodley and Deenesh Khoosal). With these efforts, attention was more directly drawn to the injustice of mental health care being more coercive and less therapeutic for black and minority ethnic groups. Even this sentence, despite decades of evidence, is still disputed by some commentators whose location of problems is not in race, ethnicity or culture, but in individual risk behaviours, social status and deprivation, and psychosocial adversity including urban environments. All of these are relevant, yet if understood as individual cognitive or behavioural risk factors, rather than products of historical and social contexts, these do not explain the patterns of disparities in the incidence, experiences and outcomes from interactions with health systems. Rather more complex and intersectional and interacting causal and preventive models are required.

Conclusion

Many young black people are ambitious, want higher education, to have professional careers, or own businesses, and are prepared to work hard to achieve their goals. But like some of their parents, they face frustrating racist 'glass ceilings', which prevent access or promotion. Yet, encouraged by the resolve of their forerunners, they determinedly fight for their rights, and pursue their dreams. The alternative is demoralisation, depression or worse. The unequal impacts of assessment and treatment in care services compounds, and may even escalate, the detrimental impacts of pre-existing levels of inequality and historical legacies.[42] Historical injustices are regrettably silenced in contemporary debate, just as crises are full of promises soon forgotten when the political and public gaze shifts.[43]

Key Summary Points

- The period 1960–2010 was a time of marked immigration into the UK from Commonwealth countries, either to fill employment gaps in the UK or to escape hostilities and conflict as many Commonwealth countries secured independence.
- The political climate of the UK; attitudes to immigration and cultural integration; the evolution of mental health sciences, including British Psychiatry and the Royal College; the emerging research evidence; and the controversies around why migrants and minorities appeared to have higher incidence rates of severe mental illness and

poorer outcomes were, and are still, all inter-related to contribute to the lives of minorities.

- In the 1970s, as a community, Black African Caribbean people of the Windrush generation were concerned about their children getting police attention; which occurred in a racist and political climate of oppression. Over sixty years later the situation has escalated and diversified, so that illegal drugs, gangs, and violent crime is now stereotyped as 'Black culture'.

- Inequalities generated by the education and criminal justice systems, early years care and employment practices are a backdrop against which the mental health systems are positioned to respond to societal harms to the marginalised.

- The powers held in psychiatric systems are often co-opted to reflect the interests, and institutional practices and attitudes, of the state. This is most evident in detentions under the powers of the mental health act and in the forensic and criminal justice systems.

Notes

1.   R. K. Merton, The Matthew effect in science: The reward and communication systems of science are considered. *Science* (1968) 159: 56–63.

2.   A. T. Geronimus et al., 'Weathering' and age patterns of allostatic load scores among blacks and whites in the United States. *American Journal of Public Health* (2006) 96: 826–33; L. Jackson, Z. Jackson and F. Jackson, Intergenerational resilience in response to the stress and trauma of enslavement and chronic exposure to institutionalized racism. *Journal of Clinical Epigenetics* (2018) 4: 7.

3.   Y. A. A. Ben-Jochannan, *Africa, Mother of Western Civilisation*. Baltimore: Black Classic Press, 1988.

4.   W. D. Jordan, *White over Black: American Attitudes toward the Negro, 1550–1812*. Chapel Hill: University of North Carolina Press and the Institute of Early American History and Culture, 1968.

5.   W. J. Wilson, *Power, Racism and Privilege: Race Relations in Theoretical and Sociohistorical Perspectives*. New York: Macmillan Co, 1973; E. Eze, *Race and the Enlightenment*. Oxford: Blackwell Publishers, 1997; E. Said, *Orientalism*. London: Penguin Books, 1991.

6.   D. Joseph, *Perfect Circles, Volume 1: An Exploration of Faith and Relationships with YHWH (Yahweh) Our Heavenly Father*. Kindle Direct Publishing, 2013; D. Joseph, *Perfect Circles, Volume 2: An Exploration of Faith and Relationships with YHWH – Unveilings and Further Profound Revelations*. Kindle Direct Publishing, 2015; R. Omonira-Oyekanmi, Black and dangerous? Listening to patients' experiences of mental health services in London, Open Democracy (website), 30 September 2014, www.opendemocracy.net/en/shine-a-l ight/black-and-dangerous-listening-to-patients-experiences-of-mental/; S. Hall, *Formations of Modernity: The West and the Rest*. Cambridge: Polity Press, 1992.

7.   M. Kohn, *The Race Gallery: The Return of Racial Science*. London: Jonathan Cape, 1995.

8.   Hall, *Formations of Modernity*.

9.   O. Wambu, *Empire Windrush: Fifty Years of Writing about Black Britain*. London Victor Gollancz, 1998.

10. B. Coard, Making black children subnormal in Britain. *Equity and Excellence in Education* (1971) 9: 49–52.

11. N. H. J. Hare, *The Miseducation of the Black Child: The Hare Plan: Educate Every Black Man, Woman and Child*. Black Think Tank, 1991.

12. Centre for Contemporary Cultural Studies, *Empire Strikes Back*. London: Routledge,1982, https://doi.org/10 .4324/9780203639948; G. John, *Taking a Stand: Gus John Speaks on Education, Race, Social Action and Civil Unrest 1980–2005*. Manchester: The Gus John Partnership, 2006.

13. M. Barker, *The New Racism: Conservatives and the Ideology of the Tribe*. London: Junction Books, 1981; A. Rattansi, Racism, 'postmodernism' and reflexive multiculturalism. In S. May, ed., *Critical*

Multiculturalism: Rethinking Multicultural and Antiracial Education, 80–1. London: The Falmer Press, 1999.

14. Ben-Jochannan, *Africa, Mother of Western Civilisation*; A. Mazrui, *The Africans: A Triple Heritage*. London: BBC Publications, 1986; I. Van Sertima, *Golden Age of the Moor*. New Brunswick, NJ: Transaction Publishers,1992; C. A. Diop, *The African Origin of Civilisation: Myth or Reality?*. Chicago: Lawrence Hill, 1978.

15. L. E. Barrett, *The Rastafarians: The Dreadlocks of Jamaica*. London and Kingston: Heinemann Educational Books, 1977.

16. A. Pilkington, *Racial Disadvantage and Ethnic Diversity in Britain*. New York: Palgrave, 2003.

17. Coard, *Making black children subnormal in Britain*.

18. *This Is Our Families: The Nailors*. Sky TV documentary, Little Gem Production, 2020.

19. Centre for Contemporary Cultural Studies, *Empire Strikes Back*.

20. Report on Brixton riots. *The Mirror*, 30 September 1985.

21. T. A. Van Djik, New(s) racism: A discourse analytical approach. In *Ethnic Minorities and the Media*. Maidenhead: Open University Press, 2000.

22. J. Coid et al., Ethnic disparities in psychotic experiences explained by area-level syndemic effects. *British Journal of Psychiatry* (2019): 1–7.

23. P.R. D. Gordon, *Daily Racism: The Press and Black People in Britain*. London: The Runnymede Trust, 1989.

24. W. MacPherson, *The Stephen Lawrence Inquiry* [MacPherson Report], Cm 4262-1, February 1999, https://assets.publishing.service.gov.uk/government/uploads/system/uploads/attachment_data/file/277111/4262.pdf.

25. V. Adebowale and M. Rao, Racism in medicine: Why equality matters to everyone. *British Medical Journal* (2020) 368: m530.

26. J. Benyon and J. Solomos, *Roots and Urban Unrest*. Oxford: Pergamon, 1987; G. Scarman, *The Scarman Report: The Brixton Disorders 10–12 April 1981*. London: Pelican Books, 1982; A. Sivanandan, *A Different Hunger: Writings on Black Resistance*. London: Pluto Press, 1982; P. Gilroy, *There Ain't No Black in the Union Jack*. London: Routledge, 2003, https://doi.org/10.4324/9780203995075.

27. Joseph, *Perfect Circles, Volume 1*.

28. Jordan, *White over Black*. F. O. Shyllon and Institute of Race Relations, *Black People in Britain, 1555–1833*. London: Institute of Race Relations and Oxford University Press, 1977.

29. G. Craig, Invisibilizing 'race' in public policy. *Critical Social Policy* (2013) 33: 712–20.

30. Van Sertima, *Golden Age of the Moor*.

31. Gilroy, *There Ain't No Black in the Union Jack*.

32. S. Fernando, *Institutional Racism in Psychiatry and Clinical Psychology: Race Matters in Mental Health*. New York: Springer, 2017; F. W. Hickling, K. McKenzie, R. Mullen et al., A Jamaican psychiatrist evaluates diagnoses at a London psychiatric hospital. *British Journal of Psychiatry* (1999) 175: 283–5.

33. *Independent Inquiry into the death of David Bennett*. Report, December 2003, http://image.guardian.co.uk/sys-files/Society/documents/2004/02/12/Bennett.pdf. See also the Sean Rigg Justice & Change campaign website: www.seanriggjusticeandchange.com.

34. D. Joseph, What happens when Baby-Father is absent or part-time?. West Indian Magazine of Caribbean Times, 1983. Joseph, *Perfect Circles, Volume 1*.

35. Joseph, *Perfect Circles, Volume 1*.

36. F. Fanon, *Black Skins, White Masks* (Penguin Modern Classics). London: Penguin,2020.

37. Ibid.

38. P. Barnett et al., Ethnic variations in compulsory detention under the Mental Health Act: A systematic review and meta-analysis of international data. *Lancet Psychiatry* (2019) 6: 305–17; K. Bhui, K. Halvorsrud and J. Nazroo, Making a difference: ethnic inequality and severe mental illness. *British Journal of Psychiatry* (2018) 213: 574–8; K. Bhui, S. Ullrich and J. W. Coid, Which pathways to psychiatric care lead to earlier treatment and a shorter duration of first-episode psychosis?. *BMC Psychiatry* (2014) 14: 72.

39. Synergi Collaborative Centre, *Ethnic Inequalities in UK Mental Health Systems*, Briefing Report, November 2017, https://synergicollaborativecentre.co.uk/wp-content/uploads/2017/11/Synergi_Report_Web.pdf.

40. Box 35.1 is adapted and extended from D. Olajide, Mental health policy. In K. Bhui and D. Olajide, eds, *Mental Health Service Provision for a Multicultural Society*. London: Saunders, 1999. See also Chapter 10, this volume.

41. G. Ellison, P. Aspinall, A. Smart et al., The ambiguities of 'race' in UK science, social policy and political discourse. *Journal of Anthropological Science* (2017) 95: 299–306; S. Salway, G. Mir, D. Turner et al., Obstacles to 'race equality' in the English National Health Service: Insights from the healthcare commissioning arena. *Social Science and Medicine* (2016) 152: 102–10.

42. A. Kapilashrami and K. Bhui, Mental health and COVID-19: Is the virus racist?. *British Journal of Psychiatry* (2020): 1–3.

43. Notes on legislation: (1) Suspected persons Stop and Search Vagrancy Act 1824 (SUS law); (2) Race Relations Act 1965, first in UK; (3) Equality Act 2010, prohibits race discrimination.

Refugees, Asylum and Mental Health in the UK

Peter Hughes and Cornelius Katona

Of troubles none is greater than to be robbed of one's native land.

Euripides, 431 BC[1]

Introduction

In 2007, there were 11.4 million refugees worldwide of which the UK had just 3 per cent. This was about 300,000 people or 0.5 per cent of the UK population.[2]

The story in the UK is one of both welcome and rejection.[3] It brings out the best and the worst of society. Refugees are traumatised by not only the experiences of their homeland and their journey but also settling in the UK.[4] They have been disbelieved, accused of embellishing their stories to get asylum and subjected to racism.[5]

Both authors could retell gruelling accounts of torture, murder and humiliation. This is not what we want to do. We want to celebrate the resilience of refugees. We therefore dedicate this chapter to all those who came to the UK seeking protection and who have made a life in the UK against the odds.

Refugees, Psychiatrists and Mental Health Services

A refugee is defined as a person who is outside of their country of origin and who has a well-founded fear of returning there on the grounds that they may be persecuted because of race, religion, nationality, membership of a particular social group or political opinion or affiliation.[6] Refugees are a marginalised and isolated group.[7] We remember their humanity and that they are normal people who have had to face extraordinary circumstances. They are us.

Refugees have been recognised as entitled to international protection. Asylum seekers are waiting for their refugee status to be established legally. Such waiting causes a great deal of anxiety.[8]

The number of refugees to the UK has steadily diminished since 1960.[9] Both before this period and in the early years covered, the UK had generally been a welcoming place in spite of the views of the hostile minority exemplified by the 'Rivers of Blood' speech by Enoch Powell in 1968.[10]

The story of refugees' mental health during the period covered in this book was less about theoretical arguments regarding psychiatric diagnosis and more about their struggles with the Home Office, getting food on the table, having a place to live and finding acceptance and work.[11] All too many refugees have told us that it was neither the problems they faced back home country nor their journey that caused them the greatest difficulty but rather the challenges of surviving day-to-day in a new country facing the machinery of government which seemed to be against them.[12]

Past mental health research has been disproportionately focused on post-traumatic stress disorder (PTSD) as a diagnosis.[13] The focus has broadened in more recent years. Refugees are now known to have a higher rate and wider range of mental health problems as well as experiencing psychosocial stress.[14] Their overall risk of mental disorder is increased fivefold and may also increase with age – particularly in the case of depression and anxiety.[15]

Working as a clinician with refugees is more often about writing supportive letters for their housing difficulties and reports for the Home Office in the context of their immigration claims rather than about identifying and treating their mental health problems. Their story is tied up with politics and resources. They have been at the bottom rung of the society they have joined and are affected disproportionately when economies are stretched.[16] This is also when racism increases. Refugee women and children are particularly marginalised and vulnerable.[17]

We avoid the word trauma as this tends to perpetuate the narrative of victimhood.[18] We want to celebrate refugees as potential or actual contributors to the society they have joined rather than as victims. Throughout recent history, the UK has benefited overwhelmingly (economically, socially and culturally) from the contribution of refugees.[19] To take one obvious example, Sigmund Freud arrived in the UK as a refugee from Austria in 1938 and lived there until his death in 1939.[20] Anna Freud, his daughter, was a pioneer in child mental health in what is now called the Anna Freud Centre in London. Lucian Freud, his grandson, was one of the greatest post-war British painters.

During the period in question, considerable development took place of organisations to support refugees and asylum seekers.[21] There has been a developing balance between specialised refugee services and mainstream (publicly funded) health and social care services. Interpreters and mediators both of language and of culture have been crucial and their role cannot be overstated.[22]

Origins

Britain is an island that used to be joined to Europe by a land bridge until 10,000 years ago.[23] The first recorded arrivals were farmers from south-east Europe. There have been waves of arrivals since – the Romans in 55 BC, the Anglo-Saxons from Europe in the fifth century AD, the Vikings in AD 789, the Normans in the eleventh century.[24] There has been uncertainty about which of them were escaping persecution and were therefore refugees. The Huguenots – French protestants who fled French persecution in the seventeenth century – were a clear example of refugees. Since then, there have been successive waves such as a quarter of a million Irish who fled the potato famine since the1850s.[25] In the early twentieth century, 120,000 Jewish people arrived, fleeing from persecution ('pogroms') in eastern Europe and Russia.[26]

The Second World War transformed UK policy due to the increased post-war need for labour. Volunteers were recruited from displaced camps in Europe to come to the UK. After the war, the largest refugee group were from Poland. By 1950, 85,000 people had arrived from Europe. Migrants also came from former colonial countries in the 1950s, again to meet labour shortage. There was a substantial influx of Hungarians fleeing persecution after the 1956 uprising against the communist regime.[27]

Table 36.1 Waves of migration: main waves 1960–2010[28]

Years of arrival in UK	Groups	Approximate figures of arrivals in UK	Reason for flight
1960s	Kenya Asians	Unknown figure	Conflict
1972	Ugandan Asians	30,000	Forced deportation
1974	Chilean/ Argentinian	5,000	Political oppression
1974–5	Cypriots (mainly Greek)	10,000	War
1979	Vietnamese	16,000	War
1980s and 1990s	Tamils of Sri Lanka	100,000	War
1983	Iranians	8,000	War/revolution
1990s	Refugees from Bosnian/ Kosovo war	5,000	War
2000s	Sierra Leone war	17,000	War

There have been several thousand asylum seekers each year during the period covered in this book (see Table 36.1), with about half having their application granted. The influx has reflected geopolitical turmoil. Examples of this include the influx of Asians from Kenya in the 1960s and of Czech refugees after the 1968 uprising. In 1972, 30,000 Ugandan Asian refugees arrived (mainly whole families), following their expulsion by Idi Amin. Several of the new arrivals had relatives already living in the UK. They spoke English and had British passports. Their arrival was planned. They moved to places where there was more housing capacity and assimilated relatively easily. The Cypriots (mainly Greek) of 1973 and 1974 similarly came as whole families with previous UK connections. As with the Asians from Uganda, many already had family connections in the UK.[29]

In 1974, political opponents of the Chilean and Argentinian dictatorships came to the UK. In 1979, the influx of 16,000 Vietnamese – mainly boat people from the Hong Kong camps – began. Some of the people granted protection in the UK had come as students but could not return when the situation in their country changed. These include many Iranians who were in the UK at the time of the 1983 Islamic Revolution.[30] In the early 2000s, many citizens of Sierra Leone left the civil war to come to the UK. About 100,000 Tamil people live in the UK – most of whom because of the prolonged Sri Lankan civil war.[31]

Many refugees came to specific areas of the UK to be within their own communities. Though this brought risks of ghettoisation, the growth of migrant communities also facilitated group support and the preservation of cultural identity. There are, for example, well-defined Vietnamese, Tamil and Somali communities in London.[32]

Although the government has been keen to encourage integration,[33] there has been an ongoing tension between integration and multiculturalism.[34] Only a small number of refugees moved from densely populated areas such as London to less populated areas.

Most of those making such moves were males in their twenties or thirties; they represent only about 10–20 per cent of refugees.[35]

There have been services focused on particular groups – for example, Polish, Vietnamese, Irish and Somali. However, this approach has changed to one of mainstreaming all into standard NHS services regardless of origin. There are some charitable organisations that support particular communities. For example, the Vietnamese mental health project helps people from their community in accessing health care.[36]

Reception

There are more than 190 different nationalities represented in the UK – reflective of its complex global history, including the arrival of migrants and refugees. They include many of the people who staff our NHS today. The history of refugees in the UK parallels the experience in other developed nations – a balance of official/community support and scepticism.[37] The tensions between embracing multiculturalism and encouraging integration are exemplified on the one hand by the development of specialised culture-specific services and on the other by encouraging incorporation into mainstream ones.[38] Irrespective of how the host society manages that balance, what is common in the refugee experience is the exposure to poverty and discrimination, compounding an existential loss of one's homeland.[39]

New arrivals' hope for the future is linked to their application for asylum and their expectation of welcome and protection. However, simply a mention of 'Lunar House' in Croydon (the headquarters of 'UK Visas and Immigration', a division of the Home Office in the UK where most new arrivals seeking asylum attend) will provoke a marked emotional reaction in refugees. This is where they wait for hours to process their papers. It symbolises a loss of control over their lives and of hope. Many reported experiencing scepticism and a dehumanising approach. They carry a substantial baggage of fear – of not being believed and of being deported. Any inconsistency may lead to them being discredited. In consequence, they may be suspicious of state and voluntary organisations.[40]

The UK is bound by two international legal instruments in its dealings with those seeking and/or granted asylum – the UN Refugee Convention of 1951 and the Protocol of 1967.[41] These established basic minimum standards for refugees and asylum seekers and enshrined the right to asylum and not to be forcibly returned if such return was to result in further state-sponsored ill treatment ('refoulement'). Additionally, the Human Rights Act 1998 provides a framework for protection of those who fall outside the Refugee Convention but whose human rights would be jeopardised by a return to their home country.

In parallel with the development of a legislative framework of protection, the history of migration and immigration in the UK is of a legal framework of increasing restrictions on entry to and domicile in the UK. The Aliens Act of 1905 and 1920 as well as successive immigration acts since 1968 have restricted the borders. From 1929 to 1939, more obstacles were put in place. Within the provisions of the 1971 Immigration Act, people can be prevented from coming to the UK based on a psychiatric diagnosis.[42]

There are also language, cultural and informational barriers to accessing health services.[43] Refugees themselves often prioritise their basic needs and status before being able to address psychological issues. Health services must be aware of culture and of the intrinsic power imbalance. The agendas between refugee and health worker may be mismatched in that the mental health worker wants to focus on mental health issues while refugees may fear being disbelieved or deported and therefore try to present information in a way that might be acceptable to the health worker and perceived as 'normal'. As a result, their accounts may appear coached and embellished, or they may appear inscrutable or ungrateful.[44]

Refugees give consistent stories of their stressful experiences and the situation impeding them. Recounting stories itself can be experienced as traumatic and may be met with disbelief. There are a minority of stories that have been 'coached'.[45] Even where this is the case (e.g. in survivors of human trafficking who have been told what to say by their traffickers and threatened with retribution to themselves or their families if they tell the truth), this does not detract from the intrinsically stressful nature of that person's experience. It is, however, challenging for UK mental health professionals to get through these defences and to be sufficiently aware of our own prejudices and countertransference. In response to this imbalance, specific refugee and trauma-focused services were developed. There remain tensions between mainstream and specialist as well as between trauma-focused and resilience-based psychological interventions.[46]

Refugee Experience

Being a refugee/migrant is intrinsically stressful.[47] There is an initial relief. This is followed by anxiety, depression, guilt, anger and fear of being returned, compounded by feelings of injustice. There is a culture shock which is increased by language difficulties.[48] The resilience of refugees is related to their experience before leaving their home country, their journey and the opportunities they have (or have not) been given to assimilate in UK. They may have what has been termed 'survivor syndrome', where they feel guilty about leaving behind their home country.[49] The asylum process also causes distress with protracted periods of uncertainty. Those who have pre-existing mental health issues may be more vulnerable, or problems may manifest later in life.[50] The experience of being a refugee has led people to become depressed.[51] Common clinical symptoms in refugees include sleep problems, restlessness, inertia and somatisation (headaches, dyspepsia and 'cardiac'-type symptoms).[52]

There has been an excess focus on mental health problems rather than on social adversity. Meeting basic needs has been shown to reduce psychiatric morbidity.[53] Mental health problems may also be missed or misidentified as PTSD.[54] There may be an incentive to diagnose PTSD to fit with the narrative of the asylum process. This can miss other diagnoses or pathologise normal distress. For example, one study in the Somali community showed that more than a third had a mental disorder but that PTSD was present in just 14 per cent.[55] There can be cross-cultural aspects to psychosis which can lead to a barrier to treatment or inappropriate treatment. Hyperarousal, anger or silence may be misinterpreted as paranoia.

Understanding a refugee's culture is crucial. Unaccompanied minors, single men, women and frail elderly are all particularly vulnerable.[56] Gaining employment is a key factor especially for men.[57] Being able to work is an important theme for refugees' well-being.[58]

Refugees and other migrants face obstacles in accessing health services, housing, employment, education and acceptance by the host community.[59] The longer the period of adjustment, the greater the increased risk of mental health difficulties.[60] They also feel more distressed when they hear of events back home.[61]

One of the authors (PH) reflects on someone he saw during this period:

A young man from Central Africa. He had torture wounds. He had the stress of his Home Office asylum application. He had poor sleep, depression. He was referred for 'depression' but the problem was poverty and isolation. His past experiences were just that – the past relative to his current struggles. Treatment consisted of referring him to the hospital football team. This taught me that the role of the psychiatrist stretches us to think beyond the narrow diagnostic perspective.[62]

Women Refugees

Women refugees are particularly vulnerable.[63] They have often been exposed to sexual and gender-based violence.[64] Adjustment is particularly difficult for those separated from their families and their children.[65] Traditional roles of childrearing and household chores may be affected by the refugee experience, with women disproportionately affected. Women have also been found to be less likely to be able to access services or have a social network than men.[66] Some women do not feel comfortable talking to a male health worker. They report that they would fear just being given medication for a mental health problem.[67]

Among women refugees, there have been some myths that they should not and could not access primary health care and in turn all health services. It is unclear whether these arose out of suspiciousness or from a misconstrued gender belief. After sexual and gender-based violence, there can be anxiety, sexual difficulties and concerns about fertility.[68] When a woman can return to a previous role as a mother this can, however, be protective. The importance of such family reunion (often very challenging to achieve) cannot be overestimated.

Interventions

The authors have been involved in interventions in third-sector settings such as the Helen Bamber Foundation and the Vietnamese Mental Health project as well as in mainstream services. Whatever the context in which interventions are delivered, the key to good mental health is achievement of settled status and meeting basic needs. The unmet needs are the loss of one's past and the injustice.[69]

A report in 2007 describes different innovative treatments for refugees with mental health problems.[70] These were started by refugees and were locally owned, which helped with their success. They included offering refugee women work, creative therapies, horticulture, crafts and psychological therapy. Mental health services have not been viewed as a support system by the women. Instead, there have been programmes for the mental health of various groups staffed by people from that community,[71] for example Somali and Vietnamese.

Employment

Programmes of employment have been a key factor in refugee integration.[72] However, until their asylum status is settled, most asylum seekers cannot work. Finding work is difficult even after refugee status has been granted. Refugee unemployment was 36 per cent in 2002 when the general UK rate was approximately 5 per cent.[73] Many remain unemployed long-term in the UK even when they are technically able to work.[74] The refugee integration and employment service was established in 2008 to help with this.[75]

The Example of Vietnamese Refugees

The Vietnamese diaspora to the UK began in the 1960s in different waves, including the boat people of the 1970s from Hong Kong camps. The Vietnamese struggled with a different culture and language. The stigma of mental illness was strong and symptoms were often concealed within the family. The old suffered from a loss of their role in their family and community.[76] Young men did better, and women did better if they could resume a domestic role at home. The most common psychiatric disorders in this group were schizophrenia or depression,[77] with the rate of schizophrenia 1.3 per cent higher than back in Vietnam. In the UK, the Vietnamese mental health project was set up to bridge the cultural gap, tackle stigma and work with families. Services included drop-in centres, advocacy and support in accessing mainstream services. The project provided a gateway from specialised to mainstream services.

The Life and Work of Helen Bamber

Helen Bamber (1925–2014),[78] with whom one of the authors of this chapter (CK) had the privilege of working closely with towards the end of her long and distinguished life, had a career in human rights, working mainly but not exclusively with asylum seekers and refugees, which spanned the whole of the period covered in this book. This brief summary of her career, and the ethical principles that underpinned her work, draws both on published material and on CK's unpublished interviews with her.

> People often ask me why I have spent most of my life concerned with the consequences of conflict and violence. The simple answer is 'why not?'. It is about the suffering of refugees. It is about the short life of compassion, how quickly it is born and how quickly it dies. It is about the stranger to whom we owe nothing. It is about how our society will be judged and how we discover our humanity. It is about love.[79]

In 1945, as a member of the British Jewish Relief Unit, Bamber entered the liberated concentration camp at Bergen-Belsen.[80] In 1961, Bamber joined Amnesty International and, in 1974, she helped establish the Medical Group within Amnesty. In this role, she was instrumental in persuading the British Medical Association to establish a Working Party on Torture. During the 1970s and 1980s, she helped develop a framework for documenting torture and inhuman or degrading treatment and was active in campaigning against torture internationally. The groups on whom she focused included the 'disappeared' in Chile, victims of the political abuse of psychiatry in the Soviet Union and people 'interrogated' by the authorities during the Troubles in Northern Ireland.

Bamber also worked therapeutically with individual victims of such torture and ill treatment. In 1985, she founded the Medical Foundation for the Care of Victims of Torture (now Freedom from Torture). In 2005, she set up the Helen Bamber Foundation to work with survivors of a broader range of extreme human cruelty such as human trafficking, domestic violence and ill treatment because of gender or sexual orientation as well as with survivors of torture.

The conventional wisdom identifies Bamber's experiences of working in the newly liberated Bergen-Belsen concentration camp in 1945 as the main driver of her future work. However, as she explained to CK, her journey into human rights started even earlier, as a Jewish child in London in the 1930s, witnessing fascist mobs and hearing Hitler's radio broadcasts.

This is not to deny the importance of what Bamber witnessed in Bergen-Belsen. As she told CK,

> I remember very clearly that there was one day in Belsen when some people ... were coming. They wanted some clothes, some provisions. And they were pretty aggressive and I said to one of the group, 'I really don't like that man very much'. And she said to me, 'We're not here to like people or not to like people. We're here for something quite different.'[81]

Bamber often spoke of the necessity of 'bearing witness' to the crimes of humanity and of distinguishing between bystanders and active witnesses. In her own words,

> sometimes I found it necessary to say to people who I knew were not going to live: 'You are giving me your testimony and I will hold it for you and I will honour it and I will bear witness to what has happened to you.'[82]

Another of Bamber's guiding principles was that survival itself was not enough – what was needed was what she called 'creative survival'. She encouraged the survivors she worked with to take part in cultural and skill-building group activities that helped them develop identities beyond that of 'survivor' while also helping them to trust and respect each other and themselves.

Bamber remained angry and energised by that anger throughout her working life but she was also a consummate diplomat. She understood that dialogue was necessary even with people and systems with whom she remained angry – and that anger and sympathy could coexist. As she told CK,

> in our relationship with decision makers here, we do find a certain sympathy. And that in many places there are people who do appear to understand. But the systems are not designed for understanding the questions people asked, the links that are not made in asking them questions.

Conclusion

Refugees have been coming to the UK for generations. The waves of refugee influx during the time period addressed in this volume reflected geopolitical turmoil during the time in question. The experience of the refugee has been intrinsically stressful with increased mental health problems. Refugees suffer from an increased rate of mental illness. This is particularly evident in women.[83] It may take much longer to get a clear health history from a refugee. Clinicians need to be aware of culture and the refugee agenda, and follow-up may be more difficult. Refugees' access to mental health services has also been problematic. Mainstreaming was the main approach but some specialist services enhanced access during this time. Some specialist services also developed within the voluntary sector – such as Freedom from Torture and the Helen Bamber Foundation.

Key Summary Points

- We want to celebrate the resilience of refugees. We therefore dedicate this chapter to all those who came to the UK seeking protection and have made a life in the UK against the odds.

- Past mental health work has been disproportionately focused on post-traumatic stress disorder (PTSD) as a diagnosis.[84] This has improved in more recent years. Refugees are now known to have a higher rate and wider range of mental health problems as well as psychosocial stress.
- Refugees need their basic needs met as well as addressing mental health problems. Interventions that have helped have been social such as access to employment,[85] combating discrimination and fostering inclusiveness. Resolving asylum uncertainty has been central to a reduction in mental health distress.
- The culture of the refugee cannot be underestimated in assessing and managing their health needs.
- One difficulty has been refugees' access to mental health services. Mainstreaming was the main approach but some specialist services enhanced access during this time. Some specialist services developed within the voluntary sector.

Notes

1. Euripides, *Medea* 653 (Tufts English edition), www.perseus.tufts.edu/hopper/text?doc+Perseus%3Atext%3A1999.01.0114%3Acard%3D645.

2. R. Baker, *The Psychosocial Problems of Refugees*. London: British Refugee Council and European Consultation on Refugees and Exiles, 1983.

3. Ibid.; D. Summerfield, Asylum seekers, refugees and mental health services in the UK. *Psychiatric Bulletin* (2001) 25: 161–3.

4. Baker, *Psychosocial Problems of Refugees*.

5. Summerfield, Asylum seekers.

6. Baker, *Psychosocial Problems of Refugees*.

7. Ibid.

8. International Rescue Committee, Migrants, asylum seekers, refugees and immigrants: What's the difference?, International Rescue Committee (website), 22 March 2019, www.rescue-uk.org/article/migrants-asylum-seekers-refugees-and-immigrants-whats-difference? gclid=EAIaIQobChMI9am5kPS16gIVWuztCh3gMg1KEAAYAiAAEgLlIfD_BwE.

9. Ibid.

10. Enoch Powell's 'Rivers of blood' speech. The full text is available online: https://anth1001.files.wordpress.com/2014/04/enoch-powell_speech.pdf.

11. Baker, *Psychosocial Problems of Refugees*.

12. Ibid.

13. G. De Jirolamo and A. C. McFarlane, The epidemiology of PTSD: A comprehensive review of the international literature. In A. Marsella, M. J. Friedman, E. T. Gerrity and R. M. Scurfield, eds, *Ethnocultural Aspects of Post-traumatic Stress Disorder*, 33–86. Washington, DC: American Psychological Association, 2003; Summerfield, Asylum seekers.

14. Baker, *Psychosocial Problems of Refugees*.

15. Ibid.

16. Ibid.; Summerfield, Asylum seekers.

17. A. Ahmad and J. Smith, *Humanitarian Action and Ethics*. London: Zed Books, 2018, pp. 181–200; Baker, *Psychosocial Problems of Refugees*.

18. Ahmad and Smith, *Humanitarian Action and Ethics*.

19. Baker, *Psychosocial Problems of Refugees*.

20. Ibid.

21. Ibid.

22. Ahmad and Smith, *Humanitarian Action and Ethics*; R. Tribe and N. Patel, Editorial special issue on refugees and asylum seekers. *The Psychologist* (2007) 20: 149–51.

23. H. Dillon and A. Smith, *Life in the UK Test Handbook: 2019 Edition*. London: Red Squirrel Publishers, 2019.

24. Ibid.

25. D. Bhugra, Migration and mental health. *Acta Psychiatrica Scandinavica* (2004) 109: 243–58.

26. Baker, *Psychosocial Problems of Refugees*.

27. Ibid.

28. Ibid.

29. Ibid.

30. Ibid.

31. R. Healey, Refugee employment experiences: The case of Tamil refugees in the UK. PhD thesis, University of Chester, 2010.

32. Baker, *Psychosocial Problems of Refugees*; De Jirolamo and McFarlane, The epidemiology of PTSD; Healey, Refugee employment experiences.

33. A. Ager and A. Strang, *The Experience of Integration: A Qualitative Study of Refugee Integration in the Local Communities of Pollockshaws and Islington*. Home Office Report No. 55/04, 2004.

34. A. Rogers and D. Pilgrim, *A Sociology of Mental Health and Illness* (5th ed.). Maidenhead: Open University Press.

35. K. Bhui, A. Abdi, M. Abdi et al., Traumatic events, migration characteristics and mental symptoms among Somali refugees. *Social Psychiatry and Psychiatric Epidemiology* (2003) 38: 35–43; De Jirolamo and McFarlane, The epidemiology of PTSD.

36. Healey, Refugee employment experiences; H. McColl and S. Johnson, Characteristics and needs of asylum seekers and refugees in contact with London Community Mental Health Teams. *Social Psychiatry and Psychiatric Epidemiology* (2006) 41: 789–95, https://doi.org/10.1007/s00127-006-0102-y.

37. Baker, *Psychosocial Problems of Refugees*; Summerfield, Asylum seekers.

38. Ager and Strang, *The Experience of Integration*.

39. Baker, *Psychosocial Problems of Refugees*.

40. Summerfield, Asylum seekers.

41. Baker, *Psychosocial Problems of Refugees*.

42. Ibid.

43. Ibid.

44. Summerfield, Asylum seekers.

45. Ibid.

46. Baker, *Psychosocial Problems of Refugees*.

47. Ibid.

48. Baker, *Psychosocial Problems of Refugees*.

49. Ibid.

50. D. Patrick and P. J. D. Heaf, *Long Term Effect of War Related Deprivation on Health: A Report on the Evidence*. London: St Thomas's Hospital Medical School, 1981.

51. Baker, *Psychosocial Problems of Refugees*; Summerfield, Asylum seekers.

52. Ahmad and Smith, *Humanitarian Action and Ethics*; Baker, *Psychosocial Problems of Refugees*; D. Giacco, A. Matanov and S. Priebe, Providing mental healthcare to immigrants: Current challenges and new strategies. *Current Opinion in Psychiatry* (2014) 27: 282–8; McColl and Johnson, Characteristics and needs of asylum seekers and refugees.

53. K. Day and P. White, Choice or circumstance: The UK as the location of asylum application by Bosnian and Somali refugees. *GeoJournal* (2002) 56: 15–26; S. W. Turner, C. Bowie, G. Dunn, L. Shapo and W. Yule, Mental health of Kosovan Albanian refugees in the UK. *British Journal of Psychiatry* (2003) 102: 444–8.

54. Ahmad and Smith, *Humanitarian Action and Ethics*.

55. Day and White, Choice or circumstance.

56. Baker, *Psychosocial Problems of Refugees*.

57. Day and White, Choice or circumstance; Healey, Refugee employment experiences.

58. Baker, *Psychosocial Problems of Refugees*; Miller et al., The relative contribution of war experiences and exile-related stressors to levels of psychological distress among Bosnian refugees. *Journal of Traumatic Stress* (2002) 15: 377–87; Turner, Bowie, Dunn, Shapo and Yule, Mental health of Kosovan Albanian refugees.

59. Baker, *Psychosocial Problems of Refugees*; Giacco, Matanov and Priebe, Providing mental healthcare to immigrants; McColl and Johnson, Characteristics and needs of asylum seekers and refugees; S. Schaecter, A study of psychosis in female migrants. *Medical Journal of Australia* (1962) 2: 458–61.

60. Baker, *Psychosocial Problems of Refugees*.

61. P. Hitch and P. Clegg, Modes of referral of overseas immigrant and native born first admission to psychiatric hospital. *Social Science and Medicine* (1980) 14: 369–74; Baker, *Psychosocial Problems of Refugees*; Patrick and Heaf, Long Term Effect of War Related Deprivation on Health.

62. Ahmad and Smith, *Humanitarian Action and Ethics*.

63. U. Eziefula, Refugee women in the UK: Factors affecting engagement with mental health services. PhD thesis, Canterbury Christchurch University, 2012; V. Patel, H. Minas, A. Cohen and M. Prince, *Global Mental Health*. Oxford: Oxford University Press, 2014.

64. Ahmad and Smith, *Humanitarian Action and Ethics*.

65. Eziefula, Refugee women in the UK.

66. Baker, *Psychosocial Problems of Refugees*; Eziefula, Refugee women in the UK.

67. Eziefula, Refugee women in the UK.

68. M. Picinelli and G. Wilkinson, Gender differences in depression: Critical review. *British Journal of Psychiatry* (2000) 177: 486–92.

69. Baker, *Psychosocial Problems of Refugees*.

70. Hitch and Clegg, Modes of referral.

71. McColl and Johnson, Characteristics and needs of asylum seekers and refugees.

72. Healey, Refugee employment experiences; Turner, Bowie, Dunn, Shapo and Yule, Mental health of Kosovan Albanian refugees.

73. Ager and Strang, *The Experience of Integration*.

74. Baker, *Psychosocial Problems of Refugees*.

75. Healey, Refugee employment experiences.

76. Baker, *Psychosocial Problems of Refugees*.

77. Ibid.

78. BBC, Bearing witness to the Holocaust. *BBC News*, 25 January 2001, http://news.bbc.co.uk/1/hi/uk/1133227 .stm.

79. BBC, Bearing witness; Helen Bamber quoted in L. Gray, *You Have breath for No More Than 99 Words: What Would They Be?* London: Darton, Longman & Todd, 2011.

80. N. Belton, *The Good Listener: Helen Bamber, a Life against Cruelty*. London: Weidenfeld & Nicolson, 1998.

81. Bamber quoted in Gray, *No More Than 99 Words*.

82. Ibid.

83. Giacco, Matanov and Priebe, Providing mental healthcare to immigrants.

84. Dillon and Smith, *Life in the UK Test Handbook*; Summerfield, Asylum seekers.

85. Healey, Refugee employment experiences.

Religion, Spirituality and Mental Health

Esther Ansah-Asamoah, Jamie Hacker Hughes, Ahmed Hankir and Christopher C. H. Cook

Introduction

Religion, spirituality and psychiatry share many ideals, including the importance of a holistic understanding of mental well-being,[1] yet in the past have clashed. This chapter explores the journey from mutual suspicion to the recognition of their positive intersection with a focus on Britain during the period 1960–2010.

Historical Context

The divisions between religion, spirituality and medicine date back to the Enlightenment period during the seventeenth and eighteenth centuries.[2] During this time, scientific communities began to develop empirical methods of explanation for behaviours and mind. While other medical fields diverged quickly, mental health continued to be closely linked with religion and spirituality until psychiatry was established as a medical discipline in the mid-nineteenth century.

From the late nineteenth century onwards, Freudian psychoanalysis understood religious belief as a form of psychopathology, attributable to the conflict between instinctual drive and intrapsychic representations of social and moral expectations: the ego and superego.[3] Freud asserted that religious belief in a monotheistic God was the result of a transference phenomenon which stemmed from childhood and that belief in God was similar to an exaggerated admiration of a father by his son in early childhood. In his book *Totem and Taboo*, he went on to say that the roots of religion arose from the need to resolve guilt through reconciliation; this need for redemption was projected onto a heavenly father.[4]

The evolution of behaviourism in the early twentieth century helped to create a gap between religion and psychology, too. Behaviourists postulated that all behaviour could be traced to physiological sources such as limbs, muscles and glands.[5] This allowed for the development of empirical studies, seeking to put psychology on par with other natural sciences, and simultaneously dismissed the importance of internal motivations.[6] Where there were once commonalities in practice, there now existed an ever-widening chasm fuelled by discord and distrust.

By the mid-twentieth century, the influence of biological psychiatry was increasing.[7] The medicalisation of mental health gradually undermined the importance of the clergy, who hitherto had been primarily responsible for the care of emotional and spiritual problems in the church community.[8] Additionally, many churchgoers perceived the rise of psychiatry/psychology as a direct 'anti-Christian' threat to biblical explanations of the human experience.[9] This disconnect may have contributed to the idea that patients' religious beliefs and spiritual concerns had no place within the realm of psychiatry and were often seen as detrimental to their psychological health. Standard psychiatric textbooks of the 1960s, such as Mayer-Gross, Slater and Roth's *Clinical Psychiatry*, perpetuated the idea that religious belief could be associated with neurotic behaviours and stated that religion was practised by 'the hesitant, the guilt-ridden, the excessively timid, those lacking clear convictions with which to face life'.[10]

Towards the end of the twentieth century, attitudes surrounding the involvement of religion and spirituality in psychiatry in the UK began to change, at least in part, in response to the transatlantic influence. This new outlook sparked an increase in research attempting to integrate religion and spirituality into the diagnosis and treatment of psychiatric problems. A seminal paper by Allport and Ross published in 1967, titled 'Personal Religious Orientation and Prejudice', highlighted the importance of considering not whether an individual is religious or not but of how important the role of that religion is in their life.[11] According to the authors, whereas 'intrinsic' religiosity provides a major motivation in life, 'extrinsic' religiosity is driven by other concerns, such as social esteem. Intrinsic religiosity, in contrast to extrinsic religiosity, has subsequently been shown in many studies to be good for mental health.

Both versions of the third edition of the *Diagnostic and Statistical Manual of Mental Disorders* (DSM-III and DSM-III-R) published in the 1980s were criticised for their inclusion of negative religious references and the implication that participation in religious activity was deviant from normal mental health.[12] The introduction of a new V code (V62.89) in DSM-IV in 1994 titled 'Religious or Spiritual Problems' went a long way to reversing this negative portrayal. The category addressed scenarios where people may seek clinical advice following mental health distress due to religious or spiritual problems, such as 'loss or questioning of faith', without the need to see this as pathological.[13] For the first time, it was widely recognised that individuals could have spiritual problems that were independent of mental disorders.

In 2001, Harold Koenig and his colleagues published the first edition of an encyclopaedic review of the scientific literature on religion and health (followed in 2012 by a second edition).[14] Increasingly, the scientific literature, largely emanating from the United States and Europe, was providing an evidence base to support the contention that spirituality and religion were important variables to be considered in the promotion of mental well-being and in understanding the causation and treatment of mental disorders.

Religion and Spirituality in Britain, 1960–2010

In Britain, the church was responding to the rising social and cultural liberalism of the 1960s. Liberal Christianity was growing in popularity while conservative Christianity was becoming sometimes associated with intolerance, despite (or perhaps reflecting) Allport and Ross's conclusions that intrinsic religiosity was associated with less prejudice.[15]

In his book *The Religious Crisis of the 1960s*, Hugh McLeod argued that secularisation in Britain created a rift within the church in the early 1960s whereby conservative Christianity was marginalised by a more liberal tradition.[16] He posited that the loss of the social significance of religious beliefs, practices and institutions paved the way for reform within the church to better reflect the changing socio-political climate. He designated 1967 as the 'turning point' by which the Christian church succumbed to the tidal wave of secularism.[17] Church attendance declined and a growing number of individuals began to designate themselves as being spiritual but not religious (SBNR) or having no religion at all.[18]

However, the secularisation hypothesis has been widely questioned. The sociologist Grace Davie, for example, has argued that secularisation does not necessarily correspond with a decline in religion in Britain but rather an evolution through which more people are choosing to keep their religious beliefs private, in effect 'believing without belonging' to an institution.[19] This hypothesis also has been questioned and there is evidence to suggest that many people are 'neither believing nor belonging'.[20]

In this context, at least in some quarters, discourse on religion has given way to an emphasis on spirituality. Although there is currently no universal definition of spirituality, in Britain 'spirituality' has often been understood as a more inclusive term, applicable to individuals of all faiths and none, focusing more on individual practices and beliefs rather that institutional affiliations.[21] In their book *The Spiritual Revolution: Why Religion Is Giving Way to Spirituality*, Heelas and Woodhead acknowledge that, while practice of traditional Christianity is declining and (they say) will continue to do so for decades to come, spirituality as a stand-alone concept has not yet overtaken traditional religion.[22] They propose instead that the decline in Christian religiosity can be attributed to an increase in 'holistic activity' in middle-aged women and a shift in British culture to favour subjective governance of life, where external obligations and objective societal roles defined by religious authorities are less important than individual experience.[23]

The decrease in religious affiliation to Christianity has also been associated with a decline in the transmittance of religiosity through generations.[24] Children and young people with religious parents are reportedly only 45 per cent likely to adopt their parents' religious affiliations. In contrast, children brought up by non-religious parents have a 95 per cent chance of being and staying non-religious themselves.[25]

Modernisation, industrialisation and globalisation have led to the increase of religious pluralism in Britain since 1960. Immigration has introduced new groups to the religious landscape. The growing number of religious communities has meant that the dominance of Christianity has begun to decrease. Religious pluralism is a controversial subject and was highly contested in the late twentieth century. Some scholars such as Steve Bruce have argued that pluralism weakened overall religious faith as it allowed for the element of choice, eventually leading to lower levels of religious participation.[26] Linda Woodhead has suggested that increasing pluralism must eventually result in a breakdown of boundaries between religious and secular groups, resulting in de-differentiation.[27] Others believe that pluralism is the result of the natural order of religious society where no religions are repressed, which is thought to generate higher levels of religious participation than religious monopolies.[28] Empirically, the beginning of the twenty-first century in Britain has seen a continued rise in pluralism accompanied by a sustained decline in Christian religious practice.

Changing Attitudes to Spirituality and Religion within Psychiatry, 1960–2010

From the 1960s through to the early 1990s, attitudes to spirituality within psychiatry began to shift. Many psychiatrists and psychologists, such as Albert Ellis, were openly dismissive of religion and spirituality through to the 1980s, maintaining that religious beliefs conferred no benefits to an individual's mental state despite being a large part of many people's lives.[29] In a paper he wrote detailing his experience as a psychiatrist in the late twentieth century,

Andrew Sims remarked that in the 1960s 'there was no sense that there could be collaboration between psychiatrists and religious leaders in the care of patients'.[30]

By the late 1980s, however, attitudes had begun to shift to a more tolerant view of the place of spirituality and religion in psychiatry.[31] Since that decade, several groups affiliated with both religion and psychiatry have begun to form. The Christian Medical Fellowship held its first breakfast meeting at a national conference of the Royal College of Psychiatrists (RCPsych) in 1986, helping to alleviate some of the stigma surrounding psychiatric practice and Christian faith. One of the early meetings of the Philosophy in Psychiatry Special Interest Group (formed in 1988) was centred on the topic of religion and psychiatry. In 1991, the patron of the RCPsych, HRH The Prince of Wales, gave a speech highlighting the importance of acknowledging the impact of religion and spirituality on patients' well-being.[32] By 1998, the message of HRH's speech had been echoed a number of times at prominent meetings attended by psychiatrists and religious leaders such as the Archbishop of Canterbury.[33] The relation between religiosity and mental illness became a quickly expanding field of study and it became clear that religion and spirituality could no longer be ignored.

By the early twenty-first century, it was generally accepted that spirituality and religion provide meaningful frameworks for living and community support systems that help individuals to cope with the stresses of daily life and mental illness. In that respect, engaging in religious and spiritual belief could positively contribute to a person's mental health and improve their outcomes following psychiatric treatment.[34] There have, however, been concerns surrounding the inclusion of spirituality in psychiatric practice as – it is alleged – it may lead to an erosion of professional boundaries between the doctor and their patient.[35]

Interest in the intersections between spirituality, religion and psychiatry resulted in the formation of the Spirituality and Psychiatry Special Interest Group (SPSIG) of the RCPsych in 1999.[36] SPSIG is concerned with the spiritual and religious affairs of both psychiatrists and their patients and aims to promote an integrative approach to mental health care by stimulating discussion within the College on matters relating to spirituality and religion and proposing revisions to the psychiatric curriculum to better reflect the advances of psychiatric and religious research.[37] In 2009, an edited volume, *Spirituality and Psychiatry*, conceived within the SPSIG, was published by RCPsych Press, providing the first critical attempt by a group of British psychiatrists and mental health professionals to address the implications of spirituality/religion for clinical practice.[38]

The General Synod of the Church of England held debates on mental health in 2003 and 2008. The president of the RCPsych and three members of the College were invited to observe the debate, which concluded with the passing of a motion to 'welcome the recognition within mental health services of the significance of spirituality for assessment and treatment, and encourage parishes to ensure that the support and care of people with mental health problems, their carers and NHS staff is a key priority for the Church's ministry'.[39] There was clearly an implicit reference here to the way in which spirituality was increasingly being seen – at the RCPsych and elsewhere – as an important part of mental health care. The work of the RCPsych SPSIG was explicitly referred to in the *Continuing Issues in Mental Health* report discussed by the Synod in 2008.[40]

In the last few decades, policies have been established within various national psychiatric associations that recognise the contributions of religion and spirituality to an individual's mental health. In the UK, the SPSIG first drafted a position statement making recommendations on practice in relation to spirituality and religion in psychiatry in October 2005.[41]

After a series of revisions, the recommendations were approved by the RCPsych as its position statement in 2011 (later revised in 2013). In 2015, the Executive Committee of the World Psychiatric Association also agreed a position statement on spirituality and religion in psychiatry which owed much to the RCPsych's position statement.[42] The impact of these policies upon clinical practice has yet to be evidenced, but a number of other national psychiatric associations have gone on to provide their own policies and guidance in relation to spirituality/religion.[43]

The Mental Health Foundation carried out a comprehensive review of the literature on the impact of spirituality on mental health in 2006.[44] They concluded it justified 'cautious optimism' about the relationship between spirituality and religion in the promotion and maintenance of good psychological health, with possible mechanisms being: locus of control and coping styles; the formation and supportive nature of social networks; promotion of healthy lifestyle choices; and, even, positive effects of the built environment.[45]

Religious Perspectives on Mental Health, 1960–2010

Conservative religious perspectives on mental health have followed a similar trajectory to that of psychiatric perspectives on religion. Early suspicion and alienation meant that religious groups were reluctant to accept the involvement of psychiatrists in treating mental health issues within their community. The anti-psychiatry movement of the 1960s and 1970s probably further contributed to negative Christian perspectives on psychiatry, too.[46] Some Christians considered mental illness a result of spiritual failings such as lack of faith, which could only be treated with pastoral counselling (see also Chapter 20).[47] This attitude weakened over the last few decades of the twentieth century but nevertheless persisted through to the early twenty-first century.

While psychiatry was coming to terms with the positive role that a religious support system could play in mental illness recovery, a study conducted in the United States by Mathew Stanford, published in 2007, found that many mentally ill individuals experienced negative interactions within their church communities when they sought counsel. Stanford found that, in a group of 293 Christian participants (mostly from the United States), 30 per cent reported feeling abandoned or dismissed by the church or told to ignore advice and medical prescriptions given by psychiatrists.[48] While we are not aware of similar research in the UK at this time, we imagine that in at least some churches here findings would have been very similar.

Increasing Influence of Service Users

In 1997, the Mental Health Foundation conducted the first nationwide service user–led survey. The study found that more than half of the service users and survivors associated positively their religious and spiritual beliefs with their mental health. People reported that their beliefs offered them comfort, a sense of purpose and guidance.[49] This research helped to realise the benefits of religion and spirituality to psychiatric treatments.

The Somerset Spirituality Project, also supported by the Mental Health Foundation, interviewed mental health service users in Somerset between late 2000 and early 2001 and found that they valued highly their religious experiences and considered them to be positive influences on their mental health. The Somerset Spirituality Project highlighted the import-ance of service users/survivors feeling supported in their spirituality within mental health services. Results from the project have been used in psychiatric training to inspire empathy and understanding towards those who are spiritually inclined (see also Chapter 13).[51]

Spiritual Crisis Network

The steadily increasing number of people who identified as SBNR in the late twentieth and early twenty-first centuries led to the establishment of support groups such as the Spiritual Crisis Network (SCN) in 2008. The SCN provide resources and counselling to individuals who have had spiritual experiences but may not be able to get the help they need or do not feel comfortable approaching a religious leader or a psychiatrist. Despite a lack of academic studies relating to spiritual crises, the SCN has developed a strategy to aid people in spiritual distress involving positive appraisals and construction of narrative frameworks.[52]

Scientific and Medical Network

The Scientific and Medical Network (SMN) is an international charity founded in 1973 which is dedicated to 'exploring and expanding the frontiers of science, medicine and spirituality'. It has a strong presence in the UK, with ten local groups. Since its conception, the SMN has encouraged scientists and medical professionals to incorporate spiritual and philosophical elements into their work, with a focus on enhancing understanding around parapsychological phenomena and how they influence the human experience and impact on mental health.[53]

Developments in Other Professions

At the same time as the developing acknowledgement of the importance of religion and spirituality to psychiatry, there have been similar developments within other mental health professions. In nursing, the Patient's Charter, introduced by the Department of Health in 1991, emphasised 'respect for privacy, dignity and religious and cultural beliefs'.[54] Greasley and colleagues, in a paper on spiritual care in mental health nursing published in 2001, defined spiritual care in mental health nursing as relating to 'the acknowledgement of a person's sense of meaning and purpose to life which may, or may not be expressed through religious beliefs or practices'.[55] They expressed, as does Sartori in a more recent paper,[56] the view that, despite an acknowledgement that spirituality is important in the care of patients, it is still an area in which few nurses feel that they meet their patients' needs.

Other professions have had similar concerns. Occupational therapists (OTs) take a holistic approach to practice in which they consider the role of the body, mind and spirit in illness.[57] Prior to the 1990s, they did not generally address spiritual issues with patients although, when surveyed, the results showed that they did recognise the importance of spirituality in health and rehabilitation.[58] In a follow-up study conducted in 2002, OTs reported an increase in spiritual discussions with their patients, indicative of an advancing acceptance of the role of religion and spirituality in health care.[59] Despite this, in a 2004 paper, 'Spirituality in occupational therapy, theory in practice?',[60] Belcham expressed concern that some OTs continued to neglect this area in their practice, for example in assessments.

Coyle and Lochner, in an article in the 2011 issue of *The Psychologist*,[61] summarised the areas where the interactions between religion and spirituality and therapeutic practice are important to clinical and other applied psychologists: the process of assessment; responses to religious or other spiritual material which may be problematic; and in the areas of training and supervision. In the latter area, as recently as 2016, Jafari found that attention to religion and spirituality in clinical and counselling psychology training programmes was still being neglected.[62]

Spirituality and Psychiatry in Other Faiths

The 2001 census conducted by the British government revealed that Britain is ethnically, culturally and religiously diverse, especially in larger cities such as Manchester, Glasgow and Birmingham. In London, for example, 8.5 per cent of inhabitants identified as Muslim, 4.1 per cent as Hindu, 2.1 per cent as Jewish and 0.8 per cent as Buddhist.[63] This section focuses on those of Islamic faith, as its adherents make up the second largest religious group in Britain.

Over the last few decades, there has been some concern that British Muslims with mental illnesses may be avoiding mainstream mental health services,[64] thus missing out on early intervention and this could be associated with poorer outcomes. Research suggests that this avoidance may be related to their religious beliefs, as many were reported to attribute their adverse experiences to supernatural causes such as 'Jinn possession' and/or 'being cursed by the evil eye of envy'.[65]

Explanatory models of mental illness strongly influence coping strategies and help-seeking behaviours, too. Bhui and colleagues conducted in-depth interviews in the UK with 116 people from 6 ethnic groups to ascertain how they cope with mental distress. The results showed that religious coping was most commonly practised by Bangladeshi Muslims and Afro-Caribbean Christians.[66]

In an effort to combat the overt distrust of mental health services within the Muslim religious community, faith leaders (Imams) have joined chaplaincy services in NHS Trusts from the early 2000s.[67] They have worked closely with other religious leaders and healers to provide ad hoc advice and pastoral support on faith related matters and mental health. The actual provision, however, of contemporary mental health services in the UK is not faith-sensitive insofar as it does not incorporate religious principles and modalities in treatment. A more holistic approach is needed that integrates spirituality/religiosity with 'conventional' psychiatry. We believe that such a model would help to break down the barriers for Muslims (and others) who urgently need mental health support.

Conclusion

Religion, spirituality and psychiatry have had a complicated relationship over the years. Early mutual mistrust meant that, despite their congruent goals, there was a marked reluctance to associate them with each other. Over the decades, against a backdrop of rapid socio-political and cultural change, religion and psychiatry in Britain began to intertwine. Many psychiatrists began to see religion as a facilitator for good mental health practice and as a community-based support system which would help to improve patient outcomes. While battling the rise of secularism and the loss of social significance through religious pluralism, the Christian church has gradually adjusted its relationship with psychiatry. Other faith groups have similarly had to come to terms with a secular provision of mental health services which has often not been understanding of the spiritual and religious concerns of patients.

Key Summary Points

- Religion, spirituality and psychiatry share many ideals, such as the importance of a holistic understanding of mental well-being,[68] yet in the past have clashed. The transitions that occurred from 1960 to 2010 have significantly shaped the contemporary relationships between religion, spirituality and psychiatry in Britain.
- Interest in the intersections between spirituality, religion and psychiatry resulted in the formation of the Spirituality and Psychiatry Special Interest Group (SPSIG) of the RCPsych in 1999. In 2009, an edited volume, *Spirituality and Psychiatry*, conceived within the SPSIG, provided the first critical attempt by a group of British psychiatrists and mental health professionals to address the implications of spirituality/religion for clinical practice.
- At the same time as the developing acknowledgement of the importance of religion and spirituality to psychiatry, there were similar developments within a number of other mental health professions.
- The General Synod of the Church of England held debates on mental health in 2003 and 2008. The president of the RCPsych and three members of the College were invited to observe the 2008 debate, which concluded with the passing of a motion to 'welcome the recognition within mental health services of the significance of spirituality for assessment and treatment, and encourage parishes to ensure that the support and care of people with mental health problems, their carers and NHS staff is a key priority for the church's ministry'.
- A more holistic approach to the treatment of mental health difficulties is needed that integrates spirituality/religiosity with 'conventional' psychiatry. We believe that such a model would help to break down the barriers to mental health services for people of strong faith and spiritual orientation who urgently need them.

Notes

1. S. Sullivan, J. M. Pyne, A. M. Cheney, J. Hunt, T. F. Haynes and G. Sullivan, The pew versus the couch: Relationship between mental health and faith communities and lessons learned from a VA/clergy partnership project. *Journal of Religion and Health* (2014) 53: 1267–82; Á. de Jesús Cortés, Antecedents to the conflict between psychology and religion in America. *Journal of Psychology and Theology* (1999) 27: 20–32.

2. Sullivan et al., The pew versus the couch.

3. J. W. Jones, *Contemporary Psychoanalysis and Religion: Transference and Transcendence.* New Haven, CT: Yale University Press, 1991.

4. S. Freud, *Totem and Taboo.* Boston, MA: Beacon Press, 1913.

5. K. Hilner, *History and Systems of Psychology: A Conceptual Approach.* Gardner Press, 1984.

6. Á. de Jesús Cortés, Antecedents to the conflict between psychology and religion in America. *Journal of Psychology and Theology* (1999) 27: 20–32.

7. G. N. Grob, The attack of psychiatric legitimacy in the 1960s: Rhetoric and reality. *Journal of the History of Behavioral Sciences* (2011) 47: 398–416.

8. Sullivan et al., The pew versus the couch; R. F. Larson, The clergyman's role in the therapeutic process: Disagreement between clergymen and psychiatrists. *Psychiatry* (1968) 31: 250–63.

9. Sullivan et al., The pew versus the couch.

10. W. Mayer-Gross, E. Slater and M. Roth, *Clinical Psychiatry* (3rd ed.). London: Bailliere Tindall & Cassell, 1969.

11. G. W. Allport and J. M. Ross, Personal religious orientation and prejudice. *Journal of Personality and Social Psychology* (1967) 5: 432–43.

12. J. T. Richardson, Religiosity as deviance: Negative religious bias in and misuse of the DSM-III. *Deviant Behavior* (1993) 14: 1–21.

13. D. Lukoff, C. R. Cloninger, M. Galanter et al., Religious and spiritual Considerations in Psychiatric Diagnosis: Considerations for the DSM-V. In P. J. Verhagen, H. M. van Praag, J. J. López-Ibor et al., eds, *Religion and Psychiatry*, 423–44. Oxford: Wiley-Blackwell, 2010.

14. H. G. Koenig, M. E. McCullough and D. B. Larson, *Handbook of Religion and Health* (1st ed.). Oxford: Oxford University Press, 2001; H. Koenig, D. King and V. Carson, *Handbook of Religion and Health* (2nd ed.). Oxford: Oxford University Press, 2012.

15. Allport and Ross, Personal religious orientation and prejudice.

16. H. McLeod, *The Religious Crisis of the 1960s*. Oxford: Oxford University Press, 2007.

17. Ibid.

18. L. Woodhead, The rise of 'no religion' in Britain: The emergence of a new cultural majority. *Journal of the British Academy* (2016) 4: 245–61; V. Ertit, Secularization: The decline of the supernatural realm. *Religions* (2018) 9: 92.

19. G. Davie, Believing without belonging: Is this the future of religion in Britain? *Sociology Compass* (1990) 37: 455–69.

20. D. Voas and A. Crockett, Religion in Britain: Neither believing nor belonging. *Sociology* (2005) 39: 11–28.

21. Royal College of Psychiatrists, *Recommendations for Psychiatrists on Spirituality and Religion*. Position Statement No. PS03/13, November 2013, www.rcpsych.ac.uk/pdf/PS03_2013.pdf.

22. P. Heelas, L. Woodhead, B. Seel, B. Szerszynski and K. Tusting, *The Spiritual Revolution: Why Religion Is Giving Way to Spirituality*. Oxford: Wiley-Blackwell, 2005.

23. Ibid.

24. Woodhead, Rise of 'no religion' in Britain; Voas and Crockett, Religion in Britain.

25. Woodhead, Rise of 'no religion' in Britain.

26. R. Stark, R. Finke and L. R. Iannaccone, Pluralism and Piety: England and Wales, 1851. *Journal for the Scientific Study of Religion* (1995) 34: 431.

27. L. Woodhead, Intensified religious pluralism and de-differentiation: The British example. *Society* (2016) 53: 41–6.

28. Stark, Finke and Iannaccone, Pluralism and Piety.

29. W. R. Breakey, Psychiatry, spirituality and religion. *International Review of Psychiatry* (2001) 13: 61–6.

30. A. Sims, Mysterious ways: Spirituality and British psychiatry in the 20th century. Online article, 2003, www.rcpsych.ac.uk/docs/default-source/members/sigs/spirituality-spsig/andrew-sims-1–11-03-mysterious-ways–spirituality-and-british-psychiatry-in-the-20th-century.pdf?sfvrsn=40adb83a_4.

31. Ibid.

32. L. Culliford, Spiritual care and psychiatric treatment. *Advances in Psychiatric Treatment* (2002) 8: 249–61.

33. Sims, Mysterious ways.

34. Koenig, King and Carson, *Handbook of Religion and Health*.

35. C. C. H. Cook, Controversies on the place of spirituality and religion in psychiatric practice. In C. C. H Cook, ed., *Spirituality, Theology and Mental Health*, 1–19. London: SCM Press, 2013.

36. Sullivan et al., The pew versus the couch; A. Powell and C. C. H. Cook, Spirituality and Psychiatry Special Interest Group of the Royal College of Psychiatrists. In *Reaching the Spirit: Social Perspectives Network Study Day Paper Nine*, 34–9. 2006.

37. Powell and Cook, Spirituality and Psychiatry Special Interest Group; C. Cook, A. Sims and A. Powell, *Spirituality and Psychiatry*. London: RCPsych Publications, 2009.

38. Cook, Sims and Powell, *Spirituality and Psychiatry*.

39. Mission and Public Affairs Council, *Continuing Issues in Mental Health*. Report No. GS1678. London: Church House, 2008, www.churchofengland.org/sites/default/files/2018–11/GS%201678.pdf

40. Ibid., p. 15.

41. C. C. H. Cook, Spirituality and religion in psychiatry: The impact of policy. *Mental Health Religion and Culture* (2017) 20: 589–94.

42. Ibid.

43. Ibid.

44. Mental Health Foundation, *The Impact of Spirituality on Mental Health*. London: Mental Health Foundation, 2006. www.mentalhealth.org.uk/sites/default/files/impact-spirituality.pdf.

45. Ibid., p. 32.

46. Breakey, Psychiatry, spirituality and religion; N. R. D. Crossley, Laing and the British anti-psychiatry movement: A socio-historical analysis. *Social Science and Medicine* (1998) 47: 877–89.

47. M. S. Stanford, Demon or disorder: A survey of attitudes toward mental illness in the Christian church. *Mental Health Religion and Culture* (2007) 10: 445–9.

48. Ibid.

49. Mental Health Foundation, *Impact of Spirituality on Mental Health*.

50. Mental Health Foundation, *Taken Seriously: The Somerset Spirituality Project*. London: Mental Health Foundation, 2002, www.mentalhealth.org.uk/sites/default/files/taken-seriously.pdf.

51. Ibid.

52. See the 'Research' section on the Spiritual Crisis Network's website: https://spiritualcrisisnetwork.uk /research.

53. See the 'About' section on the Scientific and Medical Network's website: https://explore.scimednet.org/index .php/about/.

54. S. Gilliat-Ray, Nursing, professionalism, and spirituality. *Journal of Contemporary Religion* (2003) 18: 335–49.

55. P. Greasley, L. F. Chiu and R. M. Gartland, The concept of spiritual care in mental health nursing. *Journal of Advanced Nursing* (2001) 33: 629–37.

56. P. Sartori, Spirituality 1: Should spiritual and religious beliefs be part of patient care? *Nursing Times* (2010) 106: 14–17.

57. J. S. Collins, S. Paul and J. West-Frasier, The utilization of spirituality in occupational therapy: Beliefs, practices, and perceived barriers. *Occupational Therapy in Health Care* (2002) 14: 73–92.

58. Ibid.

59. Ibid.

60. C. Belcham, Spirituality in occupational therapy: Theory in practice? *British Journal of Occupational Therapy* (2004) 67: 39–46.

61. A. Coyle and J. Lochner, Religion, spirituality and therapeutic practice. *Psychologist* (2011) 24: 264–6.

62. S. Jafari, Religion and spirituality within counselling/clinical psychology training programmes: A systematic review. *British Journal of Guidance and Counselling* (2016) 44: 257–67.

63. Office for National Statistics, Religion (2001 Census), https://data.gov.uk/dataset/17080d4d-793d-4931-925 4-a9f6c7652c3e/religion-2001-census.

64. S. Dein and S. Sembhi, The use of traditional healing in South Asian psychiatric patients in the U.K.: Interactions between professional and folk psychiatries. *Transcultural Psychiatry* (2001) 38: 243–57.

65. S. M. Razali, U. A. Khan and C. I. Hasanah, Belief in supernatural causes of mental illness among Malay patients: Impact on treatment. *Acta Psychiatrica Scandinavica* (1996) 94: 229–33.

66. K. Bhui, M. King, S. Dein and W. O'Connor, Ethnicity and religious coping with mental distress. *Journal of Mental Health* (2008) 17: 141–51.

67. M. Imran Hussain, *Evaluation of the Muslim Chaplaincy Service Calderdale and Huddersfield NHS Trust*. Huddersfield: Calderdale and Huddersfield NHS Trust, 2014, www.cht.nhs.uk/fileadmin/site_setup/contentUploads/Services/Non-clinical/Chaplaincy/R.C._Muslim_Evaluation_2014.pdf.

38 Soldiers, Veterans and Psychological Casualties: Legacies of Northern Ireland, the Falklands, Afghanistan and Iraq

Edgar Jones

Introduction

While the fifty years from 1960 did not produce a conflict on the scale of the two world wars, the UK adopted an increasingly interventionist foreign policy that drew British forces into campaigns beyond Europe. Counter-insurgency operations in Northern Ireland served as an enduring backdrop, involving 300,000 UK service personnel and resulting in 1,441 deaths between 1969 and 2006.[1] However, until the breakup of the Soviet Union in December 1991, the primary role of the British armed forces remained within NATO, protecting Western Europe from the Eastern Bloc. These long-term commitments were eclipsed when international destabilisation led to the breakup of Yugoslavia and UN peacekeeping roles followed in Bosnia, Kosovo and Macedonia. Yet, by 1997, after a decade of Conservative cuts, the defence budget as a percentage of GDP had shrunk to its lowest level in the twentieth century.[2] In July 1998, a strategic defence review conducted by New Labour identified growing risks: terrorism in particular but also drugs, ethnic and population pressures and scarce resources.[3] The government sought to create a tri-service force able to operate regularly beyond Europe on a joint and multinational basis. Designed to raise Britain's international influence, it required the military 'to punch above its weight'.[4] Deployments to Sierra Leone, Afghanistan and Iraq followed, stretching the resources of the UK armed forces to the limit. The physical and psychological casualties that were sustained created a popular support for the individual soldier but eventually eroded public support for the interventionist policy.

The Falklands War

Despite the physical challenges of the terrain and the extended supply chain, the Falklands War of spring 1982 appeared to produce little post-traumatic illness, reported as 2 per cent of all wounded.[5] Of the 9,000 ground troops deployed, 150 (1.7 per cent) were killed in action. Although sixteen psychiatric cases were evacuated to SS *Uganda*, the hospital ship, only four were diagnosed with 'battleshock', the term then used for acute stress reaction.[6] The lengthy sea voyages to and from the South Atlantic were thought to have provided time to prepare mentally for combat and to readjust to peacetime soldiering or a return to civilian life.[7] Research conducted after the war identified functional somatic presentations that elevated the rate of psychiatric casualties to 8 per cent.[8] This was significantly below the 20 per cent commonly recorded for major battles in the Second World War and was explained by the short duration of the war and the fact that British troops were highly trained regulars.[9]

Yet subsequent studies raised the possibility that the 8 per cent of all wounded did not capture the full impact of the traumatic experience.[10] In 1987, Jones and Lovett reported three delayed cases of post-traumatic stress disorder (PTSD) from members of the task force.[11] Five years after the conflict, O'Brien and Hughes compared a group of sixty-four infantry soldiers who had served in the Falklands with matched controls who had equivalent training but had remained in the UK during the conflict.[12] On the basis of self-report questionnaires, it was found that fourteen (22 per cent) met the criteria for PTSD and a further eighteen (28 per cent) had a range of these symptoms. PTSD scores were not associated with age, rank or length of service but were higher for those who had lost comrades through wounding or death or who had killed the enemy or assisted in the management of casualties. They were also likely to have experienced emotional difficulties on returning home from the war. In 1993, a study of Falklands' veterans found a 60 per cent rate of PTSD from fifty-three respondents who had completed a postal questionnaire. However, this was not a representative sample, as the investigators had sought volunteers using a networking model.[13] While the operational success of the Falklands War was unquestioned, it increasingly appeared that the cost in terms of psychiatric casualties was hidden. In 2002, this notion received support from an article published in the *Daily Mail* claiming that 264 Falklands veterans had committed suicide, more than the 237 killed in the conflict.[14] Research published by Defence Analytical Services and Advice in 2013 showed that 95 veterans had taken their own lives, which represented 7 per cent of the 1,335 who had then died since serving in the Falklands campaign.[15] A lasting effect of the war was a change to the policy for commemoration of casualties. Following pressure from relatives, the Ministry of Defence (MoD) agreed that bodies could be repatriated to the UK for burial,[16] a ritual that was to influence public opinion once campaigns in Iraq and Afghanistan proved costly.

Forward Psychiatry

Forward psychiatry, the classic method of managing breakdown on the battlefield developed during the First World War, was not employed in the Falklands. The two Navy psychiatrists with the task force remained on hospital ships throughout the campaign, so that a key element, return to unit, was prohibited under the terms of the Geneva Convention.[17] Known by the acronym PIE (proximity to the battlefield, immediacy of delivery and expectation of recovery), the procedure had been widely used in the Second World War and Korea when it returned around 30 per cent of those treated to duty.[18] However, the counter-insurgency operations in Malaya, which engaged British troops from June 1948 to July 1960, offered no obvious application for an intervention that required defined battle lines. As army psychiatrists with first-hand knowledge of forward psychiatry retired, training in its use ceased during the 1960s. The end of National Service saw the number of soldiers in the army fall from 430,000 in the mid-1950s (of whom just over half were conscripts)[19] to 157,000 by 1965.[20] It was assumed that volunteers who had joined to the armed forces as a career would be less vulnerable to breakdown.

Forward psychiatry was reintroduced in the early 1980s in response to the threat of a massed Soviet assault from the East.[21] Warsaw Pact forces had developed a tactic of concentrated bombardment to induce severe dissociation in front-line troops. Large numbers of 'battleshock' cases were predicted, requiring rapid treatment.[22] The surprise attack on the Israeli Defense Force in the Yom Kippur War was identified as a model for an invasion of Europe, and Israeli clinicians were invited to the UK to brief their British counterparts.[23] Mobile field psychiatric teams (FPTs) were formed at brigade level and attached to field ambulances, comprising two doctors and four mental health nurses, and incorporated within battlefield training. To overcome stigma and present the policy in terms that fighting units would recognise, Brigadier Peter Abraham published on 'battleshock' and briefed British troops stationed in Germany.[24]

Northern Ireland

Running from 1969 to 2006, counter-insurgency operations in Northern Ireland served as an enduring commitment and saw more than 300,000 UK service personnel deployed with 1,441 deaths.[25] The decade from 1971 to 1980, which saw the worst of the violence, raised the strength of troops in the province to 20,000. It was a period during which 330 regular soldiers and 107 members of the Ulster Defence Regiment were killed and many more injured. Nevertheless, combat stress reactions remained at a low level and were managed by community psychiatric nurses (1 per 5,000 soldiers) supported by regular clinical sessions from uniformed psychiatrists. Not until the 1980s was a full-time, army psychiatrist deployed to Northern Ireland.[26] However, a study in 2015 of veterans treated for PTSD at the inpatient facility of the mental health charity Combat Stress showed that 55 per cent had served in Northern Ireland compared with the Falklands (16 per cent), Iraq (33 per cent) and Afghanistan (17 per cent).[27] The preponderance was probably a consequence of the numbers deployed rather than a heightened incidence of traumatic events during the Troubles.

UK Recognition of PTSD

Although the American Psychiatric Association (APA) recognised PTSD in 1980, the association with Vietnam veterans delayed its acceptance in Britain. The 1986 edition of the *Oxford Textbook of Psychiatry*, for example, referred only to a 'post-traumatic syndrome' which related to 'chronic neuroses after head injury'.[28] Until the 1990s, little was published on PTSD affecting UK armed forces or civilians exposed to terrorism. However, in the late 1980s, Morgan O'Connell, a Navy psychiatrist, saw an increasing number of Falklands' veterans with chronic psychological symptoms and explored the usefulness of PTSD as a diagnosis and route to treatment. On 21 December 1988, the detonation of a terrorist bomb on board Pan Am Flight 103 from London to New York introduced Royal Air Force clinicians to the new disorder.[29] The aircraft crashed at Lockerbie, killing 259 passengers and crew, together with 11 local residents. Four RAF mountain rescue teams were sent to the site to look for possible survivors but found only the dead and body parts.[30] Gordon Turnbull, a RAF neuropsychiatrist, employed critical incident stress debriefing (CISD) to treat the teams who had not expected to encounter such devastation.[31] CISD was adopted by the military as a way of dealing with the acute effects of trauma and subsequently proposed as a way of reducing the incidence of PTSD.[32] RAF psychiatrists developed a twelve-day structured, inpatient course of group psychotherapy and day case follow-up sessions, in which psychological debriefing was the main therapeutic technique.[33]

Gulf War

In contrast to the Falklands, where the size of the battlegroup was determined by available sea transport, the Gulf War in 1990–1 saw a force of 53,400 sent to Kuwait.[34] With such numbers and the possibility of an extended land campaign, forward psychiatry had an obvious role. Two FPTs worked in conjunction with a Battleshock Recovery Unit.[35] However, a short campaign with only forty-eight deaths resulted in few psychological casualties. The most challenging health effect emerged after the conflict and was given the popular term Gulf War syndrome. Veterans in the UK and the United States succumbed to a range of common, medically unexplained symptoms that impaired their daily function. Intense media and public interest followed in part because the mystery illness was hypothesised as having a toxic cause, whether from chemical weapons, vaccinations, organophosphates, depleted uranium munitions or oil well fires. Although a major research programme failed to find a unique disease,[36] similarities were identified with post-combat syndromes from earlier wars.[37] Such was the dominance of Gulf War syndrome that no studies were conducted into rates of PTSD suffered by UK service personnel and veterans until the new millennium.[38] An investigation of troops deployed on peacekeeping duties between 1991 and 2000 found a PTSD prevalence rate of 3.6 per cent,[39] while a study carried out from 2001 to 2002 of a representative sample of UK armed forces found a probable PTSD prevalence of only 2.5 per cent.[40] These percentages were equivalent to those for the UK population as a whole (males between the ages of sixteen and sixty-four having a rate of 3.6 per cent)[41] and appeared to show a military with robust mental health. In retrospect, it is surprising that the first studies of PTSD in the UK military were conducted more than twenty years after the disorder had been recognised in DSM-III. This omission was to prove costly to the MoD because it created an opportunity for a legal case brought by veterans who had served in Northern Ireland, the Falklands, the Gulf and Bosnia for negligence in the detection and treatment of PTSD. With little or no published data on rates and outcomes, they were granted legal aid to test the validity of their claim for compensation in the Royal Courts of Justice.

Peacekeeping in Bosnia

In October 1992, British troops were deployed to Bosnia as part of the UN peacekeeping operation and remained there for more than a decade. Although casualties were low, many encountered the results of atrocities or found themselves constrained by rules of engagement when presented with ethnic conflicts. A self-report study of 4,250 UK troops deployed to Bosnia between 1991 and 1997 found that they were at greater risk of heavy drinking than those who had served in the Gulf War or those who had been serving at the time but not deployed to either theatre.[42] In part explained by their younger age, it was also attributed to exposure to dangerous, provoking or humiliating experiences with limited opportunities to express the resulting anger and frustration.

Class Action for PTSD

Amid much publicity, the class action brought by 2,000 UK veterans against the MoD came to court on 4 March 2002. With so much evidence to consider, it was not until May 2003 that Mr Justice Owen delivered his judgement. The landmark case, probably the most important public inquiry into the treatment of post-traumatic illness since the

Southborough committee of inquiry into shell shock, explored six key areas: the state of knowledge, screening for vulnerability, treatment, forward psychiatry, detection together with military culture and stigma.[43] Although the MoD was not found negligent, the judge identified a need to monitor developments in screening, detection and treatment. The MoD was reminded of the need to incorporate new knowledge into training, policy and practice.[44] Compared with the United States and Israel, the UK armed forces had limited research capacity in military psychiatry, a function both of size and of institutional culture. Following the case, the MoD funded a major research programme at the Institute of Psychiatry and the King's Centre for Military Health Research (KCMHR) was set up in 2004, subsuming the Gulf War Illnesses Unit that had opened in 1996.

Treatment

The validation of cognitive behavioural therapy (CBT) for PTSD was the significant innovation in treatment during the period. However, the randomised controlled trials conducted in the early 1990s were of victims of sexual assault.[45] With large numbers of Vietnam veterans diagnosed with PTSD, US clinicians researched new treatments during the 1980s,[46] though the first UK study of trauma-focused CBT for service personnel was not published until 1995.[47] While it was subsequently shown that cognitive processing therapy and prolonged exposure therapy for PTSD in military and veteran populations achieved meaningful symptom reduction, 60 per cent to 72 per cent of subjects continued to meet the criteria for PTSD after treatment. Further, non-response and drop-out rates were high, suggesting a need for better ways of engaging with veterans.[48]

Afghanistan and Iraq

The campaigns in Afghanistan and Iraq did not produce a syndrome characterised by medically unexplained symptoms akin to that associated with the Gulf War. As a result, the main research focus was on PTSD and latterly on rates of common mental disorders and alcohol abuse. Between March 2003 and May 2011, 120,000 UK service personnel were deployed to Iraq, of whom 179 were killed. Operations overlapped with the campaign to defeat the Taliban in Afghanistan and this too proved a lengthy and challenging commitment, ending in December 2014 with 453 lives lost. A series of cohort studies published by KCMHR revealed that the incidence of probable PTSD was lower than that recorded for US forces. The British rates were 4 per cent overall and 7 per cent for front-line units,[49] whereas studies of US troops found 13 per cent.[50] Longer tours of duty undertaken by American forces together with shorter periods between deployments, service personnel of younger age and a higher proportion of reservists were cited as the causes.[51] In July 1993, the MoD had set up the Medical Assessment Programme (MAP) to investigate the symptoms of any veteran who had served in the Gulf War. Data were gathered on the physical and mental health of self-referring, ex-service personnel. Two studies by Lee and colleagues based on 3,000 and 3,233 veterans, respectively, found no unique illness or unusual disease trends.[52] Subsequent conflicts saw the MAP's role extended to include veterans of Bosnia, Iraq and Afghanistan. A study of 150 attendees with mental health problems, who believed these were caused by their operational service, was conducted Ian Palmer, a military psychiatrist.[53] Only 15 per cent of the diagnoses were of PTSD, though 89 per cent of these cases were comorbid with depression (48 per cent) or alcohol abuse (40 per cent).

Women in the UK Armed Forces

Until 1992, women who joined the armed forces had to serve in female-only units. With their abolition, women were integrated in all branches apart from those engaged in close combat. These changes corresponded with a progressive rise in the proportion of women in the UK armed forces. In 1990, women represented 6 per cent of regular forces, rising to 8 per cent by 2000 but had only achieved 11 per cent by April 2019 and are lower in the army than in the air force or navy.[54] Not until December 2014 did the Women in Close Combat Review recommend ending the ban on women in the infantry and armoured corps. However, greater integration may have increased the risk of military sexual trauma (MST). Across the world, women in the armed forces report elevated rates of mental illness compared with their male counterparts.[55] In part, this may reflect a greater willingness to disclose psychological illness but also the experience of a higher incidence of sexual assaults.[56] To date, the MoD has not sanctioned independent study of MST on the grounds it is at a low level.[57] In 2018, according to official statistics, service police conducted 153 investigations and 21 defendants were found guilty; the victims were mainly female (82.1 per cent) and the perpetrators overwhelmingly male.[58] Yet the suggestion remains that cases are under-reported.

Conclusion

Public support for the individual soldier and media focus on the welfare of veterans raised the profile of military psychiatry during the 2000s. At the end of the decade, a new edition of the Armed Forces Covenant was informed by a review of mental health services conducted by Dr Andrew Murrison MP.[59] Under the revised Covenant, veterans were granted priority access to NHS care for conditions associated with their service, subject to clinical need. The challenge of transition to civilian life was recognised and support in the form of 'training, education and appropriate healthcare referral' was recommended.[60] However, in the years that were to follow, other clinical priorities arose as a result of continuing campaigns in Afghanistan and Iraq, notably mild traumatic brain injury and, when it was demonstrated that validated treatments for PTSD were less effective for military populations, a growing interest in moral injury. Hence, the psychological challenges of conflict continue to evolve and demand solutions.

Key Summary Points

- Because of the focus on Gulf War syndrome, the UK military were slow to investigate rates of PTSD in service and veteran populations.
- The 1998 Strategic Defence Review that led Britain into an interventionist foreign policy drew the armed forces into a series of campaigns that stretched their resources and created additional psychological stressors.
- Military psychiatry tends to advance during periods of conflict because of the attention given to psychological casualties. Although the number of health care professionals fell over the period 1960–2010 in step with reductions in the strength of the armed forces, research capacity grew driven by greater public scrutiny and the development of formal links with the King's Centre for Military Health Research.
- The 2002 Class Action at the Royal Courts of Justice into negligence in the detection and treatment of PTSD prompted the Ministry of Defence (MoD) to devote greater expenditure on research and the treatment of post-traumatic illnesses.

• The integration of progressively increasing numbers of women into the UK armed forces may have led to an elevated risk of military sexual trauma (MST).

Notes

1. Ministry of Defence, *UK Armed Forces Operational Deaths Post World War II*. Bristol: Defence Statistics Health, 2015, p. 1.

2. C. McInnes, Labour's strategic defence review. *International Affairs* (1998) 74: 823–45.

3. *The Strategic Defence Review*, Cm 3999. London: The Stationery Office, 1998.

4. D. Edgerton, *The Rise and Fall of the British Nation: A Twentieth-Century History*. London: Allen Lane, 2018, pp. 514–17.

5. J. Price, The Falklands: Rate of British psychiatric casualties compared to recent American wars. *Journal of the Royal Army Medical Corps* (1984) 130: 109–13.

6. J. Price, The Falklands: Rate of British psychiatric casualties compared to recent American wars. *Journal of the Royal Army Medical Corps* (1984) 130: 109–13.

7. M. R. O'Connell, Stress-induced stress in a psychiatrist: A naval psychiatrist's personal view of the Falklands conflict. *Stress Medicine* (1986) 2: 307–14.

8. P. Abraham, Training for battleshock. *Journal of the Royal Army Medical Corps* (1982) 128: 18–27.

9. E. Jones and S. Ironside, Battle exhaustion: The dilemma of psychiatric casualties in Normandy, June–August 1944. *The Historical Journal* (2010) 53: 109–28, 119.

10. L. Freedman, *The Official History of the Falklands Campaign, Volume 2: War and Diplomacy*. London: Routledge, 2005, pp. 628–9.

11. G. Jones and J. Lovett, Delayed psychiatric sequelae among Falklands War veterans. *Journal of the Roy College of General Practice* (1987) 37: 34–5.

12. L. S. O'Brien and S. Hughes, Symptoms of post-traumatic stress disorder in Falklands veterans five years after the conflict. *British Journal of Psychiatry* (1991) 159: 135–41.

13. R. Orner, T. Lynch and P. Seed, Long-term traumatic stress reactions in British Falklands War veterans. *British Journal of Clinical Psychology* (1993) 32: 457–9.

14. A. Rees, Suicide of Falkland veterans. *Daily Mail*, www.dailymail.co.uk/news/article-94492/Suicide-Falklands-veterans.html.

15. Defence Analytical Services and Advice, *A Study of Deaths amongst UK Armed Forces Personnel deployed to the 1982 Falklands Campaign: 1982–2012*. Bristol: Ministry of Defence, 2013, p. 2.

16. E. Jones, Trans-generational transmission of traumatic memory and moral injury. *Military Behavioral Health* (2018) 6: 134–9.

17. M. R. O'Connell, Psychiatrist with the task force. In P. Pichot, P. Berner, R. Wolf and K. Thau, eds, *Psychiatry: The State of the Art*, Vol. 6. New York: Plenum Press, 1985, pp. 511–13.

18. E. Jones and S. Wessely, 'Forward psychiatry' in the military: Its origins and effectiveness. *Journal of Traumatic Stress* (2003) 16: 411–19.

19. R. Vinen, *National Service, Conscription in Britain 1945–1963*. London: Allen Lane, 2014, p. 256.

20. Hansard, Armed Forces, House of Commons debate, 14 December 1964, Vol. 404, Cols. 37–161, Frederick Mulley, Minister of Defence for the Army.

21. S. Noy, Division-based psychiatry in intensive war situations. *Journal of the Royal Army Medical Corps* (1982) 128: 105–16, 112–13.

22. P. Abraham, Training for battleshock. *Journal of the Royal Army Medical Corps* (1982) 128: 18–27.

23. S. Noy, Division-based psychiatry in intensive war situations. *Journal of the Royal Army Medical Corps* (1982) 128: 105–16.

24. Abraham, Training for battleshock.

25. Ministry of Defence, *Operational deaths post World War II*, p. 1.

26. A. P. Finnegan, P. A. Cumming and M. E. Piper, Critical incident stress debriefing following the terrorist bombing at Army headquarters Northern Ireland. *Journal of the Royal Army Medical Corps* (1998) 144: 5–10.

27. D. Murphy, G. Hodgman, C. Carson et al., Mental health and functional impairment outcomes following a 6-week intensive treatment programme for UK military veterans with post-traumatic stress disorder (PTSD): A naturalistic study to explore dropout and health outcomes at follow-up. *BMJ Open* (2015) 5: e007051.

28. M. Gelder, D. Gath and R. Mayou. *Oxford Textbook of Psychiatry*. Oxford, Oxford University Press, 1986, p. 317.

29. L. S. O'Brien. *Traumatic Events and Mental Health*. Cambridge, Cambridge University Press, 1998, pp. 70–3.

30. G. Turnbull, *Trauma, From Lockerbie to 7/7: How Trauma Affects Our Minds and How We Fight Back.* London: Corgi, 2011, pp. 21–2.

31. J. T. Mitchell, When disaster strikes: The critical incident stress debriefing process. *Journal of Emergency Medical Services* (1983) 8: 36–9.

32. A. Dyregrov, Caring for helpers in disaster situations: Psychological debriefing. *Disaster Management* (1989) 2: 25–9.

33. W. Busuttil, G. J. Turnbull, L. A. Neal et al., Incorporating psychological debriefing techniques within a brief group-psychotherapy program for the treatment of post-traumatic stress disorder. *British Journal of Psychiatry* (1995) 167: 495–502.

34. H. Lee and E. Jones, *War and Health: Lessons from the Gulf War*. Chichester: John Wiley, 2007.

35. A. B. Gillham and I. Robbins, Brief therapy in a battleshock recovery unit: Three case studies. *Journal of the Royal Army Medical Corps* (1993) 139: 58–60.

36. C. Unwin, N. Blatchley, W. Coker et al., Health of UK servicemen who served in the Persian Gulf War. *Lancet* (1999) 353: 169–78.

37. E. Jones, R. Hodgins Vermaas, H. McCartney et al., Post-combat syndromes from the Boer War to the Gulf: A cluster analysis of their nature and attribution, *British Medical Journal* (2002) 324: 321–4.

38. E. J. F. Hunt, S. Wessely, N. Jones, R. J. Rona and N. Greenberg. The mental health of the UK Armed Forces: Where facts meet fiction. *European Journal of Psychotraumatology* (2014); 5, https://doi.org/10.3402/ejpt .v5.23617.

39. N. Greenberg, A. Iversen, L. Hull, D. Bland and S. Wessely, Getting a peace of the action: Measures of posttraumatic stress in UK military peacemakers. *Journal of the Royal Society of Medicine* (2008) 101: 78–84.

40. R. J. Rona, M. Jones, C. French, R. Hooper and S. Wessely, Screening for physical and psychological illness in the British Armed Forces: I: The acceptability of the programme. *Journal of Medical Screening* (2004) 11: 148–53.

41. S. McManus, P. Bebbington, R. Jenkins and T. Brugha, eds, *Mental Health and Wellbeing in England: Adult Psychiatric Morbidity Survey 2014*. Leeds: NHS Digital, 2016, p. 114.

42. A. Iverson, A. Waterdrinker, N. T. Fear et al., Factors associated with heavy alcohol consumption in the UK armed forces: Data from a health survey of Gulf, Bosnia, and Era Veterans. *Military Medicine* (2007) 172: 956–61.

43. R. Jay and J. Glasson, The PTSD litigation. *Journal of Personal Injury Law* (2004) 2: 120–30.

44. T. McGeorge, J. Hacker Hughes and S. Wessely, The MOD PTSD decision: A psychiatric perspective. *Occupational Health Review* (2006) 122: 21–8.

45. E. B. Foa, B. O. Rothbaum, D. S. Riggs and T. B. Murdock, Treatment of posttraumatic stress disorder in rape victims: A comparison between cognitive-behavioral procedures and counselling. *Journal of Consulting and Clinical Psychology* (1991) 59: 715–23.

46. T. M. Keane, J. A. Fairbank, J. M. Caddell and R. T. Zimering, Implosive (flooding) therapy reduces symptoms of PTSD in Vietnam combat veterans. *Behaviour Therapy* (1989) 20: 245–60.

47. J. I. Bisson and N. Jones, Taped imaginal exposure as a treatment for PTSD reactions. *Journal of the Royal Army Medical Corps* (1995) 14: 20–4.

48. M. M. Steenkamp, B. T. Litz, C. W. Hoge and C. R. Marmar, Psychotherapy for military related PTSD: A review of randomised controlled trials. *JAMA* (2015) 314: 489–500.

49. N. T. Fear, M. Jones, D. Murphy et al., What are the consequences of deployment to Iraq and Afghanistan on the mental health of the UK armed forces. *Lancet* (2010) 375: 1783–97.

50. C. W. Hoge, C. A. Castro, S. C. Messer et al., Combat duty in Iraq and Afghanistan, mental health problems. *New England Journal of Medicine* (2004) 351: 13–22.

51. J. Sundin, N. T. Fear, A. Iversen et al., Mental health outcomes in US and UK military personnel returning from Iraq. *British Journal of Psychiatry* (2014) 204: 200–7.

52. H. A. Lee, R. Gabriel, J. P. G. Bolton, A .J. Bale and M. Jackson, Health status and clinical diagnosis of 3,000 UK Gulf War veterans. *Journal of the Royal Society of Medicine* (2002) 95: 491–7; H. A. Lee, A. J. Bale and R. Gabriel, Results and investigations on Gulf War veterans. *Clinical Medicine* (2005) 5: 166–72.

53. I. P. Palmer, UK extended Medical Assessment Programme: The first 150 individuals seen. *Psychiatrist* (2012) 36: 263–70.

54. N. Dempsey, *UK Defence Personnel Statistics*. Briefing Paper CBP7930. London, House of Commons Library, 2019, p. 6.

55. T. C. Smith, M. Zamorski, B. Smith et al., The physical and mental health of a large military cohort: Baseline functional health status of the millennium cohort. *BMC Public Health* (2007) 7: 340.

56. N. P. Mota, M. Medved, J. Wang et al., Stress and mental disorders in female military personnel: Comparisons between the sexes in a male dominated profession. *Journal of Psychiatric Research* (2012) 46: 159–67.

57. L. R. Godier-McBard and M. Fossey, Addressing the knowledge gap: Sexual violence and harassment in the UK armed forces. *Journal of the Royal Army Medical Corps* (2018) 164: 362–4.

58. M. Wigston, *Report on Inappropriate Behaviours*. London: Ministry of Defence, 2019, pp. 8–9.

59. A. Murrison, *Fighting Fit: A Mental Health Plan for Servicemen and Veterans*. London: Ministry of Defence, 2010.

60. Ministry of Defence, *The Armed Forces Covenant*. London: Ministry of Defence, 2011, p. 8.

Epilogue: Mind, State, Society and 'Our Psychiatric Future'

George Ikkos and Nick Bouras

'Today . . . it is part of morality not to be at home in one's home.'

T. W. Adorno[1]

Referring to work by his friend and close collaborator the early twentieth-century cultural critic Walter Benjamin, the musicologist, sociologist and philosopher Theodor W. Adorno wrote that it 'settled at the cross-roads of magic and positivism. That place is bewitched.'[2] The same might be said about contemporary psychiatry. This is an observation not a reprimand, not least because of the need to maintain hope even in the face of seemingly hopeless clinical situations where the stakes are remarkably high indeed. Arguably, this is where psychiatry should be with its laudable commitment to science confronting the indeterminacy of human action. The fact that the membership of the Spirituality Special Interest Group (SIG) of the Royal College of Psychiatrists (RCPsych) is only third to that of the Philosophy and Transcultural SIG, signals the same challenge. Perhaps 'bewitched' is too strong a word but sometimes it feels right given the heated controversies that often surround mental health.

Psychiatry and Redemption

Messianic fantasies are usually tempered with age, but one would expect to find their spark in youth. At the beginning of our half-century 1960–2010 both society and psychiatry were young. They were young in the sense that baby boomers tilted demography towards youth; the demand for rigorous application of the scientific method in psychiatry was also young; and the loud clamour for deinstitutionalisation and community care had just began.

Throughout psychiatry, grand solutions have been conceived, ideologies trumpeted, policies formed and laws enacted. Some key examples are asylums as therapeutic institutions; the magic bullets of biological psychiatry; deinstitutionalisation and care in the community; and normalisation and recovery. Each has made positive contributions yet, by their own assessments, their efforts have been only partially redeemed. The big psychiatric hospitals have mostly closed but that now is 'better' is expressed with various degrees of uncertainty, if at all, by contributors to this volume. It could and should have been better.

'Culture Is the Subject's Nature'

Since the 'decade of the brain', enormous strides have been made in neuroscience.[3] It has illuminated the exquisite complexity and plasticity of our neurobiology but this enlightenment has not been translated into advances in treatments to the same extent as in other medical specialties. The RCPsych secured funds from the Wellcome Trust and the Gatsby Foundation in 2018 to create a Neuroscience Board. Its purpose is to focus 'on the exciting advances in basic and clinical neuroscience, so that trainees are better equipped to provide mental health care in the future'. This is necessary and welcome. Psychiatrists together with psychologists are the custodians of the clinical understanding and application of neuroscience in mental health and illness, though not exclusively so.

Paradoxically, while illuminating the nature of the psychophysiological mechanisms that mediate them, neuroscience has foregrounded the importance of psychological and social processes in mental health and illness.[4] Unless this is taken fully on board, twenty-first-century neuroscience in psychiatry risks remaining therapeutically elusive, as it has been since the 1990s, the 'decade of the brain'. In 2015, Thomas Insel reached a bleak verdict on his thirteen-year term as director of the US National Institute of Mental Health where he invested $20 billion into research on biological psychiatry: 'I don't think we moved the needle in reducing suicide, reducing hospitalizations, improving recovery for the tens of millions of people who have mental illness.'[5] This may or may not change. If it does change, the question is by how much and how soon?

Affect, not the brain, is the primary object of the clinical medical expertise of psychiatrists.[6] Our contributors show unambiguously that social changes have had an overwhelmingly greater impact on psychiatry and mental health services than biomedical research. We consider it likely that social changes will continue to outpace neuroscience advances in terms of the impact on the prevalence of disorders and clinical practice. As this book goes to print, the world has experienced a global pandemic from Covid-19, with enormous and uncertain long-term social effects, though we would argue that, with the enhanced role of IT and telemedicine, we have already moved further away from community and towards meta-community psychiatry and mental health.[7] Consequently, we concur with those advocating enhanced training in the social sciences and greater integration with public health for psychiatrists.[8]

The importance of the history of psychiatry in psychiatric training has also recently been advocated.[9] There is a strong case for the RCPsych to establish a Social Sciences and History of Psychiatry Board to perform a similar function to the Neuroscience Board in updating and safeguarding the curriculum for the future. This should include leading representatives from these other disciplines as well as Mad Studies. The aim would be to provide robust foundations and the ability to keep up with evolving literature for our professionals, in a manner analogous to neuroscience. Similarly, we need a continually developing responsiveness to service users and carers. Most psychiatrists cannot be at the cutting edge of basic research in either the social sciences or the neurosciences. Yet they should be able to keep up with major developments in the literature and translate in a mature and timely fashion what is relevant into their practice.

The importance of public mental health is increasingly understood.[10] The profession will do well to engage more actively in the public sphere and be expected, trained and funded to do so. Moves in this direction should go beyond epidemiology and health services management to engage deeply with social theory and subjectivity.[11] This requires engaging with anthropology too, with its outstanding record of 'thick description' of peoples and cultures and fine conceptual analysis and investigation of personal meaning, including in severe mental illness.[12] This has implications for medical schools and psychiatric training schemes in terms of the qualities they seek in their recruits.

The Mental Health Workforce

When it comes to NHS policy, we suggest building further on the remarkable changes in mental health nursing. As a profession, it is naturally poised to maintain the right balance in making the 'biopsychosocial' model a tangible reality, especially for those with more severe impairments and disabilities. It has no need to privilege 'bio' or 'psycho' or 'social'. Skills in the whole range should be supported, continuous professional development strengthened and clinical quality actively facilitated and judiciously assured. The proposal does not intend the marginalisation of other mental health professions such as psychiatry and psychology. On the contrary, we believe it will help them fulfil their mission in terms of cultivating their special strengths. Pluralist understanding and multidisciplinary services are essential. None of the professions will succeed, however, unless there is full service-user and carer engagement, adequate provision of resources and effective recruitment and retention strategies. At present, these lag unacceptably behind.

Industrial therapy (and work) aside, the shadowy presence, even absence, of action-oriented therapies in this volume reflects a significant historical gap in mental health services development. Occupational therapy is the most obvious but others such as art, drama, dance and the like are also relevant. Such neglect flies in the face of our increasing understanding of central nervous system (CNS) plasticity and the importance of meaningful personal enterprise and practical action in both health and disease.

Conclusion

Foes and friends and even practitioners sometimes caricature psychiatry as a towering monolith. However, psychiatry is what psychiatrists do; patients, carers and colleagues experience; and the broader community understands, expects and funds. We believe that *Mind State and Society: Social History of Psychiatry and Mental Health in Britain 1960–2010* demonstrates that what Wittgenstein wrote about language applies to some extent to psychiatry too: '[it] can be seen as an ancient city: a maze of little streets and squares, of old and new houses, and of houses with additions from various periods; and this surrounded by a multitude of new boroughs with straight regular streets and uniform houses.'[13] In our city (*polis*), some find a home, others refuge and care, and still others experience neglect, oppression or abuse. In writing its history, chapter authors have also contributed to psychiatry's philosophy: ontology and ethics; resources for humility, professionalism and citizenship (*politics*).

Notes

1. T. W. Adorno, Asylum for the homeless, in *Minima Moralia*, trans. E. P. Jephcott, London: Verso, 2005.

2. Letter from Adorno to Walter Benjamin, quoted in L. De Cauter, *The Dwarf in the Chess Machine: Benjamin's Hidden Doctrine*. Rotterdam: nai010 Publishers, 2018, p. 12.

3. The quote given in this section's title is from E. Viveiros de Castro, *Cosmological Perspectivism in Amazonia and Elsewhere: Four Lectures given in the Department of Social Anthropology, University of Cambridge, February–March*, Masterclass Series 1. Hau Books, 1998, https://haubooks.org/cosmological-perspectivism-in-amazonia/.

4. T. Fuchs, *Ecology of the Brain*. Oxford: Oxford University Press, 2018.

5. G. Henriques, Twenty billion fails to 'move the needle' on mental illness: Thomas Insel admits to misguided research paradigm on mental illness. *Psychology Today*, 23 May 2017, www.psychologytoday.com/us/blog/theoryknowledge/201705/twenty-billion-fails-move-the-needlemental-illness.

6. G. Ikkos, Psychiatric expertise. *British Journal of Psychiatry* (2015) 207(5): 399, http://dx.doi.org/10.1192/bjp.bp.115.169946.

7. N. Bouras, G. Ikkos and T. Craig, From community to meta-community mental health care, www .thelancet.com/action/showPdf?pii=S2215-0366%2820%2930307–2.

8. N. Rose. *Our Psychiatric Future*. London: Polity, 2018.

9. G. Ash, C. Hilton, R. Freudenthal, T. Stephenson and G. Ikkos, History of psychiatry in the curriculum? History is part of life and life is part of history: Why psychiatrists need to understand it better. *The British Journal of Psychiatry* (2020), https://doi.org/10.1192/bjp.2020.64.

10. D. Bhugra and K. Bhui, *Oxford Textbook of Public Mental Health*. Oxford: Oxford University Press, 2018.

11. A. Rogers and D. A Pilgrim, *Sociology of Mental Health and Illness*, 6th ed. New York: Open University Press, 2021.

12. M. Engelke, *Think Like an Anthropologist*, London: Penguin, 2017; T. M. Luhrman and J. Marrow, *Our Most Troubling Madness: Case Studies in Schizophrenia across Cultures*. Oakland, CA: University of California Press, 2016.

13. L. Wittgenstein, *Philosophical Investigations*, sec. 1 8, p. 8. Quoted in J. F. Lyotard, *The Post-Modern Condition: A Report on Knowledge*. Manchester: Manchester University Press, 1984, p. 21.

Index